Textbook of Small Animal Pathophysiology

Stephan Neumann
Institute of Veterinary Medicine
University of Goettingen
Goettingen
Germany

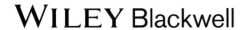

Registered Offices
John Wiley & Sons, Inc., 111 River Street, Hoboken, NJ 07030, USA
John Wiley & Sons Ltd, The Atrium, Southern Gate, Chichester, West Sussex, PO19 8SQ, UK

For details of our global editorial offices, customer services, and more information about Wiley products visit us at www.wiley.com.

Wiley also publishes its books in a variety of electronic formats and by print-on-demand. Some content that appears in standard print versions of this book may not be available in other formats.

Library of Congress Cataloging-in-Publication Data applied for
Hardback ISBN: 9781119824619

Cover Design: Wiley
Cover Images: cat © SciePro/Shutterstock, dog © SEBASTIAN KAULITZKI/SCIENCE PHOTO LIBRARY/Getty Images, organ renderings – Courtesy of Stephen Neumann

Set in 9.5/12.5pt STIXTwoText by Straive, Pondicherry, India

Printed in Singapore
M118051_260724

Contents

Preface *x*
Abbreviations *xii*

Part I   General Pathological Mechanisms *1*

1   **Inflammation** *3*

2   **Sepsis and Cytokine Storm** *14*

3   **Fibrosis** *19*

4   **Degeneration** *24*

5   **Obesity** *27*

6   **Ischaemia, Hypoxia** *32*

7   **Cell Death** *36*

8   **Neoplasia** *40*

9   **Infections** *46*

10   **Ageing** *53*

11   **Pain** *58*

12   **Hypothalamus Function** *61*

Part II   General Clinical Manifestations (Alphabetical) *65*

13   **Abdominal Enlargement** *67*

14   **Ataxia** *70*

15   **Constipation** *74*

16   **Cough** *78*

17   **Diarrhoea** *81*

18   **Dyschezia** *87*

19   **Dysphagia** *90*

20   **Dyspnoea** *93*

21   **Effusions** *97*

22   **Fatigue** *104*

23   **Fever** *106*

24   **Inappetence** *110*

25   **Jaundice** *113*

26   **Oedema** *116*

27   **Polyphagia** *119*

28   **Pruritus** *122*

29   **Regurgitation** *124*

30   **Seizure** *126*

31   **Shock** *130*

32   **Syncope** *133*

33   **Urinary Disorders** *138*

34   **Vomiting** *143*

35   **Weight Loss** *147*

Part III   **Pathophysiology of Organ Systems** *151*

36   **Cardiac System, Hypertension** *153*

36.1   **Physiological Functions and General Pathophysiology of Organ Insufficiency** *153*

36.2   **Congenital Cardiac Diseases** *161*

36.3   **Atrioventricular Valvular Diseases** *167*

36.4   **Cardiomyopathy, Hypertrophic** *172*

36.5   **Cardiomyopathy, Dilated** *176*

36.6   **Heart Arrhythmia**   *181*

36.7   **Pericardial Disease**   *184*

36.8   **Hypertension**   *190*

37   **Respiratory System**   *195*

37.1   **Physiological Functions and General Pathophysiology of Organ Insufficiency**   *195*

37.2   **Brachiocephalic Syndrome**   *200*

37.3   **Acute Respiratory Distress Syndrome (ARDS)**   *203*

37.4   **Asthma (Feline Lower Respiratory Tract Disease)**   *207*

37.5   **Chronic Obstructive Bronchitis**   *210*

37.6   **Pneumonia**   *213*

37.7   **Idiopathic Lung Fibrosis**   *217*

38   **Gastrointestinal System**   *220*

38.1   **Physiological Functions and General Pathophysiology of Organ Insufficiency**   *220*

38.2   **Megaoesophagus**   *226*

38.3   **Gastritis/Ulceration**   *229*

38.4   **Gastric Dilatation-Volvulus Syndrome**   *233*

38.5   **Enteritis/Inflammatory Bowel Disease**   *237*

38.6   **Intestinal Lymphangiectasias**   *243*

38.7   **Intestinal Obstruction**   *249*

39   **Hepatobiliary System**   *253*

39.1   **Physiological Functions and General Pathophysiology of Organ Insufficiency**   *253*

39.2   **Acute Hepatic Failure**   *261*

39.3   **Chronic Hepatitis; Liver Fibrosis and Cirrhosis**   *266*

39.4   **Portosystemic Shunts/Hepatoencephalopathy**   *272*

39.5   **Feline Hepatic Lipidosis**   *277*

39.6   **Cholangiohepatitis**   *280*

40 **Exocrine Pancreas** *284*

40.1 **Physiological Functions and General Pathophysiology of Organ Insufficiency** *284*

40.2 **Acute Pancreatitis** *287*

40.3 **Chronic Pancreatitis** *292*

40.4 **Exocrine Pancreas Insufficiency** *296*

41 **Urinary System** *300*

41.1 **Physiological Functions of the Kidneys and General Pathophysiology of Organ Insufficiency** *300*

41.2 **Glomerulonephritis/Nephrotic Syndrome** *305*

41.3 **Tubular Disease/Fanconi Syndrome** *310*

41.4 **Acute Renal Failure** *313*

41.5 **Chronic Kidney Disease** *321*

41.6 **Urinary Tract Infection** *327*

41.7 **Urolithiasis** *330*

42 **Electrolyte System and Acid-Base Balance** *335*

42.1 **Acid-Base Balance** *335*

42.2 **Hypo-/Hypernatraemia** *340*

42.3 **Hypo-/Hyperkalaemia** *344*

43 **Endocrine System** *349*

43.1 **General Physiology** *349*

43.2 **Pituitary Gland** *352*

43.2.1 **Acromegaly** *352*

43.2.2 **Pituitary Dwarfism** *356*

43.2.3 **Diabetes Insipidus** *359*

43.3 **Thyroid Gland** *362*

43.3.1 **Physiology of the Thyroid Gland** *362*

43.3.2 **Hyperthyroidism** *365*

43.3.3 **Hypothyroidism** *369*

43.4 **Parathyroid Gland** *374*

43.5 **Endocrine Pancreas** *379*

43.5.1 **Physiology of Endocrine Pancreas** *379*

43.5.2 **Diabetes Mellitus** *382*

43.5.3 **Diabetic Ketoacidosis** *387*

43.5.4 **Insulinoma** *390*

43.6 **Adrenal Gland** *393*

43.6.1 **Physiology of the Adrenal Gland** *393*

43.6.2 **Hyperadrenocorticism** *397*

43.6.3 **Hypoadrenocorticism** *402*

43.6.4 **Hyperaldosteronism** *405*

43.6.5 **Pheochromocytoma** *409*

44 **Reproduction System** *413*

44.1 **Pyometra** *413*

44.2 **Prostate Diseases** *417*

45 **Nerve System** *420*

45.1 **Brain Tumours** *420*

45.2 **Idiopathic Epilepsy** *423*

45.3 **Intervertebral Disc Disease** *426*

45.4 **Peripheral Neuropathy** *429*

46 **Joints** *431*

46.1 **Arthritis** *431*

46.2 **Osteoarthritis** *434*

47 **Haematology** *437*

47.1 **Physiological Functions of Red Blood Cells** *437*

47.2   **Erythrocytosis**   *441*

47.3   **Anaemia**   *444*

47.4   **Coagulation Disorders**   *450*

47.5   **Hypercoagulability**   *454*

48   **Infectious Diseases**   *457*

48.1   **Feline**   *457*

48.1.1   **Feline Leukaemia Virus Infection**   *457*

48.1.2   **Feline Infectious Peritonitis**   *461*

48.1.3   **Feline Immunodeficiency Virus Infection**   *466*

48.2   **Canine**   *471*

48.2.1   **Distemper**   *471*

48.2.2   **Canine Parvovirus**   *475*

48.3   **Bacterial Diseases**   *480*

48.3.1   **Anaplasmosis**   *480*

48.3.2   **Borreliosis**   *484*

48.3.3   **Ehrlichiosis**   *488*

48.3.4   **Leptospirosis**   *491*

48.4   **Protozoal Infections**   *495*

48.4.1   **Babesiosis**   *495*

48.4.2   **Giardiasis**   *499*

48.4.3   **Leishmaniasis**   *503*

49   **Common Immune-mediated Diseases**   *507*

49.1   **Autoimmunity**   *507*

49.2   **Lupus Erythematosus**   *510*

49.3   **Myasthenia Gravis**   *514*

50   **Common Clinical Biochemical Parameters (Alphabetical)**   *517*

50.1   **Alanine Aminotransferase (ALT)**   *517*

50.2   **Albumin**   *518*

50.3   **Alkaline Phosphatase (ALP)**   *520*

50.4   **Ammonia**   *522*

50.5   **Aspartate Aminotransferase (AST)**   *523*

50.6   **Bile Acids**   *524*

50.7   **Bilirubin**   *525*

50.8   **Calcium**   *526*

50.9   **Cholesterol**   *528*

50.10   **Creatinine**   *529*

50.11   **Creatine Kinase**   *530*

50.12   **Glucose**   *531*

50.13   **Glutamate Dehydrogenase (GLDH)**   *532*

50.14   **Lipase**   *533*

50.15   **Phosphorus**   *534*

50.16   **Potassium**   *535*

50.17   **Sodium**   *537*

50.18   **Total Protein**   *539*

50.19   **Urea**   *541*

Index   *542*

Preface

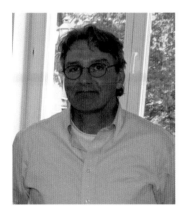

This book was written to summarise the mechanisms of canine and feline disease in one book. Although the author believes that understanding the mechanisms of disease is essential to understanding the course, diagnosis, treatment and prognosis of disease, there are only few books that have focused on the mechanisms. This was the motivation for writing this book. Not all mechanisms presented in this book have been directly investigated in dogs and cats. Some of the findings originate from studies of other species and have been adapted to the conditions in dogs and cats. This is comparable to the human medical literature on this topic. The book is structured in such a way that first the general disease mechanisms are presented. In the second part of the book, the development of the clinical symptoms is explained. Finally, in the third part of the book, the mechanisms of important diseases in dogs and cats are presented. The chapters are structured in such a way that first the disease is defined and then aetiological factors are presented. The main causes are described. In the section on pathogenesis, the mechanisms by which the aetiology leads to the disease are described. Finally, the diagnostic possibilities are briefly summarised. The section on pathophysiology explains how the symptoms typical of the respective disease develop. Each chapter ends with a summary of therapeutic options. Knowledge of the mechanisms of diseases is constantly changing as a result of increasing knowledge. Accordingly, the explanations in the book reflect current knowledge.

This book is dedicated to all those who have accompanied me on my professional journey and have been my contact and support in hours of joy and pause.

I have written this book with great enthusiasm and would be delighted if you would read it with the same pleasure.

Stephan Neumann
Göttingen, April 2023

Further Reading

Besides the literature given at the end of each chapter, the following publications provided basic information for the realisation of this book:

Black, V.L., Murphy, K.F., Payne, J.R., and Hall, E.J. (2022). *Notes on Canine Internal Medicine, 4th ed*, 7e. New York: Wiley.

Blanco, A. (2022). *Medical Biochemistry*, 2e. St. Louis: Elsevier.

Blum, H.E. and Müller-Wieland, D. (2020). *Klinische Pathophysiologie*, 11. Auflage. Stuttgart: Thieme Verlag.

Bojarb, M.J. (2010). *Mechanisms of Disease in Small Animal Surgery*, 3e. Jackson: Teton New Media.

Cui, D. (2011). *Atlas of Histology: With Functional and Clinical Correlations*, 1e. Philadelphia: Wolters Kluwer.

Ettinger, S.J., Feldman, E.C., and Cote, E. (2017). *Textbook of Veterinary Internal Medicine*, 8e. St. Louis: Elsevier.

Feldman, E.C., Nelson, R.W., Reusch, C.E., and Scott-Moncrieff, J.C.R. (2015). *Canine and Feline Endocrinology*, 4e. Philadelphia: Elsevier.

Gough, A. and Murphy, K. (2015). *Diagnosis in Small Animal Medicine*, 2e. New York: Wiley.

Greene, C.E. (2006). *Infectious Diseases of the Dog and Cat*, 3e. St. Louis: Elsevier.

Hartmann, H. and Meyer, H. (1994). *Klinische Pathologie der Haustiere*, 1. Auflage. Stuttgart: Gustav Fischer Verlag.

Harvey, R.A. and Ferrier, D.R. (2011). *Lippincott's Illustrated Reviews: Biochemistry*, 5e. Philadelphia: Wolters Kluwer.

Huether, S.E. *Understanding Pathophysiology*, 7e. St. Louis: Elsevier.

Kaneko, J.J., Harvey, J.W., and Bruss, M.L. (2008). *Clinical Biochemistry of Domestic Animals*, 6e. Burlington: Academic Press.

Kierszenbaum, A.L. and Tres, L.L. (2020). *Histology and Cell Biology. An Introduction to Pathology*, 5e. Philadelphia: Elsevier.

Klein, B.G. (2020). *Cunningham's Textbook of Veterinary Physiology*, 6e. Philadelphia: Elsevier.

Kumar, V., Abbas, A.K., and Fausto, N. (2005). *Pathologic Basis of Disease*, 7e. Philadelphia: Elsevier.

Nelson, R.W. and Couto, G. (2014). *Small Animal Internal Medicine*, 5e. St. Louis: Elsevier.

Rastogi, S.C. (2007). *Animal Physiology*, 4e. New Delhi: New Age International (P) Limited, Publishers.

Schmidt, R.F., Lang, F., and Heckmann, M. (2010). *Physiologie des Menschen*, 31. Auflage. Berlin: Springer Verlag.

Silbernagl, S. and Lang, F. (2019). *Taschenatlas Pathophysiologie*, 6. Auflage. Stuttgart: Thieme Verlag.

Sjaastad, O.V., Sand, O., and Hove, K. (2016). *Physiology of Domestic Animals*, 3e. Oslo: Scandinavian Veterinary Press.

Stockham, S.L. and Scott, M.A. (2002). *Fundamentals of Veterinary Clinical pathology*, 1e. Ames: Iowa State Press.

Sturgess, K. (2013). *Notes on Feline Internal Medicine*, 2e. New York: Wiley.

Tilley, L.P., Smith, F.W.K., Sleeper, M.M., and Brainard, B. (2021). *Blackwell's Five-Minute Veterinary Consult. Canine and Feline, 7th ed*, 7e. New York: Wiley.

Ware, W.A. (2011). *Cardiovascular Disease in Small Animal Medicine*, 2e. London: Manson Publishing.

Zachary, J.F. (2017). *Pathologic Basis of Veterinary Disease*, 6e. St. Louis: Elsevier.

Abbreviations

ACh	Acetylcholin	**LH**	Luteinisation hormone
ACTH	Adrenocorticotropic hormone	**LPS**	Lipopolysaccharides
ADH	Antidiuretic hormone	**MAPK**	Mitogen-activated protein Kinase
ALP	Alkaline phosphatase	**MG**	Myasthenia gravis
ANP	Atrial natriuretic peptide	**MHC**	Major histocompatibility complex
APC	Antigen presenting cells	**MMP**	Matrix metalloproteinase
ARDS	Acute Respiratory Distress Syndrome	**MPS**	Mononuclear phagocytic system
ATP	Adenosine triphosphate	**Na**	Sodium
cAMP	cyclic Adenosine monophosphate	**NGF**	Nerve growth factor
BALT	Bronchus-Associated Lymphoid Tissue	**NK-cells**	Natural killer cells
BCS	Body condition score	**NO**	Nitric oxide
BMP	Bone morphogenic protein	**PAF**	Platelet-activating factor
CCK	Cholecystokinin	**PAMPS**	Pathogen-associated molecular pattern molecules
CFU	Colony forming units		
CKD	Chronic kidney disease	**PRP**	Pattern-recognition receptors
CNS	Central nervous system	**PTH**	Parathormone
COB	Chronic obstructive bronchitis	**RAAS**	Renin-Angiotensin-Aldosterone System
CRH	Corticotropin-releasing hormone	**ROS**	Reactive oxygen species
CRP	C-reactive protein	**SIBO**	Small intestine bacterial overgrowth
DAGPC	Dystrophin-associated glycoprotein complex	**SIRS**	Systemic inflammatory response syndrome
DAMPS	Danger-associated molecular patterns	**SLE**	Systemic lupus erythematosus
DIC	Disseminated intravascular coagulation	**SMAD**	Small mothers against decapentaplegic
ECM	Extracellular matrix	**TAP**	Trypsinogen activation peptide
EGF	Epidermal growth factor	**TGF**	Transforming growth factor
FeLv	Feline leukaemia virus	**TLR**	Toll-like receptor
FGF	Fibroblast growth factor	**TRPM8**	Transient receptor potential cation channel subfamily M (melastatin) member 8
FIP	Feline infectious peritonitis		
FIV	Feline immunodeficiency virus	**TRPV 1**	Transient receptor potential cation channel subfamily V member 1
FSH	Follicle stimulating hormone		
GH	Growth hormone	**TSH**	Thyroid-stimulating hormone
GnRH	Gonadotropin-releasing hormone	**UTI**	Urinary tract infection
HPA	Hypothalamic–pituitary–adrenal axis	**VEGF**	Vascular endothelial growth factor
IBD	Inflammatory bowel disease	**VLDL**	Very-low-density lipoproteins
IGF	Insulin-like growth factor	**vWF**	von Willebrand factor
LE	Lupus erythematosus		

Part I

General Pathological Mechanisms

1

Inflammation

Definition

Inflammation is by definition a defensive reaction of the body with the aim of eliminating the trigger of the inflammation and repairing the damage caused, either by restoring the tissue of origin (restitutio) or by a replacement tissue, the scar (reparatio).

Trigger

Inflammation is triggered by any stimuli, called 'noxae', that overcome the organism's defence-compensation mechanisms. By definition, a *noxious agent* is a substance or event that causes damage to a biological organism. The noxious agent can be divided according to its origin into internal and external, and according to its structure into physical, chemical or biological triggers (Table 1.1).

Defence Cascade of the Body

Numerous defence mechanisms exist to protect an organism. These are particularly effective at the 'contact surfaces' between the organism and the environment. There, the penetration of the noxious agent is prevented by mechanical as well as biological defence mechanisms.

The **skin** prevents the penetration of the noxious agent under physiological conditions due to its structural design. For this purpose, the skin consists of different layers with different functions (Figure 1.1).

The outer layer of the skin, the epidermis, is made up of the layers – stratum corneum, lucidum, granulosum, spinosum and basale from the outside inwards. The main cell type in the epidermis is the keratinocyte. This differentiates in the stratum basale from epidermal stem cells. In the stratum spinosum, the cells begin to remodel with an increase in volume and a change in shape and width. In the further course, keratohyalin grains are formed in the stratum granulosum, and further remodelling processes take place. The cells become flattened, the nucleus is lost, shrinkage occurs due to fluid loss, and finally cornification takes place. Eventually, no more keratinocytes can be detected in the stratum corneum. Keratinocytes become corneocytes. The cornification process builds up a mechanical protection for the skin. In addition, penetration of a noxious substance is ensured by a close connection between the keratinocytes through tight-junctions. The tight-junctions consist of connections of transmembrane proteins, such as claudin and occludin. Intracellularly, these proteins are connected to the cytoskeleton. The tight-junctions connect the cells into a bandage that forms a barrier to the paracellular penetration of a noxious agent.

In addition, defence cells such as Langerhans cells are localised in the epidermis.

These are tissue macrophages that are capable of phagocytosis but also differentiate into antigen-presenting cells after contact with an antigenically active noxious agent, which can initiate an immune response.

Finally, the extracellular matrix in the epidermis forms a molecular association that can prevent the penetration of a noxious agent. The molecules of the extracellular matrix include, for example, keratins and collagens as structural proteins

Textbook of Small Animal Pathophysiology, First Edition. Stephan Neumann.
© 2025 John Wiley & Sons Ltd. Published 2025 by John Wiley & Sons Ltd.

Table 1.1 Common causes of inflammation in dogs and cats.

Physical	Chemical	Biological	Infectious agents
Heat	Environmental toxins		Viruses
Cold	Endogenous toxins	Tumours	Bacteria
		Degenerations	Fungi
			Parasites

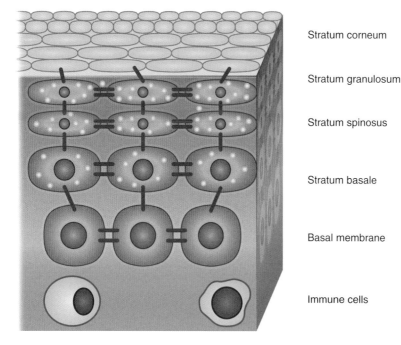

Stratum corneum

Stratum granulosum

Stratum spinosus

Stratum basale

Basal membrane

Immune cells

Figure 1.1 Structure of the outer skin and development of keratinocytes.

Table 1.2 Components of the epidermal extracellular matrix with function.

Molecule	Function
Keratin	Intermediate filament, structural element of keratinocytes
Collagen	Tight protein of the ECM, adhesion molecule
Elastin	Elastic protein of the ECM
Fillagrin	Structural protein
Ceramide	Hydrophobic protection

and ceramides, which are lipids composed of a sphingosine molecule and fatty acids that provide protection against hydrophilic noxae (Mitamura et al. 2021) (Table 1.2).

The **mucous membranes** of the body form the inner boundary layer between the organism and the environment. The microscopic structure of the mucous membranes already reflects defence competences. This includes the contact of the mucosal cells through tight-junctions. These form a tight connection between the cell membrane of neighbouring cells through proteins such as occludin. This prevents the paracellular penetration of extracorporeal noxae.

Another superficial defence mechanism is the synthesis of mucins. Mucins are glycoproteins that are synthesised by goblet cells and form a protective layer several micrometres thick on the mucosa. In the process, defence functions of the mucins develop due to their gel-like structure, which enables mechanical protection of the underlying mucosal cells. Chemically, for example, bicarbonate residues of the mucins can bind and inactivate acids, and biologically, mucins can prevent bacteria from invading by binding them.

Cells localised in the mucosa (Paneth cells) secrete lysozyme or defensins to inactivate germs. The latter are differentiated into α-, β- and θ-defensins based on their molecular structure (Lehrer and Ganz 2002).

The effects of defensins are antimicrobial and immunomodulatory. The former effect is based on their positive molecular charge, which enables a charge-dependent interaction with the negatively charged bacterial cell wall, especially the lipopolysaccharides (Scott and Hancock 2000). The binding of the defensins results in pore formation. The consequence is a depolarisation of the bacterial cell membrane and thus a breakdown of the membrane potential and lysis of the cell (Scott and Hancock 2000; Sahl et al. 2005).

In addition, defensins show immunomodulatory functions. Defensins have a chemotactic effect on dendritic cells and memory T cells, and thus represent a link between innate and adaptive immune responses. In addition, some defensins act chemotactically on monocytes and macrophages, and in some cases induce mast cell activation and degranulation. As a result, histamine and prostaglandins are released, which promote the migration of neutrophilic granulocytes. Degranulation of the recruited neutrophilic granulocytes in turn releases defensins again, resulting in a positive feedback loop (Yang et al. 2002).

The secretion of lysozyme is another defence mechanism against bacterial invasion of the mucous membranes. Lysozyme is an enzyme that cleaves murein. Murein is a peptidoglycan and a component of the bacterial cell wall. Due to the hydrolytic cleavage of murein, the bacterial cell wall loses its selective permeability and rupture of the bacterial cell wall occurs due to increased water influx.

Another defence mechanism in the mucosa is the mucosa-associated lymphoid system located in the lamina propria, which is called 'gut associated lymphoid tissue' (GALT) in the gastrointestinal tract and bronchial associated lymphoid tissue (BALT) in the respiratory tract. This system includes numerous cells of the non-specific and specific defence response, such as macrophages and lymphocytes (Figure 1.2).

Figure 1.2 Building up the defence system of the mucous membrane.

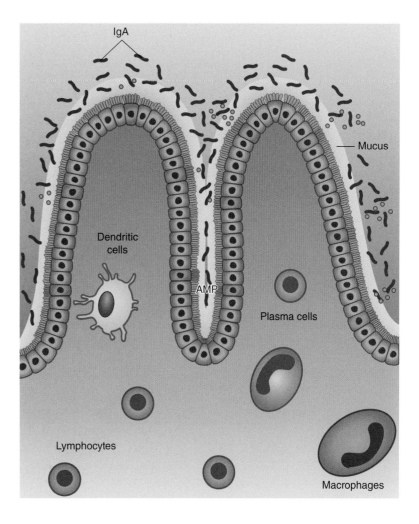

Player of the Inflammation

The inflammatory process is maintained by some so-called 'inflammatory cells'. These combine some properties that predispose them to fulfil the definitional task of inflammation. This states that inflammation is a reaction of the body that serves to eliminate a noxious agent and its consequences.

The following cells are involved in the inflammatory process:

Neutrophilic granulocytes originate from the leukocyte pool of the bone marrow and are distributed throughout the blood. The residence time in the blood is a few hours (6–12 hours). Subsequently, the neutrophilic granulocytes leave the blood capillaries under the influence of chemoattractive substances. These are released as part of the local inflammatory process. The process of neutrophilic granulocyte emigration from the blood vessels takes place via adhesion and transmigration. Integrin-mediated, the neutrophilic granulocytes adhere to the surfaces of the endothelial cells. In the process, the cells change their shape from roundish to an amoeboid cell shape. The cells can now migrate trans- and paracellularly through the vascular endothelial layer.

In the area of inflammation, the neutrophilic granulocytes have different functions. The ability to phagocytose allows the cells to take up and lyse the noxious agent (e.g. bacteria). For this process, the noxious agent is taken up by membrane invagination and the resulting vesicle combines with the granular structures of the granulocyte. In particular, molecules of the so-called 'primary granules' are responsible for the process of phagocytosis; these include myeloperoxidases, defensins and lysozyme.

Beyond the process of phagocytosis, neutrophilic granulocytes are able to maintain the inflammatory process through the secretion of prostaglandins, leukotrienes and proinflammatory cytokines (TNF-α, IL-1, IL-6). At the same time, they link the innate immunity with the adaptive immunity e.g. via macrophage-inflammatory-protein 1 (MIP-1) (Salazar-Mather and Hokeness 2003). Antigen presentation by neutrophilic granulocytes has also been described, underlining that neutrophilic granulocytes link the two immune systems (Appelberg 2007). A special form of defence by neutrophilic granulocytes occurs when they form neutrophilic extracellular traps (NETs) as part of specialised cell death (NETosis). These are networks formed by neutrophilic granulocyte chromatin and proteins such as elastase, cathepsin or histones. All NETs have an antibacterial effect by binding and inactivating bacteria (Muñoz et al. 2019) (Figure 1.3).

Monocytes and tissue macrophages represent the mononuclear phagocyte system and are part of the innate immune system. Monocytes are distributed throughout the blood and differentiated into macrophages with different functions after emigration into the surrounding tissue. The process of emigration is comparable to that of neutrophilic granulocytes and is composed of rolling, adhesion and para- or transcellular migration (Gerhardt and Ley 2015).

Macrophages are capable of phagocytosis and they link the innate and acquired immune systems by presenting antigen. In addition, they control the course of the inflammatory response.

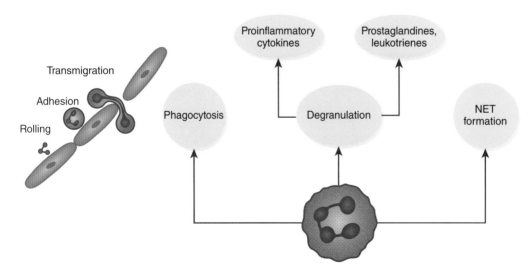

Figure 1.3 Defence mechanism by neutrophilic granulocytes.

Phagocytosis is a process in which particles in the form of large molecules (e.g. proteins), prokaryotic or eukaryotic cells are taken up and 'digested' by the phagocytosing cells. Of the inflammatory cells, primarily macrophages and neutrophilic granulocytes are capable of phagocytosis. The phagocytosis process can take place after prior opsonisation of the particle or without it. If opsonisation takes place, the particle is opsonised before phagocytosis, e.g. by IgG or complement (C3). Particles labelled in this way react with specific receptors (FcR, CR) of the phagocyte. In non-opsonised phagocytosis, a reaction takes place through the particle's own surface molecules (e.g. saccharides). Phagocytosis begins with the attachment of the particles to receptors on the cell membrane. The particle–receptor connection initiates the signal transduction for phagocytosis. Subsequently, polymerisation of cytoskeletal actin occurs, causing the cell membrane to develop pseudopodial protrusions, enclosing the particle and invaginating it into the cell interior. The invagination process results from depolymerisation of the basal actin filaments. Eventually, the particle is pinched off and a vesicle is formed. In this process, part of the cell membrane is used for vesicle formation and after the vesicle is strangulated, the lipid double membrane closes again. Inside the cell, the vesicle is now called a 'phagosome', which fuses with a primary lysosome released from the Golgi apparatus to form a secondary lysosome. The lysosome contains an acidic environment inside with numerous digestive enzymes. Proteins and polysaccharides are broken down into amino acids and monosaccharides by the lysosomal enzymes and can diffuse out of the secondary lysosome into the cell interior. The remaining, indigestible components of the secondary lysosome can fuse with the cell membrane again and be released into the environment (Rosales and Uribe-Querol 2017).

In addition, protein components of the antigen will be bound to molecules of the major histocompatibility complex II (MHC II). These complexes reach the cell surface, are attached to the cell membrane and can be presented to other cells in this way (Savina and Amigorena 2007; Roche and Furuta 2015).

The control of the inflammatory process by macrophages is governed by numerous cytokines secreted by the macrophages. These include proinflammatory cytokines such as IL-1, IL-6 and TNF-α. But anti-inflammatory cytokines such as IL-10 or TGF are also synthesised. Through their diverse functions and the formation of numerous mediators, macrophages essentially control the local inflammatory process (Figure 1.4).

Eosinophilic granulocytes are easily recognised by their eosinophilic cell granules. Their formation takes place predominantly in the bone marrow. In circulation, the eosinophilic granulocytes only move for a few hours before emigrating into the tissue. This process is similar to the processes already described for neutrophilic granulocytes and monocytes. The preferred tissues for emigration are those of the gastrointestinal tract and the respiratory tract. In the tissues, the eosinophilic granulocytes undergo apoptosis after a few days, unless they are previously activated by cytokines (e.g. IL-5).

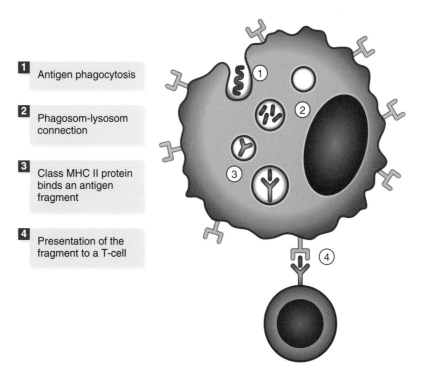

Figure 1.4 Antigen presentation by macrophages.

1 Antigen phagocytosis

2 Phagosom-lysosom connection

3 Class MHC II protein binds an antigen fragment

4 Presentation of the fragment to a T-cell

The functional roles of eosinophilic granulocytes are cytotoxic effects, tissue remodelling and immune cell interaction. Eosinophilic granulocytes are capable of phagocytosis of e.g. bacteria or antigen–antibody complexes. However, their effectiveness is less than that of neutrophilic granulocytes. By secreting growth factors (e.g. TGF-β, VEGF), the eosinophilic granulocytes play a role in the healing process of the inflammation. The secretion of growth factors usually implies connective tissue proliferation in the sense of fibrosis. Finally, eosinophilic granulocytes may interact with other immune cells of the innate and acquired immune system (Rothenberg and Hogan 2006; Wechsler et al. 2021).

Basophilic granulocytes are particularly rare in the blood and have a half-life of only a few hours. They then migrate into the tissue, where they remain for a few weeks. After activation by IgE, for example, degranulation occurs with the release of heparin and histamine. In this way, local blood circulation is promoted, which supports the inflammatory process or allergic reactions (Stone et al. 2010) (Figure 1.5).

Lymphocytes morphologically belong to the mononuclear cells and develop from lymphatic stem cell lineage. The majority of lymphocytes are located in the bone marrow and lymphoid organs. The life span of lymphocytes is function-dependent and ranges from a few days to several years. The lymphocytes represent the specific defence and can be divided into three main groups, depending on the respective tasks. These can be classified morphologically on the basis of specific CD-surface molecules (cluster of differentiation).

The CD3-positive T cells, like the macrophages, represent the cellular immune response in the area of inflammation.

CD4-positive T helper cells support the immune response of T- and B-lymphocytes through secretion of cytokines and via direct interaction with surface molecules of the target cells. They are stimulated by antigen-presenting cells and can be differentiated into two subtypes TH1 and TH2 cells with different functions. TH1 lymphocytes secrete, for example, IFN-γ, TNF-β and IL-2, and thereby regulate the inflammatory response by stimulating the phagocytotic activity of macrophages and cytotoxic T cells. In addition, the differentiation of B-lymphocytes into plasma cells is supported.

TH2 cells essentially secrete IL-4, 5, 9 and 13 and trigger the maturation and differentiation of B-lymphocytes. IL-4 induces isotype switching from IgM to IgG and IgE, while IL-5 increases IgA synthesis.

The CD8-positive T cells act cytotoxically against extracellular and intracellular bacteria as well as virus-infected cells. They are activated by antigenic peptides presented by the MHC I molecules present on all nucleated somatic cells. By releasing granules with cytotoxic molecules (e.g. perforin), and receptor induction of the target cells, the cytotoxic cells can induce apoptosis of the target cell.

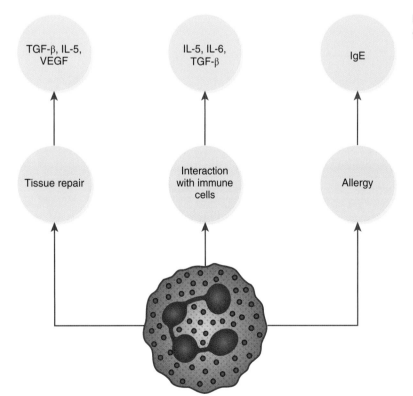

Figure 1.5 Function of the eosinophilic granulocytes.

Figure 1.6 Function of the lymphocytes.

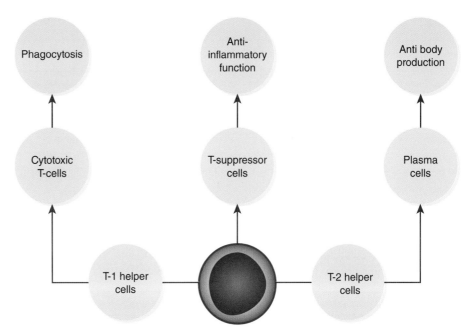

CD4-positive T-suppressor cells suppress the immune response and serve to finalise the inflammatory process.

The B cells produce and secrete specific antibodies and can also present antigen. Activation of the B-lymphocytes takes place via antigen binding to surface receptors. The complex of receptor and antigen is taken up by the cell and proteolysed, forming peptides that are bound to MHC II molecules to be presented on the B-lymphocyte surface. CD4-positive T helper cells recognise the structures and stimulate the differentiation and clonal expansion of B-lymphocytes into antibody-producing plasma cells. The antibodies, in turn, bind to the antigen and can directly inactivate it by forming insoluble complexes or neutralise it by activating the complement system. Antigen–antibody complexes are also more likely to be taken up by phagocytes.

Another lymphocyte subpopulation is the natural killer (NK) cell. Like the T cells, they belong to the cellular defence system. Their primary function is to recognise and eliminate virus-infected or neoplastic body cells. In contrast to the T and B cells, the NK cells do not recognise foreign antigens, but modified endogenous cells on the basis of the expression pattern of the MHC molecules. Active NK cells secrete cytotoxic (including perforin, granzymes and TNF-β) and various regulatory (including IFN-γ, IL-1, IL-5, IL-8, IL-10 and GM-CSF) cytokines that initiate destruction of the malignant degenerated or virus-infected target cell (Freitas and Rocha 2000; LeBien and Tedder 2008) (Figure 1.6).

Course of the Acute Inflammation

The inflammatory process is initiated by the receptor binding of molecules of the inflammatory trigger. These are called 'pathogen-associated molecular patterns' (PAMPs) for external triggers or danger-associated molecular patterns (DAMPs) for internal triggers. They react with so-called 'germline-encoded pattern-recognition receptors' (PRRs), which also include toll-like receptors (TLRs). This is followed by intracellular signal transduction via various pathways (NF-κ B, MAPK, JAK-Stat) and increased gene expression of inflammatory mediators (cytokines, chemokines) (Fioranelli et al. 2021).

The pattern of mediators and chemokines can be influenced by the type of pathogen. For example, the reaction of glycan components of the *Staphylococcus aureus* cell wall with TLR2 induces the secretion of CXCL-8 by dendritic cells; this induces the migration of neutrophilic granulocytes into the area. The reaction of lipopolysaccharides of *Escherichia coli* with TLR leads to the secretion of CXCL-10, which induces migration of T cells into the area (Luster 2002) (Table 1.3).

The time course of inflammation begins with vasodilation and an increase in the permeability of the blood vessels.

Vasodilation is caused by leucocyte mediators, such as bradykinin. This is structurally an oligopeptide and functionally a tissue hormone. It binds to endothelial cell receptors in the vessel wall and initiates a change in smooth muscle tone.

The consequence of vascular dilatation is increased intravascular hydrostatic pressure. This increases the pressure gradient to the surrounding tissue and promotes an increase in the permeability of the vessel wall.

Table 1.3 Cytokines, resource, effect.

Cytokines	Source	Effect
IL-1	Macrophages	Stimulation of macrophages and T lymphocytes, acute phase reaction
IL-2	Activated Th1 lymphocytes	Proliferation of B cells and activated T cells
IL-5	Th2 lymphocytes, mast cells	Formation of eosinophilic granulocytes
IL-6	Activated Th2 lymphocytes, macrophages, somatic cells	Acute phase reaction, B cell proliferation
IL-8	Macrophages, somatic cells, neutrophilic granulocytes	Chemoattractant for neutrophils and T cells
IL-10	Activated Th2 lymphocytes, macrophages	Inhibits cytokine production, promotes B cell proliferation and antibody production, suppresses cellular immunity
IFN-α IFN-β	Macrophages, neutrophilic granulocytes, somatic cells	Antiviral effects, induction of MHC I activation of NK cells and macrophages
IFN-γ	Activated Th1 lymphocytes, NK cells	Induces MHC I + II activates macrophages, neutrophilic granulocytes, NK cells, antiviral effects
TNF-α	Macrophages, mast cells	Inflammation induction, phagocytosis

In addition, the increase in permeability is achieved by the leukocytes penetrating the endothelial cell wall of the vessel transcellularly or mostly paracellularly, attracted by chemokines. For this purpose, the expression of transcellular endothelial cell adhesion molecules is influenced under the influence of inflammation, and leukocytes are also able to enzymatically cleave the cell-to-cell adhesion molecules, and therefore migrate into the surrounding tissue (Reglero-Real et al. 2016). In the tissue, leukocytes follow chemokine gradients and can orient themselves in different chemoattractive fields (Foxman et al. 1997).

The inflammatory reaction is essentially controlled by different mediators. In addition to cytokines, which are messenger substances that enable the interaction between the cells of the inflammatory cascade, some mediators serve as initiators of the inflammatory reaction.

These include eicosanoids that are formed by activating several enzyme systems in the arachidonic acid metabolism. Arachidonic acid is formed from phospholipids of the cell membranes under the influence of phospholipase A2. This in turn can be converted to prostaglandins, prostacyclin and thromboxanes under the catalysis of cyclooxygenases (COX). The lipoxygenases serve to synthesise leukotrienes from arachidonic acid. Eicosanoids can be formed in all cells of the body with the exception of erythrocytes. There are specific differences. In the thrombocytes, thromboxanes are formed almost exclusively. The vascular endothelial cells, on the other hand, produce mainly prostacyclins. The eicosanoids have hormone-like properties. They act as second messengers via cyclic AMP (cAMP). Unlike hormones, however, eicosanoids are formed locally and are not transported via the bloodstream to the site of their effect. Eicosanoids are not stored in the body. They have a half-life of a few minutes (Table 1.4).

In addition, inflammatory cytokines induce the secretion of acute phase proteins, which include over 40 proteins classified by function into transport proteins (e.g. ceruloplasmin), coagulation and fibrinolysis proteins (e.g. prothrombin, fibrinogen), complement system proteins (e.g. complement C3), antiproteases (e.g. α1-antitrypsin) and immune proteins (e.g. prothrombin, fibrinogen) and immunoactive proteins (e.g. CRP, SAA). The synthesis of acute phase proteins takes place in different organs, such as the liver (Ceron et al. 2005) (Table 1.5).

Table 1.4 Some eicosanoids with effect.

Eicosanoid	Effect
Prostaglandin	Pain response
Prostacyclin	Vasodilation, inhibition of platelet aggregation
Leukotriene	Leukocyte chemotaxis, adhesion of leukocytes to vascular endothelium, increase of capillary permeability
Thromboxane	Vasoconstriction, platelet aggregation

Table 1.5 Some acute phase proteins.

Name	Source	Effect
C-reactive protein (CRP)	Predominantly hepatocytes, also lymphocytes, macrophages	Opsonisation and activation of the complement system
Serum amyloid A (SAA)	Hepatocytes, adipocytes	Activation of inflammatory cells, and MMP
Haptoglobin	Hepatocytes	Binding of free haemoglobin
Ceruloplasmin		Iron oxidation

The acute phase proteins fulfil different functions in the course of the inflammation.

C-reactive protein (CRP) belongs to the opsonins that activate the complement system. It binds to phosphocholine, a component of bacterial cell membranes, among other things. The binding activates the complement system and the macrophage function.

Serum amyloid A (SAA) is involved in immune cell chemotaxis and activation of matrix metalloproteinases.

Haptoglobulin and ceruloplasmin and other metal-binding molecules serve the bacterial defence via the binding of iron by withholding iron from the bacterial metabolism (Figure 1.7).

After the initiation of the **inflammatory** process, the process follows a similar pattern. This is initially characterised by an infiltration of neutrophilic granulocytes. Due to their phagocytosis activity, these are able to eliminate the inflammatory triggers. This is followed by a phase with increased activity of lymphocytes and monocytes, which represents an essential link between innate and acquired immunity. Finally, the increase of eosinophilic granulocytes in the inflammatory area completes the response.

The termination of the inflammatory response is controlled by various mediators and cytokines, such as IL-10, and serves to protect the tissue.

The interleukin prevents the production of various cytokines, inhibits phagocytosis and weakens the microbicidal activity of neutrophilic granulocytes. In addition, their migration is reduced. IL-10 prevents the differentiation of immature dendritic cells and thus inhibits inflammatory responses. IL-10 inhibits INF-γ and TNF production by NK cells. It also induces lysis of infected cells (Mocellin et al. 2004) (Figure 1.8).

Figure 1.7 Induction of the acute phase response.

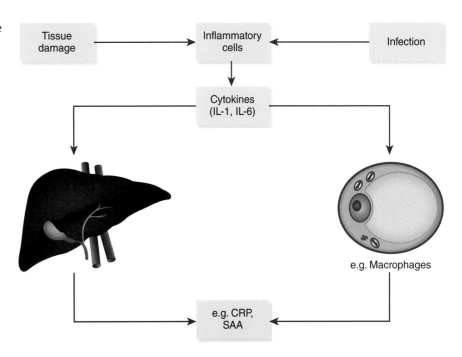

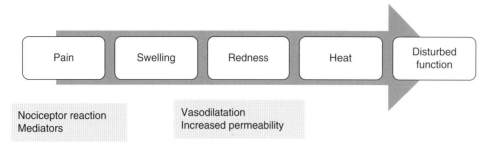

Figure 1.8 Overview of the inflammatory reaction.

Clinically, acute inflammation proceeds with the reactions described as cardinal symptoms: pain, redness, swelling and heat. These changes can be explained by the inflammatory process described, which is accompanied by increased blood flow, the formation of mediators and an increase in vascular permeability. In sum, a disturbance of tissue or organ function also develops in the inflamed area; this is called 'functio laesa'. This induces major clinical consequences of the acute inflammation and includes pain, destruction of tissue architecture and metaplasia.

An acute inflammatory event can develop into a chronic process. This results predominantly from a persistent inflammatory stimulus or an insufficient anti-inflammatory response after the elimination of the noxious agent has been completed. The process of chronic inflammation extends over several weeks or months. The result is a tissue remodelling that prevents a restitutio and thus a restoration of the initial tissue situation. In such a case, chronic inflammation leads to a fibrotic remodelling of the tissue.

References

Appelberg, R. (2007). Neutrophils and intracellular pathogens: beyond phagocytosis and killing. *Trends in Microbiology* 15 (2): 87–92. https://doi.org/10.1016/j.tim.2006.11.009.

Ceron, J.J., Eckersall, P.D., and Martýnez-Subiela, S. (2005). Acute phase proteins in dogs and cats: current knowledge and future perspectives. *Veterinary Clinical Pathology* 34 (2): 85–99. https://doi.org/10.1111/j.1939-165x.2005.tb00019.x.

Fioranelli, M., Roccia, M.G., Flavin, D., and Cota, L. (2021). Regulation of inflammatory reaction in health and disease. *International Journal of Molecular Sciences* 22 (10): 5277. https://doi.org/10.3390/ijms22105277.

Foxman, E.F., Campbell, J.J., and Butcher, E.C. (1997). Multistep navigation and the combinatorial control of leukocyte chemotaxis. *The Journal of Cell Biology* 139 (5): 1349–1360. https://doi.org/10.1083/jcb.139.5.1349.

Freitas, A.A. and Rocha, B. (2000). Population biology of lymphocytes: the flight for survival. *Annual Review of Immunology* 18: 83–111. https://doi.org/10.1146/annurev.immunol.18.1.83.

Gerhardt, T. and Ley, K. (2015). Monocyte trafficking across the vessel wall. *Cardiovascular Research* 107 (3): 321–330. https://doi.org/10.1093/cvr/cvv147.

LeBien, T.W. and Tedder, T.F. (2008). B lymphocytes: how they develop and function. *Blood* 112 (5): 1570–1580. https://doi.org/10.1182/blood-2008-02-078071.

Lehrer, R.I. and Ganz, T. (2002). Defensins of vertebrate animals. *Current Opinion in Immunology* 14 (1): 96–102. https://doi.org/10.1016/s0952-7915(01)00303-x.

Luster, A.D. (2002). The role of chemokines in linking innate and adaptive immunity. *Current Opinion in Immunology* 14 (1): 129–135. https://doi.org/10.1016/s0952-7915(01)00308-9.

Mitamura, Y., Ogulur, I., Pat, Y. et al. (2021). Dysregulation of the epithelial barrier by environmental and other exogenous factors. *Contact Dermatitis* 85 (6): 615–626. https://doi.org/10.1111/cod.13959.

Mocellin, S., Panelli, M., Wang, E. et al. (2004). IL-10 stimulatory effects on human NK cells explored by gene profile analysis. *Genes and Immunity* 5 (8): 621–630. https://doi.org/10.1038/sj.gene.6364135.

Muñoz, L.E., Boeltz, S., Bilyy, R. et al. (2019). Neutrophil extracellular traps initiate gallstone formation. *Immunity* 51 (3): 443–450.e4. https://doi.org/10.1016/j.immuni.2019.07.002.

Reglero-Real, N., Colom, B., Bodkin, J.V., and Nourshargh, S. (2016). Endothelial cell junctional adhesion molecules: role and regulation of expression in inflammation. *Arteriosclerosis, Thrombosis, and Vascular Biology* 36 (10): 2048–2057. https://doi.org/10.1161/ATVBAHA.116.307610.

Roche, P.A. and Furuta, K. (2015). The ins and outs of MHC class II-mediated antigen processing and presentation. *Nature Reviews Immunology* 15 (4): 203–216. https://doi.org/10.1038/nri3818.

Rosales, C. and Uribe-Querol, E. (2017). Phagocytosis: a fundamental process in immunity. *BioMed Research International* 2017: 9042851. https://doi.org/10.1155/2017/9042851.

Rothenberg, M.E. and Hogan, S.P. (2006). The eosinophil. *Annual Review of Immunology* 24: 147–174. https://doi.org/10.1146/annurev.immunol.24.021605.090720.

Sahl, H.G., Pag, U., Bonness, S. et al. (2005). Mammalian defensins: structures and mechanism of antibiotic activity. *Journal of Leukocyte Biology* 77 (4): 466–475. https://doi.org/10.1189/jlb.0804452.

Salazar-Mather, T.P. and Hokeness, K.L. (2003). Calling in the troops: regulation of inflammatory cell trafficking through innate cytokine/chemokine networks. *Viral Immunology* 16 (3): 291–306. https://doi.org/10.1089/088282403322396109.

Savina, A. and Amigorena, S. (2007). Phagocytosis and antigen presentation in dendritic cells. *Immunological Reviews* 219: 143–156. https://doi.org/10.1111/j.1600-065X.2007.00552.x.

Scott, M.G. and Hancock, R.E. (2000). Cationic antimicrobial peptides and their multifunctional role in the immune system. *Critical Reviews in Immunology* 20 (5): 407–431.

Stone, K.D., Prussin, C., and Metcalfe, D.D. (2010). IgE, mast cells, basophils, and eosinophils. *The Journal of Allergy and Clinical Immunology* 125 (2 Suppl 2): S73–S80. https://doi.org/10.1016/j.jaci.2009.11.017.

Wechsler, M.E., Munitz, A., Ackerman, S.J. et al. (2021). Eosinophils in health and disease: a state-of-the-art review. *Mayo Clinic Proceedings* 96 (10): 2694–2707. https://doi.org/10.1016/j.mayocp.2021.04.025.

Yang, D., Biragyn, A., Kwak, L.W., and Oppenheim, J.J. (2002). Mammalian defensins in immunity: more than just microbicidal. *Trends in Immunology* 23 (6): 291–296. https://doi.org/10.1016/s1471-4906(02)02246-9.

2

Sepsis and Cytokine Storm

Sepsis is an excessive, systemic inflammatory reaction, due to an infectious event, which can lead to organ dysfunction or organ failure. The course of the disease and the prognosis can be negatively influenced by the massive release of cytokines as hypercytokinaemia or 'cytokine storm'.

The onset of sepsis is associated with the binding of microbial molecules to receptors of the inflammatory cells (e.g. toll-like receptor). This results in the expression of proinflammatory cytokines. This activates both the inflammatory cascade and the coagulation cascade. The activation of the coagulation cascade results in the formation of microthrombi, which can lead to organ damage through ischaemia and hypoxia. As a result of the consumption of coagulation factors, a bleeding tendency develops. This, in turn, can further impair the supply of organs and lead to organ dysfunction.

On the other hand, activation of the inflammatory cascade leads to irritation of the blood vessel epithelia. This can lead to vasodilation and permeability changes of the vessels. In extreme cases, a relative blood deficiency develops, resulting in shock.

All organ systems are affected by the vascular changes. The symptoms that develop are (Table 2.1).

In connection with sepsis or severe non-septic diseases, there may be an acute massive release of cytokines (Figure 2.1).

Cytokines are polypeptides that play a central role in intercellular communication and are essential for mediating and regulating immunological responses. Their mode of action is to bind to surface receptors to activate signal transduction cascades. This ultimately leads to altered cellular gene expression, which influences metabolic activity, cell differentiation, proliferation, migration and apoptosis.

Different cytokines can activate the same signal transduction cascade; conversely, the cytokine can act as a pleiotropic molecule on different cell types and elicit different responses.

Cytokines are polypeptides with molecular weights of approximately 15–25 kDa. They are usually not stored as pre-formed molecules but secreted when needed. Usually, they are only transiently expressed; however, constitutive forms have also been found. Cytokines are secreted in pico- to nanomolar concentrations. This is sufficient because cytokine receptors have a very high affinity for their ligands. In contrast to hormones, cytokines act over much shorter distances – autocrine or paracrine, but also endocrine (e.g. IL-1). Although the mode of action of some cytokines is similar to that of hormones, cytokines can act on a wider range of target cells than hormones. The biggest difference is probably that cytokines are not produced by specialised cells in glands responsible for them.

The effect of cytokines is mediated by membrane-bound surface molecules on the target cells, the so-called 'transmembrane proteins'. The extracellular signals are converted into intracellular impulses by binding on a receptor, which results in the transcription of new genes. Functionally, cytokines are divided into growth factors, interferons, chemokines and interleukins.

Cytokines can also be classified according to structural features: The α-helical cytokines consist of four α-helices. IL-2-12 as well as INF-α, -β and -γ are counted among this group. The next group includes cytokines with a β-leaflet structure. It is represented, for example, by the TNF family and the IL-1 family. There are also short-chain α/β-cytokines, which include the EGF family, the insulin-related cytokines and the chemokines. The chemokines are again divided into four groups: the C-chemokines (lymphotactin), CC-chemokines (MCP, RANTES), the CXC-chemokines (IL-8, NAP-2) and the CX3C-chemokines (fractalkines). In addition, a fourth group is described: the mosaic structure cytokines. The family of heregulins or HGF are assigned to this group.

Table 2.1 Clinical consequences of sepsis.

Central nervous system	Cardiovascular system	Respiratory system	Gastrointestinal system	Hepatobiliary system	Urinary tract	Endocrine system
Lethargy	Tachycardia	Tachypnoea	Diarrhoea	Cholestasis	Uraemia	Pituitary dysfunction
Reduced mental status	Decreased vascular resistance	Respiratory distress syndrome Hypoxaemia	Ileus	Azotaemia	Oliguria	
					Proteinuria	

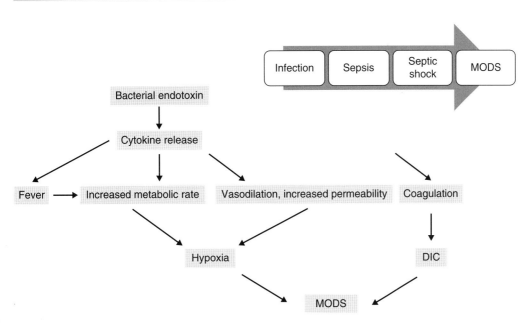

Figure 2.1 Pathophysiology of sepsis.

A classification according to the type of immune response in which they are secreted is also possible. Type I cytokines are those secreted by TH-1 lymphocytes as part of the cellular immune response. They include IFN-γ and IL-2 and also IL-12, which is released by antigen-presenting cells and promotes the differentiation of TH-1 cells. Type II cytokines are released by TH-2 lymphocytes during humoral immune responses. Typical representatives are IL-4, IL-5, IL-10 and IL-13.

In the inflammatory process, cytokines can be categorised into pro- and anti-inflammatory forms, depending on their effect. Those that initiate and stimulate inflammatory processes are, for example, TNF-α, IL-1, IL-2, IL-6, IFN-γ, macrophage colony-stimulating factor (M-CSF) and granulocyte macrophage colony-stimulating factor (GM-CSF). Classic anti-inflammatory factors are IL-4, IL-13, IL-10 or TGF-β.

The cytokine storm that develops in sepsis leads significantly to an increase in the proinflammatory cytokines TNF-α; IL-1 and IL-6. These are characterised in more detail below.

TNF-α is a mediator of inflammatory responses. As such, it increases the cytotoxicity and phagocytosis of neutrophilic granulocytes and macrophages, causing their adhesion to the endothelium and the production of superoxide. In interaction with IL-1, TNF-α is responsible for many endothelial remodelling processes that lead to an increase in permeability. It prevents anti-coagulatory mechanisms and supports thrombotic processes by decreasing the expression of thrombomodulin, which can lead to the formation of venous thrombosis, vasculitis and intravascular disseminated coagulopathy. The ability of TNF-α to stimulate the synthesis of PGI_2, nitric oxide and PAF causes vasodilation, leukocytosis and increased vascular permeability. TNF-α is able to induce the production of MHC antigen on endothelial cells to transform them into APC. Furthermore, TNF-α plays a significant role in defence against bacteria and parasites, and modulation of the immune response through its ability to activate phagocytosis and recruitment of leukocytes. Granulocytes stimulated by TNF-α show increased microbicidal activity through increased production of superoxide anions and degranulation. TNF-α also increases the toxicity of eosinophilic granulocytes and macrophages.

Interleukin-1 is the most important proinflammatory cytokine alongside TNF-α and IFN-γ. It is present in the form of two subtypes, IL-1α and IL-1β, mainly produced by monocytes, macrophages, endothelial cells and fibroblasts.

Signal transduction at the cellular level is initiated after binding to an IL-1 receptor molecule. There are two cellular receptors for IL-1 – IL-1 receptor I (IL-1RI) and IL-1 receptor II (IL-1RII). The binding of IL-1 to the former receptor is followed by signal transduction, whereas binding to the latter is not. The IL-1RII is also called the 'bait receptor' for IL-1, since its mode of operation causes a drop in the IL-1 level, which then leads to no subsequent reaction due to the lack of intracellular signal transduction. Both receptor subtypes are not only cell-bound, but also circulate in the blood and intercept IL-1 there.

IL-1 has a fever-inducing effect in the organism, stimulates lymphocyte activity and promotes the release of acute phase proteins of the liver, as well as the production of collagenases and prostaglandins, and leukocyte diapedesis.

Canine IL-6 consists of 187 amino acids. IL-6 is produced by activated macrophages, T and B cells, endothelial cells, fibroblasts, keratinocytes and mesangial cells. The main suppliers are resident monocytes and macrophages in the acute phase of inflammation, and T cells in chronic inflammatory processes. The synthesis and release of the cytokine is mainly stimulated by IL-1, TNF-α, TGF-β, bacterial and viral infections, as well as endotoxins and liposaccharides (LPS).

The membrane-bound IL-6 receptor consists of an α- and a β- subunit; and is mainly expressed on hepatocytes, neutrophilic granulocytes, monocytes, macrophages and some leukocytes.

To initiate the intracellular signalling cascade, the receptor interacts with the tyrosine kinases of the Janus family.

Important functions of the B cells are influenced by IL-6, such as the growth of certain B cell series, and, together with IL-4 and -5, the B cell differentiation into plasma cells is controlled. In interaction with IL-2 and IL-5, IL-6 is also involved in IgM and IgA synthesis. In addition to B cells, T cells are also controlled. These are activated by IL-6 and can be converted into cytotoxic T cells.

In terms of the inflammatory response, IL-6 is one of the main stimulators of the acute phase response. The acute phase response is a systemic immune system response to infection, trauma, inflammation and tissue injury. It is characterised by fever, increased tissue permeability, an increase in peripheral leukocyte count and synthesis of acute phase proteins by the liver. Acute phase proteins include, for example, fibrinogen, α-1-antitrypsin, α-1-chymotrypsin, haptoglobulin and C-reactive protein. Together with IL-1 and TNF-α, IL-6 causes not only the acute phase reaction but also the development of fever by stimulating the thermoregulatory centre in the brain and subsequent increase in the set point (Figure 2.2).

In a cytokine storm, there is a massive release of mainly proinflammatory cytokines into the blood. This results in the activation of inflammatory cells in various organs and the initiation of organ dysfunction or failure. The following organ dysfunctions and clinical symptoms are described:

Lungs

- Pulmonary oedema
- Dyspnoea, hypoxaemia
- Acute respiratory distress syndrome (ARDS)

Figure 2.2   Effects of TNF-α, IL-1, IL-6.

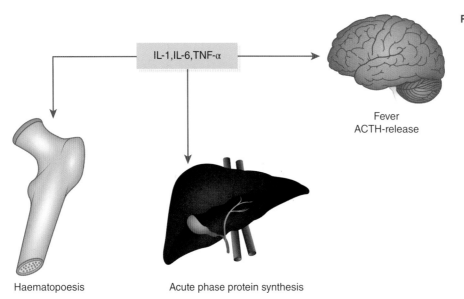

IL-1, IL-6, TNF-α

Fever
ACTH-release

Haematopoesis

Acute phase protein synthesis

Liver

- Hepatomegaly
- Elevated liver enzymes – Increased hepcidin
- Hypoalbuminaemia
- Liver injury
- Cholestasis
- Liver failure

Kidneys

- Acute renal dysfunction or injury
- Renal failure

Vascular and lymphatic systems

- Cytopenia, anaemia, leukocytosis
- Coagulopathy
- Hyperferritinemia, increase in other acute phase reactants (e.g. CRP, D-dimer)
- Elevated cytokines (e.g. IL-1, IL-6, interferon-γ) and growth factors (e.g. VEGF)
- Endothelial damage and vascular permeability
- Capillary leak syndrome
- Vasodilatory shock
- Spontaneous haemorrhage
- Lymphadenopathy

Nervous system

- Confusion
- Aphasia
- Seizures

Constitutional symptoms

- Fever
- Anorexia
- Fatigue

Heart

- Hypotension
- Tachycardia
- Cardiomyopathy

Gastrointestinal system

- Nausea
- Vomiting
- Diarrhoea
- Ascites

Skin

- Rash
- Oedema

The cytokine storm resulting from sepsis develops due to the cytokine reaction after dissemination of a local bacterial infection. The consequence is an excessive activation of leukocytes, primarily neutrophilic granulocytes, monocytes and macrophages. These can produce more cytokines after contact with antigens. The cytokine storm also activates cells of the adaptive immune system, mainly Th-1 cells. These secrete high concentrations of interferon-γ and activate macrophages. This results in cytokine-induced direct tissue destruction.

This leads to a reaction of the leukocytes in the sense of leukocytosis or leukopenia as a sign of excessive leukocyte release with depletion of the depots. Thrombocytopenia also develops as a result of the cytokine reaction. All factors together lead to DIC with vascular thrombosis or a bleeding tendency due to consumption of clotting factors. This, in turn, can lead to hypoxaemia via vasodilation and hypotension. This induces tissue or organ failure. The organs affected are the kidneys via prerenal renal failure and the liver via reduced blood flow with cholestasis. Finally, the lungs may develop ARDS.

All affected patients are febrile because cytokines such as IL-1 or IL-6 act directly on the temperature regulation centre and induce a setpoint shift there.

The hypothalamus regulates core body temperature. This nerve cell region receives afferent signals from thermoreceptors in the skin and is, additionally, able to measure the core body temperature itself. Based on this information, the setpoint is controlled in two different directions. Substances that cause fever are called 'pyrogens'. Exogenous pyrogens are microbial toxins, metabolic products or the microorganisms themselves. A classic example is the lipopolysaccharide endotoxin of gram-negative bacteria.

The cytokines IL-1, IL-6 and TNF act as endogenous pyrogens. The synthesis and release of cytokines is triggered not only by microbial pathogens, but also by inflammation.

The pyrogens cause an increased production of prostaglandin E2 (PGE2) in the hypothalamic endothelium and in the periphery. This binds it to the EP2 receptor of glial cells, which secrete cAMP. This transmitter leads to an increase in the thermoregulatory setpoint.

Further Reading

Angus, D.C. and van der Poll, T. (2013). Severe sepsis and septic shock. *The New England Journal of Medicine* 369 (9): 840–851. https://doi.org/10.1056/NEJMra1208623.

Bosmann, M. and Ward, P.A. (2013). The inflammatory response in sepsis. *Trends in Immunology* 34 (3): 129–136. https://doi.org/10.1016/j.it.2012.09.004.

Chousterman, B.G., Swirski, F.K., and Weber, G.F. (2017). Cytokine storm and sepsis disease pathogenesis. *Seminars in Immunopathology* 39 (5): 517–528. https://doi.org/10.1007/s00281-017-0639-8.

Fajgenbaum, D.C. and June, C.H. (2020). Cytokine storm. *The New England Journal of Medicine* 383 (23): 2255–2273. https://doi.org/10.1056/NEJMra2026131.

Iba, T. and Levy, J.H. (2020). Sepsis-induced coagulopathy and disseminated intravascular coagulation. *Anesthesiology* 132 (5): 1238–1245. https://doi.org/10.1097/ALN.0000000000003122.

Karki, R. and Kanneganti, T.D. (2021). The 'cytokine storm': molecular mechanisms and therapeutic prospects. *Trends in Immunology* 42 (8): 681–705. https://doi.org/10.1016/j.it.2021.06.001.

Pool, R., Gomez, H., and Kellum, J.A. (2018). Mechanisms of organ dysfunction in sepsis. *Critical Care Clinics* 34 (1): 63–80. https://doi.org/10.1016/j.ccc.2017.08.003.

Tisoncik, J.R., Korth, M.J., Simmons, C.P. et al. (2012). Into the eye of the cytokine storm. *Microbiology and Molecular Biology Reviews: MMBR* 76 (1): 16–32. https://doi.org/10.1128/MMBR.05015-11.

3

Fibrosis

Definition

Fibrosis is a process characterised by a pathological proliferation of connective tissue in tissues and organs. There is an excessive increase in extracellular matrix (ECM). The cause is tissue damage triggered by different stimuli, which can recur or take a chronic course. Despite the variety of different stimuli in different tissues and organs, the response to these stimuli is the same. It can lead to physiological restriction or even loss of organ function. Physiologically, fibrosis is part of any temporary wound healing.

Cells of Fibrosis Initiation

While fibrotic remodelling is controlled by connective tissue cells, such as myofibroblasts, the initiation of fibrosis is a consequence of the function of inflammatory cells. Macrophages, neutrophilic granulocytes, natural killer cells and T and B lymphocytes are involved in the pathogenesis of fibrosis.

Macrophages can differentiate into M-1 and M-2 macrophages during the inflammatory response depending on cytokine influences. The former are formed under the influence of IFN-γ and TNF-α, while the latter are formed in response to IL-4, IL-10, IL-13 and TGF-β. Both macrophage types are involved in fibrosis. The M-1 macrophages produce proinflammatory cytokines and chemokines that promote myofibroblast activation and differentiation. However, they can also modulate fibrosis through the synthesis of matrix metalloproteinases (MMPs), as MMPs can degrade the ECM and contribute to the resolution of fibrosis. M-2 macrophages show anti-inflammatory properties and play an anti-fibrotic role in fibrosis.

Neutrophilic granulocytes are involved in fibrosis through different mechanisms. For example, neutrophilic granulocytes secrete elastase, which has a proteolytic effect on proteins of the ECM (e.g. elastin and collagen type IV). In this way, the enzyme contributes to remodelling in the fibrotic area. In addition, endocytosis of neutrophilic granulocyte elastase by fibroblasts increases α-smooth muscle actin (α-SMA) expression, promoted cell proliferation and improved migration and contractility of these cells.

Natural killer (NK) cells also influence fibrotic remodelling by eliminating activated myofibroblast precursor cells. This happens, for example, with activated Ito cells, the myofibroblast precursors in the liver. Accordingly, the NK cells initiate an anti-fibrotic effect.

Of the cells of the adaptive immune system, Th1 cells are thought to have anti-fibrotic activity and Th2 cells are thought to have fibrotic activity (Figure 3.1, Table 3.1).

Course of the Fibrosis

Fibrosis initiation in an inflammatory process is triggered by proinflammatory cytokines of activated inflammatory cells.

The mechanism will be explained using the function of IL-6 as an example. IL-6 is secreted by numerous inflammatory cells during the course of the inflammatory cascade. These include lymphocytes and macrophages. IL-6 in turn acts on a

Textbook of Small Animal Pathophysiology, First Edition. Stephan Neumann.
© 2025 John Wiley & Sons Ltd. Published 2025 by John Wiley & Sons Ltd.

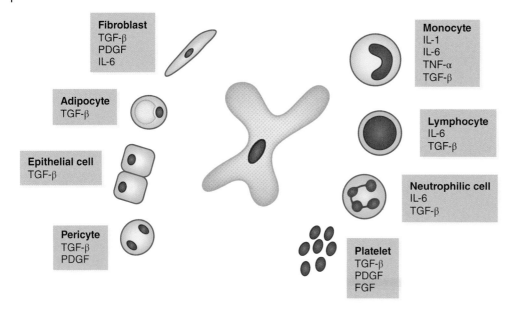

Figure 3.1 Inflammatory cells with their influence on the myofibroblasts.

Table 3.1 Functional cells of fibrosis.

Cell	Function in fibrosis
Macrophages	Promotion of fibrosis
	Degradation of the ECM
Neutrophils	Promotion of fibrosis
	Elastase formation
NK cells	Promotion of fibrosis
	Suppression of fibrosis

Source: Adapted from Huang et al. (2020).

variety of different cells that play a role in the inflammatory process, such as macrophages, T-lymphocytes, endothelial cells and fibroblasts. IL-6 action is mediated by receptor binding of the cytokine and subsequent signal transduction by gp130. Cells lacking a receptor cannot mediate IL-6 action. However, IL-6 can also be bound intravascularly by soluble IL-6 receptors, which can then activate gp130 as a complex even in cells without an IL-6 receptor. Through this mechanism, fibroblast migration into the inflammatory arena is also initiated (Rose-John 2012).

Another mechanism of fibroblast activation takes place via the activation of pattern recognition receptors (PRRs) that react to microbial pathogen-associated molecular patterns (PAMPs). This mechanism is described in Chapter 1, but also occurs in the activation of fibroblasts (Akira and Takeda 2004; Johnson et al. 2020).

Initiated, tissue fibrosis often proceeds according to the laws of wound healing.

Wound healing is divided into the phases of haemorrhage, inflammation, proliferation and remodelling. Each phase is dominated by specific cells that facilitate the molecular remodelling process via cytokines and growth factors. The bleeding phase is dominated by platelets, which initiate the coagulation cascade and the formation of a fibrin network.

Platelets also synthesise numerous 'active substances' such as growth factors and cytokines. Through these, the phase of inflammation is initiated, which is characterised by migration of mononuclear cells such as monocytes and lymphocytes. Phagocytic and proteolytic properties of these cells help to break down and remove necrotic material.

In the subsequent proliferative phase, after a few days, capillaries sprout and fibroblasts migrate, which form a granulation tissue rich in capillaries and cells and stimulate the formation of ECM.

The fibroblasts are converted into myofibroblasts, which are capable of producing large amounts of collagen. In addition, this cell type contributes to wound contraction due to its contractile property. The wound is finally closed by immigration of new cells.

In the final step, remodelling occurs and the collagens gain stability through cross-linking. Once wound healing is complete, collagen synthesis is reduced back to a basal level and the myofibroblasts are removed by apoptosis (Diegelmann and Evans 2004).

In wound healing, it is important to ensure a balance between the build-up and degradation of ECM. For example, matrix can be degraded by endogenous metalloproteinases (MMPs). If the build-up of ECM predominates, fibrosis develops.

Although the cellular processes in fibrotic tissue are comparable to those in wound healing, the proliferative reaction in fibrosis leads to a pathological remodelling of the tissue. An essential step is the proliferation of fibroblasts and their differentiation into myofibroblasts. The latter develop from mesenchymal, endothelial or epithelial cells as well as pericytes, fibrocytes and fibroblasts.

The differentiation of epithelial cells or endothelial cells into myofibroblasts with a mesenchymal character is called 'epithelial–mesenchymal transformation' (EMT) or 'endothelial–mesenchymal transformation' (EndMT). In this process, the gene expression of the cells changes. Due to the reduced transcription of adhesion molecules, the cells lose their polarity and cell–cell contact. They take on a mesenchymal phenotype and are able to migrate across the basement membrane into the extracellular space. There, as the main effector cells in fibrosis, they are responsible for the secretion of profibrotic cytokines and MMPs as well as the excessive synthesis of various collagens or fibronectin. Furthermore, myofibroblasts are characterised by contractile properties as well as the expression of α-SMA.

In advanced stages, the excessive accumulation of ECM results in tissue hypoxia, which in turn is associated with cell loss and further fibrogenesis (Weiskirchen et al. 2019).

An essential growth factor of fibrosis is transforming growth factor-β (TGF-β). From the TGF family, TGF-β1 is particularly important for fibrosis. It is a 25 kDa homodimeric protein. TGF-β1 is mainly synthesised by platelets, macrophages, fibroblasts and myofibroblasts as an inactive precursor. After secretion, the inactive precursor of TGF-β1 is probably activated by different proteases such as plasmin or cathepsin (Yin et al. 2012). Activated TGF-β1 can act on the target cells via different TGF receptors. After receptor binding, signal transduction takes place via the SMAD-MAPK pathway. This results in increased gene activation with the synthesis of profibrotic molecules.

Stimulation of TGF-β1 can initiate the synthesis of fibronectin, laminin and collagen types I, II and IV of the ECM. Increased synthesis of proteoglycans, glucosaminoglycans and chondroitin sulphate also takes place. Finally, controlling glycoproteins, such as thrombospondin, osteopontin, osteonectin and tenaskin are also increased in expression. At the same time, TGF-β1 inhibits the expression of MMPs and plasminogen activators (Okuda et al. 1990; Tomooka et al. 1992).

The MMPs, which are important for the degradation of ECM, maintain the physiological balance between the formation and degradation of connective tissue components. In fibrotic tissue, both the expression and activity of the MMPs and their natural inhibitors are pathologically altered.

Besides TGF-β, the cytokines platelet-derived growth factor (PDGF) and connective tissue growth factor (CTGF) have a profibrotic effect via receptor tyrosine kinases. The vasoactive peptides angiotensin-II (AT-II) and endothelin-1 (ET-1), which act via G-protein-coupled receptors, or high glucose serum concentrations also promote fibrosis (Leask and Abraham 2004; Rodríguez-Pascual et al. 2014) (Figure 3.2).

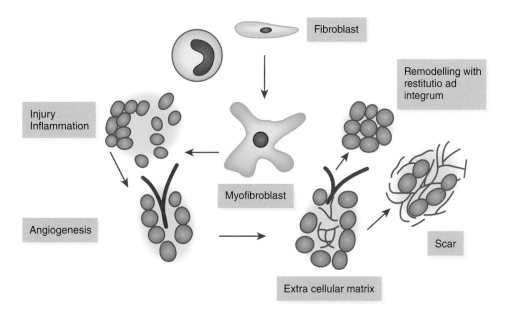

Figure 3.2 Mechanism of tissue fibrosis.

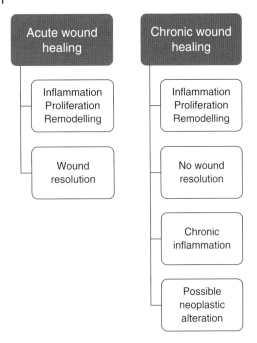

Figure 3.3 Relation between fibrosis and tumour (Rybinski et al. 2014).

Fibrosis as a consequence of chronic inflammation does not develop equally in all tissues. In dogs and cats, it is described particularly in the liver, kidneys, lungs and skin. The consequence of fibrosis is tissue or organ dysfunction. This results in clinical consequences that are organ specific. Within the organ, however, fibrosis leads to comparable consequences.

On the one hand, tissue fibrosis changes the connection with blood vessels. Vessels are displaced by fibrosis. This leads to thrombosis of the vessels with the need to form collateral vessels. This can lead to reduced tissue supply and hypoxia. In addition, the reduced removal of CO_2 can contribute to an accumulation in the tissue and formation of metabolic acidosis. This, in turn, also leads to cellular dysfunction.

Another consequence is the widening of resorption pathways. For example, pulmonary fibrosis leads to a widening of the alveolar-erythrocytic exchange pathway. As a result, less oxygen is absorbed and CO_2 is released. This leads to an accumulation of carbonic acid in the organism with metabolic acidosis as a consequence.

In the liver sinusoids, the resorption pathways between sinus blood and hepatocytes also lengthen. This can contribute to a reduced absorption of nutrients.

Another consequence of fibrosis is the continuous initiation of an inflammatory reaction. This is given by the disturbed homeostasis in the fibrotic tissue and thus a perpetual induction of the defence against noxious agents.

Finally, fibrotic remodelling processes are to be considered precancerous.

For example, in humans, chronic fibrosis, such as cirrhosis of the liver, of various aetiologies, is associated with an increased risk of cancer. Both fibrotic and tumour tissue are characterised by hyperproliferation of their cells. Although carcinoma cells show transformative mutations that fibrotic tissue lacks, a large population of myofibroblasts is present at the tumour stroma as carcinoma-associated fibroblasts. These myofibroblasts initiate tumour progression or chronic fibrosis through paracrine effects on surrounding cells by producing numerous growth factors, inflammatory cytokines, proteolytic enzymes and ECM proteins (Figure 3.3).

References

Akira, S. and Takeda, K. (2004). Toll-like receptor signalling. *Nature Reviews Immunology* 4 (7): 499–511. https://doi.org/10.1038/nri1391.

Diegelmann, R.F. and Evans, M.C. (2004). Wound healing: an overview of acute, fibrotic and delayed healing. *Frontiers in Bioscience: A Journal and Virtual Library* 9: 283–289. https://doi.org/10.2741/1184.

Huang, E., Peng, N., Xiao, F. et al. (2020). The roles of immune cells in the pathogenesis of fibrosis. *International Journal of Molecular Sciences* 21 (15): 5203. https://doi.org/10.3390/ijms21155203.

Johnson, B.Z., Stevenson, A.W., Prêle, C.M. et al. (2020). The role of IL-6 in skin fibrosis and cutaneous wound healing. *Biomedicine* 8 (5): 101. https://doi.org/10.3390/biomedicines8050101.

Leask, A. and Abraham, D.J. (2004). TGF-beta signalling and the fibrotic response. *FASEB Journal: Official Publication of the Federation of American Societies for Experimental Biology* 18 (7): 816–827. https://doi.org/10.1096/fj.03-1273rev.

Okuda, S., Languino, L.R., Ruoslahti, E., and Border, W.A. (1990). Elevated expression of transforming growth factor-beta and proteoglycan production in experimental glomerulonephritis.Possible role in expansion of the mesangial extracellular matrix. *The Journal of Clinical Investigation* 86 (2): 453–462. https://doi.org/10.1172/JCI114731.

Rodríguez-Pascual, F., Busnadiego, O., and González-Santamaría, J. (2014). The profibrotic role of endothelin-1: is the door still open for the treatment of fibrotic diseases? *Life Sciences* 118 (2): 156–164. https://doi.org/10.1016/j.lfs.2013.12.024.

Rose-John, S. (2012). IL-6 trans-signaling via the soluble IL-6 receptor: importance for the pro-inflammatory activities of IL-6. *International Journal of Biological Sciences* 8 (9): 1237–1247. https://doi.org/10.7150/ijbs.4989.

Rybinski, B., Franco-Barraza, J., and Cukierman, E. (2014). The wound healing, chronic fibrosis, and cancer progression triad. *Physiological Genomics* 46 (7): 223–244. https://doi.org/10.1152/physiolgenomics.00158.2013.

Tomooka, S., Border, W.A., Marshall, B.C., and Noble, N.A. (1992). Glomerular matrix accumulation is linked to inhibition of the plasmin protease system. *Kidney International* 42 (6): 1462–1469. https://doi.org/10.1038/ki.1992.442.

Weiskirchen, R., Weiskirchen, S., and Tacke, F. (2019). Organ and tissue fibrosis: molecular signals, cellular mechanisms and translational implications. *Molecular Aspects of Medicine* 65: 2–15. http://dx.doi.org/10.1016/j.mam.2018.06.003.

Yin, M., Soikkeli, J., Jahkola, T. et al. (2012). TGF-β signaling, activated stromal fibroblasts, and cysteine cathepsins B and L drive the invasive growth of human melanoma cells. *The American Journal of Pathology* 181 (6): 2202–2216. https://doi.org/10.1016/j.ajpath.2012.08.027.

4

Degeneration

Definition

The term 'degeneration' refers to functional and morphological changes in a cell, tissue or organ that represent deterioration compared to full physiological capacity.

Aetiology

The triggers of degenerative changes are multiple. In most cases, there is a chronic disease process in which the cellular metabolism is changed. In addition to the cellular changes, changes are also implied in the tissue or organ.

Cellular Disturbances in Degeneration

Degenerative processes develop through sublethal disturbances of cell metabolism and are characterised by morphological cell alteration, e.g. in the sense of vacuole formation. In a metabolically disturbed cell, the mechanisms of metabolism do not change in principle, but the metabolic processes run incompletely. Processes and structures that are affected are:

Energy generation
Enzyme systems
Transport processes and
Organelle or cell membrane structures

An important primary causality of degenerative cell change is based on reduced **energy production**. Cellular energy production is associated with the synthesis of ATP. This is particularly effective in the context of oxidative phosphorylation and thus associated with aerobic glycolysis. Insufficient supply of substrates, reduced oxygen supply or disturbances of the biochemical processes due to enzyme inhibition disrupt the energy production of the cell.

Consequences of a reduced energy supply in the cell are the intracellular accumulation of water and electrolytes. Here, the reduced availability of ATP leads to the dysfunction of the energy-dependent sodium pump in the plasma membrane. This results in an influx of sodium and water into the cell. The result is water retention, which can be visualised microscopically as turbid swelling (mitochondria), vacuolar degeneration (mitochondria and endoplasmic reticulum) and hydropic degeneration (cytoplasm). Endoplasmic reticulum swelling leads to ribosome detachment and disrupts protein synthesis. Mitochondrial swelling causes uncoupling of oxidative phosphorylation, which further impairs ATP synthesis.

Alterations also occur in the intracellular concentrations of other electrolytes (especially K^+, Ca^{2+} and Mg^{2+}), which are maintained by energy-dependent activity of the plasma membrane. These electrolyte abnormalities can lead to impaired electrical activity and **enzyme inhibition** (Figure 4.1).

Due to the increasingly anaerobic glycolysis in cellular hypoxia, more lactate is formed. The lactic acid causes a decrease in the intracellular pH. This leads to consequences in all cellular compartments. In the nucleus, acidic pH can cause condensation of chromatin and thereby disrupt gene expression. Intracellular membranes of cell organelles can change their permeability at a lower pH value and, for example, result in an intracellular release of hydrolytic enzymes from lysosomes.

Textbook of Small Animal Pathophysiology, First Edition. Stephan Neumann.
© 2025 John Wiley & Sons Ltd. Published 2025 by John Wiley & Sons Ltd.

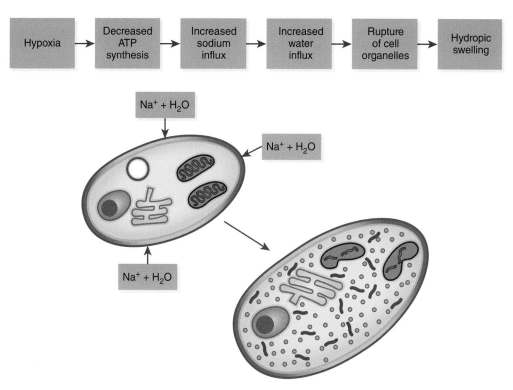

Figure 4.1 Hydropic swelling due to water retention.

Numerous cellular enzymes have an optimal activity in the neutral range. A reduction of the pH value restricts the activity, resulting in, e.g. a reduction in protein biosynthesis. A lack of structural proteins leads to a permeability disorder of the cell membrane and damage to the cell organelles and to disturbed **transport processes** within the cell. Furthermore, important lipoproteins for the removal of neutral fats are no longer provided. Reduced transport and reduced fatty acid oxidation due to oxygen deficiency lead to fatty degeneration of the cell (Figure 4.2).

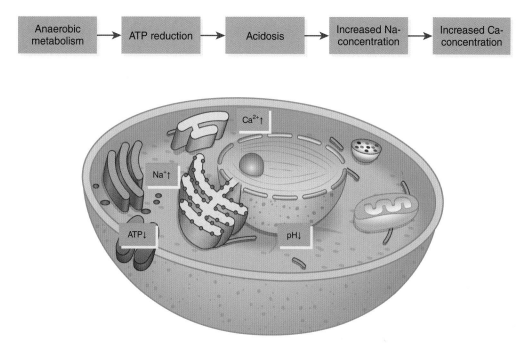

Figure 4.2 Consequences of decreased cell pH.

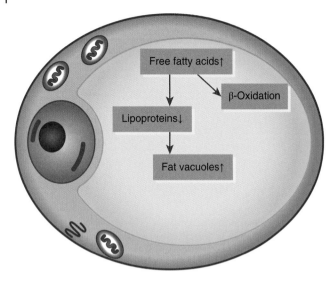

Figure 4.3 Disturbances of lipid metabolism in hepatocellular fatty degeneration.

Another degenerative pathomechanism is the increased synthesis of free radicals and thus the increase in oxidative stress. Free radicals are highly unstable particles with an unpaired electron in their outer shell. This makes free radicals extremely reactive. A frequent consequence of oxidative stress is lipid peroxidation of the cell membrane with functional damage and **morphological changes**.

Degenerative Tissue Changes

Fatty degeneration, deposition of metabolites and connective tissue structural changes are frequent consequences of degenerative processes in the tissue or organ.

Fatty degeneration is caused by an accumulation of triglycerides in the cells and often takes place in the liver. The liver has a central function in fat metabolism. Free fatty acids are supplied to the hepatocytes by the sinusoid. In the hepatocytes, the triglycerides are used for energy supply via β-oxidation or they are released into the plasma by binding in lipoproteins. Degenerated liver cells synthesise fewer proteins for lipoprotein synthesis, which increases the concentration of triglycerides in the hepatocytes. At the same time, β-oxidation is reduced. Both lead to the accumulation of triglycerides in the hepatocytes. These accumulate in vacuoles, which in the chronic course usually confluence to form a large vacuole (Figure 4.3).

Connective tissue remodelling processes are another form of a degenerative process in the tissue. These often arise from a primary inflammatory process, but are not initially inflammatory in genesis. Fibrotic remodelling processes occur increasingly in the liver, kidneys, lungs and joints. Although the remodelling is not inflammatory, degenerative processes can in turn have an inflammation-inducing effect and be accompanied by recurrent inflammation.

The clinical consequences of the degenerative processes are initially associated with a reduction in cellular function and thus organ performance. Cats with hepatolipidosis, for example, may develop hepatoencephalic syndrome due to reduced detoxification capacity of the liver.

Degenerative remodelling processes in the kidney disrupt the function of the nephron. Both glomerular filtration and tubular reabsorption can be impaired. In addition to disturbances of the water balance, disturbances of the acid-base balance and electrolyte balance develop, as well as a reduced excretion of toxins. These can accumulate and cause the clinical picture of uraemia.

In the lungs, the degenerative remodelling of the alveoli is associated with a restricted gas exchange surface. Reduced oxygen uptake and CO_2 release are the result. Hypoxia in turn causes restrictions in cellular energy production. Reduced CO_2 expiration induces respiratory acidosis.

Osteoarthrotic remodelled joints show a restricted 'range of motion', take less load and also lead to secondary atrophy of the associated muscles due to the restricted joint function.

Further Reading

Andreone, B.J., Larhammar, M., and Lewcock, J.W. (2020). Cell death and neurodegeneration. *Cold Spring Harbor Perspectives in Biology* 12 (2): a036434. https://doi.org/10.1101/cshperspect.a036434.

Di Pasqua, L.G., Cagna, M., Berardo, C. et al. (2022). Detailed molecular mechanisms involved in drug-induced non-alcoholic fatty liver disease and non-alcoholic steatohepatitis: an update. *Biomedicine* 10 (1): 194. https://doi.org/10.3390/biomedicines10010194.

French, S.W. (2000). Mechanisms of alcoholic liver injury. *Canadian Journal of Gastroenterology = Journalcanadien de gastroenterologie* 14 (4): 327–332. https://doi.org/10.1155/2000/801735.

Ota, T. (2021). Molecular mechanisms of Nonalcoholic Fatty Liver Disease (NAFLD)/Nonalcoholic Steatohepatitis (NASH). *Advances in Experimental Medicine and Biology* 1261: 223–229. https://doi.org/10.1007/978-981-15-7360-6_20.

Yan, T., Feng, Y., and Zhai, Q. (2010). Axon degeneration: mechanisms and implications of a distinct program from cell death. *Neurochemistry International* 56 (4): 529–534. https://doi.org/10.1016/j.neuint.2010.01.013.

5

Obesity

Definition

Obesity is defined as an excessive increase in fat tissue in the body resulting from a positive energy balance.

Fat Metabolism

Fat Absorption

Fats are absorbed as basic nutritional substances through food. Due to their low water solubility, their absorption is complex. In the intestinal lumen, the fats ingested with food (triacylglycerols and cholesterol) become absorbable through partial degradation and very fine emulsification.

The partial degradation is due to the lipase secreted via pancreatic secretion, which cleaves the triacylglycerol compounds with the formation of β-monoacylglycerols and fatty acids. Complete cleavage into glycerol and fatty acids occurs only to a small extent, and only small amounts of diacylglycerols occur as reaction products. The monoacylglycerols enable the formation of micelles in the presence of bile acids. Additional lipids such as fatty acids, cholesterol and fat-soluble vitamins can be included in the micelles.

It is assumed that the entire micelle comes into contact with the brush border of the mucosa, disintegrates there and the various components of the micelle are absorbed individually. The uptake of fatty acids, monoacylglycerols, cholesterol and fat-soluble vitamins into the mucosa cell occurs by simple diffusion.

In this context, the 'Fatty Acid Binding Protein' plays a role.

This is a cytoplasmic protein that binds fatty acids and accelerates the cellular uptake of fatty acids. In the mucosa cell, re-esterification of the absorbed fatty acids occurs, resulting in the formation of triacylglycerols. Subsequently, triacylglycerol and cholesterol esters associate with apolipoprotein B-48, forming chylomicrons that enter the bloodstream via the lymph.

Fat Transport

Lipoproteins are spherical particles consisting of lipid and protein molecules.

Their task is to transport the hydrophobic plasma lipids, especially triglycerides and cholesterol, in the plasma.

Lipoproteins consist of a hydrophobic core and contain, depending on the density class, a varying proportion of cholesterol esters and triacylglycerols. This hydrophobic core is surrounded by a single phospholipid layer, which forms the link to the hydrophilic surface of the lipoproteins. The surface of the lipoproteins consists predominantly of hydrophilic, non-esterified cholesterol and of proteins.

The apoproteins, which are also located on the surface of the lipoproteins, are not only responsible for the structural stability of the lipoproteins, they also play an extremely important role in the regulation of lipid transport and lipoprotein metabolism.

Textbook of Small Animal Pathophysiology, First Edition. Stephan Neumann.
© 2025 John Wiley & Sons Ltd. Published 2025 by John Wiley & Sons Ltd.

According to their density, lipoproteins are divided into five main groups: Chylomicrons, very-low-density lipoproteins (VLDLs), intermediate-density lipoproteins (IDL), low-density lipoproteins (LDL) and high-density lipoproteins (HDLs).

Proteins are always involved as vehicles in **lipid transport** in the body. Albumin, which can bind and transport a variety of substances in serum, is also involved to some extent in the transport of free fatty acids. Apart from albumin and some specific lipid transport proteins, such as retinol-binding proteins, the transport of lipids mainly takes place in the form of lipoproteins.

The triglycerides ingested through food are transported to the fat and muscle tissues, where they are converted into fatty acids. The cholesterol that is also absorbed through food is supplied to the liver, where it is either used for bile acid biosynthesis, incorporated into biomembranes or secreted back into the bloodstream as lipoprotein-bound cholesterol (VLDL). Alternatively, the cholesterol absorbed by the liver can also be excreted as free cholesterol via the bile, with some remaining in the enterohepatic circulation.

Intracellularly, the ingested cholesterol is used, among other things, for the synthesis of cell membranes. In some organs, cholesterol can be the basic component of cell-specific products. Thus, in the gonads and in the adrenal cortices, cholesterol is used for the synthesis of steroid hormones. In the hepatocytes, cholesterol is used for the synthesis of bile acids.

Mechanism of Obesity

Internal and external factors are held responsible for the accumulation of fat in adipocytes (Figure 5.1).

A distinction is made as to whether the fat accumulates in the subcutaneous fat tissue or in the visceral fat tissue. An influence of genetics, age and gender has been described. Other factors result from an increased availability of fatty acids and glycerides or their reduced clearance. Cytokines, especially proinflammatory cytokines, seem to play a role. A connection between obesity and chronic inflammation is seen. Another influencing factor is liver metabolism, for example, through increased lipoprotein synthesis. Other hormones, such as cortisol or growth hormone, also have an effect on the accumulation of fat.

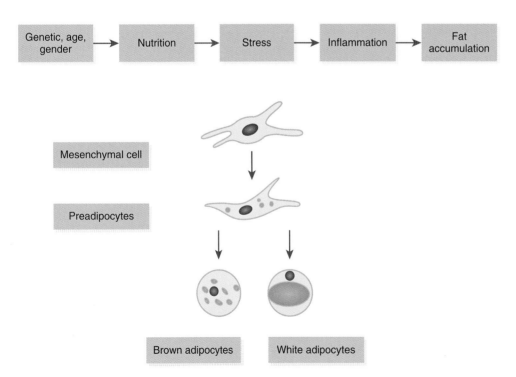

Figure 5.1 Mechanism of fat accumulation.

Consequences of Obesity

The multiple consequences of obesity result from the functions of adipose tissue in addition to fat accumulation. These include, in particular, hormonal and inflammatory factors.

The fatty tissue influences a wide variety of hormones and cytokines (Figure 5.2).

These in turn influence an equally large number of physiological processes (Figure 5.3).

The adipose tissue can influence other organs through increased or decreased secretion of mediators. Table 5.1 lists some secretion products with their respective functions.

Diabetes types I and II are distinguished as disorders of glucose metabolism. In normal-weight organisms, insulin binds to the insulin receptor in muscle, fat and liver tissues. This receptor belongs to the group of tyrosine kinases. The binding with insulin leads to a phosphorylation of tyrosine residues, which causes the activation of a glucose transport protein and

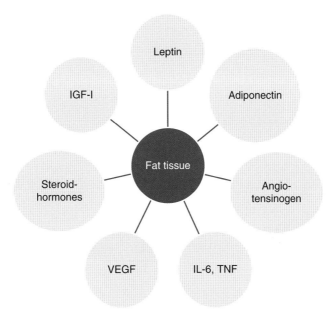

Figure 5.2   Hormones and cytokines produced by adipose tissue.

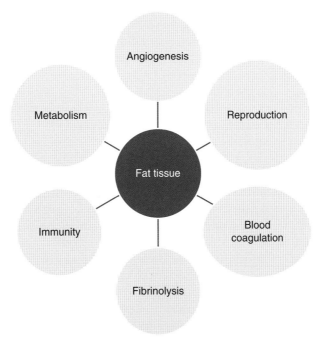

Figure 5.3   Influence of fat on different physiological mechanisms.

Table 5.1 Mediators from the adipose tissue.

Hormone	Function
Leptin	Signals to the brain about body fat stores, regulates appetite and energy expenditure
Adiponectin	Protective role in the pathogenesis of type II diabetes and cardiovascular disease
TNF	Affects insulin receptor signalling, possible cause of the development of insulin resistance in obesity
IL-6	Lipid and glucose metabolism, regulates body weight

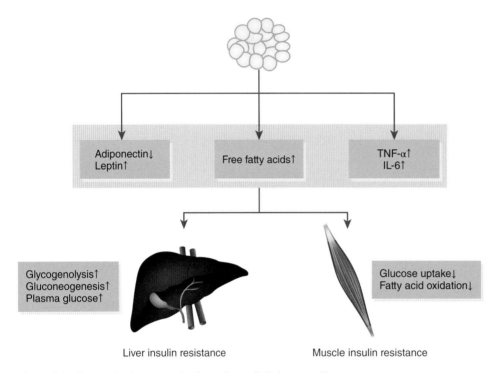

Figure 5.4 Connection between obesity and type II diabetes mellitus.

its incorporation into the cell membrane. As a result, glucose transport into the cell is increased. In the case of obesity, insulin resistance develops due to the binding of proinflammatory cytokines and palmitic acid to the receptor with subsequent phosphorylation of serine residues. This influences signal transduction and reduces the activation of glucose transport proteins.

The consequence is the development of type II **diabetes mellitus**. This is also accompanied by an increased infiltration of macrophages into the fatty tissue. The consequence is increased secretion of proinflammatory cytokines (IL-6, TNF-α) which is accompanied by increased secretion of fatty acids. In addition, the secretion of leptin increases. In turn, adipokine secretion decreases. This leads to increased insulin resistance in the hepatocytes. As a result, hepatic gluconeogenesis increases. Both lead to type II diabetes mellitus (Figure 5.4).

The connection between obesity and **cardiovascular diseases** has been known for a long time. The cause of the development of left ventricular hypertrophy, a frequent cardiogenic concomitant disease in obesity, is seen as the increased oxygen demand associated with an increase in fat mass and muscle mass. This leads to an increase in erythrocyte mass and thus in blood volume. The left ventricular hypertrophy can, therefore, be explained by the increased cardiac force that is necessary to transport the blood with an expanded intravascular volume and a constant heart rate.

Hypertension as a consequence of obesity is related to the cardiogenic consequences. It is also explained by the influence of adipose tissue on the secretion of renin and angiotensin. This increases systemic blood pressure via the renin-angiotensin-aldosterone system (RAAS). Structural changes in the area of the nephrons, in obesity, could also have an effect on blood pressure by influencing the juxta-glomerular apparatus (Figure 5.5).

Figure 5.5 Obesity and hypertension.

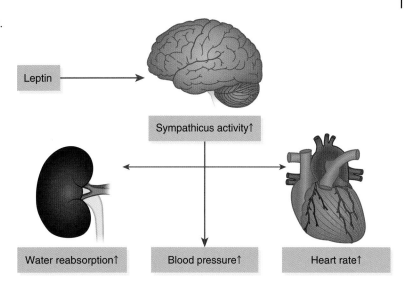

Finally, a link is seen between obesity and the development of **neoplasms.**

In particular, the endocrine functions of adipose tissue are held responsible for increased tumourigenesis. Insulin like growth factor (IGF) is produced by fat cells and is considered a strongly proliferative growth factor, which at the same time exerts a negative influence on apoptosis. On this basis, tumour growth can be supported. At the same time, the local IGF concentration increases if the increased IGF secretion by the adipose tissue is not accompanied by increased synthesis of the IGF-binding proteins that transport IGF. This increased local proliferative IGF function is also seen as a tumour-genetic factor.

Other hormone effects through secretion from the adipose tissue, such as sex hormones could also influence tumourigenesis. Last but not least, the increased secretion of growth factors such as vascular endothelial growth factor (VEGF) increases tumour proliferation.

Further Reading

Basen-Engquist, K. and Chang, M. (2011). Obesity and cancer risk: recent review and evidence. *Current Oncology Reports* 13 (1): 71–76. https://doi.org/10.1007/s11912-010-0139-7.

Calle, E.E. and Thun, M.J. (2004). Obesity and cancer. *Oncogene* 23 (38): 6365–6378. https://doi.org/10.1038/sj.onc.1207751.

Ceschi, M., Gutzwiller, F., Moch, H. et al. (2007). Epidemiology and pathophysiology of obesity as cause of cancer. *Swiss Medical Weekly* 137 (3–4): 50–56. https://doi.org/10.4414/smw.2007.11435.

Harvey, I., Boudreau, A., and Stephens, J.M. (2020). Adipose tissue in health and disease. *Open Biology* 10 (12): 200291. https://doi.org/10.1098/rsob.200291.

Koenen, M., Hill, M.A., Cohen, P., and Sowers, J.R. (2021). Obesity, adipose tissue and vascular dysfunction. *Circulation Research* 128 (7): 951–968. https://doi.org/10.1161/CIRCRESAHA.121.318093.

Koliaki, C., Liatis, S., and Kokkinos, A. (2019). Obesity and cardiovascular disease: revisiting an old relationship. *Metabolism, Clinical and Experimental* 92: 98–107. https://doi.org/10.1016/j.metabol.2018.10.011.

Pischon, T., Nöthlings, U., and Boeing, H. (2008). Obesity and cancer. *The Proceedings of the Nutrition Society* 67 (2): 128–145. https://doi.org/10.1017/S0029665108006976.

Powell-Wiley, T.M., Poirier, P., Burke, L.E. et al. (2021). Obesity and cardiovascular disease: ascientific statement from the American Heart Association. *Circulation* 143 (21): e984–e1010. https://doi.org/10.1161/CIR.0000000000000973.

Stolarczyk, E. (2017). Adipose tissue inflammation in obesity: a metabolic or immune response? *Current Opinion in Pharmacology* 37: 35–40. https://doi.org/10.1016/j.coph.2017.08.006.

6

Ischaemia, Hypoxia

Importance of Oxygen

Oxygen is an element involved in the composition of biological molecules. An essential biochemical function of oxygen is the uptake of electrons in the mitochondrial respiratory chain and thereby the generation of ATP, the essential cellular energy carrier.

The process of electron transfer is localised at the inner mitochondrial membrane. It is preceded by the formation of NADH and FADH in the citric acid cycle, which represents a central element of the intermediate metabolism.

The **citric acid cycle** consists of eight biochemical reactions that take place in the mitochondria of eukaryotic organisms. Overall, the citric acid cycle shows catabolic and anabolic functions, including the synthesis of molecules that serve to produce energy.

The starting molecule for the citric acid cycle is acetyl-CoA, which comes from the breakdown of carbohydrates, fats and proteins. In the citric acid cycle, acetyl-CoA is degraded to CO_2, releasing energy. Part of the energy released is stored by so-called 'electron carriers' NAD^+ and FAD by accepting electrons. By accepting the electrons, the carriers are reduced to $NADH + H^+$ and $FADH_2$.

The eight reaction steps can be divided into a degrading part and a regenerating part. In the degrading part, succinyl-CoA is synthesised from acetyl-CoA via intermediate steps (citrate, isocitrate, alpha-ketoglutarate), whereby two molecules of $NADH + H^+$, as well as two molecules of CO_2 are formed by oxidation of NAD^+ ($NAD^+ + 2H^+ + 2e^-$). In the regenerating part, succinyl-CoA is again combined with acetyl-CoA via intermediates (succinate, fumarate, malate, oxaloacetate), which is again fed into the citric acid cycle. In the process, electron carriers are again formed in the form of a molecule of $FADH_2$ ($FAD + H^+ + e^-$), as well as a molecule of $NADH + H^+$.

The electron carriers now transport the electrons to the inner mitochondrial membrane, where the electrons are transferred to O_2 together with hydrogen protons. For this purpose, the electrons are transferred from the carriers to a total of four so-called 'complexes', which function as redox systems and can accept and release electrons. The last, fourth complex finally transfers the electrons, together with hydrogen protons, to oxygen. Water is formed and, through the formation of the energy-rich compound ATP from ADP and phosphorus, the most important energy carrier for biochemical processes.

The Physiological Way of Oxygen

Oxygen is absorbed during the breathing process and finally reaches the alveoli via the upper and lower airways. There is a local oxygen partial pressure of approximately 100 mmHg. This is the driving force for the diffusion of oxygen into the pulmonary capillaries, where the partial pressure is about 37 mmHg. To do this, oxygen must pass through the surfactant, the alveolar membrane, the basement membrane of the epithelium, the interstitial space between the alveolar epithelium and the capillary membrane, the basement membrane of the capillary and finally the capillary endothelium.

Textbook of Small Animal Pathophysiology, First Edition. Stephan Neumann.
© 2025 John Wiley & Sons Ltd. Published 2025 by John Wiley & Sons Ltd.

A very small proportion (<5%) of the oxygen transported in the blood is dissolved. The majority is bound to haemoglobin. The amount of bound oxygen depends on its partial pressure. In arterial blood, the partial pressure of oxygen is approximately 100 mmHg, in which case approximately 95% of the oxygen is bound to haemoglobin. A complete saturation of haemoglobin with oxygen is not achieved because small amounts of blood have no alveolar flow through pulmonary shunts, or small amounts of haemoglobin are occupied by other molecules (e.g. methaemoglobin).

Haemoglobin consists of four polypeptide chains, as well as a porphyrin complex with a centrally located divalent iron molecule (Fe^{2+}). Oxygen forms a reversible compound with the iron atom without changing the charge state of the iron. In this way, oxygen is transported into the capillaries.

Capillary oxygen transfer also follows a difference between the oxygen partial pressures in the capillary and the mitochondrion. In the mitochondrion, an oxygen partial pressure of at least 1 mmHg is required to enable oxidative metabolism. However, at a capillary oxygen partial pressure lower than 25 mmHg, the cells generate more energy via anaerobic glycolysis (Brahimi-Horn and Pouysségur 2007; Larsen 2016).

Definition of *Hypoxia, Ischaemia*

Generally, a decreased oxygen concentration is called *hypoxia*. Aetiologically, hypoxia can occur at any point of oxygen transport. 'Hypoxaemic hypoxia' describes a reduced oxygen concentration in the blood, which is caused by a reduced oxygen uptake from the alveolus. This can be caused by hypoventilation resulting in a lowered alveolar oxygen partial pressure or alveolar diffusion disorders. A reduced haemoglobin concentration leads to a reduction in oxygen transport capacity and is called 'anaemic hypoxia'. In most cases, reductions in red blood cells are caused by various forms of anaemia. Ischaemic hypoxia describes the reduced cellular oxygen supply due to reduced tissue perfusion. This is caused by reduced cardiac activity and vascular occlusion. Finally, hypoxia can also occur at the cellular level due to the blockage of the mitochondrial respiratory chain, which is caused by intoxications (Table 6.1).

Hypoxia can be classified according to its time course as acute or chronic, and according to its extent as mild to severe.

Depending on the course and extent, hypoxia can lead to serious cell changes with cell death or induce adaptive reactions of the entire organism. An example of the latter is adaptation to higher altitudes, where the lack of oxygen in the air leads to increased erythropoiesis. The pathophysiological consequences of hypoxia can be acute or chronic.

Acute Hypoxia

Acute hypoxia induces the most serious consequences at the cellular level. These are essentially based on a reduced intracellular ATP synthesis. A lack of ATP affects, among other things, the ATP-dependent Na^+/K^+ pump, with the consequence of a reduced sodium efflux. This causes a destabilisation of the membrane resting potential and a depolarisation of the cell membrane. This in turn leads to a polarisation-dependent opening of calcium channels, which induces an increased calcium influx and increases the cellular calcium concentration.

The consequences of an increased cellular calcium concentration are multiple. Intra-mitochondrially, the complexes of the respiratory chain are affected, resulting in an increased synthesis of reactive oxygen species (ROS). This increases the oxidative stress in the cell. At the same time, intramitochondrial glutathione is lost, which reduces oxidative stress as a 'radical scavenger'. As a result, mitochondrial membrane damage and organelle dysfunction occur (Hardie 2003; Starkov et al. 2004).

Table 6.1 Clinical causes of hypoxaemia.

Disease	Mechanism
Respiratory diseases	Decreased oxygen uptake
Haemoglobinopathies/anaemia	Reduced transport capacity
Peripheral circulation disorders	Decreased oxygen release
Intoxication of the respiratory chain	Reduced aerobic glycolysis

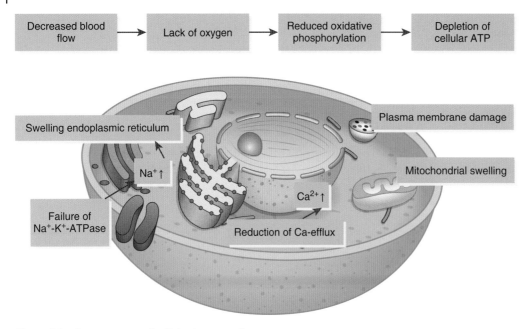

Figure 6.1 Consequences of cellular hypoxaemia.

Other consequences of an increased cellular calcium concentration are the increases in activity of lipases, protease and endonucleases. All of these lead to progressive cellular dysfunction.

A final consequence of hypoxia, based on the described consequences, is cell death. This can take place as necrosis, apoptosis or autophagy. Presumably, the speed of the decline and the final concentration of intracellular ATP determine the type of cell death (Eguchi et al. 1997) (Figure 6.1).

Chronic Hypoxia

In contrast to acute hypoxia, which focuses on changes in electron transport, chronic hypoxia induces the expression of different genes. Mediators of gene regulation are HIF transcription factors (hypoxia-inducible factors). These bind to the promoter region of the target gene. A total of more than 200 target genes of the HIF family have currently been described; these influence erythropoiesis, angiogenesis and metabolism (Kaur et al. 2005; Loor and Schumacker 2008).

Chronic hypoxia induces the synthesis of erythropoietin, mainly in peritubular, interstitial cells of the renal cortex, but also in some species to a small percentage in the liver. Erythropoietin reaches the bone marrow via the blood, where it prevents the apoptosis of precursor cells of erythropoiesis and induces their proliferation in this way (Lacombe and Mayeux 1999). In addition, iron metabolism is supported, for example, by the increased expression of iron transport proteins (Wenger 2000).

Another consequence of chronic hypoxia is angiogenesis, which describes vascular sprouting from already existing vessels. HIF mediated, different angiogenic factors are formed, for example vascular endothelial growth factor (VEGF), platelet-derived growth factor (PDGF) and interleukin-8 (Rankin and Giaccia 2008).

The hypoxic influence on cell metabolism is due to the switch from oxidative phosphorylation to anaerobic glycolysis, which leads to reduced ATP synthesis and increased lactate formation. This leads to the development of cellular acidosis, which initially has protective properties because it suppresses energy-consuming intracellular processes and ROS production (Yao and Haddad 2004). Secondly, the increased AMP induces the activity of AMP-activated protein kinase (AMPK). This has the task of adapting the metabolism in the cells to the changed oxygen supply. In the process, different metabolic pathways are activated. The uptake of glucose, the β-oxidation of fatty acids and gluconeogenesis are stimulated. At the same time, energy-consuming, anabolic processes such as the synthesis of fatty acids or proteins are inhibited (Hardie et al. 2006). (Figure 6.2).

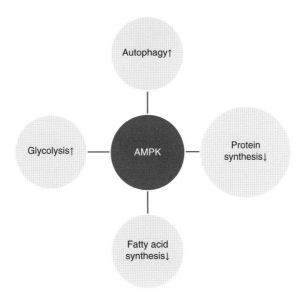

Figure 6.2 Catabolic consequences of AMPK activation.

References

Brahimi-Horn, M.C. and Pouysségur, J. (2007). Oxygen, a source of life and stress. *FEBS Letters* 581 (19): 3582–3591. https://doi.org/10.1016/j.febslet.2007.06.018.

Eguchi, Y., Shimizu, S., and Tsujimoto, Y. (1997). Intracellular ATP levels determine cell death fate by apoptosis or necrosis. *Cancer Research* 57 (10): 1835–1840.

Hardie, D.G. (2003). Minireview: the AMP-activated protein kinase cascade: the key sensor of cellular energy status. *Endocrinology* 144 (12): 5179–5183. https://doi.org/10.1210/en.2003-0982.

Hardie, D.G., Hawley, S.A., and Scott, J.W. (2006). AMP-activated protein kinase--development of the energy sensor concept. *The Journal of Physiology* 574 (Pt 1): 7–15. https://doi.org/10.1113/jphysiol.2006.108944.

Kaur, B., Khwaja, F.W., Severson, E.A. et al. (2005). Hypoxia and the hypoxia-inducible-factor pathway in glioma growth and angiogenesis. *Neuro-Oncology* 7 (2): 134–153. https://doi.org/10.1215/S1152851704001115.

Lacombe, C. and Mayeux, P. (1999). The molecular biology of erythropoietin. *Nephrology, Dialysis, Transplantation : Official Publication of the European Dialysis and Transplant Association – European Renal Association* 14 (Suppl 2): 22–28. https://doi.org/10.1093/ndt/14.suppl_2.22.

Larsen, R. (2016). Physiology of respiration. *Anaesthesia and Critical Care for the Specialist Nurse* 696–708. https://doi.org/10.1007/978-3-662-50444-4_52.

Loor, G. and Schumacker, P.T. (2008). Role of hypoxia-inducible factor in cell survival during myocardial ischemia-reperfusion. *Cell Death and Differentiation* 15 (4): 686–690. https://doi.org/10.1038/cdd.2008.13.

Rankin, E.B. and Giaccia, A.J. (2008). The role of hypoxia-inducible factors in tumorigenesis. *Cell Death and Differentiation* 15 (4): 678–685. https://doi.org/10.1038/cdd.2008.21.

Starkov, A.A., Chinopoulos, C., and Fiskum, G. (2004). Mitochondrial calcium and oxidative stress as mediators of ischemic brain injury. *Cell Calcium* 36 (3–4): 257–264. https://doi.org/10.1016/j.ceca.2004.02.012.

Wenger, R.H. (2000). Mammalian oxygen sensing, signalling and gene regulation. *The Journal of Experimental Biology* 203 (Pt 8): 1253–1263. https://doi.org/10.1242/jeb.203.8.1253.

Yao, H. and Haddad, G.G. (2004). Calcium and pH homeostasis in neurons during hypoxia and ischemia. *Cell Calcium* 36 (3–4): 247–255. https://doi.org/10.1016/j.ceca.2004.02.013.

Further Reading

Brahimi-Horn, M.C., Chiche, J., and Pouysségur, J. (2007). Hypoxia signalling controls metabolic demand. *Current Opinion in Cell Biology* 19 (2): 223–229. https://doi.org/10.1016/j.ceb.2007.02.003.

Dunn, J.-O.C., Mythen, M.G., and Grocott, M.P. (2016). Physiology of oxygen transport. *BJA Education* 16 (10): 341–348.

7

Cell Death

Definition

Cell death is defined as an irreversible functional and morphological alteration of cells associated with their destruction. Different forms of cell death are distinguished.

Apoptosis

Apoptosis, or programmed cell death, is considered a physiological event and serves to keep the number of cells in the tissue constant and to eliminate cells from the system that are pathologically altered.

In the context of the immune response, apoptosis regulates the elimination of defence cells that recognise the body's own structures and thus display an autoimmune character. Cytotoxic T lymphocytes can also eliminate virus-infected cells through the mechanism of apoptosis.

Causes

The causalities described for the initiation of cellular apoptosis are diverse and depend, in their inducing effect, also on cellular factors such as cell type, differentiation state or phase in the cell cycle. Principle causalities are an increased concentration of reactive oxygen species (ROS), a drop in the cellular ATP concentration and mitochondrial disorders with formation of pre-apoptotic proteins. In addition, apoptosis develops through DNA damage. For example, the tumour suppressor gene p53 induces the repair of DNA damage. If this is not possible, the protein induces apoptosis.

Depending on the causality, extrinsic apoptosis is distinguished from intrinsic apoptosis.

Extrinsic apoptosis is induced by factors outside the cells. These include cytokines, such as tumour necrosis factor (TNF) or apoptosis-inducing factor (TRAIL). Via receptor coupling (Fas ligand), the intracellular formation of caspases is induced, which in turn activate intracellular nucleases.

Intrinsic apoptosis is controlled by the release of mitochondrial cytochrome C and activates caspases in this way. Caspases, as an essential control molecule of apoptosis, belong to the family of aspartate-specific cysteine proteases, since they cleave their substrates after an aspartate residue and there is a cysteine in the active centre. The caspases exist intracellularly as inactive procaspases and activate by cleavage. Activated caspases are able to activate other procaspases and induce autocatalysis in this way.

Mechanisms

The mechanism of apoptosis is divided into different phases. First, the contact with neighbouring cells is broken by destruction of the cytoskeleton. This also leads to cell shrinkage. In the cell nucleus, chromatin is cleaved by specific endonucleases, which are present in the cytosol in an inactive state and are selectively activated by caspases via a cleavage reaction. As a result, cell fragments are formed which are separated into individual so-called 'apoptotic bodies' by cell membrane folding. The apoptotic bodies are surrounded by the cell membrane and are phagocytosed by neighbouring cells or macrophages. These recognise the bodies to be phagocytosed by rearrangements of membrane components. For example, phosphatidylserine molecules are rearranged from the inner to the outer membrane during the formation of apoptotic bodies.

Textbook of Small Animal Pathophysiology, First Edition. Stephan Neumann.
© 2025 John Wiley & Sons Ltd. Published 2025 by John Wiley & Sons Ltd.

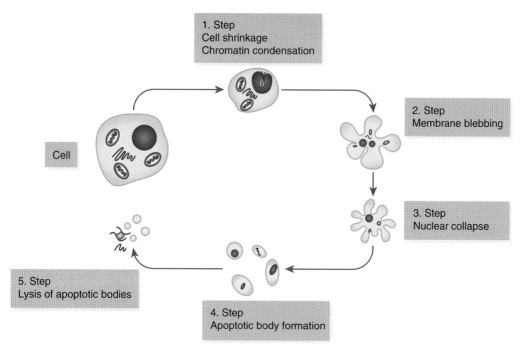

Figure 7.1 Apoptosis, process.

Table 7.1 Structural proteins influenced by caspases during apoptosis.

Protein	Function
Actin microfilament forming protein	Structure of the cytoskeleton
Spectrin-actin cross-linking protein	Structure of the cytoskeleton
β-catenin	Cell-to-cell contact
Gelsolin	Microfilament
Rabaptin	Intracellular transport processes
Laminin	Intermediate filaments

The process of body formation improves phagocytosis by reducing the size of the cell. Through an outward K^+ and Cl^- shift, as well as contraction of the cytoskeletal components, the fragments are further reduced in size and improve the possibilities of phagocytosis (Figure 7.1, Table 7.1).

Diseases that are associated with an increased apoptosis frequency have been described, especially for humans. These include degenerative diseases, chronic inflammatory diseases and autoimmune diseases. A reduced apoptosis frequency is observed in hyperplastic and neoplastic diseases.

Necrosis

Necrosis is also called 'accidental cell death'. It is a form of cell death caused by cell damage.

Causes

In contrast to apoptosis, necrosis is pathological cell death. This is caused by non-compensable nutrient and oxygen deficiency, as well as strong physical influencing factors such as radioactive radiation. The triggers associated with cell necrosis are listed in Table 7.2.

Table 7.2 Trigger of cell necrosis and the mechanism.

Cause	Mechanism
Hypoxia	Disruption of the cellular energy supply
Physical factors, injuries, heat, cold	Disruption of morphological cell integrity, destruction of the cytoskeleton
Infectious agents	Energetic and morphological cell destruction
Defence cells	Cytotoxicity

Mechanisms

The mechanism of necrosis differs from that of apoptosis essentially in that in necrosis there is membrane destruction, as a result of which components are released from the cell. This induces an inflammatory reaction, which is prevented in apoptosis by the formation of bodies. The morphological changes that form during necrosis are swelling of the cell and swelling of the cell nucleus as initial events, followed by dissolution of the cell nucleus or fragmentation of the cell nucleus (karyolysis, karyorrhexis).

The formation of vacuoles is possible, but there is an increased leakage of cell components through the destroyed cell membrane, which triggers an inflammatory reaction of the surrounding tissue.

Oxygen deficiency is a major trigger of necrosis. This leads to a lack of ATP, which causes the energy-dependent sodium pump in the plasma membrane to become insufficient. This is followed by an influx of water and calcium ions.

This leads to cell swelling and detachment of ribosomes from the endoplasmic reticulum. Increased cytosolic calcium and oxidative stress also lead to mitochondrial damage. Cytosolic calcium can also lead to the activation of several cytosolic enzymes, including phospholipases and proteases, which lead to the degradation of both membranes (including lysosomal membranes) and proteins.

In the process, cellular proteins are released, which, as so-called 'DAMPs', initiate the formation of cytokines, such as IL-1, from neighbouring inflammatory cells via receptor action. This release triggers an inflammatory response that attracts leukocytes and nearby phagocytes to clear the dead cells and their products through phagocytosis. Initially, neutrophils rapidly infiltrate the tissue site, followed by monocytes.

Necrosis occurs in numerous diseases. These include circulatory disorders, inflammation and neoplasia. The occurrence of necrosis is often associated with severe disease symptoms due to the associated inflammatory response and the release of cellular components that can exert toxic effects (Figure 7.2).

Although a distinction is made in principle between apoptosis and necrosis, both processes sometimes take place in parallel.

Necroptosis

A special form of cell death is necroptosis. In direct contrast to unregulated necrosis, necroptosis represents a regulated version of the necrotic cell death pathway. As with necrosis, necroptosis is caspase-independent. However, analogous to apoptosis, necroptosis is triggered by the binding of TNF-α to Fas ligands at their respective cell surface receptors, which is also observed in classical extrinsic apoptosis induction. Ligand binding to surface receptors of the TNF family triggers signal transduction, resulting in activation of protein kinases. These induce the formation of proteins that are incorporated into the cell membrane and cause the release of intracellular molecules, which is the initial event for the development of an inflammatory reaction.

Apoptosis → Phagocytosis

Necrosis → Inflammation and lysis

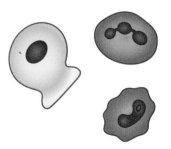

Figure 7.2 Comparison of apoptosis and necrosis.

Autophagy

Another form of cellular degradation is autophagy. Here, the degradation of damaged cellular material takes place within the affected cell. In autophagy, cellular material is taken up into a specialised organelle, the autophagosome. This fuses with lysosomes, creating so-called 'autophagolysosomes'. The cytosolic material from the autophagosomes is degraded by the enzymes of the lysosomes.

Autophagosomes are formed de novo from the so-called 'phagophore', which presumably originate from the endoplasmic reticulum.

Pyroptosis

Pyroptosis is a type of programmed cell death that is initiated by inflammatory stimuli, such as pathogen-associated molecular patterns (PAMPs) and damage-associated molecular patterns (DAMPs). Biochemically, pyroptosis is characterised by the activation of caspase-1 or -4/-5/-11, which cleave gasdermin D to form membrane pores and induce cell lysis. This process leads to the release of proinflammatory cytokines and DAMPs, which can activate additional immune cells and contribute to the inflammatory response. Pyroptosis is a critical part of the innate immune response to pathogens, but excessive or dysregulated pyroptosis can contribute to a variety of inflammatory and autoimmune diseases.

Further Reading

Chu, Q., Gu, X., Zheng, Q. et al. (2021). Mitochondrial mechanisms of apoptosis and necroptosis in liver diseases. *Analytical Cellular Pathology (Amsterdam)* 2021: 8900122. https://doi.org/10.1155/2021/8900122.

Galluzzi, L., Kepp, O., Chan, F.K., and Kroemer, G. (2017). Necroptosis: mechanisms and relevance to disease. *Annual Review of Pathology* 12: 103–130. https://doi.org/10.1146/annurev-pathol-052016-100247.

Green, D.R. and Llambi, F. (2015). Cell death signaling. *Cold Spring Harbor Perspectives in Biology* 7 (12): a006080. https://doi.org/10.1101/cshperspect.a006080.

Li, P., Dong, X.R., Zhang, B. et al. (2021). Molecular mechanism and therapeutic targeting of necrosis, apoptosis, pyroptosis, and autophagy in cardiovascular disease. *Chinese Medical Journal* 134 (22): 2647–2655. https://doi.org/10.1097/CM9.0000000000001772.

Nikoletopoulou, V., Markaki, M., Palikaras, K., and Tavernarakis, N. (2013). Crosstalk between apoptosis, necrosis and autophagy. *Biochimica et Biophysica Acta* 1833 (12): 3448–3459. https://doi.org/10.1016/j.bbamcr.2013.06.001.

8

Neoplasia

Definition

Neoplasms are characterised by unregulated cell growth of transformed cells. In the process, tumour cells show numerous morphological and physiological changes. Depending on the type of growth, its speed and tendencies to metastasise, benign neoplasms can be distinguished from malignant forms.

Causes

The causes of neoplasia in dogs and cats, like those of other mammalian species or humans, can be grouped into:

Inheritance

Breed-specific predispositions are known for a variety of tumours (Davis and Ostrander 2014). In dogs, mesenchymal tumours, in particular, occur more frequently in specific breeds. For example, osteosarcoma is overrepresented in the Great Dane, Rottweiler or Irish Wolfhound. Other tumour entities that are overrepresented include malignant histiocytosis in the Bernese Mountain Dog or Flat-coated Retriever and mast cell tumour in Retriever species (Michell 1999;Mendoza et al. 1998;Dobson 2013).

Breed predispositions for certain tumours have also been described in cats. For example, mammary carcinoma occurs more frequently in Siamese cats (Egenvall et al. 2010).

Physico-Chemical Causes

Physical triggers of tumours are all forms of radiation. Radioactive substances (α, β, γ radiation) as well as X-rays or ultraviolet radiation can cause cells to undergo neoplastic transformation. This involves direct damage to the genome by the high-energy radiation or damage to the organelles by the non-specific formation of reactive radicals (Shim et al. 2014).

Ultraviolet light, for example, can link neighbouring pyrimidine bases (cytosine and thymine) to form a pyrimidine dimer. Correspondingly mutated regions lose their function. If, for example, tumour suppressor genes (p53) are affected, a neoplastic transformation can develop from this. The development of squamous cell carcinomas on unpigmented ear margins in cats is an example of a neoplastic transformation presumably triggered by ultraviolet light.

Chemical substances can be directly or indirectly carcinogenic. The indirect form occurs as a result of biochemical transformation of chemical substances in cell metabolism. Some chemical substances can initiate neoplastic transformation by forming covalent bonds with regions in the genome. Other substances act as promoters and stimulate clonal replication of the 'initiated cells' (Slaga1983).

Textbook of Small Animal Pathophysiology, First Edition. Stephan Neumann.

Infections

Neoplastic transformation as a result of infection has been described for parasitic diseases, bacterial infections and viral infections. Neoplasia as a consequence of parasite infestation has been described, for example, for *Spirocerca lupi* (Porras-Silesky et al. 2021). For this and other neoplasia-causing parasites, the chronic inflammatory reaction to the parasite or its excretory and secretory products is seen as the triggering mechanism.

Similar to parasitic diseases, bacterial infections are rarely accompanied by tumour formation. The significance of *Heliobacter pylori* as a cause of adenocarcinomas of the stomach wall is not certain in small animals. The mechanism of neoplastic transformation in bacterial infections, as in some parasitic diseases, is considered to be the chronic inflammatory process (Amieva and Peek 2016).

From an epidemiological point of view, neoplastic transformations resulting from viral infections are more significant. Both RNA and DNA viruses can trigger neoplastic transformation. In the case of RNA viruses, retroviruses are known to trigger tumours. Retroviruses influence the expression of proteins involved in cell proliferation or maturation or they disable tumour suppressor genes. Similar mechanisms also lead to neoplastic transformation in DNA virus infections.

Neoplastic Transformation

The causalities described lead to neoplastic transformation via various successively occurring phases, namely initiation, promotion and progression. Initiation, the transformation of a cell into a neoplastic form, is at the beginning. As already explained in the causalities, initiation usually takes place as a result of an alteration of the genetic information.

Increased activity of oncogenes and suppression of tumour suppressor genes seem to be important prerequisites for neoplastic transformation.

Oncogenes arise from proto-oncogenes through mutation, proliferation or dysregulation as a result of chemical activation, physical action or infection by RNA viruses. Proto-oncogenes are gene sequences that encode specific, mostly proliferative proteins. Proto-oncogenes include genes for growth factors, for growth factor receptors and for proteins of growth-associated intracellular signal transduction. If mutation of a proto-oncogene occurs, the cell often stops growing and undergoes apoptotic cell death and is eliminated in this way. However, it is possible that growth is promoted by the mutation of the proto-oncogene, for example, if the mutation causes a chromosomal shift in a promoter region. Promoters are DNA segments that regulate gene expression. After an oncogene has developed from a proto-oncogene, proteins are formed that are components of growth factor signalling pathways. They mainly include growth factors, growth receptors, protein kinases and transcription factors. Increased synthesis of growth factors or their receptors leads to proliferative autostimulation of the transformed cell (Martínez-Reyes and Chandel 2021).

In addition to alterations of proto-oncogenes, disorders of tumour suppressor genes can also lead to neoplastic transformation. Tumour suppressor genes encode proteins that can suppress uncontrolled cell division. As in the example of the tumour suppressor gene p53, these are transcription factors that are initially inactive in the cell nucleus. After initiation of neoplastic transformation due to DNA damage, the inactive p53 molecules can be activated by phosphorylation. After activation, the p53 molecules bind to promoter regions and implicate the synthesis of further tumour suppressor proteins. These finally initiate apoptosis via the activation of Bcl-2-associated X protein (BAX) molecules present in the cytosol (Chen 2016; Kaiser and Attardi 2018).

The initiation phase is followed by the promotion phase. Promoters can influence tumour formation after the completion of neoplastic transformation without having a carcinogenic effect themselves. Promoters induce a growth-promoting effect via receptor activation on the tumour cells or growth-promoting effects on the microenvironment (Slaga 1983). Various endogenous growth factors have been described as tumour promoters. These include epidermal growth factor (EGF), transforming growth factor (TGF) and insulin-like growth factor (IGF). The functions of the IGF system in tumourigenesis are based on an increase in proliferation, an inhibition of apoptosis and effects on cell transformation through the synthesis of various regulatory proteins. The IGF system controls tumour cell survival and influences clonal expansion and metastasis of tumour cells. Overall, the components of the IGF system exert their impacts through both direct and indirect effects. The direct effects are mediated via IGF-1 and the IGF-1 receptor and the signal transduction pathway it activates, leading to an increase in mitogenesis, cell cycle progression and protection against various apoptotic stresses.

Finally, the progression phase describes the tumour development from the transformed cell to morphologically manifest tumour tissue. It is characterised by an increased growth rate and a tendency to metastasise (Lisovska and Shanazarov 2019) (Figure 8.1).

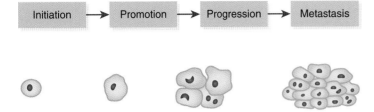

Figure 8.1 Oncogenesis initiation, promotion, progression.

Metastasis

The process of metastasis can be divided into four phases:

I) Invasion phase: Tumour tissue grows into a blood vessel. To do this, structures such as the basement membrane and the endothelial cell layer must be destroyed by proteolytic enzymes synthesised by the tumour.

II) Embolisation phase: Intravascular tumour cells are transported further via the blood vessels, they embolise. As a rule, only a few of the tumour cells survive, but these are capable of developing metastases. In the blood vessel, tumour cells are enclosed by platelets and fibrin, which protects them from lytic defence reactions.

III) Tumour implantation: Tumour implantation is initiated by the adhesion of tumour cells in the area of the vascular endothelia.

IV) Vessel penetration: The tumour cells penetrate the vessel wall and implant themselves in the neighbouring tissue.

The onset and development of metastases depend on the formation of new blood vessels (neoangiogenesis) and the general metabolic situation in the respective organ. Depending on the location of the primary tumour, a distinction can be made between recurring but not fixed metastatic pathways of malignant tumours. In lymphogenic metastasis, the regional lymph nodes are in the foreground. Haematogenous metastasis primarily involves organs with a good blood supply, such as the lungs. Finally, tumours can also spread locally directly by 'smear' or intracanalicularly (Valastyan and Weinberg 2011) (Figure 8.2).

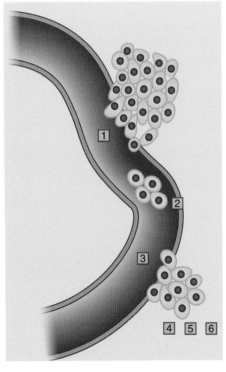

1. Invasion: Cancer cells acquire the ability to invade nearby tissues by breaking down the extracellular matrix (ECM) through the secretion of enzymes like matrix metalloproteinases (MMPs). This allows them to detach from the primary tumour mass. Cancer cells enter nearby blood vessels or lymphatic vessels.

2. Circulation: Once In the bloodstream or lymphatic system, cancer cells travel through the vessels, surviving various challenges such as shear forces, immune surveillance, and interaction with other blood components.

3. Adhesion and Extravasation: Cancer cells arrest in capillaries of distant organs. Here, they adhere to the endothelial lining and extravasate from the vessels, infiltrating the target tissue.

4. Micrometastasis formation: Extravasated cancer cells establish macrometastasis by proliferating and evading immune detection within the new tissue microenvironment.

5. Angiogenesis at secondary site: Micrometastases release signals that induce angiogenesis, the formation of new blood vessels, to provide oxygen and nutrients essential for tumour growth.

6. Formation of macrometastasis: Some macrometastasis develop into macrometastasis, larger tumour masses that continue to grow and can eventually cause clinical symptoms.

Figure 8.2 Mechanism of metastasis.

Pathophysiology

The pathophysiological consequences of tumours are manifold. Besides local processes and the formation of metastases, systemic processes are often a consequence of the synthesis of active metabolites by the tumour cells.

Local Processes

Local processes are caused by tumour expansion and the reaction of the surrounding tissue.

Tumour expansion results from the more or less continuous growth of the tumour tissue. Neighbouring tissue is displaced in the process. Due to the expansion and possibly a reduction of the blood supply in the surrounding area, atrophy of the neighbouring structures develops. These can become functionally impaired or non-functional. Pressure atrophy has particular consequences when surrounding tissue cannot avoid the tumour growth, as is the case in the brain, for example. Increasing tumour growth in the brain leads to seizures or coma due to progressive neurological dysfunction.

Other local consequences of neoplasia are described. For example, dilatation or intussusception of the intestine in the case of an intestinal wall tumour. These occur in dogs and cats predominantly as adenocarcinomas or lymphomas. An intestinal dilatation develops towards the stomach, as in the case of a foreign body. On the one hand, the dilatation impairs the blood supply to the wall, and on the other hand, it leads to a disturbance of the resorption processes because the enteric chyle contact surface is reduced. The impaired peristalsis also leads to reduced mixing of the chyle and limited digestion. The impaired peristalsis can also lead to intussusception of the intestine. Renal tumours are less common in dogs and cats and are usually lymphomas in cats. Urinary retention may develop due to the reduction of urine flow in the collecting tubes or renal pelvis. In slow progression, this leads to atrophy of the renal parenchyma and hydronephrosis. As the kidney function is given in the case of an unaffected contralateral kidney, kidney failure does not always occur. Bronchial tumours may lead to collapse of the bronchus and atelectasis of the allocated lung parenchyma. Lung tumours are more common in dogs than in cats and are usually adenocarcinomas. Liver tumours can lead to bile duct obstruction with subsequent jaundice if the liver parenchyma architecture is destroyed. This is rarely observed in dogs and cats.

Tumour growth can also influence the local vascular supply. As veins are more sensitive to pressure due to their thinner wall structure, local venous outflow disorders develop first. This leads to oedema formation and local acidosis in the affected tissues. In the case of arterial obstruction, ischaemia also develops. Cellular consequences of ischaemia are hypoxia, disturbance of cellular energy production, disturbance of cellular transport processes, with accumulation of water in the cell; at the same time, enzyme systems are inhibited by the cellular acidosis after hypoxia. In the overall consequence, this can lead to local necrosis of the neighbouring tissue. This in turn is associated with a local inflammatory response. The inflammation can lead to further tissue alteration with morphological remodelling, also in the sense of fibrosis, which additionally hinders the blood supply in the tumour area. Another local consequence can be tumour haemorrhage. This develops when tumour growth leads to an increasingly unstable architecture in the neoplastic tissue complex. This can lead to erosion of the vessel walls and bleeding.

Systemic Processes

Systemic consequences of a neoplastic process also result, for example, from local impairment of neighbouring tissue. As already shown in the case of the brain, progressive tumour growth can have a lasting effect on brain structures and induce systemic consequences. Systemic effects of a tumour process can also arise through the increased synthesis of tumour cell products. These include, for example, the synthesis of ACTH or cortisol in the various forms of Cushing's disease, which usually results from an adrenal or, more frequently, pituitary neoplasia. Tumours of the adrenal medulla, pheochromocytomas, induce hypertension due to increased synthesis of adrenergic substances.

A special form of systemic tumour consequences is the paraneoplastic syndrome.

Paraneoplastic Syndrome

Paraneoplastic syndromes are symptoms or complexes that are attributed to metabolic activity of tumours. The biological basis for many paraneoplastic syndromes is not fully understood. Biologically active substances such as peptide hormones, growth factors and cytokines or their biochemically active analogues are often secreted. In addition, a paraneoplastic

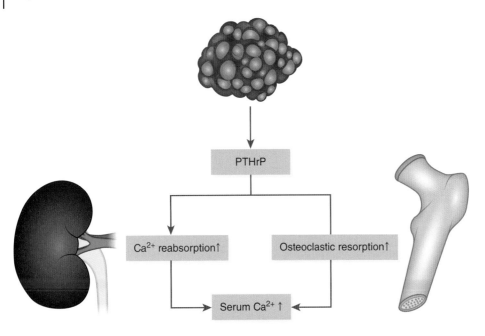

Figure 8.3 PTHrP effect.

syndrome occurs due to the reaction of the immune system to tumour cells and the formation of immune complexes. Autoimmune reactions can develop from this. The paraneoplasias are divided into different categories:

Paraneoplasticendocrinopathies
Disorders of the haematopoietic system
Neuromuscular syndromes

The prevalence of paraneoplastic syndromes is relatively common, especially in the dog, whereas there are few reports in cats. Cachexia, anaemia and hypercalcaemia appear to be most common in dogs (Tumielewicz et al. 2019).

Hypercalcaemia develops in connection with a tumour via different mechanisms. The most frequently described is hypercalcaemia as a result of anal sac carcinoma. This goes back to the synthesis of a parathyroid hormone-like peptide (PTHrP). PTHrP is also physiologically produced in the organism, but unlike parathormone, it has a more paracrine effect. Through increased expression in certain tumours (anal sac carcinomas, lymphomas), PTHrP also becomes systemically active. In bone, osteoclastic bone resorption is increased; in addition, the hormone effect increases renal Ca reabsorption.

Other mechanisms of neoplastic-induced hypercalcaemia are the effects of tumour cell products, such as cytokines, arachidonic acid metabolites or thrombin. They lead, via osteoclasts, to local bone lysis and the activation of metalloproteinase. The result is a decomposition of the bone with consecutive releases of calcium (Figure 8.3).

Disorders of the haematopoietic system in tumours result from the tumour haemorrhages already described. These result from vascular erosions during progressive tumour growth with necrosis of the tumour parenchyma. These are haemorrhage anaemias that are initially non-regenerative and can be regenerative after a few days. However, disturbed homeostasis can also occur in tumour diseases as a result of tumour-induced consumption coagulopathy. This induces regenerative anaemia, in principle. Invasion of tumour cells into the bone marrow cause non-regenerative anaemia through myelodestructive processes.

Neuromuscular disorders have been described in dogs with thymoma in the sense of paraneoplastic myasthenia gravis. Circulating antibodies occupy the acetylcholine (ACh) receptors of the postsynaptic membrane. As a result, the development of an action potential at the postsynaptic membrane is reduced or inhibited, leading to muscle weakness.

Tumour Cachexia

Neoplasms influence the metabolism through various factors. Overall, they produce a catabolic metabolic state with reduction of the body condition up to cachexia.

Cachexia due to reduction of muscle and fat tissue is a common condition in advanced cancer. The mechanism can be seen as the release of biologically active mediators and the initiation of proteolytic catabolism. Proteolytic activity in tumour tissue can synthesise peptides that have lipolytic effects. Cathepsins, proteolytically acting enzymes, are produced by tumour cells and degrade cell organelles or components of the extracellular matrix. Furthermore, in connection with neoplasia, the ubiquitin-proteasome pathway is activated, which contributes to a catabolic metabolic state via increased proteolysis (Rubin 2003).

Ubiquitin-directed proteolysis involves several steps. First, ubiquitin is bound to a carrier protein by reaction with ATP under the catalysis of the ubiquitin-activating enzyme (E1) and transferred from this to the target protein. This step is repeated several times so that, finally, a polyubiquitin-protein complex is formed. In the next step, this is broken down into amino acids and peptides by the proteinase 26S proteasome, an enzyme that cleaves peptide bonds.

Another mechanism by which tumours cause cachexia is anorexia. This can be caused directly by neoplastic mediators or by proinflammatory cytokines synthesised during tumour-associated inflammation. Tumour necrosis factor plays a central role in this.

References

Amieva, M. and Peek, R.M. Jr. (2016). Pathobiology of *Helicobacter pylori*-induced gastric cancer. *Gastroenterology* 150 (1): 64–78. https://doi.org/10.1053/j.gastro.2015.09.004.

Chen, J. (2016). The cell-cycle arrest and apoptotic functions of p53 in tumor initiation and progression. *Cold Spring Harbor Perspectives in Medicine* 6 (3): a026104. https://doi.org/10.1101/cshperspect.a026104.

Davis, B.W. and Ostrander, E.A. (2014). Domestic dogs and cancer research: a breed-based genomics approach. *ILAR Journal* 55 (1): 59–68. https://doi.org/10.1093/ilar/ilu017.

Dobson, J.M. (2013). Breed-predispositions to cancer in pedigree dogs. *ISRN Veterinary Science* 2013: 941275. https://doi.org/10.1155/2013/941275.

Egenvall, A., Bonnett, B.N., Häggström, J. et al. (2010). Morbidity of insured Swedish cats during 1999–2006 by age, breed, sex, and diagnosis. *Journal of Feline Medicine and Surgery* 12 (12): 948–959. https://doi.org/10.1016/j.jfms.2010.08.008.

Kaiser, A.M. and Attardi, L.D. (2018). Deconstructing networks of p53-mediated tumor suppression in vivo. *Cell Death and Differentiation* 25 (1): 93–103. https://doi.org/10.1038/cdd.2017.171.

Lisovska, N. and Shanazarov, N. (2019). Tumour progression mechanisms: insights from the central immune regulation of tissue homeostasis. *Oncology Letters* 17 (6): 5311–5318. https://doi.org/10.3892/ol.2019.10218.

Martínez-Reyes, I. and Chandel, N.S. (2021). Cancer metabolism: looking forward. *Nature Reviews Cancer* 21 (10): 669–680. https://doi.org/10.1038/s41568-021-00378-6.

Mendoza, S., Konishi, T., Dernell, W.S. et al. (1998). Status of the p53, Rb and MDM2 genes in canine osteosarcoma. *Anticancer Research* 18 (6A): 4449–4453. PMID: 9891508.

Michell, A.R. (1999). Longevity of British breeds of dog and its relationships with sex, size, cardiovascular variables and disease. *The Veterinary Record* 145 (22): 625–629. https://doi.org/10.1136/vr.145.22.625.

Porras-Silesky, C., Mejías-Alpízar, M.J., Mora, J. et al. (2021). *Spirocerca lupi* proteomics and its role in cancer development: an overview of spirocercosis-induced sarcomas and revision of helminth-induced carcinomas. *Pathogens (Basel, Switzerland)* 10 (2): 124. https://doi.org/10.3390/pathogens10020124.

Rubin, H. (2003). Cancer cachexia: its correlations and causes. *Proceedings of the National Academy of Sciences of the United States of America* 100 (9): 5384–5389. https://doi.org/10.1073/pnas.0931260100.

Shim, G., Ricoul, M., Hempel, W.M. et al. (2014). Crosstalk between telomere maintenance and radiation effects: a key player in the process of radiation-induced carcinogenesis. *Mutation Research Reviews in Mutation Research* S1383-5742(14) 00002-7 10.1016/j.mrrev.2014.01.001. Advance online publication. https://doi.org/10.1016/j.mrrev.2014.01.001.

Slaga, T.J. (1983). Overview of tumour promotion in animals. *Environmental Health Perspectives* 50: 3–14. https://doi.org/10.1289/ehp.83503.

Tumielewicz, K.L., Hudak, D., Kim, J. et al. (2019). Review of oncological emergencies in small animal patients. *Veterinary Medicine and Science* 5 (3): 271–296. https://doi.org/10.1002/vms3.164.

Valastyan, S. and Weinberg, R.A. (2011). Tumour metastasis: molecular insights and evolving paradigms. *Cell* 147 (2): 275–292. https://doi.org/10.1016/j.cell.2011.09.024.

9

Infections

Infections with viral, bacterial or parasitic pathogens lead to a confrontation between the defence mechanisms of the macro-organism (organism) and the pathogen, and can finally result in pathogen elimination or an infectious disease.

The different levels of the body's own defence have already been presented in Chapter 1. They are composed of non-specific mechanisms of mechanical defence, such as the skin or mucous membrane structure, and of non-specific or specific defence mechanisms of the immune system.

For each type of pathogen, there are specific factors that originate from the pathogen and specific defence mechanisms that determine the course of an infection or infectious disease. Pathogen-specific factors are described by the terms 'pathogenicity', which means disease-causing property, and 'virulence', which describes the extent of the disease-causing properties.

Based on the respective distribution, local infections that are limited to one organ system are distinguished from systemic infections with involvement of different organ systems. Different infections are differentiated in their clinical manifestations.

In subclinical infection, the potency of the immune system predominates and thus prevents the disease from breaking out. In latent infection, there is a balance between the pathogen and the immune system. Should one side dominate, either the pathogen is killed or the disease breaks out. Occult infections are neither directly nor indirectly detectable. In the case of clinically manifest infections, there is a clinical symptomatology depending on the organ system affected (Figure 9.1).

Virus

Viruses are infectious agents that require cellular structures of the macro-organism for their multiplication. This also creates an essential damaging mechanism in a viral infection. In principle, viruses consist of genetic information in the form of DNA or RNA. This is surrounded by a protein structure, the capsid, which protects the genetic information. In the case of enveloped viruses, the capsid is also surrounded by an envelope consisting of a lipid bilayer with integrated surface proteins (Figure 9.2).

The central disease-causing mechanism of a viral infection is the intracellular replication of the virus, which can be inconsequential or result in cell death or neoplastic transformation.

The following principles are adopted for viral infections:

1) Many viral infections are subclinical.
2) The same disease syndrome can be caused by a variety of viruses.
3) The disease symptomatology is determined by both viral and host factors.

Pathogenesis of Viral Diseases

To induce a disease, viruses must enter the body, reach their target cells, invade them and eventually multiply.

Specific steps involved in viral pathogenesis are the following:

Textbook of Small Animal Pathophysiology, First Edition. Stephan Neumann.
© 2025 John Wiley & Sons Ltd. Published 2025 by John Wiley & Sons Ltd.

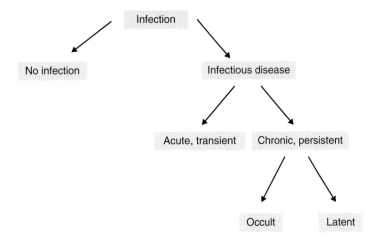

Figure 9.1 Course of an infection.

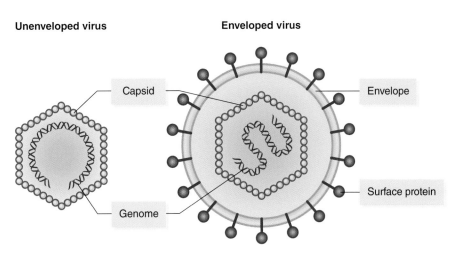

Figure 9.2 Schematic virus structure.

Viral invasion of the host
Virus replication
Virus spread
Cell injury
Host immune response
Viral clearance or establishment of infection and viral excretion

Most viral infections are induced when the pathogen adheres to and penetrates the external body surface or mucous membranes. The most common entry site is the mucous membrane of the respiratory or gastrointestinal tract.

Some viruses, such as calici or parvoviruses, induce an infectious disease at the entry site and do not usually spread systemically. Most viruses, however, use the entry site for symptomless primary replication, which is followed by virus spread. The mechanisms of virus spread vary. The most common route is spread via the bloodstream. The presence of viruses in the blood is called 'viraemia'. Viruses can be present freely in the blood plasma or spread via certain cell types, usually leukocytes. Viruses show cell tropism, which means that certain cells are primarily infected. These are reached via haematogenous or lymphogenous spread.

Cellular tropism is due to the presence of specific cell surface receptors for the respective virus. Receptors are components of the cell surface with which a region of the virus surface (capsid or envelope) specifically interacts and can trigger an infection.

The level of cell surface receptor expression and post-translational modifications influence the ability of viruses to infect different cell types. For example, influenza virus infection requires cellular proteases to cleave virally encoded haemagglutinin in order for the virus to infect new cells. In addition, cellular expression of a glycolytic enzyme (neuraminidase) is necessary to release newly formed viruses.

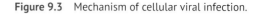
Figure 9.3 Mechanism of cellular viral infection.

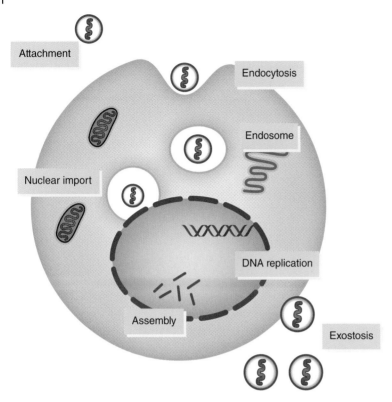

The course of a typical viral cell infection begins with the binding of the virus particle to cellular surface receptors. Through invagination of the cell membrane, the virus is taken up intracellularly with the cell membrane as a so-called 'endosome'. Through the process of uncoating, viral DNA or RNA is released and can be integrated into the cellular genomic DNA. In the case of RNA viruses, the RNA must first be converted into DNA by an enzyme, reverse transcriptase. After viral DNA has been integrated into the cellular DNA, it can synthesise viral proteins through translation. During assembly, the virus is assembled from the individual components and released from the cell as a finished virus by exocytosis.

The destruction of virus-infected cells and the organism's reaction to such cells is responsible for the development of the disease. Some tissues, such as the intestinal epithelium, can regenerate quickly and compensate for extensive damage better than other tissues, such as the brain. Clinical diseases caused by viral infections are the result of a complex series of events, many of which are still unknown.

The final stage of pathogenesis is the shedding of infectious viruses. This is a necessary step for a viral infection to spread. The excretion of viruses occurs at different stages of the disease, depending on the particular pathogen (Figure 9.3).

Immune Response of the Host

The immune response to a viral infection is initially mediated by interferons (IFNs), which inhibit viral replication. They are produced very rapidly (within hours) in response to viral infections. IFNs also modulate humoral and cellular immunity and have broad regulatory activities related to cell growth.

There are several types of IFNs, which can be differentiated into three groups: IFN-α, IFN-β and IFN-γ. Both IFN-α and IFN-β are considered type I or viral IFNs; IFN-γ is type II or immune IFN. Viral infection is a strong inducer of IFN-α and IFN-β production; RNA viruses are stronger inducers of IFN than DNA viruses. IFN-γ is not produced exclusively in response to viral infection, but is also stimulated by mitogens. IFNs are detectable shortly after viral infection, but their concentration decreases as soon as antibodies are detectable. This temporal relationship suggests that IFN plays a primary role in the host's non-specific defence against viral infection.

Interferon is secreted and binds to cell receptors, causing an antiviral state by inducing the synthesis of proteins that inhibit viral replication. Several pathways appear to be involved, including: (i) a dsRNA-dependent protein kinase (PKR) that phosphorylates and inactivates a cellular initiation factor (eIF-2), preventing the formation of the initiation complex required for viral protein synthesis; (ii) an oligonucleotide synthetase (2-5A synthetase) that activates a cellular endonuclease; (iii) an RNase that degrades mRNA; (iv) a phosphodiesterase that inhibits peptide chain elongation; and (v) nitric oxide synthetase induced by IFN-γ in macrophages, which induces the synthesis of nitric oxide (NO) with various roles in immune responses, including activity against viruses.

In contrast, viruses can block the induction of IFN expression, PKR protein kinase or IFN-induced signal transduction. Or they neutralise IFN-γ by inducing the synthesis of soluble IFN receptors.

Both humoral and cellular components of the adaptive immune response are involved in the control of viral infections. Viruses elicit a tissue response that differs from the response to pathogenic bacteria. While polymorphonuclear leukocytes form the major cellular response to acute inflammation by pyogenic bacteria, infiltration with mononuclear cells and lymphocytes characterises the inflammatory response to viral infection.

Virus-encoded proteins serve as targets for the immune response. Virus-infected cells can be lysed by cytotoxic T lymphocytes as a result of recognition of viral polypeptides on the cell surface. Humoral immunity protects the host from reinfection by the same virus. Neutralising antibodies to capsid proteins block the initiation of viral infection, presumably at the binding or entry stage. Secretory IgA antibody is important for protection against viral infections of the respiratory or gastrointestinal tract.

The pathophysiological consequences of a viral infection depend on the particular virus. However, there are also general symptoms associated with many viral infections, such as malaise and inappetence. In this process, different cytokines, especially proinflammatory cytokines such as IL-1, IL-6 and TNF-α, are produced by the macro-organism in response to the viral infection. These induce the non-specific infection symptoms by directly influencing the central nervous system (CNS), especially the hypothalamus.

Bacteria

Bacteria differ from viruses in their size and metabolism. Although they are considered prokaryotes, which means they do not have a cell nucleus, they already show cellular structures, such as a cell membrane, cell organelles and also their own metabolism (Figure 9.4).

Pathogenesis of Bacterial Infections

Different pathogenic bacteria use similar mechanisms to cause infectious diseases. These include the ability to adhere to cells, penetrate the cell membrane and damage them. In addition, pathogenic bacteria are characterised by a successful evasion of the body's defences.

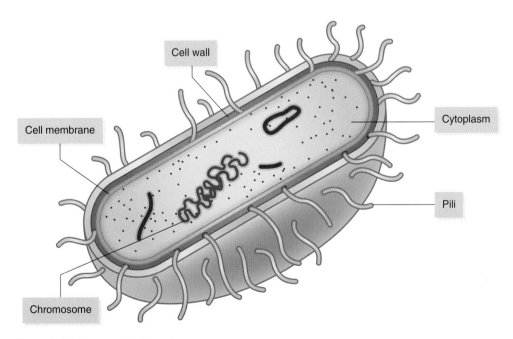

Figure 9.4 Anatomy of a bacterium.

The role that different mechanisms play in the pathogenesis of an infection depends on the bacterial species, the site of entry, the immune status of the host and similar factors. The following factors influence the pathogenesis of a bacterial infection.

Capsule

Some bacteria synthesise polysaccharides with a high molecular weight (exopolysaccharides) to create a shell around the cell wall, this extracellular layer is called a 'capsule'. The capsule is an important virulence factor. It provides protection from the body's defence mechanisms, e.g. phagocytosis, by preventing opsonising antibodies from being recognised by defence cells, such as macrophages. This 'frustrated phagocytosis' leads to an increased inflammatory response as the macrophages and neutrophils produce more inflammatory cytokines to clear the bacteria. The increased inflammatory response leads to increased tissue damage as more neutrophilic granulocytes and macrophages are recruited to the site of infection.

An example of a pathogen that synthesises a capsule is *Pseudomonas aeruginosa*.

Cell Wall

Bacteria can be divided into gram-positive and gram-negative pathogens based on their cell wall structure. The cell wall contains components that play a role in the development of septic shock as virulence factors.

Septic shock is the consequence of synthesis and release of cytokines and other mediators by inflammatory cells. A major bacterial trigger for septic shock is lipopolysaccharide (LPS), this is also called 'endotoxin'. It is found in the outer membrane of gram-negative bacteria. The released LPS acts, for example, on the CD14 receptor on the surface of macrophages. By binding to the receptor, LPS induces the secretion of numerous proinflammatory cytokines and activates the complement and coagulation cascades.

Gram-positive pathogens do not synthesise LPS but produce cytokine secretions via components of the bacterial wall, such as peptidoglycans and teichoic acids, leading to septic shock. Gram-positive bacteria that can trigger septic shock include *Staphylococcus aureus* and streptococci.

Toxins

Release of toxins is another mechanism by which bacteria damage the organism. These are components of the bacteria and are either secreted (exotoxins) or released during lysis (endotoxins). The latter includes LPS, which is a component of the outer membrane of gram-negative bacteria. The toxic component of LPS is lipid A. Endotoxins are usually released during the lysis of bacteria and develop toxic properties through the activation of cells of the defence system, predominantly macrophages. In addition, they are able to activate both the coagulation and complement systems. Finally, endotoxins induce the formation and secretion of proinflammatory cytokines (e.g. TNF-α, IL-1, IL-6).

Further toxic properties of bacteria, often caused by exotoxins include membrane damage. The toxins can disturb the membrane potential physically, through pore formation and chemically through interaction with components of the cell membrane. As a result, cell lysis can occur.

Toxins that are secreted by bacteria and cause intracellular damage are called 'intracellular toxins'. Different mechanisms have been described. By activating adenylate cyclase, bacterial toxins can induce the formation of the second messenger cAMP, in some cells this leads to an increased excretion of chloride ions with the consequence of cellular water loss and cell lysis. Diarrhoeal pathogens, in particular, can damage enterocytes in this way and cause secretory diarrhoea.

Other bacterial toxins inhibit protein biosynthesis and can thus destroy the structure of the cytoskeleton.

Adhesins

An important step in the interaction between bacteria and cells of the organism and a prerequisite for colonisation is the adhesion of the pathogen to the cell surfaces. Adhesion is made possible by the bacterial synthesis of specific polypeptides or polysaccharides called 'adhesins'. One form of adhesins is fimbriae or pili, which are hair-like structures that protrude from the bacterial surface and are more common in gram-negative bacteria. Another form is microbial surface components recognising adhesive matrix molecules (MSCRAMM).

The adhesins bind to surface structures of the cells of the organism, such as surface immunoglobulins, glycolipids, glycoproteins and extracellular matrix proteins (such as fibronectin and collagen). In addition to bacterial fixation, the mechanism of adhesion can initiate pathological biochemical processes, such as toxin secretion, host cell invasion and activation of cellular signalling cascades.

Invasion

The spread of pathogens in the body is called 'invasion' and can take place extracellularly and intracellularly. In extracellular invasion, the bacteria penetrate the tissue by secreting enzymes that degrade structures of the organism, such as hyaluronidases or collagenases (proteoglycan degradation in connective tissue).

Intracellular invasion occurs when bacteria invade and multiply in cells of the organism. This can happen in phagocytosing and non-phagocytosing cells. In phagocytosing cells, the uptake takes place via the phagocytosis process and is accordingly uncomplicated. The bacteria are present intracellularly in phagosomes. However, multiplication in phagocytosing cells is a complex process because the bacteria must prevent their own lysis. To do this, bacteria can protect themselves intracellularly by preventing the fusion of the phagosome with the phagocytic lysosomes. In some bacteria, phagosome–lysosome fusion occurs, but bacterial destruction is prevented by inhibition of the lysosomal components.

In contrast, in non-phagocytic cells, the uptake of the bacteria is the challenging process. This is mediated by different mechanisms, zipper-like, trigger-like and caveoli.

In the zipper-like mechanism, the bacteria attach themselves to the cell membrane and are enclosed by it, in the sense of a zipper mechanism. The resulting vesicle is called a 'phagosome'. Bacteria that use this mechanism are, for example, *Yersinia pseudotuberculosis*.

In trigger-like uptake, the inoculation process of the bacteria is triggered by an induced signal transduction that originates from the bacteria. Injection of bacterial messenger substances into the cell triggers reformation of the actin scaffold, which results in protrusion of the cell membrane and enclosure of the bacterium with subsequent intracellular uptake. This type of intracellular uptake takes place, for example, in salmonellae.

The last known form of intracellular invasion by bacteria is the caveoli-mediated form. In this case, the bacteria are taken up by membrane invasion in a similar way to phagosomes, but in this case there is no formation of a phagolysosome resulting in bacterial lysis. This principle is followed by viruses or, in the case of bacteria, by mycobacteria, for example.

Reproduction and Protection from the Body's Own Defences

Bacteria use several mechanisms to protect themselves from the body's own defence mechanisms. The formation of a capsule has already been described; this is predominantly composed of polysaccharides and grants the bacteria protection against factors of the immune system, such as antibodies or complement. Furthermore, through the expression of coagulases, bacteria have a mechanism with the help of which they can fragment fibrin in order to protect themselves from contact with immune cells or antibodies through the fragments that coat the bacterium. *Staphylococcus aureus* is one bacterium that uses this mechanism. The third mechanism by which bacteria can protect themselves from the immune system is the expression of Fc receptors in the bacterial wall. Antibodies bind to these receptors with their Fc region, which has no immunological function and thus protects the bacterium from access by antibodies.

Finally, bacteria are able to induce the formation of immune-incompetent T cells or antibodies, e.g. through the formation of LPS.

Parasites

The damaging mechanisms of parasitic forms are as variable as the forms themselves, but there are some basic cross-species factors that are focused on here.

Induction of an Immune Response

A parasite infestation induces a typical immune reaction, the purpose of which is to eliminate the parasite. The consequences of this immune reaction can be visible clinical symptoms. The initial response of the macro-organism to the parasite is carried by the innate immune system. Parasites also have pathogen-associated molecular patterns (PAMPs) that react with receptors (PRR), leading to cytokine secretion by non-specific defence cells. Dendritic cells, for example, secrete IL-12, IL-18 and TNF-α under the influence of parasitic PAMPs. Natural killer cells secrete IFN-γ. Subsequently, other immunological effector cells are activated. The cytokine-dependent activation causes an increase in phagocytosis activity in macrophages and the increased formation of reactive oxygen species (ROS). Other effector cells, such as eosinophilic granulocytes, empty their granules.

The acquired immune system reacts to the parasite infestation with a time delay of several days. T helper cells direct the respective reaction, which depends on the type of parasite infestation. In the case of intracellular parasite infestation, Th1 cells secrete IFN-γ, which attracts macrophages and other cytotoxic cells. Upon activation, Th2 cells secrete IL-4, which stimulates B cells and increases antibody production. In addition, mast cells and eosinophilic granulocytes are stimulated to divide and degranulate. This form of immune response develops more frequently in extracellular parasites, primarily helminths.

Since parasitic infections produce different stages that also parasitise in different tissue compartments, they also activate different defence mechanisms depending on the phase.

In the case of large parasites, mostly helminths, different defence systems are required to attack the parasite. A classical approach is antibody-dependent cellular cytotoxicity. Here, the parasites are marked by antibodies in order to be fought more effectively by effector cells, such as macrophages or eosinophilic granulocytes. These can attack the parasite directly through mediators in their granules, but also generate increased intestinal peristalsis and mucus production in order to get rid of the parasite more quickly.

The confrontation between the immune system and the parasite serves to eliminate the pathogen, but also produces collateral damage in the host organism. An excessive inflammatory reaction, for example, can cause lasting damage to the tissue of the host organism.

The formation of immune complexes from antibodies and parasite antigen also produce damage to the host organism. Deposited immune complexes produce an inflammatory reaction and can lead to circulatory disturbances in the affected capillaries. This process produces disturbances in small capillaries due to reduced blood flow, and in the kidneys, glomerulonephritis is caused by stenosis of the glomerular capillaries.

Finally, parasites can suppress the immune system, one mechanism being the depletion of defence cell production due to the ongoing inflammatory response.

Variation of the Host Cell

Intracellular forms of parasites (e.g. coccidia, toxoplasma) are able to change the cells morphologically and metabolically. Intracellular cyst formation or variations of the cellular cytoskeleton are caused by intracellular parasites in that parasitic molecules, for example, as transcription factors, influence cellular gene expression and thus protein biosynthesis in their own favour. *Toxoplasma gondii*, for example, secretes phosphatases that influence cellular gene expression as transcription factors.

In addition, there are other mechanisms that are independent of the cell nucleus, as shown by morphological alterations of nucleus-less erythrocytes after infection with *Plasmodium falciparum*. Here, a cytoplasmic network is formed by the parasite.

Endocrine Influences

Endocrine consequences of a parasitic infestation have been described, in particular, for the intermediate hosts of tapeworms. Here, the influence on the parasitic cycle seems to be in the foreground. Due to the reduction of male sex hormones and the subsequent feminisation, some metacestodes (e.g. *Taenia crassiceps*) improve their growth conditions. The immune response in the female organism tends to be of the Th2 type, which creates better living conditions for parasites than a dominant Th1 type found in males. The mechanism consists of parasite-induced IL-6 expression in the testicular tissue of the intermediate host. IL-6 induces the expression of aromatase P-450, which transforms testosterone into oestradiol.

Further Reading

Brun, A. (2022). An overview of veterinary viral diseases and vaccine technologies. *Methods in Molecular Biology (Clifton, N.J.)* 2465: 1–26. https://doi.org/10.1007/978-1-0716-2168-4_1.

Getts, D.R., Chastain, E.M., Terry, R.L., and Miller, S.D. (2013). Viral infection, antiviral immunity, and autoimmunity. *Immunological Reviews* 255 (1): 197–209. http://dx.doi.org/10.1111/imr.12091.

Selbitz, H.-J., Truyen, U., and Valentin-Weigand, P. (2015). *Tiermedizinische Mikrobiologie*. Infektion- und Seuchenlehre: Enke Verlag.

Zeisel, M.B., Crouchet, E., Baumert, T.F., and Schuster, C. (2015). Host-targeting agents to prevent and cure hepatitis C virus infection. *Viruses* 7 (11): 5659–5685. https://doi.org/10.3390/v7112898.

10

Ageing

Molecular Aspects of Ageing

Many insights into the ageing process have come from studies on non-mammals. However, today it is assumed that the knowledge gained can also be transferred to higher organisms.

The general ageing process begins at the cellular level. All functional units of the cell are affected, from the cell nucleus to the cell membrane and beyond that the extracellular matrix (ECM). Ageing processes are accompanied by a reduction in cellular self-organisation, resulting in a disturbed stress response, the deposition of misexpressed molecules and disturbed autophagy.

Cell Ageing and Telomere Length

Telomeres are non-coding, single-stranded ends of chromosomes. They act like protective caps at the ends of the chromosomes, which become shorter with each cell division. Factors that accelerate shortening are oxidative stress and increased telomerase activity, for example in neoplastic transformation. If the telomeres shorten, the genes they protect can be damaged with the consequence that the affected cells reduce their division rate and their regenerative capacity (Bernadotte et al. 2016; Zhu et al. 2019).

Cell Ageing and Transcription and Translation

The cellular ageing process leads to disturbances in the nuclear cell organisation, through disturbances in transcription with misreading of genes or formation of structurally altered mRNA. Cellular ageing also leads to morphological alterations of the nuclear pore complex through which the mRNA leaves the cell nucleus. As a result, mRNA information cannot adaptively lead to protein expression with the consequence of a delayed or insufficient cellular response.

Protein expression is another critical area of cellular ageing where morphologically, usually misfolded, or functionally altered proteins disrupt protein homeostasis (proteostasis). Under physiological conditions, misfolded proteins are eliminated by chaperones (e.g. heat shock proteins) by being taken up, chaperone-mediated, by lysosomes. This process is disturbed with increasing cell age. The result is deposits of misfolded proteins (Choi et al. 2017; Uyar et al. 2020).

Cell Ageing and Mitochondrial Function

With increasing cell age, mitochondrial DNA reduces. At the same time, reactive oxygen species (ROS) increase, resulting in increasing oxidative damage. Mitochondria show impaired function with age, such as reduced oxidative capacity and oxidative phosphorylation, and thus reduced ATP production. In addition, mitophagy, an autophagy process that removes dysfunctional mitochondria, decreases with age. (Chistiakov et al. 2014).

Textbook of Small Animal Pathophysiology, First Edition. Stephan Neumann.
© 2025 John Wiley & Sons Ltd. Published 2025 by John Wiley & Sons Ltd.

Cell Ageing and the Cytoskeleton

The cytoskeleton comprises a multitude of structural proteins that give the cell a shape, but are also responsible for intracellular transport processes, as well as the connection between cells and the cell and the ECM. Alterations of the cytoskeleton, which increase with increasing cell age, are consequences of age-related impaired protein expression (see Cell Ageing and Transcription and Translation). Disorders of the cytoskeleton in turn induce apoptosis (Gourlay and Ayscough 2005; Amberg et al. 2012).

Ageing and Extracellular Matrix

The ECM forms the structural environment of the cells and is also a distributor of cellular activity. Essential structural proteins of the ECM are collagens and elastin. Both molecules can be morphologically altered by ageing processes and thus be functionally limited (Birch 2018) (Figure 10.1).

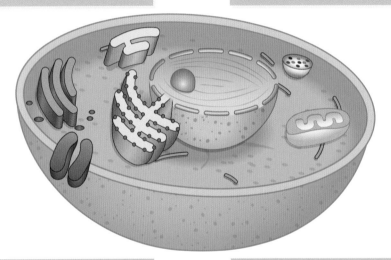

Senescence-associated secretory phenotype (SASP):
Senescent cells secrete a variety of pro-inflammatory cytokines, growth factors, and proteases, contributing to chronic inflammation and tissue dysfunction.

Telomere shortening:
Telomeres are protective caps at the ends of chromosomes that shorten with each cell division. When telomeres become critically short, cells may enter a state of senescence or apoptosis (cell death)

Cellular communication:
Signaling between cells, including paracrine and endocrine factors, influences the aging process and contributes to tissue dysfunction.

Mitochondrial dysfunction:
Impaired mitochondrial function, including reduced energy production and increased reactive oxygen species (ROS) generation, can lead to cellular damage and senescence.

Figure 10.1 Overview of cell ageing mechanisms.

Ageing in the Dog

The cellular changes described lead overall to a reduced function and adaptation of the cell, from which the increase in diseases in old age can be explained. This so-called 'old-age morbidity' reflects an increase in morbidity with increasing age, but varies from breed to breed. The incidence of disease in dogs older than 15 years increases fivefold compared to one-year-old dogs (Dankert 1998). The incidence of disease also increases system-specifically with age. An increase in diseases of the cardiovascular system, the endocrine system and tumour diseases are in the foreground. Parasitosis and malformations, on the other hand, are observed more frequently in young dogs (Salzborn 2003). The increase in cardiovascular diseases in dogs reflects the reduced organ adaptation in old age (Guglielmini 2003). For example, the length of the contraction period, as well as the rigidity of the ventricular musculature, increases with age (Templeton et al. 1979). This, in conjunction with increased peripheral resistance, leads to disturbances in peripheral blood flow (Haidet et al. 1996). In addition, a reduced response of the heart to impulses from the β-adrenergic system is seen with increasing age (Haidet 1993). The increase in the incidence of endocrine diseases in old age is partly attributed to age-related changes in the hypothalamic-pituitary axis. Among other things, there is an age-related reduction in the number of cells in both organs (Thamer et al. 2012). The age-related changes lead to a loss of reserve capacity and to a reduced adaptive capacity (Boari and Aste 2003). The increase in tumorous diseases can be explained by tumorigenesis, according to which the number of preneoplastic alterations increases with age.

Ageing in the Cat

Typical age-related processes in cats are described for almost all organ systems. Cats are often classified into the age groups: young (<3 years), adult (3–8 years), old (8–12 years) and senior (>12 years). A reduction of cognitive abilities is described in cats from an age of >10 years (Landsberg et al. 2010). Age-related skin changes lead to a thinner and slightly greasy coat in cats (Bellows et al. 2016). A decrease in body condition score has been described especially for senior cats (Vogt et al. 2010). In addition to these general changes, renal and endocrine diseases, in particular, occur in old cats.

The prevalence of chronic kidney disease in senior cats increases up to 80% (Marino et al. 2014). The most common pathological change is tubulointerstitial fibrosis, which eventually leads to impaired renal function resulting in chronic renal failure (Chakrabarti et al. 2013; Lawler et al. 2006). Such remodelling processes can be triggered by a variety of systemic diseases, the prevalence of which increases with age (Brown et al. 2016). Hyperthyroidism is also considered a classic age-related disease of the cat (Ray et al. 2021). It is assumed that the cumulative exposure to potential causalities of hyperthyroidism over a lifetime is the reason for its occurrence at an advanced age. For example, bisphenol A, a plasticiser used in ready-to-eat cat food packaging, has been found to affect thyroid metabolism at different levels (Kim and Park 2019).

Clinical-Pathological Changes in Old Age

The age-related changes described above lead to age-associated laboratory changes. (Radakovich et al. 2017). This shows that between adult and geriatric patients, urea concentrations increased and creatinine concentrations decreased. Possible explanations are seen in subtle gastrointestinal bleeding, which is more likely in geriatric patients and leads to increased protein concentration in the gastrointestinal tract, which results in increased ammonia absorption, which leads to increased urea synthesis in the liver. The reduction in creatinine concentrations is interpreted as a consequence of decreasing muscle mass with age (Hall et al. 2015).

Increased liver enzymes are also observed with increasing age. Reactive hepatitis or degenerative hepatopathies could be the cause. These are causally related to numerous comorbidities of different organ systems, such as cardiovascular, respiratory, endocrine, gastrointestinal and urinary. Disorders can trigger degenerative changes within the hepatocytes via different mechanisms. Possible triggers are hypoxia, increased concentration of ROS and increased inflammatory mediators.

Changes in plasma proteins show decreased albumin concentrations and increased globulin concentrations with age. This could be evaluated as a consequence of subclinical inflammatory processes in old age, especially if albumin is evaluated as a negative-acute phase protein (Ceron et al. 2005).

The increase in degenerative changes in the kidney in cats of advanced age cause laboratory changes based on reduced kidney function. (Miele et al. 2020).

References

Amberg, D., Leadsham, J.E., Kotiadis, V., and Gourlay, C.W. (2012). Cellular ageing and the actin cytoskeleton. *Sub-cellular Biochemistry* 57: 331–352.

Bellows, J., Center, S., Daristotle, L. et al. (2016). Aging in cats: common physical and functional changes. *Journal of Feline Medicine and Surgery* 18 (7): 533–550.

Bernadotte, A., Mikhelson, V.M., and Spivak, I.M. (2016). Markers of cellular senescence. Telomere shortening as a marker of cellular senescence. *Aging* 8 (1): 3–11.

Birch, H.L. (2018). Extracellular matrix and ageing. *Sub-cellular Biochemistry* 90: 169–190.

Boari, A. and Aste, G. (2003). Diagnosis and management of geriatric canine endocrine disorders. *Veterinary Research Communications* 27 (Suppl 1): 543–554.

Brown, C.A., Elliott, J., Schmiedt, C.W., and Brown, S.A. (2016). Chronic kidney disease in aged cats: clinical features, morphology, and proposed pathogeneses. *Veterinary Pathology* 53 (2): 309–326.

Ceron, J.J., Eckersall, P.D., and Martýnez-Subiela, S. (2005). Acute phase proteins in dogs and cats: current knowledge and future perspectives. *Veterinary Clinical Pathology* 34 (2): 85–99.

Chakrabarti, S., Syme, H.M., Brown, C.A., and Elliott, J. (2013). Histomorphometry of feline chronic kidney disease and correlation with markers of renal dysfunction. *Veterinary Pathology* 50 (1): 147–155.

Chistiakov, D.A., Sobenin, I.A., Revin, V.V. et al. (2014). Mitochondrial aging and age-related dysfunction of mitochondria. *BioMed Research International* 2014: 238463.

Choi, S.W., Lee, J.Y., and Kang, K.S. (2017). miRNAs in stem cell aging and age-related disease. *Mechanisms of Ageing and Development* 168: 20–29.

Dankert, D. (1998). Life expectancy and incidence of disease in the old dog. Diss Munich.

Gourlay, C.W. and Ayscough, K.R. (2005). The actin cytoskeleton in ageing and apoptosis. *FEMS Yeast Research* 5 (12): 1193–1198.

Guglielmini, C. (2003). Cardiovascular diseases in the ageing dog: diagnostic and therapeutic problems. *Veterinary Research Communications* 27 (Suppl 1): 555–560.

Haidet, G.C. (1993). Effects of age on beta-adrenergic-mediated reflex responses to induced muscular contraction in beagles. *Mechanisms of Ageing and Development* 68 (1–3): 89–104.

Haidet, G.C., Wennberg, P.W., Finkelstein, S.M., and Morgan, D.J. (1996). Effects of aging per se on arterial stiffness: systemic and regional compliance in beagles. *American Heart Journal* 132 (2 Pt 1): 319–327.

Hall, J.A., Yerramilli, M., Obare, E. et al. (2015). Relationship between lean body mass and serum renal biomarkers in healthy dogs. *Journal of Veterinary Internal Medicine* 29 (3): 808–814.

Kim, M.J. and Park, Y.J. (2019). Bisphenols and thyroid hormone. *Endocrinology and metabolism (Seoul, Korea)* 34 (4): 340–348. https://doi.org/10.3803/EnM.2019.34.4.340.

Landsberg, G.M., Denenberg, S., and Araujo, J.A. (2010). Cognitive dysfunction in cats: a syndrome we used to dismiss as 'old age'. *Journal of Feline Medicine and Surgery* 12 (11): 837–848.

Lawler, D.F., Evans, R.H., Chase, K. et al. (2006). The aging feline kidney: a model mortality antagonist? *Journal of Feline Medicine and Surgery* 8 (6): 363–371.

Marino, C.L., Lascelles, B.D., Vaden, S.L. et al. (2014). Prevalence and classification of chronic kidney disease in cats randomly selected from four age groups and in cats recruited for degenerative joint disease studies. *Journal of Feline Medicine and Surgery* 16 (6): 465–472.

Miele, A., Sordo, L., and Gunn-Moore, D.A. (2020). Feline aging: promoting physiologic and emotional well-being. *The Veterinary Clinics of North America. Small Animal Practice* 50 (4): 719–748.

Radakovich, L.B., Pannone, S.C., Truelove, M.P. et al. (2017). Hematology and biochemistry of aging-evidence of 'anemia of the elderly' in old dogs. *Veterinary Clinical Pathology* 46 (1): 34–45.

Ray, M., Carney, H.C., Boynton, B. et al. (2021). 2021 AAFP feline senior care guidelines. *Journal of Feline Medicine and Surgery* 23 (7): 613–638.

Salzborn, C. (2003). Disease incidence in the dog. Diss Munich.

Templeton, G.H., Platt, M.R., Willerson, J.T., and Weisfeldt, M.L. (1979). Influence of aging on left ventricular hemodynamics and stiffness in beagles. *Circulation Research* 44 (2): 189–194.

Thamer, I.K., Ja'afar, H.A., and Mahood, A.K.S. (2012). Morphological and hormonal studies related to ageing changes of hypothalamo-pituitary gland in rabbits. *Iraqi Journal of Medical Sciences* 10 (2).

Uyar, B., Palmer, D., Kowald, A. et al. (2020). Single-cell analyses of aging, inflammation and senescence. *Ageing Research Reviews* 64: 101156.

Vogt, A.H., Rodan, I., Brown, M. et al. (2010). AAFP-AAHA: feline life stage guidelines. *Journal of Feline Medicine and Surgery* 12 (1): 43–54.

Zhu, Y., Liu, X., Ding, X. et al. (2019). Telomeres and its role in the aging pathways: telomere shortening, cell senescence and mitochondria dysfunction. *Biogerontology* 20 (1): 1–16.

Further Reading

DiLoreto, R. and Murphy, C.T. (2015). The cell biology of ageing. *Molecular Biology of the Cell* 26 (25): 4524–4531.

11

Pain

Definition

Pain is a complex reflex sensory perception. The reflex is triggered by pain receptors, the nociceptors, but processed in the brain and finally perceived. Pain is considered a protective reflex, but can be a disease problem in its own right, especially in a chronic state.

The development of pain in the periphery begins with the stimulation of peripheral nociceptors, 'free' nerve endings or sensory nerve fibres (Figure 11.1).

Triggers of nociceptor stimulation are physical (thermal) and chemical stimuli as well as inflammatory mediators. These generate impulses in the sense of action potentials at the pain receptors. Due to the nociceptor effect of the stimulus, a change in the membrane potential proportional to the stimulus strength occurs. This potential change leads, above a threshold value, to the activation of voltage-dependent ion channels and the development of an action potential.

The impulse reaches the spinal cord via different nerve fibres (Aβ-, Aδ- or C-fibres) and is transmitted there via synaptic connections to neurons, which conduct the impulse to the 'pain centre' in the brain via ascending nerve tracts.

The sensation of pain in inflammatory processes is initiated by mediators such as proinflammatory cytokines (IL-1, IL-6, TNF-α), bradykinin, serotonin, histamine, prostaglandins and leukotrienes.

The release of substance P from the peripheral nerve endings is also important for the maintenance of peripheral sensitisation. In combination with vasoactive substances, such as bradykinin, histamine or serotonin, this can trigger vasodilation with increased vascular permeability and thus maintain regional sensitivity.

The sensation of pain occurs in the brain, involving numerous brain systems. These include the brain stem, the thalamus and areas in the cortex. The sensation of pain can be modified via inhibitory nerves. These are activated by serotonin and noradrenaline and release γ-hydroxybutyric acid (GABA) and glycine as transmitters. The transmitter effect hyperpolarises the neurons, making them less sensitive to nociceptive stimuli. Endogenous opiates also influence the modulation of pain sensation.

The stimulus response to the pain is conducted via descending efferent nerve pathways to the site of stimulus generation (Figure 11.2).

Classification of Pain

Pain can be differentiated according to the type, the place of origin and the duration.

The **type of** pain origin can be physiological, pathological or neuropathic. Physiological nociceptor pain arises from tissue damage in connection with physical or thermal stimuli. Its function corresponds to the protective mechanism that is supposed to emanate from a pain sensation.

Pathological nociceptor pain is triggered as a result of pathological organ changes, such as inflammation. Here, the inflammatory mediators induce the sensation of pain.

If the pain is associated with damage to the peripheral nerves or the central nervous system, it is called 'neuropathic pain'. Possible causes are nerve damage due to operations, injuries of other origin or tumour infiltration.

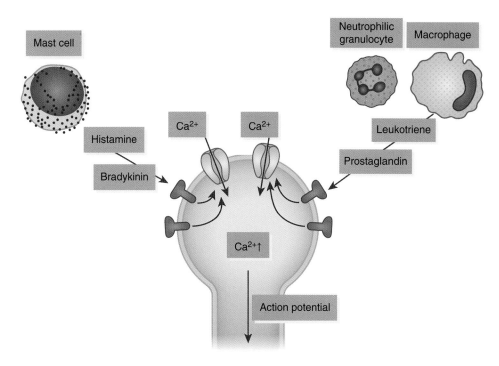

Figure 11.1 Irritation of the nociceptors.

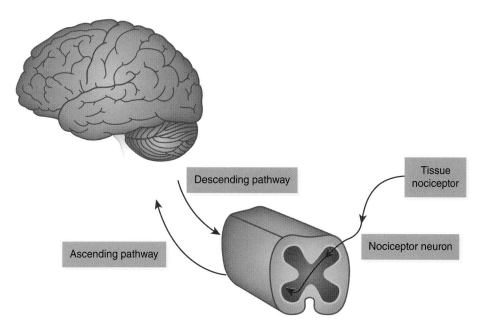

Figure 11.2 Pain reflex arc.

Based on the **site of origin**, pain can be divided into somatic (surface pain and deep pain) and visceral pain. Irritation of nociceptors in the skin triggers somatic surface pain. This is felt as bright. Somatic deep pain is produced in muscles, ligaments, joints and connective tissue and is characterised as dull.

If the pain originates from the internal organs, it is called 'visceral pain'. The sensation can be bright or dull, depending on the organ affected.

Finally, pain can be divided into acute and chronic pain according to **duration**. Acute pain is temporary and lasts as long as the causative disorder exists. Chronic pain is present when the sensation of pain lasts for a period of several months. Chronic pain can develop into an independent clinical picture.

Influence of Pain on the Organism

Physiological pain has a protective function by enabling the animal to respond to damaging environmental influences.

However, pain is also a stressor that induces the organism's adaptation to a stressful situation through neuronal, metabolic, immunological and endocrine processes. This process, in which the organism adapts to the stress-induced situation, was coined by Selye (1946) with the term 'general adaptation syndrome'. However, in the case of severe and persistent pain or poor compensation, the acquired adaptation is lost and distress occurs.

Part of a stress reaction is the activation of the sympathetic nervous system and the increased release of catecholamines from the adrenal medulla. This leads to an increase in respiratory rate, heart rate and blood pressure through vasoconstriction. This in turn results in hypoperfusion of peripheral organs.

Further consequences of the stress reaction are hormonal changes through activation of the hypothalamo-pituitary-adrenergic system. This leads to increased secretion of adrenocorticotrophic hormone (ACTH) and catecholamines and subsequently of cortisol, renin, aldosterone, antidiuretic hormone (ADH) and glucagon. At the same time, insulin secretion decreases.

The consequences are changes in the water and electrolyte balance as well as the mobility of the energy reserves in the sense of a catabolic metabolic state.

Clinically, there is weight loss, reduced wound healing and general fatigue.

Reference

Selye, H. (1946). The general adaptation syndrome and the diseases of adaptation. *The Journal of Clinical Endocrinology & Metabolism* 6: 117–230. https://doi.org/10.1210/jcem-6-2-117.

Further Reading

Armstrong, S.A. and Herr, M.J. (2022). Physiology, nociception [Updated 1 May 2023]. In: *StatPearls* [Internet]. Treasure Island (FL): StatPearls Publishing https://www.ncbi.nlm.nih.gov/books/NBK551562/.

Baral, P., Udit, S., and Chiu, I.M. (2019). Pain and immunity: implications for host defence. *Nature Reviews Immunology* 19 (7): 433–447. https://doi.org/10.1038/s41577-019-0147-2.

Baronio, M., Sadia, H., Paolacci, S. et al. (2020). Molecular aspects of regional pain syndrome. *Pain Research & Management* 2020: 7697214. https://doi.org/10.1155/2020/7697214.

Chen, J.S., Kandle, P.F., Murray, I. et al. (2022). Physiology,pain. In: *StatPearls*. Treasure Island (FL): StatPearls Publishing https://www.ncbi.nlm.nih.gov/books/NBK539789.

Jänig, W. (2014). Neurobiologie viszeraler Schmerzen [Neurobiology of visceral pain]. *Schmerz (Berlin, Germany)* 28 (3): 233–251. https://doi.org/10.1007/s00482-014-1402-x.

Matsuda, M., Huh, Y., and Ji, R.R. (2019). Roles of inflammation, neurogenic inflammation, and neuroinflammation in pain. *Journal of Anesthesia* 33 (1): 131–139. https://doi.org/10.1007/s00540-018-2579-4.

Pinho-Ribeiro, F.A., Verri, W.A. Jr., and Chiu, I.M. (2017). Nociceptor sensory neuron-immune interactions in pain and inflammation. *Trends in Immunology* 38 (1): 5–19. http://dx.doi.org/10.1016/j.it.2016.10.001.

Sneddon, L.U. (2018). Comparative physiology of nociception and pain. *Physiology (Bethesda, Md.)* 33 (1): 63–73. https://doi.org/10.1152/physiol.00022.2017.

12

Hypothalamus Function

Functions

An important neuro-hormonal switch point is the hypothalamus. It is a small brain structure that is assigned to the diencephalon and is located in a region between the optic chiasm, pituitary gland, third cerebral ventricle and thalamus. The tissue itself can be differentiated into a medial and lateral portion with different nuclear areas.

The functions of the hypothalamus can be summarised in the maintenance of the internal milieu, the homeostasis. In detail, the hypothalamus influences different physiological mechanisms (Table 12.1).

The information is sent to the hypothalamus via vegetative afferents, hormones or other mediators. As a result, the hypothalamus can secrete hormones directly or via the pituitary gland (Figure 12.1).

The Control Circuits in Detail

Thermoregulation

Maintaining a certain **body temperature** is an essential prerequisite for homeostasis in the body of warm-blooded animals. Biochemical processes are temperature-dependent and would no longer be able to take place effectively in the event of falling or rising temperatures. These include enzyme functions, fluidity properties at the cell membrane, diffusion processes and osmosis. Oxygen binding to haemoglobin is also temperature-dependent. Furthermore, mechanical functions in the organism, such as the gliding ability of myofibrils or tendons, are also temperature-dependent.

The maintenance of the body temperature in a narrow temperature range is disturbed by numerous processes. In principle, different mechanisms of regulation are available. These are essentially controlled by the activity of the hypothalamus.

The information regarding the peripheral body temperature is perceived via receptors. 'Cold receptors' are activated by opening temperature-dependent ion channels in the cell membrane and thus generating an action potential. One described cold-dependent ion channel is the transient receptor potential cation channel subfamily M (melastatin) member 8 (TRPM8). This is expressed in sensory neurons. At temperatures lower than 26–28°C, the channel opens and ion flow becomes possible (Bautista et al. 2007; Dhaka et al. 2007).

The sensation of warmth is perceived by different receptors. One, the transient receptor potential cation channel subfamily V member 1 (TRPV 1), is additionally counted among the pain receptors. Heat stimulation is made possible by allowing high temperatures (>42°C) to open the channel and thus generate an action potential (Yarmolinsky et al. 2016).

Temperature information from the receptors is transmitted via sensory afferents to the preoptic region in the hypothalamus. There, regulatory mechanisms are initiated to compensate for the temperature deviations. A distinction is made between cooling and heating measures.

Possibilities of heat generation are thermogenesis of brown adipose tissue.

In addition to direct sympathetic activation, this is regulated by the hormone noradrenaline. Noradrenaline acts via G-protein-coupled β-receptors on the fat cells. As a result, adenylate cyclase is activated and cAMP is formed as a second messenger. This activates protein kinase A, which activates lipases via phosphorylation. The fats degraded under the influence of the lipases provide their energy via β-oxidation and the respiratory chain, whereby heat is generated (Morrison et al. 2012).

Table 12.1 Physiological mechanisms influenced by the hypothalamus.

Function	Afferentic system
Thermoregulation	Thermoreceptors peripheral and central
Volume and osmoregulation	Osmoreceptors peripheral and central
Metabolism	Vagus nerve, hormones (ghrelin, insulin, glucagon, leptin)
Stress (fight-or-flight)	Nociceptor
Immune defence	Cytokines

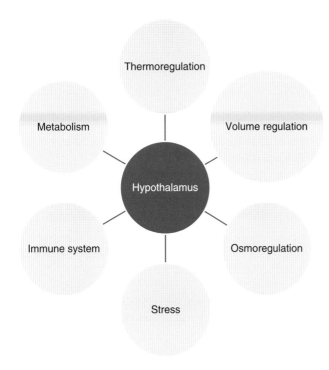

Figure 12.1 Physiological processes regulated by the hypothalamus.

Another temperature-regulating mechanism is skin circulation. Vasodilation and vasoconstriction increase or decrease the release of heat through the skin surface. In the process, heat can be released or conserved. Another form of heat dissipation via the skin takes place through sweating. The small domestic animals compensate for the lack of sweat glands by the 'dead space respiration' of panting.

'Sweating' utilises the heat release that occurs when water is transformed into water vapour. The water originates from eccrine sweat glands that are distributed over the body. In dogs and cats, sweat glands are located in the area of the paws.

When 'panting', water evaporates on the surfaces of the mucous membranes of the respiratory system and the oral cavity, including the tongue, and heat is dissipated from the body.

Finally, the organism has a mechanism at its disposal through which heat can be generated by 'shivering'. Here, the production of heat that arises in connection with repeated muscle contractions is used to compensate for heat losses in the organism (Figure 12.2).

Volume and Osmoregulation

The 'thirst centre' is located in the hypothalamus. Information about the water balance reaches the hypothalamus after peripheral osmoreceptors have registered the osmolality of the blood plasma. These are localised in various places in the organism, such as the juxtaglomerular apparatus of the kidney, the hypothalamus, the digestive tract or the portal vein. The receptors generate impulses through action potentials that develop through ionic flows. The latter depend on the opening and closing of ion channels. In the context of osmolality detection, the trigger is a 'cell shrinkage' in a hypertonic environment or a 'cell swelling' in a hypotonic environment. Both lead to the generation of impulses that are delivered to the hypothalamus via afferent nerve pathways.

The hypothalamic response to changes in osmolality is essentially based on the release of antidiuretic hormone (ADH). ADH is a peptide hormone that is produced by the hypothalamus and released via the posterior pituitary lobe after activation of the prohormone by proteolytic cleavage of the active hormone. ADH is transported via the blood to the kidneys. There, it causes increased expression of aquaporin proteins in the cells of the collecting ducts. The cells of the collecting ducts are only partially open to water penetration. ADH causes the formation of aquaporins via a membrane receptor and cAMP as second messenger. These are incorporated into the cell membrane as water-permeable tubules and thus enable water and urea reabsorption in the collecting tube. The increased reabsorption of urea can increase the osmotic gradient in the renal parenchyma, which also leads to increased water reabsorption in Henle's loop (Larsen et al. 2014).

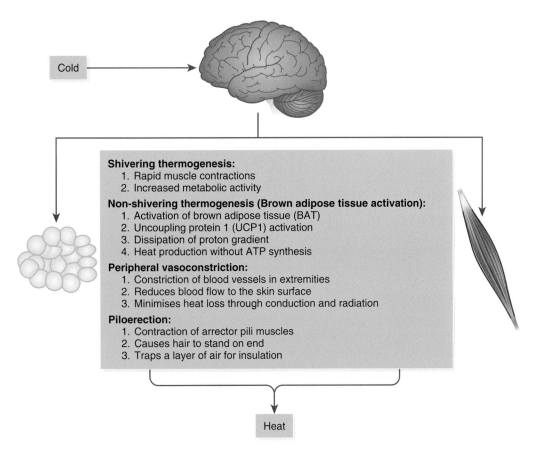

Cold

Shivering thermogenesis:
  1. Rapid muscle contractions
  2. Increased metabolic activity
Non-shivering thermogenesis (Brown adipose tissue activation):
  1. Activation of brown adipose tissue (BAT)
  2. Uncoupling protein 1 (UCP1) activation
  3. Dissipation of proton gradient
  4. Heat production without ATP synthesis
Peripheral vasoconstriction:
  1. Constriction of blood vessels in extremities
  2. Reduces blood flow to the skin surface
  3. Minimises heat loss through conduction and radiation
Piloerection:
  1. Contraction of arrector pili muscles
  2. Causes hair to stand on end
  3. Traps a layer of air for insulation

Heat

Figure 12.2 Regulation of body temperature.

Metabolism

The influence of the hypothalamus on metabolism results essentially from its regulation of food intake. For this purpose, a 'hunger and satiety centre' is located in the hypothalamus. Impulses for the regulation of food intake are transmitted to the hypothalamus via afferent nerve pathways from peripheral chemoreceptors of the intestine or the liver. A further flow of information exists through hormones or metabolites that act on the hypothalamus. These include insulin, cholecystokinin, leptin or glucose.

Stress and the Immune System

The importance of the hypothalamus in the stress response and the control of the immune response is closely linked and will therefore be presented together.

Stress is, by definition, a mental and physical reaction of the body caused by specific external stimuli. The hypothalamus is involved in the reaction to different stress stimuli (stressors). These can arise neurogenically, such as anxiety. This is an unsettling of the emotional life due to internal or external triggers. Physiological stress is the result of disturbances of the internal milieu, e.g. disturbances of the water balance or hypoxia. Inflammation mediates stress through the release of cytokines.

Hypothalamic reaction to the stressor effect is, among other things, the formation of adrenocorticotrophic hormone (ACTH), prolactin or sympathetic stimulation. The consequences are adjustments in metabolism, blood pressure and the immune system. Specifically, stress affects the pituitary gland via the hypothalamus and the release of corticotropin-releasing hormone (CRH). ACTH is formed there, which peripherally induces the formation of glucocorticoids in the adrenal cortex. This results in protein and fat breakdown and increased gluconeogenesis. The aim is to provide energy. Through the formation of aldosterone, electrolyte and water reabsorption in the kidneys is promoted, thereby increasing blood pressure. Sympathetic response reduces digestive activity and increases heart rate. Stress produces immunosuppression. This comes into play especially in the case of chronic stress. Described mechanisms are based on a disturbance of the balance between

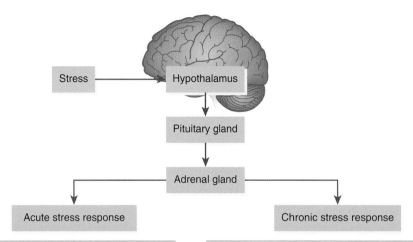

Figure 12.3 Control of stress.

Th-1 and Th-2 cells. Corticoids can weaken Th-1 cells, which secrete mainly IL-2, IL-12 and IFN-γ and thus stimulate the cellular immune response. Th-2 cells, on the other hand, secrete mainly IL-4, IL-6 and IL-10 and thus stimulate humoral immune responses (Soto-Tinoco et al. 2016) (Figure 12.3).

References

Bautista, D.M., Siemens, J., Glazer, J.M. et al. (2007). The menthol receptor TRPM8 is the principal detector of environmental cold. *Nature* 448 (7150): 204–208. https://doi.org/10.1038/nature05910.

Dhaka, A., Murray, A.N., Mathur, J. et al. (2007). TRPM8 is required for cold sensation in mice. *Neuron* 54 (3): 371–378. https://doi.org/10.1016/j.neuron.2007.02.024.

Larsen, E.H., Deaton, L.E., Onken, H. et al. (2014). Osmoregulation and excretion. *Comprehensive Physiology* 4 (2): 405–573. https://doi.org/10.1002/cphy.c130004.

Morrison, S.F., Madden, C.J., and Tupone, D. (2012). Central control of brown adipose tissue thermogenesis. *Frontiers in Endocrinology* 3 (5): 5. https://doi.org/10.3389/fendo.2012.00005.

Soto-Tinoco, E., Guerrero-Vargas, N.N., and Buijs, R.M. (2016). Interaction between the hypothalamus and the immune system. *Experimental Physiology* 101 (12): 1463–1471. https://doi.org/10.1113/EP085560.

Yarmolinsky, D.A., Peng, Y., Pogorzala, L.A. et al. (2016). Coding and plasticity in the mammalian thermosensory system. *Neuron* 92 (5): 1079–1092. https://doi.org/10.1016/j.neuron.2016.10.021.

Further Reading

Nakamura, K. (2011). Central circuits for body temperature regulation and fever. *American Journal of Physiology. Regulatory, Integrative and Comparative Physiology* 301 (5): R1207–R1228. https://doi.org/10.1152/ajpregu.00109.2011.

Tan, C.L. and Knight, Z.A. (2018). Regulation of body temperature by the nervous system. *Neuron* 98 (1): 31–48. https://doi.org/10.1016/j.neuron.2018.02.022.

Part II

General Clinical Manifestations (Alphabetical)

13

Abdominal Enlargement

Definition

An enlargement of the abdomen is a visible increase in volume of the abdominal cavity. This is most definitely seen in lean dogs.

Aetiology

Enlargement of the abdomen results either from enlargement of one or more organ parenchyma or from the accumulation of fluid or gas in the abdomen or abdominal organs. The differential diagnoses are listed below:

Effusions	Organ enlargement	Reduced muscle tone
Blood	Liver	Cushing's disease
Urine	Stomach	
Bile	Spleen	
Transudate	Uterus	
Modified transudate	Urinary bladder	
Exudate		

The effusions are dealt with in Chapter 21.

Organ Enlargement

Pathogenesis

Enlargement of abdominal organs can be acute or chronic and affect one or more organs. Not every organ enlargement is externally recognisable.

Acute enlargement is usually accompanied by gas accumulation, as increases in parenchyma are usually chronic. Gas accumulation is possible in the **stomach** or intestinal area. Externally recognisable is gastric torsion or gastric dilatation. Dilatation of the **intestine** in the form of paralytic ileus is not externally visible. Another acute abdominal organ enlargement can be a congested **urinary bladder**. This enlargement is also not visible externally.

Chronic organ enlargements are mostly caused by an increase in parenchyma. In the **liver**, generalised organ enlargements can be the result of an accumulation of fat, as in hepatic lipidosis, primarily in cats. Other diffuse liver diseases, such as accumulation of glycogen or cells of a round cell tumour (lymphoma) lead to generalised enlargement. Focal changes in the liver associated with organ enlargement are more commonly tumour diseases. Epithelial and mesenchymal tumours

Textbook of Small Animal Pathophysiology, First Edition. Stephan Neumann.
© 2025 John Wiley & Sons Ltd. Published 2025 by John Wiley & Sons Ltd.

Table 13.1 Abdominal organ enlargements.

	Acute	Chronic
Stomach	x	
Intestine	x	
Liver		x
Spleen		x
Kidneys		x
Urinary bladder	x	
Uterus		x
Fat accumulation		x
Acromegaly		x

lead to focal enlargement of the liver. Liver parenchymal enlargements may be visible externally. This is especially true if the extent is advanced or the animal is in a reduced nutritional state.

Enlargements of the **spleen** occur diffusely or focally. Diffuse enlargements can be splenic congestions; these also develop acutely. Infiltrative diseases of the spleen also lead to diffuse enlargement of the organ. Splenic tumours, predominantly haemangiosarcomas, enlarge the spleen focally. Splenic enlargements are also rarely externally recognisable.

Enlargement of the **kidneys** that is not externally visible can be seen in infiltrative diseases, such as lymphoma.

Finally, chronic organ enlargement is possible with uterine inflammation. The accumulation of purulent secretions or mucus can lead to a considerable enlargement of the uterus. However, the enlargement is not visible externally. Enlargement of the uterus due to pregnancy would be a physiological chronic enlargement of the organ, which may also be visible externally.

Generalised organ enlargement is possible in growth hormone excess (see Chapter 43.2.1).

Abdominal enlargement can also be the result of diffuse abdominal fat accumulation. In dogs, in particular, depot fat tends to be deposited abdominally rather than subcutaneously. Abdominal fat deposits are more common around the umbilical, in the mesentery or perirenally (Table 13.1).

Pathophysiologic Consequences

Influenced organs	Clinical symptoms	Clinical pathological alterations
Abdominal cavity	Pain	Acidosis
	Ischaemia	

Depending on the cause and extent of the enlargement, the pain can be a pathophysiological consequence of the enlargement of the abdominal organs. Pain receptors are localised both visceral and parietal. Organ enlargements associated with significant pain are the acute enlargements associated with gastric torsion and dilatation, intestinal dilatation and urinary bladder obstruction. Here, the visceral nociceptors are essentially irritated (Struller et al. 2017).

A further consequence may result from vascular compression due to organomegaly. This has been described as vascular compression syndrome in various localisations. The result can be ischaemic consequences of various organs. In gastric torsion, for example, the dilated stomach presses against the diaphragm. The consequence is reduced inspiration and, as a result, reduced expansion of the alveoli. This results in generalised hypoxia. This affects various internal organs, such as the liver, kidneys or spleen. At the same time, the enlarged stomach reduces venous return to the heart by compressing the caudal vena cava. This reduces cardiac output and also leads to generalised hypoxia.

Hypoxia causes an energy deficiency at the cellular level. This is due to reduced intracellular ATP synthesis as a result of the switch to anaerobic glycolysis. A lack of ATP affects, among other things, the ATP-dependent Na^+/K^+ pump, with the consequence of a reduced sodium efflux. This causes water accumulation in the cell, as well as disturbances of the membrane balance. This opens calcium channels and leads to increased calcium influx.

The consequences of an increased cellular calcium concentration are multiple. These include increased formation of reactive oxygen species (ROS). This results in mitochondrial membrane damage and organ dysfunction.

Other consequences of increased cellular calcium concentrations include increases in destructive enzyme activities. All of these lead to progressive cellular dysfunction.

Another consequence of restricted breathing during abdominal enlargement is reduced carbon expiration. This leads to an increase in CO_2 blood concentration and, thus, respiratory acidosis.

The clinical consequences of acidosis depend on the degree and duration. Overall, the cardiovascular and respiratory systems as well as metabolism, are most frequently affected. Through its overall depressive effects on cardiac activity, acidosis leads to a reduction in cardiac contractility and a reduction in cardiac output. At the same time, peripheral resistance decreases due to arterial vasodilation. This in turn reduces the blood flow to peripheral organs, such as the liver and kidneys and can cause organ insufficiencies there. The effect is intensified by a reduced responsiveness of the cardiovascular system to catecholamines. A major triggering factor is hyperkalaemia, which occurs in acidosis due to a dislocation of potassium ions from the cell. At the same time, acidosis impairs cellular energy production and thus ATP synthesis. The reduced energy production is caused by insulin resistance in acidosis, which leads to a reduced influx of glucose into the cells. Chronic acidosis also has a catabolic effect by increasing protein breakdown and demineralising bone.

Reduced Muscle Tone

Pathogenesis

A special form of abdominal enlargement is possible as a result of the reduction of abdominal muscle tension. The reduction of abdominal muscle tension reduces the resistance to the abdominal organs, which leads secondarily to a relative enlargement of the abdomen. Cushing's disease often shows abdominal enlargement, the genesis of which is a consequence of steroid hepatitis with liver enlargement and reduction of abdominal muscle tone. The latter is caused by increased muscle catabolism in Cushing's disease.

Reference

Struller, F., Weinreich, F.J., Horvath, P. et al. (2017). Peritoneal innervation: embryology and functional anatomy. *Pleura and Peritoneum* 2 (4): 153–161. https://doi.org/10.1515/pp-2017-0024.

Further Reading

Zahid, M., Nepal, P., Nagar, A., and Ojili, V. (2020). Abdominal vascular compression syndromes encountered in the emergency department: cross-sectional imaging spectrum and clinical implications. *Emergency Radiology* 27 (5): 513–526. https://doi.org/10.1007/s10140-020-01778-1.

14

Ataxia

Definition

Ataxia is defined as a lack of coordination in the movement of the limbs, head and trunk.

Physiology of Movement Coordination

The coordination of locomotion takes place hierarchically in the spinal cord segments via spinal reflex arcs and in the brain. In the brain, the vestibular apparatus and the cerebellum are particularly involved in the coordination of movement.

At the spinal cord segment level, spinal reflexes play a role in movement coordination. They are triggered by the activation of reflex arcs consisting of sensory neurons, interneurons and motor neurons. These reflexes enable the body to react quickly to external stimuli without the brain being directly involved. Receptors for the reflex arcs are for example:

Muscle spindles: These are specialised muscle fibres surrounded by a connective tissue capsule and arranged parallel to the working muscles. They can measure the muscle length and its stretching speed.

Tendon organs: These are strain sensors that measure the tension state of the muscles. They are located at the transition from muscle tendon to muscle.

Afferent nerve pathways originate from these sensors and transport the impulses to the spinal cord. There the impulses enter the spinal cord via the dorsal horn and connect via a synapse with an efferent nerve, which leaves the spinal cord via the ventral horn and transmits the impulse to the skeletal muscles (Figure 14.1).

In addition to this simple organisation of statics and movement, the cerebellum and the vestibular apparatus are particularly involved in locomotion as central brain components. Impulses reach the central brain structures via ascending nerve tracts from the spinal cord and from higher centres of the brain. The latter act as impulse generators for locomotion.

The cerebellum is a structure in the back of the brain and consists of two hemispheres. It contains multiple grooves and folds. The surface of the cerebellum is covered by a thin layer of grey matter known as the 'cerebellar cortex'. Below the cerebellar cortex is a layer of white matter called the 'cerebellar centre'. The centre contains axons that transmit signals to and from other parts of the brain. The importance of the cerebellum in relation to locomotion is in the coordination of movement, not in its initiation. The cerebellum receives sensory impulses from ascending neural pathways, from the vestibular apparatus and the cortex.

The vestibular apparatus is another central nervous structure involved in movement coordination. It consists of three arcades and the otolith organs. The arcades are filled with a sodium-rich fluid (endolymph) and detect head movements in different directions. The otolith organs consist of the utriculus and sacculus, which are able to sense linear acceleration and changes in gravity.

The sensory cells of the vestibular apparatus are located in maculae, in the utriculus and sacculus, and in cristae at the base of the arcades. The sensory cells are equipped with hair cells that are vibrated by the movement of the fluid or otoliths. The hair cells send signals to the brain via the vestibular nerve. Information from the vestibular apparatus is sent to the brainstem, cerebellum, spinal cord and cerebrum. In the brainstem, the vestibular nuclei are located near the vomiting centre. This explains nausea or vomiting in disorders of the vestibular apparatus.

Textbook of Small Animal Pathophysiology, First Edition. Stephan Neumann.
© 2025 John Wiley & Sons Ltd. Published 2025 by John Wiley & Sons Ltd.

Figure 14.1 Simple reflex arc.

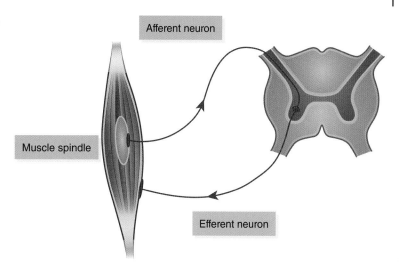

Afferent neuron

Muscle spindle

Efferent neuron

Aetiology

Ataxia can be the result of direct disturbances of the control structures for locomotion. In addition, indirect metabolic causalities can lead to ataxia. While the former disorders are described in dogs and cats, hypoglycaemia and hypocalcaemia as metabolic disorders are more common in dogs. Hypoglycaemia is often a consequence of insulinoma or Addison's disease, both of which are rare in cats. Hypocalcaemia is described as eclampsia in the bitch after birth; this clinical picture is also less common in the cat.

Neurological	Metabolic
Sensory (D/C)	Hypoglycaemia (D)
Cerebellar (D/C)	Hypokalaemia (D/C)
Vestibular (D/C)	Hypocalcaemia (D)

D – Dog, C – Cat

Pathogenesis

Diseases of different genesis can lead to clinical pictures of sensory, cerebellar and vestibular ataxia. Metabolic ataxias are to be distinguished from these.

Sensory ataxias result from proprioception deficits and lead to reduced correction of the limb after reflex activation. They are mostly ataxias that develop as a result of upper motor neuron dysfunction. In these disorders, ascending afferent pathways in the spinal cord are impeded from transmitting the impulse to the brain. The cause can be diseases that have a compressive effect on the nervous system in the spinal cord or restrict its blood supply. These include discopathies or extra- and intramedullary tumours, as well as spinal cord ischaemias of various origins.

Cerebellar ataxias are coordination weaknesses usually associated with hypermetria and intention tremor. Their genesis is based on diseases of the cerebellum. In cerebellar abiotrophy, there is a hereditary premature death of cerebellar nerve fibres, mostly Purkinje fibres in the cerebellar cortex. Breed predispositions have been described for West Highland White Terriers, Kerry Blue Terriers and others. Cerebellar hypoplasia develops more frequently after intrauterine infections with panleukopenia virus in cats and herpes virus in dogs. Other causes include inflammation or neoplasia involving the cerebellum.

Vestibular ataxia shows head tilt, nystagmus and possibly strabismus in addition to coordination disorders. Peripheral vestibular syndrome is differentiated from central vestibular syndrome. Peripheral vestibular syndrome is caused by diseases in the area of the middle ear. These are polyps or inflammations with empyema formation in the bulla. Central vestibular syndrome develops from diseases in the area of the brain stem. Accordingly, those affected also show disturbances in proprioception, as well as depressive behaviour. Nystagmus tends to be horizontal in peripheral vestibular syndrome and vertical in central vestibular syndrome.

Causes of vestibular syndrome are listed in Table 14.1. Conditions associated with vestibular syndrome are:

Table 14.1 Causes of vestibular diseases.

Peripheral vestibular	Central vestibular
Anomalies	Neoplasia (e.g. glioma)
Hypothyroidism	Thiamine deficiency
Neoplasia (Neurofibroma Cranial nerves; Osteosarcoma Petrous temporal bone)	Viral infection (distemper, feline infectious peritonitis, rabies)
Otitis media	Protozoal infection (Toxoplasma, Neospora)
Trauma	Mycotic infection (*Cryptococcus neoformans*, Histoplasmosis, Blastomycosis)
Toxins (e.g. aminoglycosides)	Trauma
Idiopathic	Toxins (e.g. Metronidazole)

Metabolically induced ataxias are primarily due to disturbances of the energy balance caused by hypoglycaemia or disturbances of the electrolytes.

The influence of **hypoglycaemia** on the nervous system and thus on movement results essentially from the dependence of the nervous system on continuous glucose supply. Due to its active metabolism, the brain utilises up to 25% of the free glucose in the organism. The glucose is taken up by the astrocytes from the capillaries via insulin-dependent and -independent transporters. In the case of hypoglycaemia, there is a reduced supply of glucose to the nervous system. The lack of glucose is accompanied by an excess of excitatory amino acids (e.g. glutamate, aspartate). The reason for this is a lower concentration of acetate in cases of hypoglycaemia. As a result, oxaloacetate is not passed on to the citric acid cycle, but serves the increased synthesis of aspartate and glutamate. Glutamate, in turn, is an important excitatory neurotransmitter. This acts at the postsynaptic membrane. There, glutamate binds to glutamate receptors. Ionotropic and metabotropic receptor types have been described. The ionotropic receptors are ion channels that open after transmitter binding and allow sodium and calcium influx. Metabotropic receptors are G-protein coupled and act indirectly on ion channels via a second messenger. The increased glutamate concentration during hypoglycaemia leads to increased activity of excitatory nerves via the mechanisms described.

Increased excitatory activity in the brain can lead to different effects depending on which regions are affected and how strong the activity is. Possible consequences can be seizures, hyperactivity or movement disorders (Figure 14.2).

The influence of potassium on nerve function is based on the fact that potassium is responsible for the resting potential at the nerve cell membrane. Changes thus lead to disturbed excitation. More often than hyperkalaemia, hypokalaemia is associated with neurological dysfunctions and ataxia.

Hypokalaemia can have a significant influence on the nerve cell membrane, as potassium plays a critical role in the maintenance of the resting potential of nerve cells. The resting potential is the state of the neuron when it is not transmitting any signals. Potassium ions, which have a high concentration inside the cell, move out of the cell to maintain the negative resting potential. When the concentration of extracellular potassium drops, the movement of potassium out of the cell changes, which can result in depolarisation of the nerve cell membrane. This depolarisation can lead to a reduction in nerve cell excitability and decreased nerve conduction velocity.

Hypocalcaemia produces a similar effect. This can also lead to ataxia. Hypocalcaemia can have a significant effect on the nerve cell membrane as calcium plays a critical role in the transmission of nerve impulses. Calcium ions are involved in the release of neurotransmitters, which are the chemicals that allow communication between nerve cells. When the concentration of extracellular calcium drops, the ability of the nerve cell to release neurotransmitters can be impaired, leading to a reduction in nerve impulse transmission. Additionally, calcium is important for the maintenance of the resting potential of nerve cells. Hypocalcaemia facilitates sodium transport, as the normal inhibition by Ca^{2+} of sodium movement through voltage-gated sodium channels is lost. Thus, low Ca^{2+} levels result in hyperexcitability of the neurons.

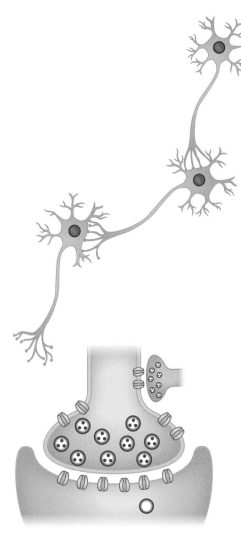

Synthesis of Excitatory Amino Acids:

1. **Glutamate Synthesis:** Glutamate is the primary excitatory neurotransmitter in the central nervous system. It is synthesised from the amino acid glutamine through a reaction catalysed by the enzyme glutaminase.

2. **Aspartate Synthesis:** Aspartate is another excitatory amino acid that is synthesised from oxaloacetate, an intermediate in the citric acid cycle.

3. **Transport and Release:** Excitatory amino acids like glutamate and aspartate are released from presynaptic nerve terminals into the synaptic cleft upon neuronal stimulation.

Consequences of Increased Excitatory Amino Acids:

1. **Excitotoxicity:** Excessive release of glutamate and other excitatory amino acids can lead to excitotoxicity, a process in which overactivation of excitatory receptors results incell damage and death.

2. **Neuronal Hyperexcitability:** Increased excitatory amino acids can lead to neuronal hyperexcitability.

3. **Calcium Influx:** Overstimulation of excitatory receptors leads to excessive calcium influx into neurons. Elevated intracellular calcium levels trigger various detrimental processes, including mitochondrial dysfunction, activation of enzymes that degrade cell structures, and initiation of apoptosis.

Figure 14.2 Synthesis and consequence of increased excitatory amino acids.

Further Reading

Akbar, U. and Ashizawa, T. (2015). Ataxia. *Neurologic Clinics* 33 (1): 225–248. https://doi.org/10.1016/j.ncl.2014.09.004.

Kornegay, J.N. (1991). Ataxia, head tilt, nystagmus. Vestibular diseases. *Problems in Veterinary Medicine* 3 (3): 417–425.

Kuo, S.H. (2019). Ataxia. *Continuum (Minneapolis, Minn.)* 25 (4): 1036–1054. https://doi.org/10.1212/CON.0000000000000753.

Marsden, J.F. (2018). Cerebellar ataxia. *Handbook of Clinical Neurology* 159: 261–281. https://doi.org/10.1016/B978-0-444-63916-5.00017-3.

Rossmeisl, J.H. Jr. (2010). Vestibular disease in dogs and cats. *The Veterinary Clinics of North America. Small Animal Practice* 40 (1): 81–100. https://doi.org/10.1016/j.cvsm.2009.09.007.

Thomas, W.B. (2000). Vestibular dysfunction. *The Veterinary Clinics of North America. Small Animal Practice* 30 (1): 227. -viii. https://doi.org/10.1016/s0195-5616(00)50011-4.

15

Constipation

Definition

Constipation is an acute or chronic disorder of defaecation.

Physiological Basics

Peristalsis is the coordinated, rhythmic contraction of the muscles in the gastrointestinal tract that moves food through the digestive system. The process of peristalsis is controlled by both hormones and the nervous system. Hormones, such as gastrin and secretin, are released in response to food entering the stomach and small intestine, respectively. These hormones stimulate the release of digestive enzymes and the contraction of smooth muscles in the gut, which contributes to the process of peristalsis.

The nervous system also plays a crucial role in controlling peristalsis. The enteric nervous system is a complex network of neurons that is present in the gut. The enteric nervous system can operate independently of the central nervous system and is responsible for regulating the contraction and relaxation of the smooth muscles in the gastrointestinal tract. The enteric nervous system receives input from sensory nerves in the gut that detect the presence of food and stretch receptors in the walls of the gastrointestinal tract. This information is integrated and processed by the enteric nervous system, which then initiates the appropriate contractions of the smooth muscles in the gut to move food along the digestive tract. The central nervous system can also influence peristalsis through the sympathetic and parasympathetic nervous systems. The sympathetic nervous system, which is activated during times of stress, can inhibit peristalsis, while the parasympathetic nervous system, which is activated during rest and digestion, can stimulate peristalsis.

Aetiology

The possible causes of constipation can be distinguished into dietary causes, mechanical disorders of ingesta passage, as well as functional disorders of ingesta passage and hormonal causes. All these causes have in common that the food is not or only slowly transported. The result is usually an increase in the viscosity of the food, which aggravates the process.

Mechanical obstruction	Neuromuscular diseases	Endocrine diseases
Neoplasia (D,C)	Polyneuropathy (D,C)	Hypothyroidism (D)
Perirectal diseases (D)		Hyperparathyroidism (D)
Enlarged prostate (D)		

D – Dog, C – Cat

Textbook of Small Animal Pathophysiology, First Edition. Stephan Neumann.
© 2025 John Wiley & Sons Ltd. Published 2025 by John Wiley & Sons Ltd.

Pathogenesis

The most common causes of constipation in dogs and cats are obstructions of the intestinal tract, which can occur in the small or large intestine. More frequently, obstructions are localised in the small intestine due to mechanical disturbances such as foreign bodies or tumours. Therefore, the pathogenesis of small intestinal obstruction will be presented.

The obstruction can be partial or complete. In both cases, due to the obstruction, dilatation of the intestine develops with the sequestration of water and electrolytes. Absorption is reduced in this area and stasis develops in venous vessels due to the dilatation. By increasing permeability, secretion of water into the intestinal lumen develops. At the same time, chloride secretion into the intestinal lumen increases, resulting in metabolic alkalosis due to loss of chloride ions.

At the site of obstruction, the intestinal mucosa is compressed, which leads to ischaemia. The consequence is a reduced supply of oxygen to the intestinal wall cells, which leads to a low synthesis of ATP. The cellular consequences are hierarchical:

1) cellular acidosis;
2) loss of sarcoplasmic membrane potential;
3) cellular swelling;
4) cytoskeleton disorganisation;
5) reduction of adenosine-5′-triphosphate (ATP);
6) reduction of glutathione, of α-tocopherol;
7) increasing expression of leukocyte adhesion molecules;
8) secretion of cytokines/chemokines
   - Tumour Necrosis Factor (TNF-α)
   - Interleukins (IL-) -1, 6, 8

In addition to the mechanical causes of constipation, the functional causes also essentially affect the function of intestinal peristalsis. Electrolyte disorders, such as hypercalcaemia, lead to impaired permeability at the cell membrane of intestinal nerve cells. The result can be reduced excitability, which can lead to reduced peristalsis. Due to permanent water removal from the ingesta, its viscosity increases with a slowed transport time. Thickened ingesta eventually acts as a mechanical obstruction with the consequences described above (Figure 15.1).

Endocrine diseases, such as hypothyroidism, also cause a reduction in peristalsis and thus a prolongation of transit time via nervous and myogenic effects. A slowing of the transit time has been observed in patients with hypothyroidism (Shafer et al. 1984).

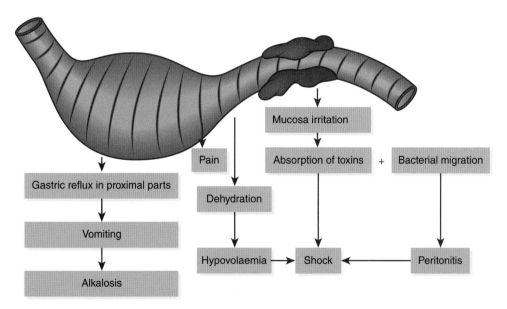

Figure 15.1 Pathological consequences at the obstruction site.

Pathophysiologic Consequences

Influenced organs	Clinical symptoms	Clinical pathological alterations
Gastrointestinal system	Dehydration	PCV increased
	Shock	Total protein increased
	Diarrhoea	
	Haematochezia (Melena)	
	Peritonitis	

The consequences of the obstruction result, on the one hand, from the shifts of water and electrolytes in the prestenotic region. **Dehydration** occurs due to the reduced water reabsorption and increased secretion. This can be seen clinically in signs, such as reduced mucosal moisture, reduced skin turgor and reduced urine volume. Haematologically, haematocrit and total protein increase. This can affect blood flow velocities and lead to hyperviscosity. In chronic cases, the consequences of hyperviscosity can be heart failure due to increased cardiac work, as well as increased peripheral pressure. In acute cases, the slowed flow velocity can be accompanied by stasis and activate the coagulation system, which can lead to thrombosis and emboli. In addition, reduced blood flow in the renal glomeruli is a possible trigger for reduced glomerular filtration, and in the brain, it is a trigger for central nervous symptoms such as headaches.

Dehydration can also develop into hypovolaemia with **shock**. This is further triggered in intestinal obstruction, where vasoactive bacterial toxins can pass through the intestinal wall due to intestinal wall ischaemia.

The measurement of **PCV** and **total protein** allows various interpretations. Besides dehydration, in which both parameters are elevated in the serum, other disease mechanisms can be interpreted. Table 15.1 summarises the differential diagnoses of both parameters:

Other consequences of constipation can trigger **diarrhoea** or **haematochezia**. The former is more common with partial obstruction. In these cases, water and electrolytes sequestered in the intestinal lumen can pass through the obstruction and affect faecal consistency. *Haematochezia* is, by definition, the detection of fresh blood in the faeces. This is more commonly associated with bleeding in distal segments of the bowel. Bleeding in the proximal sections usually results in black-coloured faeces, or **melena**. The bleeding is caused by increased permeability of the intestinal blood vessels in the obstructed region. Due to the dilatation of the intestinal wall, vascular ruptures can also lead to haemorrhage.

The black colour of the faeces in haemorrhages in the proximal small intestine is caused by the synthesis of haematin from haemoglobin by the bacterial intestinal flora. This results in an oxidation of Fe^{2+} to Fe^{3+}. The process of melena formation depends on the duration of the blood passage in the intestinal tract. A minimum time of eight hours is necessary for sufficient oxidation.

In the case of intestinal rupture during constipation, peritonitis develops. The translocation of bacteria into the peritoneal cavity causes a reaction of mesothelial cells and sessile mast cells and macrophages. Mesothelial cells belong to the mesothelium, a squamous epithelium of serous membranes. Mesothelial cells are connected by tight-junctions and thus

Table 15.1 Interpretation of altered PCV and total protein.

PCV	TP	Interpretation
↑	↑	Dehydration
↑	N or ↓	Spleen contraction; polycythaemia; dehydration + hypoproteinaemia
N	↑	Hyperglobulinaemia; anaemia + dehydration
N	N	Normal; dehydration + anaemia + hypoproteinaemia, acute haemorrhage
↓	N	Anaemia (non blood loss) + normal hydration
↓	↑	Anaemia + dehydration; anaemia + hyperproteinaemia
↓	↓	Blood loss; anaemia + hyperproteinaemia; overhydration

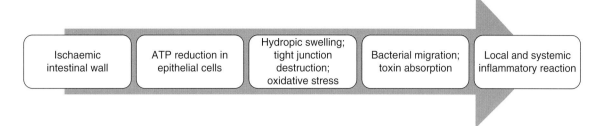

Figure 15.2 Consequences of constipation.

form an epithelial barrier. Substance transport is possible transcellularly or paracellularly. In addition to substance transport and barrier function, the mesothelial cells are capable of phagocytosis and antigen presentation. After bacterial contact, proinflammatory cytokines are released from the sessile defence cells of the peritoneal cavity. These attract polymorphonuclear neutrophilic granulocytes. Due to the release of vasoactive substances, such as histamine, bradykinin or prostaglandins and leukotrienes, vascular dilatation develops with an increase in vascular permeability and exudation into the abdominal cavity. Peritonitis can lead to sepsis, septic shock and multi-organ failure due to translocation of the bacteria into the systemic vascular system (Figure 15.2).

Reference

Shafer, R.B., Prentiss, R.A., and Bond, J.H. (1984). Gastrointestinal transit in thyroid disease. *Gastroenterology* 86 (5 Pt 1): 852–855.

Further Reading

Delibegovic, S. (2007). Pathophysiological changes in peritonitis. *Medicinski arhiv* 61 (2): 109–113.
Dimski, D.S. (1989). Constipation: pathophysiology, diagnostic approach, and treatment. *Seminars in Veterinary Medicine and Surgery (Small Animal)* 4 (3): 247–254.
Whitehead, K., Cortes, Y., and Eirmann, L. (2016). Gastrointestinal dysmotility disorders in critically ill dogs and cats. *Journal of Veterinary Emergency and Critical Care (San Antonio, Tex.: 2001)* 26 (2): 234–253. https://doi.org/10.1111/vec.12449.

16

Cough

Definition

Cough is a sudden expiratory movement caused by the respiratory muscles and is a reaction to irritation of the airways.

Physiological Basics

The cough reflex is one of the respiratory defence mechanisms to protect the airways and alveoli from foreign material including infectious agents and noxious gases. It belongs to the non-specific defence mechanisms which, together with the innate and adaptive immune system, protect the organism against aerogenic disease triggers. The cough reflex acts as a complement to the mucociliary clearance, which removes the smallest particles in the air we breathe ($<5\,\mu m$). The mechanism is based on the binding of the particles to a mucus phase located on the surface of the bronchial mucosa. The mucus is synthesised by cells of the bronchial epithelium (Goblet cells) and consists of a slightly viscous and a highly viscous phase. The light viscous phase is the lower-lying phase on the epithelial cells; it makes up about 95% of the mucus. The low viscosity is achieved by the excretion of water in a chloride symport, which is released from the epithelial cells by a sodium antiport. The upper highly viscous phase traps particles from the respiratory air. These bind to the mucus. The mucus also contains defence substances, such as defensins, lysozyme or immunoglobulin A. Cilia of the epithelial cells move with a slow aboral movement in the low-viscosity mucus layer and can thus transport the viscous mucus with the particles towards the larynx. A fast counter-rotating ciliary movement enables the continuous transport of mucus. In the pharynx, the mucus is swallowed or coughed up.

Accordingly, the cough reflex is a physiological reflex. Certain diseases are able to trigger the reflex arc and are accompanied by cough as a clinical symptom (Figure 16.1).

Aetiology

Coughs are caused by irritation of receptors in the respiratory tract. The receptors are not equally distributed throughout the entire respiratory system. In particular, the deep airways, the bronchioles and the alveoli do not have corresponding receptors, which means that triggering factors in these regions only lead to coughing when they are more extensive. Triggers can be foreign particles, mucus or inflammatory secretions that cause coughing. In the case of chronic cough, the trigger is the inflammation-related irritation of the mucous membrane.

Textbook of Small Animal Pathophysiology, First Edition. Stephan Neumann.
© 2025 John Wiley & Sons Ltd. Published 2025 by John Wiley & Sons Ltd.

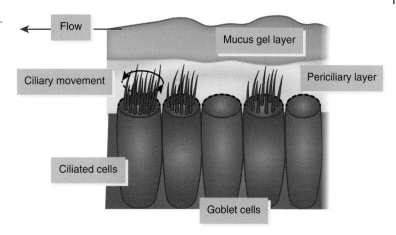

Figure 16.1 Mucociliary clearance.

Respiratory	Cardiac
Larynx	Lung oedema (D)
Laryngitis (D)	
Laryngeal paralysis (D)	
Trachea	
Tracheitis (D/C)	
Tracheal collapse (D)	
Bronchi	
Bronchitis (D/C)	
Bacterial infection (*Bordetella*, *Mycoplasma*) (D/C)	
Parasites *Aelurostrongylus* (C) *Angiostrongylus* (D)	
Asthma (C)	
Foreign bodies (D/C)	
Tumours (D)	
Thoracic wall	

D – Dog, C – Cat

Pathogenesis

Cough is an explosive form of exhalation. Its mechanism begins with inspiration, followed by a forceful exhalation against the closed glottis. By suddenly opening the glottis, the exhaled air with particles is explosively ejected from the oral cavity. The cough stimulus is initiated by stimulation of three different receptors. These include the rapidly adopting receptors (RARs), which are located subepithelially in the area of the air-conducting pathways close to the bronchial veins. They are primarily mechano-sensitive and can be irritated by increased venous pressure, increased mucus production or oedema. Similar to RARs, slow adopting receptors (SARs) are distributed throughout the respiratory tract and are mechano-sensitive. To be distinguished from these are 'C-fibres', which react less to mechanical stimuli than chemical stimuli, e.g. inflammatory mediators, such as histamine or bradykinin. In all cases, the nervous impulses are conducted via afferent fibres of the vagus nerve to the cough centre in the brainstem. From there, the impulse goes via efferent nerve fibres to the respiratory muscles.

Cough due to allergic reactions is subject to two different pathomechanisms. The exogenous pathway corresponds to the mechanisms already described, in that physical and chemical stimuli act on receptors, such as transient receptor potential vanilloid 1 (TRPV1) and transient receptor potential ankyrin 1 (TRPA1). In addition, there is another pathway; this is mediated by ATP. The release of ATP follows a calcium influx into the bronchial epithelia triggered, for example, by allergens. This induces an increased release of ATP via pannexin channels. ATP, in turn, causes the opening of

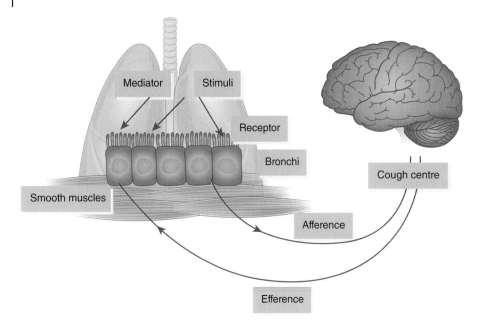

Figure 16.2 Pathways of the cough.

Sodium channels via receptors on the cell surface with the formation of an action potential. This is finally transmitted via the vagus nerve to the cough centre.

Cough due to cardiac disease occurs only in the dog. This is also an indication that the pathogenesis of cough in dogs and cats is not completely congruent. The mechanism by which cough is induced in cardiac disease is, on the one hand, compression of bronchi by cardiac enlargement. This is the case with atrial enlargement in mitral valve regurgitation. The enlarged atrium compresses the main bronchi and triggers the reflex by mechanical irritation of the cough receptors. In left heart failure, blood congests in the lungs. This leads to venous congestion and increased venous permeability. The result is exudation of blood plasma into the pulmonary alveoli and the development of alveolar pulmonary oedema (Hsieh and Beets 2020) (Figure 16.2).

Pathophysiologic Consequences

The consequences of coughing usually develop in the chronic phase. Unproductive, chronic coughing can cause further inflammation of the air-conducting organs to develop. This results from the strong air movement during coughing. The strained thoracic muscles can also be painful, especially during a chronic cough. Shortness of breath and limited performance are possible consequences.

Reference

Hsieh, B.M. and Beets, A.K. (2020). Coughing in small animal patients. *Frontiers in Veterinary Science* 6: 513. https://doi.org/10.3389/fvets.2019.00513.

Further Reading

Lee, K.K., Davenport, P.W., Smith, J.A. et al. (2021). Global physiology and pathophysiology of cough: part 1: cough phenomenology – CHEST guideline and expert panel report. *Chest* 159 (1): 282–293. https://doi.org/10.1016/j.chest.2020.08.2086.

Zhang, M., Sykes, D.L., Sadofsky, L.R., and Morice, A.H. (2022). ATP, an attractive target for the treatment of refractory chronic cough. *Purinergic Signalling* 18 (3): 289–305. https://doi.org/10.1007/s11302-022-09877-z.

17

Diarrhoea

Definition

Diarrhoea is, by definition, a more frequent defaecation of faeces that has changed in consistency.

Physiological Basics

The physiological principles of digestion are described in Chapter 38. Since disorders of intestinal motility and absorption processes at the intestinal mucosa are particularly responsible for the genesis of diarrhoea, these processes will be explained here in summary.

Intestinal motility in the small intestine is controlled by the autonomic nervous system, which is represented by Meissner's and Auerbach's plexus. These are influenced by nerve pathways from the gastrointestinal mucosa and the central nervous system. The small intestine peristaltic mechanism involves rhythmic contractions of the circular and longitudinal muscles that push ingesta forward and mix it with digestive juices. The contractions are initiated by the enteric nervous system, which coordinates the activity of the smooth muscles. The contractions also help to facilitate the absorption of nutrients from the ingesta.

The absorption of the different nutrients takes place after digestion by enzymes in the intestinal lumen. Proteins are absorbed as amino acids or oligopeptides. The absorption occurs mainly in the duodenum and jejunum.

Amino acids are transported across the apical membrane of the enterocytes by specific carrier proteins through 'active transport'. This requires energy in the form of ATP. Once inside the enterocytes, the amino acids are transported across the basolateral membrane and enter the bloodstream of the portal venous system. This occurs through facilitated diffusion or active transport, depending on the specific amino acid and its concentration gradient. Once in the bloodstream, the amino acids are transported to the liver, where they can be used for energy production or to build new proteins.

Carbohydrates are broken down into their simplest form, glucose, fructose and galactose; they are transported across the apical membrane of the enterocytes by specific transporter proteins. Glucose and galactose are transported via a sodium-dependent transporter, while fructose is transported via a facilitated diffusion mechanism. Once inside the enterocytes, glucose, fructose and galactose are transported across the basolateral membrane and enter the bloodstream through a facilitated diffusion mechanism.

Fatty acids and glycerol are transported across the apical membrane of the enterocytes by a process called 'micelle formation'. The fatty acids and glycerol are incorporated into micelles, which are small aggregates of lipids that can be absorbed by the enterocytes. Once inside the enterocytes, the fatty acids and glycerol are reassembled into triglycerides and packaged into chylomicrons, which are lipoprotein particles that can be transported through the lymphatic system and into the bloodstream.

Textbook of Small Animal Pathophysiology, First Edition. Stephan Neumann.
© 2025 John Wiley & Sons Ltd. Published 2025 by John Wiley & Sons Ltd.

Aetiology

Diarrhoea can be caused by diseases of the gastrointestinal tract or by extra-gastrointestinal causes. Depending on the duration of the diarrhoea, periods of less than a week are referred to as acute diarrhoea, and periods of more than two weeks as chronic diarrhoea.

Acute	Chronic
• Intestinal	• Intestinal
• Diet	• Diet
– Intolerance (D/C)	– Intolerance (D/C)
– Hypersensitivity (D)	– Hypersensitivity (D)
• Enteritis	• Inflammatory bowel diseases
– Haemorrhagic gastroenteritis (D)	– Gastrointestinal-lymphoma (C)
– Infectious (D/C)	• Extraintestinal
• Extraintestinal	– Exocrine pancreas insufficiency (D)
– Pancreatitis (D/C)	– Pancreatitis (D/C)
– Renal failure (D/C)	– Liver diseases (D/C)
• Endocrine disease	– Renal diseases (D/C)
– Hypoadrenocorticism (D)	• Endocrine disease
	– Hyperthyroidism (C)

D – Dog, C – Cat

Pathogenesis

The various aetiologies lead to diarrhoea via different mechanisms. A distinction is made between the following mechanisms:

Osmotic diarrhoea
Secretory diarrhoea
Exudative diarrhoea
Intestinal motility disorder

Osmotic diarrhoea occurs due to an increased concentration of osmotically active molecules in the intestinal lumen. These build up an osmotic gradient between the intestinal lumen and the extraintestinal area and prevent water reabsorption by the enterocytes. The causes are usually osmotically active molecules that remain in the intestinal lumen due to insufficient breakdown (maldigestion, malabsorption). These can be part of the food or result from insufficient activity of digestion. The latter can result from reduced microbial breakdown or reduced activity of digestive enzymes on the enterocyte membrane.

Secretory diarrhoea is the result of increased secretion of water and electrolytes across the enterocyte membrane. This process leads to a net loss of water and thus to diarrhoea. In addition to a hydrostatic pressure increase in the intestinal mucosa as a result of venous congestion in the case of right heart insufficiency or disturbed lymphatic drainage, another cause is increased chloride secretion. This is usually the result of bacterial toxin action.

Ion Transport at the Enterocyte Membrane

The resorption processes at the enterocyte membrane are made possible by different transport mechanisms. Molecules are moved passively or actively as part of a transport or cotransport. Examples are sodium/glucose cotransport. Through this active transport mechanism, sodium ions are taken up together with glucose molecules through the luminal enterocyte membrane (Wright et al. 2011). The sodium/hydrogen antiport exchanges sodium ions for hydrogen ions, thereby

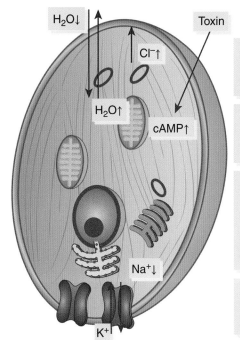

Bacterial toxins can directly affect ion transport in the intestine. For example, they increase cAMP levels, leading to chloride and water secretion.

Chloride (Cl⁻) secretion: Chloride ions are actively secreted into the intestinal lumen by channels. This creates an osmotic gradient, drawing water into the lumen.

Sodium (Na⁺) absorption: Dysfunctional sodium absorption can contribute to secretory diarrhoea. Sodium absorption via sodium-potassium ATPase and sodium-glucose cotransporters creates an osmotic gradient favouring water absorption. Disruption of these mechanisms can lead to increased fluid secretion.

Water absorption: In normal conditions, water is efficiently absorbed across the intestinal epithelium. Disruption of ion transport and osmotic gradients can impair water absorption.

Figure 17.1 Mechanism of secretory diarrhoea.

Table 17.1 Gut pathogenic microorganism causing acute diarrhoea.

	Virus	**Bacteria**	**Protozoa**
Dog	Parvovirus	*Salmonella* spp.	Giardia
		E. coli	
Cat	Feline immunodeficiency virus	*Campylobacter* spp.	Giardia
		Clostridium perfringens	Trichomonas
		Clostridium difficile	

Source: Adapted from Squires (2003).

maintaining electroneutrality (Kato and Romero 2011). Another mechanism is the chloride ion/bicarbonate antiport, in which chloride ions are exchanged for bicarbonate ions at the luminal enterocyte membrane.

Bacterial toxins can trigger secretory diarrhoea by disturbing these transport mechanisms. Numerous toxins act on the chloride channels of the cryptic enterocytes, which is why this mechanism will be presented as an example.

Escherichia coli can secrete heat-labile and heat-stable toxins. The toxins induce active chloride ion secretion at the luminal enterocyte membrane. They act via cAMP as a second messenger, which induces the influx of chloride ions at the basement membrane based on Na-K/Cl symport (Figure 17.1).

Exudative diarrhoea is caused by inflammation of the intestinal wall. As a result, the permeability of the mucosa increases. At the same time, the inflammation increases the local hydrostatic pressure, which leads to an increased leakage of interstitial fluid and blood plasma into the intestinal lumen. This process leads to a loss of serum proteins through the intestinal mucosa.

Finally, **intestinal motility** may be disturbed, causing more frequent intestinal transit.

Table 17.1 lists the intestinal pathogens that are considered to cause diarrhoea.

Pathophysiologic Consequences

Influenced organs	Clinical symptoms	Clinical pathological alterations
Gastrointestinal system	Diarrhoea	PCV increased
Cardiovascular system	Dehydration	Total protein increased
		Hypokalaemia
		Hypoalbuminaemia
		Hypocholesterinaemia

Major consequences of diarrhoea are the loss of water and the electrolytes dissolved in the water. Depending on the type of diarrhoea, water loss is particularly high in secretory and exudative diarrhoea. The consequence of increased water loss is an increased haemoconcentration.

Clinical consequences of **dehydration** have been described as inappetence, concentrated urine and seizure disorders.

Isotonic dehydration is the type of dehydration most commonly caused by diarrhoea. It occurs when the net losses of water and sodium are in the same proportion as they normally are in the extracellular fluid. The main features of isotonic dehydration are:

There is a balanced deficit of water and sodium;
Serum sodium concentration is normal (130–150 mmol/l);
Serum osmolality is normal (275–295 mOsmol/l);

Isotonic dehydration is manifested first by thirst and then by decreased skin turgour, tachycardia, dry mucous membranes, sunken eyes and oliguria. The signs of isotonic dehydration occur when the fluid deficit approaches 5% of body weight. When the fluid deficit approaches 10% of body weight, the dehydration becomes severe, and anuria, hypotension, a weak and very rapid pulse, cool extremities, decreased consciousness and other signs of hypovolaemic shock appear. A fluid deficit exceeding 10% of body weight rapidly leads to death from circulatory collapse. Laboratory diagnosis of haemoconcentration in dehydration is most readily apparent from an increased **PCV** and **total protein concentration**.

During diarrhoea, a large amount of bicarbonate can be lost in the faeces. If the kidneys continue to function normally, much of the lost bicarbonate is replaced by the kidneys and no serious base deficit develops. However, this compensatory mechanism fails when kidney function deteriorates, as happens with poor renal blood flow due to hypovolaemia. Then the base deficit and acidosis develop. Acidosis also results from excessive production of lactic acid when patients have hypovolaemic shock. The features of base deficit acidosis include:

A reduced serum bicarbonate concentration (sometimes <10 mmol/l);
A lowered arterial pH value (<7.10);
Breathing becomes deep and rapid, which helps to raise the arterial pH by causing compensatory respiratory alkalosis;
There is increased vomiting.

Patients with diarrhoea often develop **potassium deficiency** due to losses through the intestine. When potassium and bicarbonate are lost together, hypokalaemia does not usually develop. This is because the metabolic acidosis that results from the loss of bicarbonate causes potassium to move from the intracellular space to the extracellular space in exchange for hydrogen ions, keeping serum potassium levels in a normal or even elevated range. However, if metabolic acidosis is corrected by administration of bicarbonate, this shift is rapidly reversed and severe hypokalaemia may develop. This can be prevented by replacing potassium and correcting the baseline deficit at the same time. The signs of hypokalaemia may be:

General muscle weakness;
Cardiac arrhythmias;
Paralytic ileus, especially if medicines are taken that also affect peristalsis.

Exudative diarrhoea, in particular, is associated with a loss of blood plasma. Accordingly, consequences also develop due to hypoproteinaemia. Hypoproteinaemia leads to a reduced synthesis of lipoproteins in the liver. This in turn reduces the concentration of fats transported in the blood, which causes **hypocholesterolaemia** (Figures 17.2, 17.3).

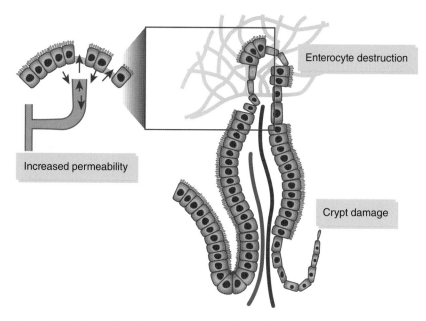

Figure 17.2 Illustration of destruction in exudative diarrhoea.

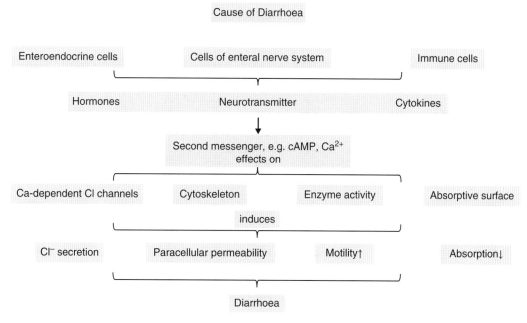

Figure 17.3 Overview of molecular mechanisms of diarrhoea.

References

Kato, A. and Romero, M.F. (2011). Regulation of electroneutral NaCl absorption by the small intestine. *Annual Review of Physiology* 73: 261–281. https://doi.org/10.1146/annurev-physiol-012110-142244.

Squires, R.A. (2003). An update on aspects of viral gastrointestinal diseases of dogs and cats. *New Zealand Veterinary Journal* 51 (6): 252–261. https://doi.org/10.1080/00480169.2003.36379.

Wright, E.M., Loo, D.D., and Hirayama, B.A. (2011). Biology of human sodium glucose transporters. *Physiological Reviews* 91 (2): 733–794. https://doi.org/10.1152/physrev.00055.2009.

Further Reading

Busch, K., Wehner, A., Dorsch, R. et al. (2014). Acute bloody diarrhoea as a presenting sign in a dog with primary hypoadrenocorticism [Acute haemorrhagic diarrhoea as a presenting sign in a dog with primary hypoadrenocorticism]. *Veterinary Practice. Issue K, Small Animals/Pets* 42 (5): 326–330.

Ewald, N., Rödler, F., and Heilmann, R.M. (2021). Chronic enteropathies in cats – diagnostic and therapeutic approach. *Veterinary Practice. Issue K, Small Animals/Pets* 49 (5): 363–376.

Gianella, P., Pietra, M., Crisi, P.E. et al. (2017). Evaluation of clinicopathological features in cats with chronic gastrointestinal signs. *Polish Journal of Veterinary Sciences* 20 (2): 403–410. https://doi.org/10.1515/pjvs-2017-0052.

Gookin, J.L., Breitschwerdt, E.B., Levy, M.G. et al. (1999). Diarrhea associated with trichomonosis in cats. *Journal of the American Veterinary Medical Association* 215 (10): 1450–1454.

Hoelzer, K. and Parrish, C.R. (2010). The emergence of parvoviruses of carnivores. *Veterinary Research* 41 (6): 39. https://doi.org/10.1051/vetres/2010011.

Jergens, A.E. (2012). Feline idiopathic inflammatory bowel disease: what we know and what remains to be unraveled. *Journal of Feline Medicine and Surgery* 14 (7): 445–458. https://doi.org/10.1177/1098612X12451548.

Levitt, D.G. and Levitt, M.D. (2017). Protein losing enteropathy: comprehensive review of the mechanistic association with clinical and subclinical disease states. *Clinical and Experimental Gastroenterology* 10: 147–168. https://doi.org/10.2147/CEG. S136803.

Marks, S.L., Rankin, S.C., Byrne, B.A., and Weese, J.S. (2011). Enteropathogenic bacteria in dogs and cats: diagnosis, epidemiology, treatment, and control. *Journal of Veterinary Internal Medicine* 25 (6): 1195–1208. https://doi.org/10.1111/j.1939-1676.2011.00821.x.

Norsworthy, G.D., Scot Estep, J., Kiupel, M. et al. (2013). Diagnosis of chronic small bowel disease in cats: 100 cases (2008-2012). *Journal of the American Veterinary Medical Association* 243 (10): 1455–1461. https://doi.org/10.2460/javma.243.10.1455.

Pilla, R. and Suchodolski, J.S. (2020). The role of the canine gut microbiome and metabolome in health and gastrointestinal disease. *Frontiers in Veterinary Science* 6: 498. https://doi.org/10.3389/fvets.2019.00498.

Suchodolski, J.S., Markel, M.E., Garcia-Mazcorro, J.F. et al. (2012). The fecal microbiome in dogs with acute diarrhea and idiopathic inflammatory bowel disease. *PLoS One* 7 (12): e51907. https://doi.org/10.1371/journal.pone.0051907.

Tangtrongsup, S. and Scorza, V. (2010). Update on the diagnosis and management of Giardia spp. infections in dogs and cats. *Topics in Companion Animal Medicine* 25 (3): 155–162. https://doi.org/10.1053/j.tcam.2010.07.003.

Unterer, S. and Busch, K. (2021). Acute hemorrhagic diarrhea syndrome in dogs. *The Veterinary Clinics of North America. Small Animal Practice* 51 (1): 79–92. https://doi.org/10.1016/j.cvsm.2020.09.007.

Volkmann, M., Steiner, J.M., Fosgate, G.T. et al. (2017). Chronic diarrhea in dogs – retrospective study in 136 cases. *Journal of Veterinary Internal Medicine* 31 (4): 1043–1055. https://doi.org/10.1111/jvim.14739.

Weese, J.S. (2011). Bacterial enteritis in dogs and cats: diagnosis, therapy, and zoonotic potential. *The Veterinary Clinics of North America. Small Animal Practice* 41 (2): 287–309. https://doi.org/10.1016/j.cvsm.2010.12.005.

Werner, M., Suchodolski, J.S., Lidbury, J.A. et al. (2021). Diagnostic value of fecal cultures in dogs with chronic diarrhea. *Journal of Veterinary Internal Medicine* 35 (1): 199–208. https://doi.org/10.1111/jvim.15982.

Westermarck, E. (2016). Chronic diarrhea in dogs: what do we actually know about it? *Topics in Companion Animal Medicine* 31 (2): 78–84. https://doi.org/10.1053/j.tcam.2016.03.001.

Yao, C. and Köster, L.S. (2015). *Tritrichomonas foetus* infection, a cause of chronic diarrhea in the domestic cat. *Veterinary Research* 46 (1): 35. https://doi.org/10.1186/s13567-015-0169-0.

18

Dyschezia

Definition

Dyschezia refers to difficulty in defaecation.

Physiological Basics

The physiology of defaecation begins with the accumulation of faeces in the distal colon. Intestinal peristalsis transports the faeces to the rectal area. When there is an increase in volume in the rectum, mechanoreceptors in the rectal wall are stimulated and initiate defaecation. This takes place through increased peristalsis in the rectum with simultaneously relaxed sphincters. The inner sphincter consists of smooth muscles and cannot be influenced voluntarily. The external sphincter, on the other hand, consists of striated muscles and is therefore subject to voluntary control to a certain extent. This means that defaecation can be partially suppressed even during the process. At the same time, defaecation is supported by a contraction of the abdominal muscles. Dogs and cats adopt a squatting position for this purpose. The neuronal control of defaecation is controlled by a higher centre in the area of the medulla oblongata and a lower centre in the area of the second to fourth sacral segments (Figure 18.1).

Aetiology

The causes of difficult defaecation result essentially from stenoses in the region of the distal colon and rectum. Functional disorders are present when disturbances in intestinal peristalsis lead to constipation and thus make defaecation difficult. Further reasons are based on the unwillingness to defaecate due to painful defaecation and thus secondary constipation.

Mechanic	Functional	Constipation
Trauma (D/C)	Megacolon (D/C)	Diet (D/C)
Pelvic neoplasms (D/C)		Anal sac diseases (D)
Enlarged prostate (D)		Back pain (D/C)
Perineal hernia (D)		
Rectal stricture (D/C)		

D – Dog, C – Cat

Pathogenesis

In the case of mechanical causes of dyschezia, faeces cannot be defaecated or can only be partially defaecated by peristalsis. Usually, these animals show a more pronounced abdominal muscle contracture to increase the pressure in the abdomen. This may result in increased gas secretion (tenesmus) or smaller quantities of faeces, which are often altered in shape.

Textbook of Small Animal Pathophysiology, First Edition. Stephan Neumann.
© 2025 John Wiley & Sons Ltd. Published 2025 by John Wiley & Sons Ltd.

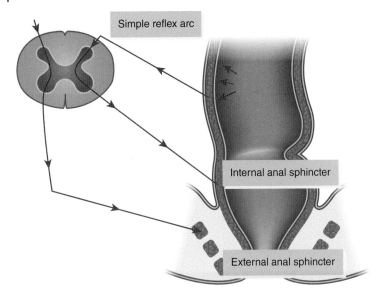

Figure 18.1 Mechanism of defaecation.
Source: Wani, R. A., Thakur, N. (2016)/Springer Nature.

In the case of functional reasons, the peristalsis is not able to transport the faeces appropriately. The faeces accumulate and constipation develops. As a result, peristalsis is further impeded. In addition, faecal stasis leads to further dehydration, which causes a hard faecal consistency. The same applies if the animals deliberately suppress defaecation due to pain during defaecation, for example, in the case of diseases in the area of the anus or back pain. Here, too, dyschezia develops due to constipation.

A special form of dyschezia develops in a perineal hernia. This is defined as a weakening of the pelvic diaphragm. As a result, faecal problems develop with constipation of faeces in the hernial sac of the rectal diverticulum. At the same time, dislocation of abdominal organs, such as the bladder or prostate may occur. The disease occurs more frequently in intact males in the second half of life. Possible breed predispositions are suspected for Pekingese, Boxer and Bouvier. Causative factors are thought to be diseases of the rectum, for example, inflammations or stenosing tumours, the effect of hormones, such as androgens or relaxin, and diseases of the prostate. In the case of hormonal imbalances, a relaxation of the diaphragma pelvis due to a hormonal imbalance is suspected. The same is discussed for a perineal hernia in connection with diseases of the prostate. Here, prostatic hypertrophy seems to cause relaxation of the muscles and connective tissue in the diaphragma pelvis due to increased secretion of relaxin. However, enlargement of the prostate may necessitate an increased abdominal press for defaecation due to stenosis of the intestinal tract, which in turn results in increased pressure on the diaphragma pelvis. Finally, neuropathies of the pudendal nerve and sacral plexus are assumed to be pathogenetic, as these lead to atrophy of the levator ani and coccygeus muscles.

Pathophysiologic Consequences

Local	Systemic
Defaecation discomfort	In case of perineal hernia urinary bladder prolapse
Haematochezia	Post-renal renal failure
Pain	

The consequences of dyschezia are initially local. Stagnant faeces can cause **pain** by irritating mechanoreceptors in the intestinal wall. Due to the increase in abdominal pressure during defaecation, small vessels in the rectal wall can burst and cause **haematochezia**. If inflammation in the bowel is the cause of the dyschezia, the local inflammatory process may also be painful. Chronic faecal problems can cause megacolon due to permanent dilatation of the colon. However, this can also be the cause of dyschezia.

A severe systemic complication follows **urinary bladder prolapse** in the context of perineal hernia. In retroflexion, the urethra is knicked and urine output is arrested or difficult. This leads to **post-renal renal failure**, which causes azotaemia or uraemia. At the same time, hyperkalaemia develops. Hyperkalaemia can lead to depolarisation of the cell membrane, which can cause altered neuronal and muscle cell function. This can result in muscle weakness, cramping and arrhythmias. High levels of potassium ions outside of cells can also lead to reduced excitability of cells and decreased neuromuscular transmission. In extreme cases, hyperkalaemia can cause cardiac arrest due to the disruption of normal heart function. Additionally, hyperkalaemia can affect the release of neurotransmitters and hormones, leading to various physiological disturbances.

Further Reading

Dimski, D.S. (1989). Constipation: pathophysiology, diagnostic approach, and treatment. *Seminars in Veterinary Medicine and Surgery (Small Animal)* 4 (3): 247–254.

Whitehead, K., Cortes, Y., and Eirmann, L. (2016). Gastrointestinal dysmotility disorders in critically ill dogs and cats. *Journal of Veterinary Emergency and Critical Care (San Antonio, Tex.: 2001)* 26 (2): 234–253.

19

Dysphagia

Definition

Dysphagia is a disorder of the act of swallowing, which can affect one or more phases of the swallowing process. Those are located in the mouth, the pharynx and the oesophagus.

Physiological Basics

The act of swallowing begins in the oral cavity with the intake and comminution of the food. The food becomes lubricious when it is salivated and can be transported to the pharynx by the movements of the tongue. By lowering the base of the tongue and pressing the back of the tongue against the hard palate, the food is pressed into the pharynx.

The pharynx then contracts and pushes the bolus of food towards the oesophagus. At the same time, the epiglottis flaps upwards to cover the opening of the larynx and prevent aspiration. As the pharynx contracts, the cricopharyngeus and thyropharyngeus muscles, which form the upper oesophageal sphincter, relax. As a result, the food bolus can enter the oesophagus. Once the bolus is in the oesophagus, the upper oesophageal sphincter closes to prevent retrograde movement of the food and the epiglottis returns to its relaxed position, allowing normal breathing.

The muscularis of the oesophageal wall of the dog is composed of striated muscle, and that of the cat is composed of striated muscle cranially and smooth muscle caudally. When the food bolus reaches the oesophagus, it is transported by peristaltic waves towards the entrance of the stomach. When the food bolus reaches the distal oesophageal sphincter, it relaxes and the bolus enters the cardiac region of the stomach.

Aetiology

Based on the swallowing phases, swallowing disorders can be etiologically differentiated into diseases of the oral cavity or the oesophagus.

Oral cavity	Oesophagus
Oral diseases (D/C)	Megaoesophagus (D)
	Obstruction(D/C)

D – Dog, C – Cat

Pathogenesis

Causes of dysphagia lead to disturbances during the swallowing process. They are divided into oral, pharyngeal, cricopharyngeal, oesophageal and gastro-oesophageal dysphagia.

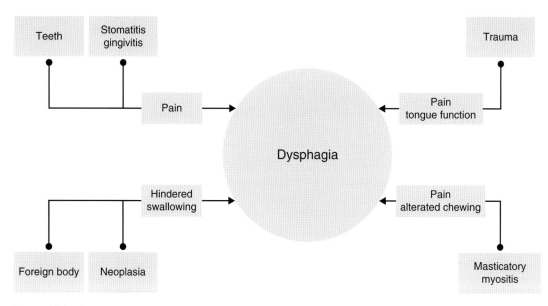

Figure 19.1 Pathogenesis of dysphagia.

The oral causes of dysphagia can be diseases of the teeth or the gingiva as stomatitis, these produce pain and thus influence the swallowing process. Trauma caused by foreign bodies or fractures in the area of the jaw bones also lead to pain, which impedes the swallowing process. In addition, trauma to the oral cavity can also influence the swallowing process itself, for example, by limiting the function of the tongue. Another process that is localised in the oral cavity are diseases of the masticatory muscles, for example, as masticatory myositis (MM). Here, pain during the chewing process is responsible for the dysphagia.

In the area of the pharynx, the swallowing process can be impaired by foreign bodies, but also by neoplasms. The same applies essentially to the oesophagus and the entrance to the stomach. In addition to these mechanical factors, functional causes are also possible. An essential factor here is the influence of the swallowing process by a megaoesophagus. Here, the swallowing process is disturbed because the peristalsis of the oesophageal muscles is impeded (Pollard 2012) (Figure 19.1).

Pathophysiologic Consequences

The pathophysiologic consequences of dysphagia result from the reduced supply of food and fluid to the organism and can lead to malnutrition or dehydration. Disorders of the process also cause aspiration of food with the consequence of aspiration pneumonia.

Influenced organ systems	Clinical symptoms	Clinical pathological alterations
Respiratory system	Pneumonia	Increased PCV
Gastrointestinal	Weight loss	Increased total protein
system	Dehydration	

Aspiration pneumonia is a major pathophysiologic consequence of dysphagia. Depending on the extent, the symptoms vary in severity. Usually, pneumonia develops in the ventral lung areas after aspiration of food. The entry of foreign material produces a massive inflammatory reaction. Bacteria present in the foreign material adhere to the respiratory epithelial cells and can lead to epithelial cell necrosis, which in turn suppresses the clearance mechanism of the bronchial apparatus, reducing local defences and promoting further infection. The neutrophilic inflammatory reaction that develops can lead to further pathological alteration. The inflammatory process results in alveolar exudation; this in turn impedes alveolar gas exchange. Hypoxia develops with the clinical consequences already described.

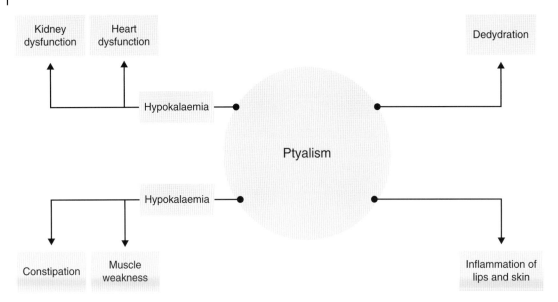

Figure 19.2 Consequences of ptyalism.

Further consequences result from the restricted intake of food or water when swallowing is difficult. This can cause weight loss or dehydration, which leads to increased packed cell volume (PCV) and total protein concentration.

Increased salivation in cases of dysphagia can also cause irritation and inflammation of the skin around the mouth, leading to infection and discomfort. Further, excessive salivation can lead to electrolyte imbalances, such as low sodium and potassium levels.

The low potassium can lead to muscle weakness, as potassium is essential for normal muscle function. Hypokalaemia can cause gastrointestinal disturbances, such as vomiting, diarrhoea and constipation. Potassium plays a critical role in regulating the heart's electrical activity. Hypokalaemia can cause abnormal heart rhythms, leading to cardiac arrhythmias and even cardiac arrest. Hypokalaemia can also cause respiratory muscle weakness and lead to breathing difficulties. Finally, hypokalaemia can cause kidney dysfunction, leading to impaired urine concentration, electrolyte imbalances, and acid-base disturbances. Hypokalaemia can cause metabolic acidosis (Figure 19.2).

Reference

Pollard, R.E. (2012). Imaging evaluation of dogs and cats with dysphagia. *ISRN Veterinary Science* 2012: 238505. https://doi.org/ 10.5402/2012/238505.

Further Reading

Downing, T.E., Sporn, T.A., Bollinger, R.R. et al. (2008). Pulmonary histopathology in an experimental model of chronic aspiration is independent of acidity. *Experimental Biology and Medicine (Maywood, N.J.)* 233 (10): 1202–1212. https://doi.org/ 10.3181/0801-RM-17.

Glazer, A. and Walters, P. (2008). Esophagitis and esophageal strictures. *Compendium (Yardley, PA)* 30 (5): 281–292.

Guilford, W.G. (1990). Megaesophagus in the dog and cat. *Seminars in Veterinary Medicine and Surgery (Small Animal)* 5 (1): 37–45.

Kogan, D.A., Johnson, L.R., Jandrey, K.E., and Pollard, R.E. (2008). Clinical, clinicopathologic, and radiographic findings in dogs with aspiration pneumonia: 88 cases (2004–2006). *Journal of the American Veterinary Medical Association* 233 (11): 1742–1747. https://doi.org/10.2460/javma.233.11.1742.

Kuyama, K., Sun, Y., and Yamamoto, H. (2010). Aspiration pneumonia: with special reference to pathological and epidemiological aspects, a review of the literature. *Japanese Dental Science Review* 46 (2): 102–111. https://doi.org/10.1016/j.jdsr.2009.11.002.

Watrous, B.J. (1983). Clinical presentation and diagnosis of dysphagia. *The Veterinary Clinics of North America. Small Animal Practice* 13 (3): 437–459. http://dx.doi.org/10.1016/s0195-5616(83)50052-1.

20

Dyspnoea

Definition

Dyspnoea refers to insufficient or difficult breathing. It can be recognised by excessive use of the respiratory muscles and an increased respiratory rate.

Physiological Basics

The main task of respiration is to supply the body with oxygen and to eliminate carbon dioxide. To ensure this task, the lungs, as the site of gas exchange, must inhale air and exhale an air-gas mixture. Since the lungs have little mobility of their own, the organism needs mechanisms for inspiration and expiration that enable air-gas movement in the lungs.

During inspiration, the thoracic space is enlarged by contraction of the diaphragmatic muscles and the intercostal muscles. This results in an outward rotation and elevation of the ribs and a flattening of the dome-shaped diaphragm of about 1 cm. The diaphragm has a higher proportion of type 1 muscle fibres , providing the energy needed for contraction through aerobic glycolysis. This results in low muscle fatigue.

The enlargement of the thorax stretches the lungs. Since there is negative pressure between the lung surface and the chest wall, the lungs must follow the movement of the chest. The inflow of room air via the airways into the lungs compensates for the pulmonary volume expansion. Lung expansion receptors in the wall of the trachea and bronchi (Hering-Breuer reflex) and muscle spindles in respiratory muscles limit inhalation and mediate inhibition of diaphragmatic activity, initiating passive exhalation. When the respiratory musculature relaxes, the thoracic space is reduced by inward rotation of the ribs and passive forward movement of the diaphragm, so that air is exhaled through the airways to compensate for the now higher intrathoracic pressure.

Breathing is controlled by neurons in the 'respiratory centre' in the formatio reticularis and medulla oblongata, which regulate both the frequency and depth of breathing. The necessary information arrives via afferents from peripherally located chemoreceptors at the aortic arch, the carotid artery as well as stretch receptors of the lungs (known as the 'Hering-Breuer reflex') and can be influenced via cortical afferents from the hypothalamus.

The increase in physiological respiratory rate associated with an increase in respiratory volume is achieved by an arterial CO_2 increase (hypercapnia) and pH decrease (acidosis) and an arterial O_2 decrease (hypoxia). In humans, it has been shown that an increase in arterial CO_2 partial pressure of 1 mmHg increases ventilation in healthy individuals by about 20–30% (Feldman et al. 2003) (Figure 20.1).

Aetiology

The causes of dyspnoea lie mainly in the respiratory tract; here different causalities can be distinguished between the upper and lower respiratory tract. Various systemic diseases can also lead to dyspnoea.

Textbook of Small Animal Pathophysiology, First Edition. Stephan Neumann.
© 2025 John Wiley & Sons Ltd. Published 2025 by John Wiley & Sons Ltd.

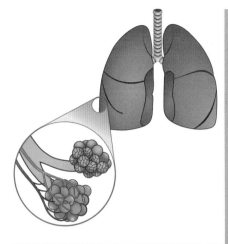

Inspiration

1. **Neural initiation:** Medullary respiratory centers in the brainstem send signals to initiate inspiration.
2. **Diaphragmatic contraction:** Phrenic nerves stimulate the diaphragm to contract.
3. **Diaphragmatic descent:** Contraction of the diaphragm causes it to move backward, expanding the thoracic cavity.
4. **External intercostal muscles:** Muscles between the ribs contract, lifting the ribcage outwards.
5. **Thoracic cavity expansion:** The expansion of the thoracic cavity lowers intrathoracic pressure.
6. **Airflow inward:** Negative intrathoracic pressure draws air through the trachea into the lungs.
7. **Alveolar expansion:** Alveoli in the lungs expand, causing a decrease in intrapulmonary pressure.

Expiration

1. **Neural control:** Medullary centers cease stimulation, leading to relaxation of inspiratory muscles.
2. **Diaphragmatic relaxation:** The diaphragm relaxes, moving forewards due to elastic recoil.
3. **Elastic recoil:** Elastic fibers in the lung tissue and chest wall passively recoil, decreasing thoracic volume.
4. **Internal intercostal muscles:** Muscles may contract to actively pull the ribcage foreward, aiding in forceful exhalation.
5. **Thoracic cavity compression:** Reduced thoracic volume increases intrathoracic pressure.
6. **Airflow outward:** Higher intrathoracic pressure forces air out of the lungs through the trachea.
7. **Alveolar compression:** Alveoli decrease in size, causing an increase in intrapulmonary pressure.

Figure 20.1 Breathing mechanism dog.

Upper respiratory tract	Lower respiratory tract	Extra respiratory diseases
Nasal diseases (D/C)	**Bronchial diseases** (D/C) Foreign body, Lungworm, Neoplasia, Feline asthma (C), Eosinophilic bronchitis (D/C)	Diaphragmatic hernia (D/C)
(Foreign body, Neoplasia, Aspergillosis)		Pleural effusion (D/C)
Laryngeal diseases	**Pulmonary diseases**	Cardiac diseases (D/C)
Neoplasia (D/C), Laryngeal paralysis (D), Everted saccules (D)	Pulmonary fibrosis (D)	Anaemia (D/C)
Tracheal diseases	Pneumonia (viral, bacterial, parasitic) (D/C)	Hyperthyroidism (C)
Neoplasia (D/C), Tracheal collapse (D)		ARDS (D/C)
		Thromboembolism (D/C)

D – Dog, C – Cat

Pathogenesis

Many causalities cause dyspnoea and thus the reduced supply of oxygen to the organism and the reduced release of carbon dioxide due to impairment of air-gas movement caused by stenotic airways. In feline lower respiratory disease (feline asthma), for example, bronchiolar stenosis develops through hypertrophy of the bronchial epithelium and bronchoconstriction (Figure 20.2).

Another pathogenesis of dyspnoea results from a functional disorder of the respiratory centre, whereby adequate gas exchange cannot be ensured. This can be a consequence of central diseases such as tumours or hydrocephalus.

Finally, dyspnoea can occur when the demand for oxygen increases or the oxygen transport capacity is insufficient. Stress, pain and fever lead to an increased oxygen demand. Reduced oxygen transport is a consequence of anaemia or cardiac insufficiency.

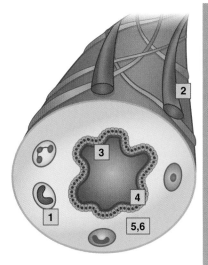

1. **Inflammatory response:** Exposure to triggering factors leads to an inflammatory response in the airways. This involves the release of inflammatory mediators, such as histamine, leukotrienes, and prostaglandins.

2. **Smooth muscle contraction:** Inflammatory mediators cause the smooth muscles surrounding the bronchi to contract excessively (bronchospasm).

3. **Airway narrowing:** As the smooth muscles contract, the diameter of the bronchi decreases, leading to narrowing of the airways. This narrowing restricts the flow of air in and out of the lungs.

4. **Mucus production:** The inflammatory response also triggers increased production of mucus in the airways. The excess mucus further contributes to airway obstruction.

5. **Decreased airflow:** The combination of bronchoconstriction and increased mucus production results in reduced airflow through the narrowed airways.

6. **Increased resistance:** Bronchospasm and airway obstruction cause increased resistance to airflow.

Figure 20.2 Mechanism of bronchoconstriction in feline lower respiratory disease.

Pathophysiologic Consequences

The pathophysiologic consequences of dyspnoea result primarily from hypoxia, as a consequence of reduced oxygen supply or hypercapnia with respiratory acidosis.

Hypoxia/hypercapnia
Tachycardia
Hyperventilation
Cyanosis
Fatigue

Clinical symptoms resulting from dyspnoea are due to an undersupply of oxygen and an increased CO_2 concentration. The immediate consequences are increased heart and lung activity stimulated by the sympathetic nervous system. This is to compensate for the acute oxygen deficiency. The simultaneous increase in CO_2 concentration in dyspnoea causes a blue colouring of the mucous membranes. Finally, both metabolic changes lead to peripheral damage in the body cells.

Hypoxia causes an energy deficiency at the cellular level. This is based on a reduced intracellular ATP synthesis due to the switch to anaerobic glycolysis. A lack of ATP affects, among other things, the ATP-dependent Na^+/K^+ pump, with the consequence of a decreased sodium efflux. This causes water accumulation in the cell, as well as disturbances of the membrane balance. This opens calcium channels and leads to increased calcium influx.

The consequences of an increased cellular calcium concentration are multiple. These include increased formation of reactive oxygen species (ROS). This results in mitochondrial membrane damage and organ dysfunction.

Other consequences of increased cellular calcium concentration are increases in destructive enzyme activities. All of these lead to progressive cellular dysfunction.

The hypoxia can additionally result in polycythaemia via erythropoietin release, but this is only likely in a chronic stage.

As a result of hypercapnia, the blood vessels in the lungs may dilate, increasing the pressure in the pulmonary arteries. This can lead to an overload of the right heart.

Centrally, CO_2 acts as a vasodilator and can induce dilation of the cerebral vessels. This can lead to an increase in intracranial pressure and an impairment of brain function. Furthermore, hypercapnia leads to acidosis due to the formation of carbonic acid. Acidosis, in turn, can lead to a number of symptoms, including fatigue, nausea, vomiting and cardiac arrhythmias (Figure 20.3).

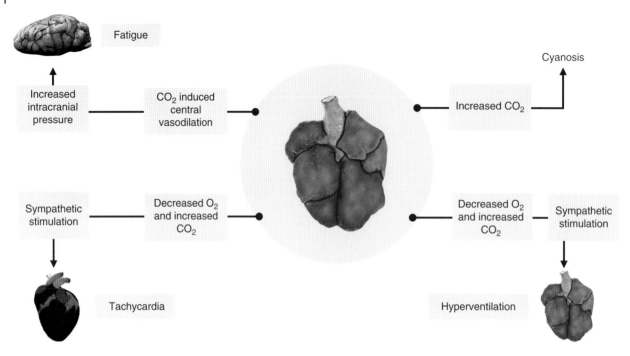

Figure 20.3 Pathophysiologic consequences of dyspnoea.

Reference

Feldman, J.L., Mitchell, G.S., and Nattie, E.E. (2003). Breathing: rhythmicity, plasticity, chemosensitivity. *Annual Review of Neuroscience* 26: 239–266. https://doi.org/10.1146/annurev.neuro.26.041002.131103.

Further Reading

O'Donnell, D.E., James, M.D., Milne, K.M., and Neder, J.A. (2019). The pathophysiology of dyspnea and exercise intolerance in chronic obstructive pulmonary disease. *Clinics in Chest Medicine* 40 (2): 343–366. https://doi.org/10.1016/j.ccm.2019.02.007.

21

Effusions

Definition

The term 'effusion' describes the accumulation of fluid in the body cavities.

Physiological Basics

Both thoracic and abdominal cavities are lined by serous membranes, the pleura or peritoneum. These lie with a visceral sheet on the internal organs and a parietal sheet on the inside of the body cavity.

Histologically, the serous membranes are composed of a layer of flat or cubic mesothelial cells, a basement membrane and a submesothelial interstitium. The total thickness varies between species, usually visceral slightly thinner than parietal and is about 50–100 μm. Blood vessels are embedded in the interstitium, which are visceral deeper than parietal and arise from the systemic blood vessels.

The mesothelial cells may be flat or cuboidal, the former containing few mitochondria or a poorly developed Golgi apparatus, while the cuboidal forms are richer in mitochondria and Golgi apparatus. The cells are connected to each other via gap junctions or desmosomes.

An essential function of the serous membranes, besides body defence, is to create a low-friction surface between the organ structures. This enables the organs to move without friction-induced shear forces destroying the surface cells. To fulfil this function, a small amount of fluid is produced as pleural or peritoneal fluid. The total amount of fluid varies from animal to animal and is on average between 0.1 and 2.0 ml/kg body weight.

The fluid is formed in the parietal interstitium and is released under the influence of hydrostatic forces. Colloid osmotic pressures counteract the release.

The fluid composition is similar to that of blood plasma, but the protein content is lower. In addition, there are a few mesothelial cells, lymphocytes and macrophages.

The resorption of the fluid takes place via active or passive transmesothelial transport, via aquaporins and transcytosis (Figure 21.1).

Aetiology

Numerous diseases are possible causes of effusion. The causalities depend very much on the type of effusion. In principle, a distinction is made between effusions in the thoracic or abdominal cavity:

Blood (thorax/abdomen)
Urine (abdomen)
Bile (abdomen)
Transudate (thorax/abdomen)
Modified transudate (thorax/abdomen)
Exudate (thorax/abdomen)

Textbook of Small Animal Pathophysiology, First Edition. Stephan Neumann.
© 2025 John Wiley & Sons Ltd. Published 2025 by John Wiley & Sons Ltd.

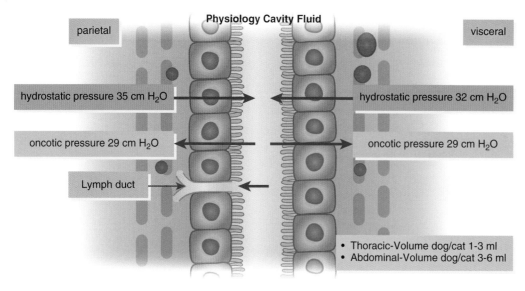

Figure 21.1 Physiology of thoracic and abdominal fluid formation.

Transudate

Pathogenesis

The main reasons for the formation of a protein-poor transudate are changes in hydrostatic and oncotic pressure within the cavity. Abdominally, changes in hydrostatic pressure are present, for example, in portal hypertension. Discharge disturbances of portal venous flow lead to an increase in pressure within the venous system and thus to leakage of blood plasma into the peritoneal area. This may result in a transudate or a modified transudate. Frequent causes of portal outflow disorders are liver changes, for example, in the sense of liver cirrhosis. This leads to a remodelling of the liver architecture with the consequence of increased vascular resistance in the sinusoids and portal vessels. Changes located cranially to the liver can also lead to portal hypertension via the liver. These include, for example, tricuspid insufficiencies. In such cases, however, telangiectasia are usually found within the liver parenchyma, which illustrate the backflow into the abdominal venous system.

In addition to an increase in hydrostatic pressure, a reduction in oncotic pressure also leads to transudate. Here, protein loss diseases, such as protein-losing enteropathy or nephropathy are causally in the foreground. Malnutrition or malabsorption would be other rarer reasons for the occurrence of a protein deficiency.

Pathophysiologic Consequences

Influenced organs	Clinical symptoms	Clinical pathological alterations
Body cavity	Ascites	Hypoproteinaemia
		Hypoalbuminaemia
		Hypocalcaemia

The main consequences of transudate are due to the underlying disease leading to a reduction in oncotic pressure. Transudate is described as a result of hypoproteinaemia due to protein-losing nephropathy. This is seen in nephrotic syndrome and may subsequently lead to renal failure, with the symptoms described there. Further loss may be seen as protein-losing enteropathy with symptoms of enteropathy, such as diarrhoea. Finally, advanced liver cirrhosis is also associated with reduced albumin synthesis and thus a reduction in oncotic pressure. In this case, symptoms of hepatopathy develop with an advanced-stage hepatic encephalopathy syndrome. The frequently observed reduction of total calcium in serum is due to the reduction of albumin. Total calcium is predominantly transported in the blood bound to albumin. A reduction in albumin concentration, therefore, also reduces the concentration of total calcium (Figure 21.2).

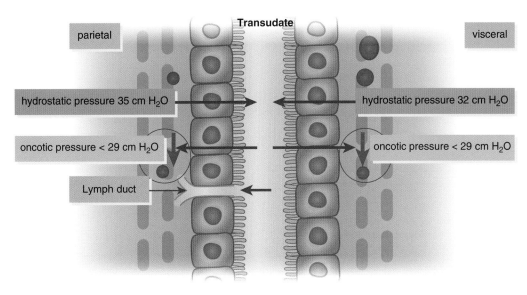

Figure 21.2 Mechanism of transudate formation.

Exudate

Pathogenesis

Exudates usually have an inflammatory or tumorous genesis. Abdominal exudates have been described in feline infectious peritonitis (FIP), abdominal lymphoma and infectious diseases leading to peritonitis. The latter is often the consequence of a perforated intestine. Intestinal bacteria are translocated into the peritoneal cavity. Their composition and quantity strongly depend on the location of the perforation. The amount ranges between 10^5 and 10^8 CFU/ml (colony-forming units) intestinal content. As a result, an inflammatory reaction occurs, which is carried by polymorphonuclear leukocytes. These are activated by resident macrophages, mesothelial cells and mast cells in the peritoneal cavity, which initiate the inflammatory cascade after initial contact with the bacteria by secreting proinflammatory cytokines. In contrast to the transudate or modified transudate, the high protein content in the exudate is remarkable. This is due to the increase in vascular permeability associated with the inflammatory process. Peritonitis also sometimes leads to a disturbance of the mesothelial integrity with the consequence of a leakage of protein-rich interstitial fluid.

Pathophysiologic Consequences

Influenced organs	Clinical symptoms	Clinical pathological alterations
Body cavity	Anorexia	Leucocytosis
	Cachexia	Left shift

The pathophysiologic consequences of exudative forms of effusion can also often be traced back to the underlying disease. The diseases often have a catabolic metabolic state in common. This is based on the energy-consuming inflammatory reaction (Figure 21.3, Table 21.1).

Abdominal Bleeding

Pathogenesis

Abdominal effusion due to haemorrhage into the abdomen is caused by traumatic rupture of vessels, rupture of tumours of different localisation or coagulation disorders. The result is a so-called 'haemoperitoneum'. Vascular ruptures are caused by blunt or sharp trauma, and are often associated with traffic accidents and biting. Iatrogenic sharp trauma is a possible

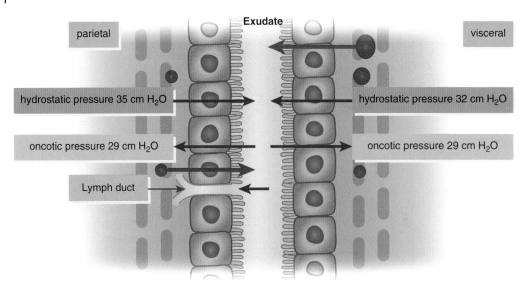

Figure 21.3 Mechanism of exudate formation.

Table 21.1 Differential diagnosis for effusions.

	Transudate	Mod. transudate	Exudate	Dog	Cat
Heart failure		xxx		xxx	xxx
Neoplasia		xxx	xxx	xxx	xxx
Pyothorax			xxx	xxx	xxx
Chylothorax		xxx		xxx	xxx
FIP			xxx		xxx
Protein loss	xxx			xxx	xxx

consequence of surgery. Here, the slipping off of a placed ligature is in the foreground. Other causes are coagulopathies of different origin. The most frequent cause in dogs is tumour haemorrhage, mostly in haemangiosarcomas of the spleen, but also in other abdominal tumours.

Pathophysiologic Consequences

Influenced organs	Clinical symptoms	Clinical pathological alterations
Cardiovascular system	Hypotension	Anaemia

The pathophysiologic consequences of abdominal haemorrhage are a drop in blood pressure with hypovolaemic shock and anaemia. Traumatic events more often lead to a rapid loss of volume into the abdomen, resulting in hypovolaemic shock.

Directly after blood is lost, PCV and protein should not be changed, because red blood cells (RBCs) and plasma are lost proportionately. But volume is decreased in total. This induces movement from extra cellular space (ECF) to the intravascular space to expand the volume. The fluid shift dilutes the plasma and PCV and total protein (TP) decrease. Especially in dogs, splenic contraction is a mechanism to diminish the erythrocyte reduction.

Erythropoetin (EPO) production will be stimulated directly, if tissue hypoxia is present, but it takes about two to three days until the first observation of reticulocytes in the blood.

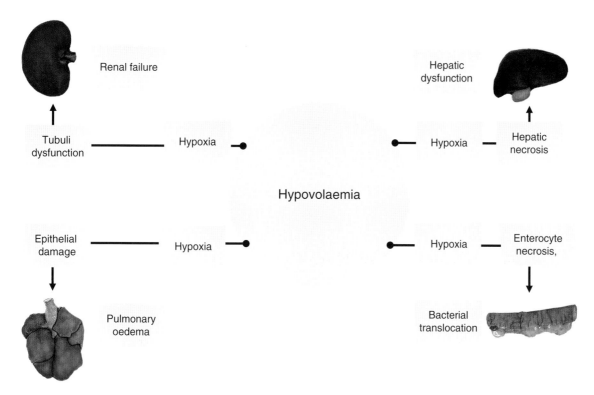

Figure 21.4 Hypoxia consequences on kidney, liver, intestine and lungs.

The consequence of hypovolaemic shock is a reduced supply of oxygen to the organs. In particular, the reduced oxygen supply leads to cellular hypoxia. This leads, among other things, to a switch from aerobic to anaerobic energy metabolism.

Anaerobic glycolysis is not only less efficient, it also leads to an increased accumulation of lactate and thus to metabolic acidosis. This, in turn, significantly disturbs cell metabolism and can lead to cell death.

The final hypoxic cell death is followed by organ dysfunction or organ failure. Both affect different organs differently.

Renally, the reduced perfusion can lead to acute renal failure. This reduces glomerular filtration and results in an increase in urinary substances (e.g. urea, creatinine) in the blood. The tubule cells are particularly sensitive to hypovolaemia, as they require a high amount of energy for their resorption capacity.

In the liver, reduced perfusion can lead to hepatocyte necrosis. The pericentral hepatocytes are particularly sensitive, as they are already in a physiologically potentially hypoxic state due to the sinusoidal supply of mixed blood.

The reduced blood supply to the intestinal wall disrupts the mucosal barrier via a dysfunction or necrosis of the enterocytes. As a result, enteric bacteria can be translocated.

Inflammatory reactions can be another consequence of hypovolaemia. In this case, the reduced blood flow in the end-stream pathway is in the foreground. In addition to capillary blood stasis with thrombus formation, hypoxic endothelial damage is followed by a release of proinflammatory mediators. This inflammatory reaction is involved in further organ dysfunction. In the lungs, hypoxia and inflammatory mediators lead to epithelial damage and thus to increased capillary permeability with alveolar pulmonary oedema (Figure 21.4).

Uroabdomen

Pathogenesis

The cause of uroabdomen is rupture of the urinary tract. Different causalities are possible. Ruptures due to trauma predominantly lead to ruptures at the confluence of the ureters with the bladder, at the apex of the bladder or at the beginning of the urethra. Iatrogenic causes are inadequately closed bladder sutures after stone removal or bladder tumour surgery, or perforation of the bladder during catheterisation. The latter leads either to a perforation in the area of the urinary bladder apex, or when catheterising urethral obstructions can lead to a perforation of the urethra. In particular, when calculi obstruct the urethra, there may be mucosal irritation due to pressure necrosis of the calculus, which facilitates perforation during catheterisation. Spontaneous ruptures of the urinary bladder have been described in chronic cystitis or with urinary bladder stones. In both cases, mucosal irritation occurs. Chronic cystitis is associated with infiltration of inflammatory cells including, mast cells, shows reduction or ulceration of the mucosal epithelium and glucosaminoglycan layer, and may be associated with fibrosis in advanced stages. All changes reduce the resistance of the bladder wall and can lead to rupture (Jones 2020).

Pathophysiologic Consequences

Influenced organs	Clinical symptoms	Clinical pathological alterations
Cardiovascular system	Lethargy	Azotaemia
Abdominal cavity	Anorexia	Metabolic acidosis
	Hypothermia	Hypercalcaemia
	Abdominal pain	Hypernatraemia
	Shock	Hyperphosphataemia
	Acute renal failure	

The main causality for the clinical symptoms of uroabdomen is the developing uraemia. Urine entering the abdomen can cause 'urinary substances' to be reabsorbed and re-enter the circulation.

The resorption of fluid from the peritoneal cavity is influenced by different forces and can lead to removal via the lymphatic vessels or, as is increasingly the case, via the capillaries. The driving forces are the intra-abdominal fluid pressure and the oncotic pressure prevailing there. Opposing forces are the interstitial hydrostatic and oncotic pressure (Stachowska-Pietka et al. 2006).

Accordingly, patients with uroabdomen develop uraemia with the clinical consequences described. Consequences such as **lethargy**, **anorexia** and **hypothermia** can be attributed to uraemic encephalopathy (Figure 21.5).

Some urinary substances act as neurotoxins on the central nervous system. Among others, such effects have been described for indoxyl sulphate, guanidine compounds, indole acid, phenols and carnitine. The mechanism by which the molecules act on the central nervous system is not fully understood. Dysbalances between inhibitory and excitatory neurotransmitters are possible. In uraemia, the cerebrospinal fluid (CSF) concentrations of glycine increase, while those of glutamine and γ-aminobutyric acid decrease.

It is possible that a disturbance in calcium metabolism due to renal hyperparathyroidism leads to neuronal disturbances, due to ion accumulation in the nerve cells.

Uraemic toxins also affect blood pressure-regulated neurons in the medulla oblongata. Changes in blood pressure also lead to reduced perfusion of neuronal areas with increased formation of reactive oxygen species and thus increased oxidative stress in the nerve cells.

Oxidative stress can alter mitochondrial function. Dysfunctional mitochondria increase oxidative stress, from which a vicious circle can develop (Olano et al. 2022).

Other reabsorbed urinary substances influence the acid-base balance, the fluid and electrolyte balance and the hormone metabolism.

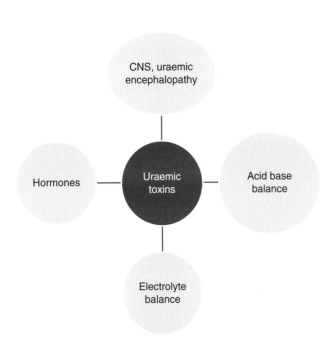

Figure 21.5 Pathophysiologic consequences of increased reabsorption of uremic toxins in uroabdomen.

Bile Peritonitis

Pathogenesis

Ruptures of the gallbladder and bile ducts are possible due to trauma, such as gunshot wounds, ruptures due to mucocele and tumour, or iatrogenic after previous surgery of the gallbladder or bile ducts (Baker et al. 2011).

Pathophysiologic Consequences

Influenced organs	Clinical symptoms	Clinical pathological alterations
Cardiovascular system	Shock	Elevated liver enzymes
Abdominal cavity	Painful abdomen	Bilirubinaemia
	Jaundice	

A major consequence is peritonitis. This results from the reaction of the peritoneum to the bile. Bile acids, in particular, are considered toxic. These can cause cell necrosis and increase the vascular permeability of the parietal vessels.

References

Baker, S.G., Mayhew, P.D., and Mehler, S.J. (2011). Choledochotomy and primary repair of extrahepatic biliary duct rupture in seven dogs and two cats. *The Journal of Small Animal Practice* 52 (1): 32–37. https://doi.org/10.1111/j.1748-5827.2010.01014.x.

Jones, E. (2020). Pathological and clinicopathological features of canine and feline bladder disease. PhD Thesis. 0000-0001-6462-1234.

Olano, C.G., Akram, S.M., and Bhatt, H. (2022). Uremic encephalopathy. In: *StatPearls*. Treasure Island (FL): StatPearls Publishing https://www.ncbi.nlm.nih.gov/books/NBK564327.

Stachowska-Pietka, J., Waniewski, J., Flessner, M.F., and Lindholm, B. (2006). Distributed model of peritoneal fluid absorption. *American Journal of Physiology. Heart and Circulatory Physiology* 291 (4): H1862–H1874. https://doi.org/10.1152/ajpheart.01320.2005.

Further Reading

Brockman, D.J., Mongil, C.M., Aronson, L.R., and Brown, D.C. (2000). A practical approach to hemoperitoneum in the dog and cat. *The Veterinary Clinics of North America. Small Animal Practice* 30 (3): 657–668. https://doi.org/10.1016/s0195-5616(00)50044-8.

Struller, F., Weinreich, F.J., Horvath, P. et al. (2017). Peritoneal innervation: embryology and functional anatomy. *Pleura and Peritoneum* 2 (4): 153–161. https://doi.org/10.1515/pp-2017-0024.

22

Fatigue

Definition

Fatigue is defined as a state of exhaustion that occurs in acute and chronic diseases of different aetiologies.

Aetiology

The causes of fatigue are manifold. Inflammatory and non-inflammatory diseases as well as tumour diseases are associated with the symptom complex.

Pathogenesis

The different causalities act via different mechanisms on the central nervous system and produce the symptom complex consisting of lethargy, inappetence and behavioural changes in the sense of withdrawal and seclusion. A distinction is made between effects emanating from proinflammatory cytokines and hormonal mechanisms.

Proinflammatory cytokines, primarily IL-1 and IL-6, are released by cells of the immune system, such as macrophages, dendritic cells and lymphocytes. They act by activating the parasympathetic nervous system (vagus nerve) or directly by transmitting the blood-brain barrier. IL-1 receptors are expressed in neurons and glial cells of the central nervous system (CNS) and allow a direct neuronal effect of the cytokine. IL-6 can be expressed in neurons under the influence of IL-1. Overall, the cytokine effects produce the symptom complex of fatigue through direct action on the neurons but also by influencing their metabolism (Quan and Banks 2007; Bluthé et al. 2000) (Figure 22.1).

Endocrine changes in fatigue syndrome are mainly related to the hypothalamic–pituitary–adrenal axis (HPA) and the thyroid hormone system. In particular, the depression of both systems negatively affects the overall metabolism. The exact mechanisms of reduction are not fully known. Proinflammatory cytokines also influence the systems here. Thus, T4 secretion and T3 action at the target cell are suppressed by proinflammatory cytokines.

Proinflammatory cytokines activate the HPA system at hypothalamic, pituitary and adrenergic levels, which leads to an increased synthesis of cortisol. However, cortisol inhibits inflammatory cell function, including cytokine production. The latter is initiated by the inhibitory effect of cortisol on the transcription factor NF-κB, the major proinflammatory transcription factor (Smoak and Cidlowski 2004; Zunszain and Anacker 2011).

In general, however, fatigue is associated with hypocortisolism. Accordingly, the cytokine effect and the HPA effect in fatigue could be two different regulatory circuits or describe a delaying effect. According to this, cortisol production would initially reflect the stress response to the disease causality, but over the time axis lead to adrenergic exhaustion by reducing the cytokine synthesis of inflammatory cells.

Another mechanism in the genesis of fatigue syndrome is oxidative stress. This arises from the increased synthesis of reactive oxygen species (ROS). Under physiological conditions, there is cellular homeostasis between mitochondrial ROS generation and the antioxidant capacities of the cell.

Textbook of Small Animal Pathophysiology, First Edition. Stephan Neumann.
© 2025 John Wiley & Sons Ltd. Published 2025 by John Wiley & Sons Ltd.

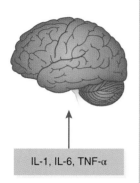

Cytokines can cross the blood-brain barrier and enter the central nervous system.

Fatigue pathways:

1. **Hypothalamus-Pituitary-Adrenal (HPA) Axis:** Cytokines can stimulate the HPA axis, leading to increased release of stress hormones.
2. **Serotonin pathway:** Cytokines can reduce the availability of tryptophan, a precursor to serotonin, affecting fatigue.
3. **Neuroinflammation:** Cytokines can cause neuroinflammation, affecting neurotransmitter function.
4. **Immune cell activity:** Cytokines divert energy towards immune response, potentially contributing to fatigue.
5. **Reduced dopamine:** Cytokines can lower dopamine levels, affecting motivation and energy.

IL-1, IL-6, TNF-α

Figure 22.1 Cytokine effects on the central nervous system.

Increased ROS generation or insufficient antioxidant protection systems lead to a shift in the redox balance, which disturbs redox signalling and damages cell structures above a certain ROS concentration. Oxidative stress, for its part, can stimulate the synthesis of proinflammatory cytokines and influence the fatigue syndrome through this mechanism.

References

Bluthé, R.M., Layé, S., Michaud, B. et al. (2000). Role of interleukin-1beta and tumour necrosis factor-alpha in lipopolysaccharide-induced sickness behaviour: a study with interleukin-1 type I receptor-deficient mice. *The European Journal of Neuroscience* 12 (12): 4447–4456.

Quan, N. and Banks, W.A. (2007). Brain-immune communication pathways. *Brain, Behaviour, and Immunity* 21 (6): 727–735. https://doi.org/10.1016/j.bbi.2007.05.005.

Smoak, K.A. and Cidlowski, J.A. (2004). Mechanisms of glucocorticoid receptor signalling during inflammation. *Mechanisms of Ageing and Development* 125 (10–11): 697–706.

Zunszain, P. and Anacker, C. (2011). Glucocorticoids, cytokines and brain abnormalities in depression. *Progress in Neuro-Psychopharmacology & Biological Psychiatry* 35 (3): 722–729.

Further Reading

Al Maqbali, M. (2021). Cancer-related fatigue: an overview. *British Journal of Nursing (Mark Allen Publishing)* 30 (4): S36–S43. doi: 10.12968/bjon.2021.30.4.S36.

Gregg, L.P., Bossola, M., Ostrosky-Frid, M., and Hedayati, S.S. (2021). Fatigue in CKD: epidemiology, pathophysiology, and treatment. *Clinical Journal of the American Society of Nephrology: CJASN* 16 (9): 1445–1455. https://doi.org/10.2215/CJN.19891220.

Nocerino, A., Nguyen, A., Agrawal, M. et al. (2020). Fatigue in inflammatory bowel diseases: etiologies and management. *Advances in Therapy* 37 (1): 97–112. https://doi.org/10.1007/s12325-019-01151-w.

Norheim, K.B., Jonsson, G., and Omdal, R. (2011). Biological mechanisms of chronic fatigue. *Rheumatology (Oxford, England)* 50 (6): 1009–1018. https://doi.org/10.1093/rheumatology/keq454.

Stanculescu, D., Larsson, L., and Bergquist, J. (2021). Theory: treatments for prolonged ICU patients may provide new therapeutic avenues for Myalgic encephalomyelitis/chronic fatigue syndrome (ME/CFS). *Frontiers in Medicine* 8: 672370. https://doi.org/10.3389/fmed.2021.672370.

23

Fever

Definition

Fever is defined as an increase in body temperature beyond normal daily variations. Often it is the result of an immune reaction associated with increased heat production. Body temperature and fever is controlled in the hypothalamus.

Physiological Basics

The body temperature fluctuates within narrow limits in the different regions of the body. The body surface is more variable than the core body temperature, which is usually kept constant. Maintaining a constant temperature is a prerequisite for the function of enzymes and thus for metabolism. There is a slight circadian variation in body temperature, whereby the temperature is somewhat lower in the morning than in the afternoon; this is related to the increased metabolism during the course of the day.

The regulation of body temperature takes place centrally in the hypothalamus. For this purpose, temperature is measured centrally and peripherally by thermoreceptors and transmitted to the hypothalamic neurons via afferents. Deviations from the optimal temperature are compensated for by different mechanisms of the temperature regulation centre.

For this purpose, circulation, metabolism, sweat production and muscle contraction can be influenced.

An **increase in body temperature** can be responded to by an increase in peripheral blood flow, this occurs by affecting arterio-venous shunts. As a result, heat can be released from the body surface. A second mechanism that starts with an increase in body temperature is the formation of sweat from eccrine sweat glands at different locations. As the fluid evaporates, heat is removed from the body through evaporative cooling. Since dogs and cats only have a few sweat glands, they use this effect by panting. In the process, cool air is passed along the mucous membrane surfaces of the upper respiratory tract, which absorbs heat and conducts it to the outside.

A **drop in body temperature** leads to peripheral vasoconstriction with the aim of reducing a loss of heat via the body surface. Corticoids and thyroid hormones increase metabolism, releasing heat. Brown adipose tissue is also capable of heat production.

In this process, under the influence of different mediators (e.g. noradrenaline, natriuretic peptides), the formation of ATP in the mitochondria is reduced in favour of heat.

In cell metabolism, various metabolic pathways produce energy and thus heat. The aerobic and anaerobic glycolysis are essential. The heat released during the metabolism of 1 mol of glucose corresponds to 2808 kJ.

Another way to produce heat in the event of a drop in body temperature is muscle tremors.

Aetiology

The main causes of fever are reactions of the immune system, either to infectious agents or to non-infectious inflammations, for example, autoimmune diseases or tumours.

Textbook of Small Animal Pathophysiology, First Edition. Stephan Neumann.
© 2025 John Wiley & Sons Ltd. Published 2025 by John Wiley & Sons Ltd.

Infection	Non-infection
Viral infection	Polyarthritis (D)
FeLV/FIV (C)	Glomerulonephritis (D/C)
FIP (C)	Lupus erythematosus (D)
Parvovirus (D/C)	Immune-mediated haemolytic anaemia (D/C)
Distemper (D)	Malignancies (D/C)
Bacterial infection (D/C)	
Gram positive	
Gram negative	
Parasites (D/C)	
Toxoplasma	
Leishmania	

D – Dog, C – Cat

Pathogenesis

Of the possible causalities, fever due to infection or sepsis is the most common. Triggering mediators for fever are called 'pyrogens'. These can be formed as exogenous pyrogens by microorganisms. They include lipopolysaccharides of the bacterial wall. Various cytokines, such as IL-1, IL-6, TNF-α or ceramides, act as endogenous pyrogens. The target organ of the pyrogens is the thermoregulation centre in the hypothalamus. This area is not separated from the vascular supply by a blood-brain barrier, so the cytokine effect takes place directly. Exogenous pyrogens produce fever through a direct neuronal effect on the thermoregulation centre, by inducing the synthesis of prostaglandins and via the cytokine pathway. After stimulation of the thermoregulation centre, prostanoids are synthesised there, which act on the preoptic nucleus of the hypothalamus and inhibit the impulse frequency of heat-reactive neurons there. The result is an increase in body temperature (Roth and De Souza 2001; Gross 2006).

The benefit of fever results from direct germ inhibition and stimulation of the defence systems. An increase in body temperature into the febrile range can significantly reduce the growth rate of bacteria (Small et al. 1986). In addition, an increase in the activity of neutrophilic granulocytes and other defence cells can be observed in fever (Rice et al. 2005).

Malignant diseases have also been described as triggers of fever. It is discussed causally that malignant diseases can promote bacterial infections due to reduced body defence and that this type of fever also develops. Furthermore, tumour necrosis in particular is associated with the synthesis of endogenous pyrogens, such as TNF-α (Toussaint et al. 2006) (Figure 23.1).

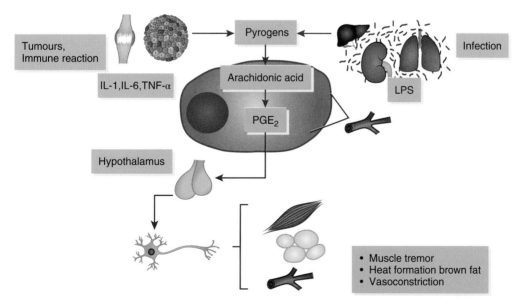

Figure 23.1 Mechanism of the fever.

Pathophysiologic Consequences

According to general observations, the protective functions of fever are lost when very high body temperatures are reached. The consequence is increased mortality (Lee et al. 2012). The damage caused by high fever is manifested at the cellular and systemic level. The cellular effects focus on structural changes of proteins and DNA molecules at high fever (>41.0°C). The former change their secondary and tertiary structure at high fever, and this is accompanied by a loss of function of the proteins. Heat shock proteins and chaperones are cellular molecules that produce a protective effect against overheating. However, their effect is insufficient if the temperature increase is persistent. Another negative effect of high fever at the cellular level is the disruption of membrane stability. Structural alteration of transmembrane transport proteins alters ion fluxes at the membrane, resulting in increased intracellular sodium concentration and decreased potassium concentration. The cell damage caused by high fever can lead to necrotic or apoptotic cell death (Walter et al. 2016).

Elevated body temperatures promote the expression of proinflammatory cytokines and subsequently of acute phase proteins. Thus, high body temperature has an inflammation-inducing effect. It is not completely clear whether the triggering factors are the causal pyrogens or whether the increase in body temperature per se can induce cytokine expression (Heled et al. 2013). In any case, the consequence is an inflammatory reaction that can show destructive as well as protective effects (see Chapter 1).

Finally, a variety of systemic consequences are associated with high body temperature.

The consequences of increased body temperature in the intestinal wall result from the cellular and local consequences described. Loss of protein function and inflammation disrupt the integrity of the intestinal wall resulting in bacterial translocation (Lambert 2004).

The renal consequences of high body temperatures can lead to acute renal failure. Described mechanisms are a temperature-dependent influence on the renal blood flow. Glomerular capillary dilation and interstitial haemorrhage occur. As a consequence, glomerular filtration is reduced and acute renal failure may develop (Vlad et al. 2010; Mustafa et al. 2007).

In the liver, high body temperature leads to increased permeability of the hepatocyte membrane with transaminase release. The mechanism corresponds to the cellular consequences of high body temperature. The same applies to the onset of myocardial and cerebral damage.

A final consequence is the influence of high body temperature on blood coagulation. Inhibited platelet aggregation and disseminated intravascular coagulopathy are observed. The hepatic consequences of high body temperature are discussed as the cause (Diehl et al. 2000) (Figure 23.2).

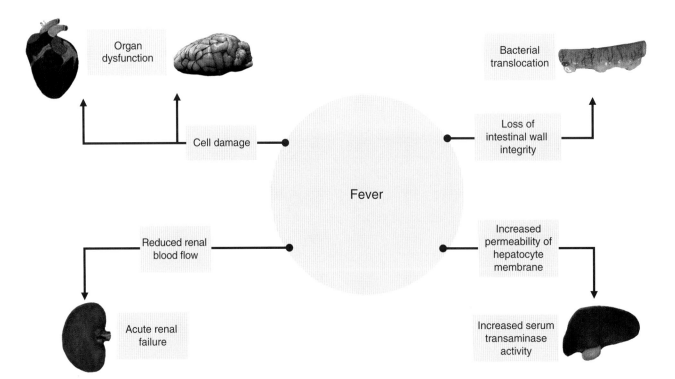

Figure 23.2 Influence of fever on various organs.

References

Diehl, K.A., Crawford, E., Shinko, P.D. et al. (2000). Alterations in hemostasis associated with hyperthermia in a canine model. *American Journal of Hematology* 64 (4): 262–270. https://doi.org/10.1002/1096-8652(200008)64:4<262:: aid-ajh5>3.0.co;2-d.

Gross, L. (2006). Anatomy of a fever. *PLoS Biology* 4 (9): e305. https://doi.org/10.1371/journal.pbio.0040305.

Heled, Y., Fleischmann, C., and Epstein, Y. (2013). Cytokines and their role in hyperthermia and heat stroke. *Journal of Basic and Clinical Physiology and Pharmacology* 24 (2): 85–96. https://doi.org/10.1515/jbcpp-2012-0040.

Lambert, G.P. (2004). Role of gastrointestinal permeability in exertional heatstroke. *Exercise and Sport Sciences Reviews* 32 (4): 185–190. https://doi.org/10.1097/00003677-200410000-00011.

Lee, B.H., Inui, D., Suh, G.Y. et al. (2012). Association of body temperature and antipyretic treatments with mortality of critically ill patients with and without sepsis: multi-centre prospective observational study. *Critical Care (London, England)* 16 (1): R33. https://doi.org/10.1186/cc11211.

Mustafa, S., Elgazzar, A.H., Essam, H. et al. (2007). Hyperthermia alters kidney function and renal scintigraphy. *American Journal of Nephrology* 27 (3): 315–321. https://doi.org/10.1159/000102597.

Rice, P., Martin, E., He, J.R. et al. (2005). Febrile-range hyperthermia augments neutrophil accumulation and enhances lung injury in experimental gram-negative bacterial pneumonia. *Journal of Immunology (Baltimore, Md.: 1950)* 174 (6): 3676–3685. 10.4049/jimmunol.174.6.3676.

Roth, J. and De Souza, G.E. (2001). Fever induction pathways: evidence from responses to systemic or local cytokine formation. *Brazilian Journal Of Medical and Biological Research = Revista brasileira de pesquisas medicas e biologicas* 34 (3): 301–314. https://doi.org/10.1590/s0100-879x2001000300003.

Small, P.M., Täuber, M.G., Hackbarth, C.J., and Sande, M.A. (1986). Influence of body temperature on bacterial growth rates in experimental pneumococcal meningitis in rabbits. *Infection and Immunity* 52 (2): 484–487. https://doi.org/10.1128/iai.52.2.484-487.1986.

Toussaint, E., Bahel-Ball, E., Vekemans, M. et al. (2006). Causes of fever in cancer patients (prospective study over 477 episodes). *Supportive Care in Cancer: Official Journal of the Multinational Association of Supportive Care in Cancer* 14 (7): 763–769. https://doi.org/10.1007/s00520-005-0898-0.

Vlad, M., Ionescu, N., Ispas, A.T. et al. (2010). Morphological changes during acute experimental short-term hyperthermia. *Romanian Journal of Morphology and Embryology = Revue roumaine de morphologie et embryologie* 51 (4): 739–744.

Walter, E.J., Hanna-Jumma, S., Carraretto, M. et al. (2016). The pathophysiological basis and consequences of fever. *Critical Care* 20: 200. https://doi.org/10.1186/s13054-016-1375-5.

Further Reading

Mota-Rojas, D., Wang, D., Titto, C.G. et al. (2021). Pathophysiology of fever and application of infrared thermography (IRT) in the detection of sick domestic animals: recent advances. *Animals: An Open Access Journal from MDPI* 11 (8): 2316. https://doi.org/10.3390/ani11082316.

24

Inappetence

Definition

Inappetence is defined as a lack of appetite, i.e. food is refused. The more severe form with complete refusal of food is called 'anorexia'.

Aetiology

Lack of appetite is usually due to a systemic disease. It is to be distinguished from swallowing difficulties of various kinds, in which the animals show appetite but cannot adequately take in or swallow the food. The latter symptoms do not belong to inappetence. The systemic diseases can originate from all organ systems, since the mechanism of inappetence is controlled by cytokines, whose synthesis is organ-independent and disease-related.

Metabolic diseases	Thoracic diseases	Abdominal diseases	Miscellaneous
Hypoadrenocorticism (D)	Heart failure (D/C)	Gastrointestinal tract (D/C)	Inflammation (D/C)
Ketoacidosis (D)	Respiratory diseases (D/C)	Liver (D/C)	Pain (D/C)
		Pancreas (D/C)	
		Kidneys (D/C)	

D – Dog, C – Cat

Pathogenesis

Inappetence or anorexia accompany disease complexes of different genesis and are partly responsible for the prognosis of the disease process. Anorexia is presumably mediated by proinflammatory cytokines whose target organ is the satiety and hunger centre. Both represent anatomical structures in the area of the hypothalamus. The arcuate nucleus and the paraventricular nucleus are described. These are reached by mediators from the periphery via the blood-brain barrier, which is permeable in the nucleus arcuatus (Kastin and Pan 2000).

Consistently, diseases associated with anorexia show increased levels of circulating proinflammatory cytokines. For example, TNF-α, IL-1 and IL-6 are elevated in heart failure, renal failure as well as in neoplastic patients (Levine et al. 1990; Kalantar-Zadeh et al. 2005; Braun and Marks 2010). Cytokines have been shown to have a direct influence on hypothalamic centres (Sonti et al. 1996). Another mode through which proinflammatory cytokines can influence neuronal activity is the synthesis of prostaglandins. These are synthesised either in endothelial cells or perivascular macrophages under the influence of cytokines, cross the blood-brain barrier and act on neuronal prostaglandin receptors (Ericsson et al. 1997; Nakamura et al. 2000).

Inflammatory cytokines from the circulation or produced locally by microglia act directly on hypothalamic neurons. The activity of anorectic neurons (pro-opiomelanocortin (POMC)) is stimulated, while the activity of orexigenic neurons (agouti-related peptide/Neuropeptide Y (AgRP/NPY)) is inhibited. This leads to reduced food intake and increased energy consumption.

Pathophysiologic Consequences

The pathophysiologic consequences of inappetence affect all organs and are thus to be considered systemic.

Influenced organ systems	Clinical symptoms	Clinical pathological alterations
Systemic	Bradycardia	Electrolyte imbalances
	Hypotension	Nutritional deficiencies
	Hypothermia	
	Bone marrow suppression	
	Neuropathy	
	Myopathy	
	Dehydration	
	Weight loss	

The clinical consequences of inappetence and anorexia have been extensively researched in human medicine. The courses of the disease are not always completely compatible between humans and dogs and cats, but numerous parallels can be found, which will now be focused on.

A very important long-term consequence is the loss of body mass. This is described in detail in Chapter 35.

In general, the following consequences are described:

Nutritional deficiencies: When dogs and cats stop eating, they may not be getting enough nutrients and energy from their food, leading to nutritional deficiencies. This can weaken their immune system, make them more susceptible to infections and affect their overall health.

Weight loss: Inappetence can cause significant weight loss in dogs and cats. This can be especially concerning in animals that are already underweight.

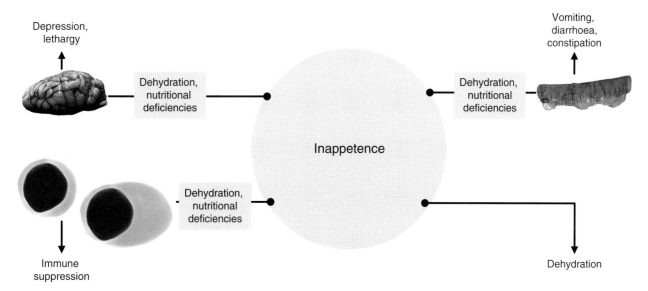

Figure 24.1 Pathophysiologic consequences of inappetence.

Dehydration: If dogs and cats are not eating, they may also be drinking less water, which can lead to dehydration. Dehydration can be very dangerous and even life-threatening, especially in young or older animals.

Gastrointestinal problems: Inappetence can also lead to gastrointestinal problems such as constipation, vomiting and diarrhoea. This can further worsen the animal's condition and lead to further health complications.

Behavioural changes: In some cases, inappetence may also lead to behavioural changes such as lethargy, depression and irritability. These changes can be due to underlying medical conditions or pain that is making it difficult for the animal to eat (Figure 24.1).

References

Braun, T.P. and Marks, D.L. (2010). Pathophysiology and treatment of inflammatory anorexia in chronic disease. *Journal of Cachexia, Sarcopenia and Muscle* 1 (2): 135–145. https://doi.org/10.1007/s13539-010-0015-1.

Ericsson, A., Arias, C., and Sawchenko, P.E. (1997). Evidence for an intramedullary prostaglandin-dependent mechanism in the activation of stress-related neuroendocrine circuitry by intravenous interleukin-1. *The Journal of Neuroscience: The Official Journal of the Society for Neuroscience* 17 (18): 7166–7179. https://doi.org/10.1523/JNEUROSCI.17-18-07166.1997.

Kalantar-Zadeh, K., Stenvinkel, P., Bross, R. et al. (2005). Kidney insufficiency and nutrient-based modulation of inflammation. *Current Opinion in Clinical Nutrition and Metabolic Care* 8 (4): 388–396. https://doi.org/10.1097/01.mco.0000172578.56396.9e.

Kastin, A.J. and Pan, W. (2000). Dynamic regulation of leptin entry into brain by the blood-brain barrier. *Regulatory Peptides* 92 (1–3): 37–43. https://doi.org/10.1016/s0167-0115(00)00147-6.

Levine, B., Kalman, J., Mayer, L. et al. (1990). Elevated circulating levels of tumor necrosis factor in severe chronic heart failure. *The New England Journal of Medicine* 323 (4): 236–241. https://doi.org/10.1056/NEJM199007263230405.

Nakamura, K., Kaneko, T., Yamashita, Y. et al. (2000). Immunohistochemical localization of prostaglandin EP3 receptor in the rat nervous system. *The Journal of Comparative Neurology* 421 (4): 543–569. https://doi.org/10.1002/(sici)1096-9861(20000612)421:4<543::aid-cne6>3.0.co;2-3.

Sonti, G., Ilyin, S.E., and Plata-Salamán, C.R. (1996). Anorexia induced by cytokine interactions at pathophysiological concentrations. *The American Journal of Physiology* 270 (6 Pt 2): R1394–R1402. https://doi.org/10.1152/ajpregu.1996.270.6.R1394.

25

Jaundice

Definition

Jaundice is defined as yellowing of the skin, mucous membranes and internal organs as a result of hyperbilirubinaemia. Jaundice usually becomes visible from a bilirubin serum concentration of 2 mg/dl.

Physiological Basics

Erythrocytes are eliminated by the cells of the mononuclear phagocyte system (MPS) in the spleen, bone marrow or liver after reaching their maximum age (dog–approximately 100 days, cat–approximately 70 days) or if they are pathologically changed.

In the process, haemoglobin is first split into haem and the globin residue. The latter is broken down to amino acids. The degradation of haem to bilirubin occurs in two steps. First, haem binds to an enzyme, haem oxygenase. This is followed by the reduction of iron III (Fe^{3+}) to iron II (Fe^{2+}), which is catalysed by cytochrome C P450 reductase. After the release of Fe^{2+}, the haem molecule is broken down into biliverdin and carbon monoxide (CO), which is exhaled through the lungs.

In the second step, the biliverdin is reduced to unconjugated bilirubin by the cytosolically localised enzyme, biliverdin reductase. Finally, bilirubin is transported freely in the blood in low concentrations, but is mainly transported to the liver bound to albumin. In the sinusoidal blood, the albumin-bilirubin complex is bound to receptors on the hepatocyte membrane and absorbed.

An ester bond between bilirubin and glucuronic acid, catalysed by uridine diphosphate-glycosyl transferase (UDP-glycosyl transferase), first produces bilirubin monoglucuronide and then bilirubin diglucuronide. The now conjugated and thus water-soluble bilirubin is released from the hepatocytes into the bile via active transport. From there, conjugated bilirubin enters the intestine and is excreted as stercobilinogen and urobilinogen or is partially transported back to the liver via the enterohepatic circulation.

Aetiology

As jaundice is a clinical syndrome of disturbed bilirubin metabolism, any factor influencing bilirubin metabolism can trigger jaundice. These include prehepatic causes in which increased bilirubin is released due to erythrocyte metabolism disorders. Hepatic causes are primarily due to disorders in the elimination of bilirubin metabolites.

Prehepatic	Intrahepatic	Posthepatic
Haemolytic anaemia (D/C)	Hepatic necrosis (D/C)	Bile duct obstruction (D/C)
Internal haemorrhage (D/C)	Hepatic lipidosis (C)	Pancreatic diseases (D/C)
Porphyria (D)	Hepatic fibrosis (D/C)	
	Hepatic cirrhosis (D)	
	Hepatic neoplasia (D/C)	

D – Dog, C – Cat

Pathogenesis

An increase in the bilirubin concentration in the blood serum can be caused by hepatopathies or haemolyses. In principle, hydrophobic bilirubin should be detected in the first instance in the case of a haemolysis-related increase in the bilirubin serum concentration (hyperbilirubinaemia) and hydrophilic bilirubin in the blood in the case of liver-related hyperbilirubinaemia. In practice, however, it has been shown that both are possible and can therefore be of little diagnostic use. Due to its colour, bilirubin produces the so-called 'icterus' at an increased blood concentration. From a serum concentration of about 2 mg/dl, this is clinically recognisable by the yellowing of the sclerae. Depending on the localisation of its development, prehepatic haemolytic jaundice is distinguished from intrahepatic jaundice and the latter from posthepatic cholestatic jaundice. Jaundice is primarily a symptom, but can also cause secondary diseases. Under the influence of an increased bilirubin concentration, pigment crystals or even pigment gallstones can form in the bile ducts. Finally, hydrophobic bilirubin shows toxic properties by inhibiting RNA and protein synthesis, as well as the inhibition of ATP-ases. The determination of bilirubin in the blood is not very suitable to reflect the nature of a liver disease.

Cholestasis, a frequent cause of hyperbilirubinaemia, leads to the retention of bile-obliging substances by halting bile excretion. The cause does not necessarily have to be the 'classic' bile stasis in posthepatic occlusive jaundice due to obstruction of the extrahepatic bile ducts; intrahepatic disorders with stagnation of bile production can also lead to cholestasis.

Pathophysiologically, the development of cholestasis or liver damage caused by cholestasis is based on a dilation of the bile ducts with a reduction in the fluidity and damage of the canalicular liver cell membrane due to bile salt action and cholesterol storage (Hyogo et al. 2000). This leads to deformations of the brush border of the cell membrane. In order to reduce the intracellular concentration of toxic bile salts, the ATP-dependent so-called 'multidrug resistance protein' (MRP) carriers are incorporated into the basolateral membrane of the liver cell (Alrefai and Gill 2007). The reduction of intracellular bile salts increases their concentration in the bile ducts; together with the increased biliary pressure in cholestasis, this leads to an increasing permeability of the intercellular tight-junctions, whereby the bile components enter the blood vessel system of the liver.

Pathophysiologic Consequences

The pathophysiologic consequences of jaundice result primarily from the underlying disease. Some clinical symptoms associated with increased retention of bile components include pruritus. This is more likely to be observed in humans than in dogs and cats as a result of cholestasis.

Bile acids are known to stimulate nerve fibres in the skin, which leads to itching. In addition, the accumulation of bile acids in the blood can lead to the release of histamine, which can also contribute to itching.

The consequences of jaundice are not only the increased concentration of bile components in the body. Their absence in the intestine is also disadvantageous.

Severe cholestasis with bile acid deficiency in the small intestine initially leads to digestive disorders and malabsorption of lipids and fat-soluble vitamins. The intraluminal deficiency of bile salts also leads to both mucosal damage of the intestinal wall and changes in the endogenous bacterial flora with overgrowth by Enterobacteriaceae. This in turn promotes bacterial translocation from the gut and results in portal bacteraemia and endotoxaemia (Figure 25.1).

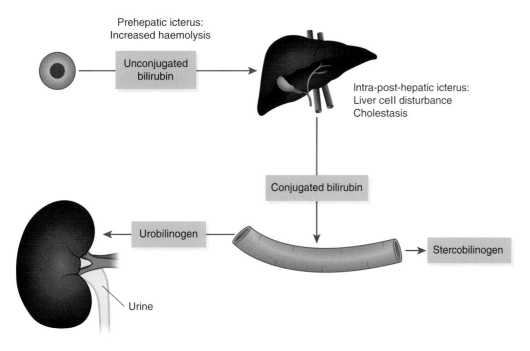

Figure 25.1 Pathophysiology of jaundice.

References

Alrefai, W.A. and Gill, R.K. (2007). Bile acid transporters: structure, function, regulation and pathophysiological implications. *Pharmaceutical Research* 24 (10): 1803–1823. https://doi.org/10.1007/s11095-007-9289-1.

Hyogo, H., Tazuma, S., and Kajiyama, G. (2000). Biliary excretory function is regulated by canalicular membrane fluidity associated with phospholipid fatty acyl chains in the bilayer: implications for the pathophysiology of cholestasis. *Journal of Gastroenterology and Hepatology* 15 (8): 887–894. https://doi.org/10.1046/j.1440-1746.2000.02221.x.

Further Reading

Ghenu, M.I., Dragoş, D., Manea, M.M. et al. (2022). Pathophysiology of sepsis-induced cholestasis: a review. *JGH Open: An Open Access Journal of Gastroenterology and Hepatology* 6 (6): 378–387. https://doi.org/10.1002/jgh3.12771.

Krell, H. and Enderle, G.J. (1993). Cholestasis: pathophysiology and pathobiochemistry. *Zeitschrift für Gastroenterologie* 31 (Suppl 2): 11–15.

26

Oedema

Definition

Oedema is swelling or fluid retention caused by an increase in interstitial fluid.

Aetiology

The causes of oedema formation are increased water retention as a result of excretory insufficiencies, for example, in renal failure. Or they are caused by an increase in hydrostatic pressure in venous insufficiency. Another reason is a reduction in vascular oncotic pressure in protein deficiency diseases or increased capillary permeability in inflammatory oedema. Finally, lymphatic drainage disorders can lead to oedema or increased interstitial osmotic pressure due to overproduction of collagen and mucopolysaccharides.

Hydrostatic	Oncotic	Inflammatory
Right heart failure (D)	Protein-loosing	
Lymphatic drainage disorder (D/C)	Enteropathy (D)	
	Nephropathy (D/C)	

D – Dog, C – Cat

Pathogenesis

Hydrostatic oedema develops when the hydrostatic pressure in the vessels increases. This can be the consequence of right heart insufficiency, where venous blood stagnates because the drainage through the right side of the heart is reduced. Blood pressure rises in the venous vessels. This can affect and reduce the removal of interstitial fluid. As a result, oedema develops. Obstructions in the venous vascular system, for example, as a result of thrombi, lead to a comparable effect.

Oncotic oedema occurs when the oncotic pressure in the vascular system decreases. This is the consequence of reduced protein synthesis, mainly albumin, in the liver. Albumin is synthesised exclusively in the liver. A deficiency of albumin lowers the oncotic pressure and leads to oedema formation. In addition to synthesis disorders, protein loss disorders can also lead to hypoproteinaemia, which lowers the oncotic pressure in the vascular system. Protein loss can occur when the renal threshold is lowered by glomerulopathies, and molecules with a mass > 50 000 KDa can pass through the glomerulum. Malabsorption and protein loss via the intestine also lead to hypoproteinaemia. If the oncotic pressure in the vascular system decreases, the hydrostatic pressure in the physiological range can cause fluid filtration into the tissue. In the tissue, the hydrostatic pressure rises and the colloid osmotic tissue pressure falls due to the diluting effect of the filtered fluid. This counteracts filtration and increases lymphatic drainage. For this reason, oedema formation is not progressive from a steady state.

Textbook of Small Animal Pathophysiology, First Edition. Stephan Neumann.
© 2025 John Wiley & Sons Ltd. Published 2025 by John Wiley & Sons Ltd.

Inflammatory oedema occurs when an inflammatory process increases vascular permeability in the area of inflammation. The result is increased fluid leakage. In addition, blood flow is increased in the area of inflammation, which can increase the hydrostatic pressure in the vessels and thus further increase leakage. However, inflammatory secretions increase colloid osmotic pressure in the interstitium, which further promotes leakage from the vessels. Finally, during the inflammatory process, increased hydrolytic enzymes are released by phagocytosing cells. These in turn lead to degradation of the surrounding tissue, which further increases the colloid osmotic pressure.

Lymphoedema develops when lymphatic drainage is interrupted. This is particularly the case when inflammation or trauma compresses or ruptures the lymph ducts. However, more than half of the local lymph ducts must be insufficient; otherwise, collaterals can continue to ensure drainage.

Finally, **myxoedema** is a special form due to increased synthesis of collagens and mucopolysaccharides by fibroblasts. These can increase water retention due to colloid osmotic forces. Myxoedema is particularly described in hypothyroidism.

Pathophysiologic Consequences

Oedema formation has different pathophysiologic consequences. These include an increase in the diffusion distance, in the case of fluid accumulation in the interstitium. This reduces the cellular supply of oxygen or nutrients. The same applies to the removal of cellular waste products. In addition, oedema can cause problems especially where there are natural limits to tissue volume increase. This includes the kidneys, for example. The fibrous kidney capsule limits swelling of the kidney. The same applies to the brain, where the skull bone limits the volume increase in brain oedema. Muscles also cannot increase much in the compartment. The consequence of the limited volume increase is an increase in tissue pressure. This can compress cells, which can lead to apoptosis or necrosis. At the very least, however, an increase in pressure leads to compression of the vessels, which further impedes supply and disposal.

Pulmonary oedema is a special form of oedema. In most cases, it is the result of an altered hydrostatic pressure caused by cardiac insufficiency. Inflammatory changes in the lung parenchyma can increase the permeability of the vessel walls through the activity of inflammatory mediators. If the alveolar capillaries are affected, pulmonary oedema results. Cadherins play a special role in increasing vascular permeability. These are glycoproteins that establish a connection between cells. The cadherins are connected intracellularly with the cytoskeleton. Destruction of the cadherins leads to an increase in permeability in blood vessels with leakage of blood cells and blood plasma (Figure 26.1).

Figure 26.1 Cell-to-cell contact via cadherins.

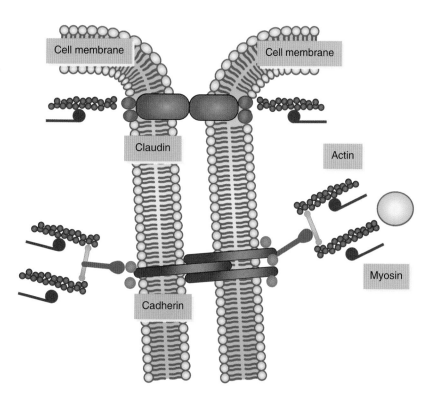

Further Reading

Davis, M.J. (1988). Microvascular control of capillary pressure during increases in local arterial and venous pressure. *The American Journal of Physiology* 254 (4 Pt 2): H772–H784. https://doi.org/10.1152/ajpheart.1988.254.4.H772.

Dongaonkar, R.M., Quick, C.M., Stewart, R.H. et al. (2008). Edemagenic gain and interstitial fluid volume regulation. *American Journal of Physiology. Regulatory, Integrative and Comparative Physiology* 294 (2): R651–R659. https://doi.org/10.1152/ajpregu.00354.2007.

Jerome, S.N., Akimitsu, T., and Korthuis, R.J. (1994). Leukocyte adhesion, edema, and development of postischemic capillary no-reflow. *The American Journal of Physiology* 267 (4 Pt 2): H1329–H1336. https://doi.org/10.1152/ajpheart.1994.267.4.H1329.

Scallan, J., Huxley, V.H., and Korthuis, R.J. (2010). Chapter 4, Pathophysiology of edema formation. In: *Capillary Fluid Exchange: Regulation, Functions, and Pathology*. San Rafael (CA): Morgan & Claypool Life Sciences.

27

Polyphagia

Definition

Polyphagia is defined as an increased food intake.

Physiological Basics

The intake of food is an essential, life-preserving activity. Food intake is controlled by the hypothalamus. A hunger centre and a satiety centre are distinguished. The two centres are triggered by different triggers. When the blood glucose concentration is elevated, more insulin is produced to lower the blood glucose concentration through cellular uptake; at the same time, the insulin activates the satiety centre.

The stretching of the stomach wall causes the release of enteral hormones, such as glucagon like peptide 1 and stimulates the satiety centre. The same applies to the secretion of cholecystokinin (CCK) after the ingestion of a fat-containing food.

Other hormones that regulate food intake are listed in Table 27.1.

Aetiology

Clinically, a distinction is made between hyperphagia and polyphagia. *Hyperphagia* is defined as an increased food intake depending on physiological processes. These include cold weather, excitement or pregnancy. Polyphagia is based on a pathomechanism. The different aetiologies cause polyphagia through increased metabolic activity or are signs of compensation for the organism in the case of disturbed digestion in the sense of malassimilation or malabsorption (Figure 27.1).

Endocrine	Metabolic	Physiological
Diabetes mellitus (D/C)	Exocrine pancreas insufficiency (D)	Exercise (D/C)
Hyperadrenocorticism (D)	Malabsorption (D/C)	Pregnancy (D/C)
Hyperthyroidism (C)		Lactation (D/C)
Acromegaly (D/C)		
Insulinoma (D)		

D – Dog, C – Cat

Pathogenesis

Increased food intake is often related to a disturbance in caloric balance. This may be the case when calories are consumed more, for example, in connection with pregnancy. In such cases, the energy consumed under normal circumstances is not sufficient to meet the needs.

Textbook of Small Animal Pathophysiology, First Edition. Stephan Neumann.
© 2025 John Wiley & Sons Ltd. Published 2025 by John Wiley & Sons Ltd.

Table 27.1 Hormones with influence on food intake.

Hormone	Synthesis	Function
Ghrelin	Gastrointestinal	Feeling hungry
Amylin	ß-cells pancreas	Sense of satiety
Leptin	Fatty tissue	Sense of satiety
Neuropeptide Y	Brain, stomach	Feeling hungry
Melanin concentrating hormone (MCH)	Brain	Feeling hungry
Serotonin	Brain, stomach	Feeling hungry

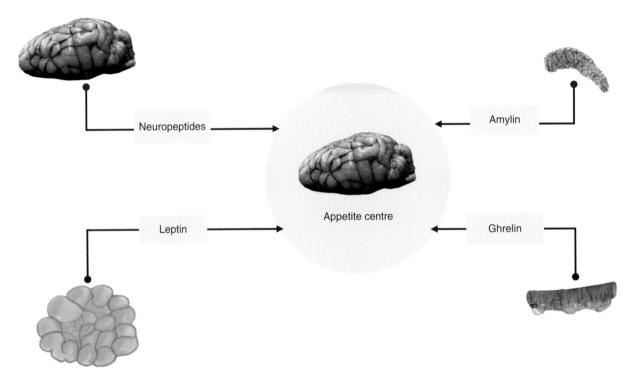

Figure 27.1 Hormonal effects on the appetite centre.

These are to be distinguished from diseases in which the demand for absorbed energy increases due to an increased metabolism. An example of this is hyperthyroidism. In the context of maldigestion, there is a reduced supply of energy via disturbed digestion, which stimulates the hunger centre; the same applies to a loss of energy, for example, due to protein losses via the kidneys and intestines. Finally, appetite can be stimulated directly by corticoids, so that an excess of hormones can lead to polyphagia.

Pathophysiologic Consequences

Influenced organ systems	Clinical symptoms	Clinical pathological alterations
Cardiovascular system	Obesity	Depending on the primary disease
Respiratory system	Exercise intolerance	
Systemic		

The pathophysiologic consequences of polyphagia develop primarily as a consequence of obesity and are described in detail in Chapter 5.

Further Reading

Barakat, B. and Almeida, M. (2021). Biochemical and immunological changes in obesity. *Archives of Biochemistry and Biophysics* 708: 108951. https://doi.org/10.1016/j.abb.2021.108951.

Camilleri, M. (2015). Peripheral mechanisms in appetite regulation. *Gastroenterology* 148 (6): 1219–1233. https://doi.org/10.1053/j.gastro.2014.09.016.

28

Pruritus

Definition

Pruritus is a sensation variation of the skin. This produces itching.

Physiological Basics

Itching has a physiological and a pathological component. Physiologically, itching serves to recognise and remove a harmful noxious substance from the skin. Pathologically, itching is an accompanying symptom of dermatological and internal diseases with loss of physiological function.

Itching is caused by an irritation of the free nerve endings, which are located at the junction of the epidermis and the dermis; they are activated by inflammatory mediators. The nerve irritation transmits an impulse to the central nervous system (CNS) via afferent nerve pathways and there, in the association centre, the sensation of pruritus develops. In addition to the peripheral triggering of pruritus, the triggering of itch via the stimulation of opiate receptors in the CNS has also been described (Schmelz 2002) (Table 28.1).

Aetiology

In addition to skin diseases, some internal diseases are also associated with pruritus.

Skin	Miscellaneous
Dermatitis (D/C)	Hypereosinophilic syndrome (C)
Immune-mediated (D/C)	Mast cell tumour (D/C)
Atopy	Hyperthyroidism (C)
Pemphigus	Hyperadrenocorticism (D)
Infection (D/C)	Hypothyroidism (D)
Bacterial	
Fungal	
Parasitic	

D – Dog, C – Cat

Pathogenesis

The actual skin diseases lead to itching via the mechanism described above. In the case of internal diseases, secondary skin changes are often the ultimate triggering factor for itching. In hyperadrenocorticism, itching is associated with calcinosis cutis. In hypothyroidism, secondary dermatitis is often associated with pruritus. In hyperthyroidism of the cat, pruritus is

Textbook of Small Animal Pathophysiology, First Edition. Stephan Neumann.

Table 28.1 Mediators of pruritus triggering.

Mediator	Mechanism
Histamine	Nerve irritation
Opioids	Opioid receptors
Cytokines (e.g. IL-2)	Mediator release
Prostaglandins	Potentiating histamine effect

Source: Ständer et al. (2003).

explained by increased behavioural activity. Neoplastic or inflammatory diseases, such as the eosinophilic syndrome of the cat and mast cell tumours are to be distinguished from this. In both cases, increased synthesis and release of mediators are the triggering factors for the itch.

Pathophysiologic Consequences

Influenced organ systems	Clinical symptoms
Skin	Dermatitis

The consequences of itching are pathologically concentrated on the skin. Destruction of the upper layers of the epidermis develops due to the recurrent mechanical irritation. This reduces the mechanical protection against infection, which can facilitate bacterial skin infection. In addition, chronic itching, in particular, can significantly affect the animal's behaviour.

References

Schmelz, M. (2002). Itch-mediators and mechanisms. *Journal of Dermatological Science* 28 (2): 91–96. https://doi.org/10.1016/s0923-1811(01)00167-0.

Ständer, S., Weisshaar, E., Steinhof, M. et al. (2003). Pruritus-pathophysiology, clinical features and therapy--an overview. *Journal der Deutschen Dermatologischen Gesellschaft = Journal of the German Society of Dermatology: JDDG* 1 (2): 105–118. https://doi.org/10.1046/j.1610-0387.2003.02023.x.

29

Regurgitation

Definition

Regurgitation is the pathological backflow of food from the oesophagus into the mouth.

Physiological Basics

The act of swallowing begins with a voluntarily controllable shift of the bolus into the pharyngeal region. This is triggered by pressing the tongue against the palate, whereby the pressure runs from the tip of the tongue to the base of the tongue. Once the bolus has reached the pharynx, the further act of swallowing is involuntary, reflexive. The nervous centre for the control of the swallowing act is located in the medulla oblongata, with afferents transmitting impulses via cranial nerves V, IX and X and efferents via cranial nerves VII, IX, X and XII. Before swallowing, the soft palate is pressed against the nasopharynx and the epiglottis closes the larynx, thus preventing the food bolus from inhalation. When the food bolus reaches the oesophagus, its sphincter relaxes and the food can enter the oesophagus. Peristaltic waves of the oesophageal muscles transport the food bolus towards the distal oesophageal sphincter. Peristalsis is triggered more strongly by solid food than by soft or liquid food. After relaxation of the distal oesophageal sphincter, the bolus can enter the stomach.

Aetiology

The causes of regurgitation can be local to the oesophagus or diseases that affect the motility of the oesophagus. These include neuronal diseases as well as systemic diseases. The diseases are much more common in dogs than in cats.

Oesophageal	Neurological	Systemic
Megaoesophagus (D)	Myasthenia gravis (D)	Hypothyroidism (D)
Oesophagus stricture (D/C)		Hypoadrenocorticism (D)
		Systemic lupus erythematosus (D)

D – Dog, C – Cat

Pathogenesis

The different aetiologies act on the oesophagus via two main mechanisms and cause regurgitation. Firstly, they can cause oesophageal obstruction, resulting in the food bolus coming to rest in front of the stenosis and being regurgitated via retracting peristalsis.

Textbook of Small Animal Pathophysiology, First Edition. Stephan Neumann.
© 2025 John Wiley & Sons Ltd. Published 2025 by John Wiley & Sons Ltd.

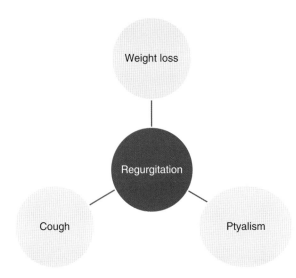

Figure 29.1 Consequences of regurgitation.

On the other hand, systemic diseases in particular lead to the symptom via oesophageal hypomotility. Immunological mechanisms are in the foreground here. In myasthenia gravis, 'autoantibodies' bind to the postsynaptic membrane and reduce the formation of a postsynaptic action potential. Other diseases such as hypothyroidism, hypoadrenocorticism and lupus erythematosus are also associated with the symptom of regurgitation. Since the diseases listed are also autoimmune events, a similar mechanism can be suspected.

Pathophysiologic Consequences

Influenced organ systems	Clinical symptoms
Respiratory system	Dysphagia
Gastrointestinal system	Cough
Neuromuscular system	Weight loss
	Ptyalism

The clinical consequences of regurgitation can include aspiration pneumonia, weight loss and oesophagitis.

Aspiration pneumonia occurs when food or liquid is inhaled into the lungs, leading to inflammation and infection. This can induce severe systemic symptoms like fever, inappetence, depressed behaviour and **cough**. The latest is the most common symptom and it is present at the early beginning of the aspiration pneumonia.

Weight loss can occur due to reduced food intake and poor absorption of nutrients from the digestive system. In consequence animals can have a reduced body condition (BCS). This can be one of the first clinical signs of the disease.

Oesophagitis is inflammation of the oesophagus that can occur as a result of prolonged exposure to food. This can induce **ptyalism**. This clinical symptom is rare compared to the described symptoms (Figure 29.1).

Further Reading

Whitehead, K., Cortes, Y., and Eirmann, L. (2016). Gastrointestinal dysmotility disorders in critically ill dogs and cats. *Journal of Veterinary Emergency and Critical Care (San Antonio, Tex.: 2001)* 26 (2): 234–253.

Mace, S., Shelton, G.D., and Eddlestone, S. (2012). Megaesophagus. *Compendium (Yardley, PA)* 34 (2): E1.

30

Seizure

Definition

Seizure is a sudden onset of uncontrolled cerebral dysfunction that can lead to convulsions and impaired consciousness.

Physiological Basics

Neuronal transmission begins with the receptor-associated formation of an action potential, which is transmitted along the axon to induce the release of a neurotransmitter at the terminal synapse. This causes the formation of an action potential on the postsynaptic membrane. In this way, impulses and thus information are transmitted neuronally. In neuronal function, excitatory and inhibitory functions can be differentiated.

Ion channels are a prerequisite for the generation of an action potential and neurotransmitters for the synaptic transmission of the impulse. Both are to be described in more detail now.

Two differently selective ion channels, the sodium and the potassium channels, are important for the development and maintenance of an action potential. Morphologically, they are transmembrane-localised protein structures composed of four subunits. The structure forms an ion-selective pore in the centre of the subunits. The distribution of ions, especially sodium localised outside the cell, creates an electrical voltage between the interior of the cell and the interstitium (resting potential). Opening of the sodium channels leads to a massive influx of sodium ions along the concentration gradient. The result is a charge reversal and the formation of an action potential. The charge is balanced by opening the potassium channels and a potassium outflow along the concentration gradient.

The resulting action potential can now be conducted continuously or saltatorily. When the action potential reaches the connection between two excitable cells, the synapse, there is a switch between electrical and chemical stimulus transmission. The action potential opens Ca^{2+} channels at the presynaptic membrane and a calcium influx follows along the concentration gradient. The increase in calcium concentration causes transmitter-loading vesicles to fuse with the presynaptic membrane and the transmitter is released into the synaptic cleft. This diffuses to the postsynaptic membrane and enables the formation of an action potential, for example, by binding to postsynaptic receptors that act as ion channels.

Neurotransmitters are distinguished as (Table 30.1):

Textbook of Small Animal Pathophysiology, First Edition. Stephan Neumann.
© 2025 John Wiley & Sons Ltd. Published 2025 by John Wiley & Sons Ltd.

Table 30.1 Neurotransmitters by chemical structure.

Substance group	Transmitter
Amino acids	Glutamate
	GABA
	Glycine
	Aspartate
Monoamines	Norepinephrine
	Adrenalin
	Dopamine
	Acetylcholine
	Serotonin
	Histamine
Peptides	Substance P
	Angiotensin
	Neurotensin

Aetiology

The causes of seizures can be differentiated into cerebral and extracerebral causalities. The latter can be metabolic disorders or toxin effects.

Cerebral	Extracerebral
Neoplasia (D/C)	Hepatoencephalopathy (D)
Trauma (D/C)	Polycythaemia (D)
Hydrocephalus (D/C)	Hypoglycaemia (D/C)
Meningoencephalitis (D/C)	Hypocalcaemia (D)
	Hyper-, hyponatraemia (D/C)

D – Dog, C – Cat

Pathogenesis

Influencing factors that can cause nervous hyperexcitability and thus lead to seizures act through an increased activity of the excitatory neurons or a reduced activity of the inhibitory neurons. Other influencing factors result from changes in the ion channels and changes in the extracellular and intracellular ion distribution.

In detail, the following factors can change neuronal excitability:

- The propagation of the action potential can be influenced by the number and distribution of the ion channels.
- Biochemical modification of receptors, such as phosphorylation of glutamate receptors, increases permeability to Ca^{2+}, leading to increased excitability.
- Activation of second messenger systems. The binding of noradrenaline to the α receptor activates cyclic guanosine monophosphate (GMP), which leads to the opening of K^+ channels mediated by G proteins, thereby reducing the formation of action potentials.
- Modulating gene expression. Gene mutations can influence the expression of ion channel proteins and thus influence their ion selectivity.

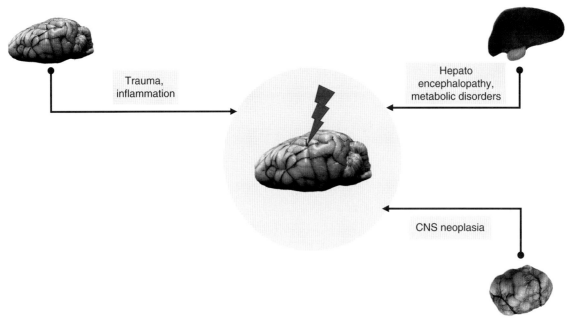

Figure 30.1   Pathogenesis of a seizure event.

- Changes in extracellular ion concentration due to variations in the volume of the extracellular space. For example, a reduced extracellular volume leads to an increased extracellular K^+ concentration. This reduces the concentration gradient for potassium, which in turn hinders the repolarisation of the cell.

In the seizure event, there is a high-frequency genesis of action potentials and a synchronisation of neuronal populations. The spread of the seizure is achieved when further neurons are activated with simultaneous cessation of inhibitory activity.

The respective symptomatology depends on the central region in which the seizure disorder is present.

A frequently affected region for seizure disorders is the hippocampus. Theoretically, a seizure can develop here when inhibitory neurons become non-functional or when neuronal reorganisation, for example, after trauma, results in increased excitatory connections.

A look at the causalities shows that the majority of seizures can be regarded as idiopathic. Possible causes for this would be mutations in the area of the sodium or potassium channels or of receptor molecules of the postsynaptic membrane.

Structural changes in the brain, such as tumour, granuloma or haematoma, cause an imbalance between the excitatory and inhibitory neurons via space development and ischaemia. This is due to the fact that inhibitory neurons react more sensitively to oxygen deficiency than excitatory neurons. The consequence of the oxygen deficiency is an insufficient supply of ATP for the Na^+-K^+ pump, which enables the nervous resting state.

Metabolic diseases cause a disturbance of the neurons with the consequence of a seizure through a reduced supply of energy-rich molecules (glucose) or influencing the extracellular ion distribution (Figure 30.1).

Pathophysiologic Consequences

The pathophysiologic consequences depend on the extent and duration of the seizure. Small seizures of a few seconds, called 'petit male', usually show no consequences on other organs or functions after the seizure. In the case of a large seizure lasting several minutes or hours, called 'grand male', consequences can occur. The main consequences are loss of water and nutrients when the animal is in a seizure. Injuries are also possible.

Influenced organ systems	Clinical symptoms	Clinical pathological alterations
Neuromuscular system	Dehydration	Increased PCV
Central nervous system		

Further Reading

Arida, R.M. (2021). Physical exercise and seizure activity. *Biochimica et Biophysica Acta. Molecular Basis of Disease* 1867 (1): 165979. https://doi.org/10.1016/j.bbadis.2020.165979.

Fordington, S. and Manford, M. (2020). A review of seizures and epilepsy following traumatic brain injury. *Journal of Neurology* 267 (10): 3105–3111. https://doi.org/10.1007/s00415-020-09926-w.

Pena, A.B. and Caviness, J.N. (2020). Physiology-based treatment of myoclonus. *Neurotherapeutics: The Journal of the American Society for Experimental NeuroTherapeutics* 17 (4): 1665–1680. https://doi.org/10.1007/s13311-020-00922-6.

Russo, M.E. (1981). The pathophysiology of epilepsy. *The Cornell Veterinarian* 71 (2): 221–247.

31

Shock

Definition

Shock is a syndrome in which the peripheral oxygen supply is insufficient due to various causes.

Aetiology

The causes of shock are divided into cardiogenic, neurogenic, hypovolaemic, anaphylactic and septic forms. Each form has different causalities; the consequence in each case is an absolute or relative reduced perfusion of the tissues with an oxygen deficiency and corresponding cellular and systemic consequences.

Cardiogenic	Neurogenic	Hypovolaemic	Anaphylactic	Septic
Heart failure (D/C)	Spinal or cerebral trauma (D/C)	Blood loss (D/C)	Immunologic reaction to allergens (D/C)	Bacterial infection (D/C)
	Inflammation (D/C)	Loss of water (D/C)		

D – Dog, C – Cat

Pathogenesis

Heart failure as a cause of **cardiogenic shock** leads to reduced perfusion of the tissue and, thus, hypoxia. The cause is a reduced cardiac output. Morphological diseases of the heart are possible, as well as functional disorders in the form of arrhythmias.

The reduction of cardiac output initially activates compensatory mechanisms. The release of catecholamines increases peripheral vascular resistance, and at the same time the activation of the renin-angiotensin-aldosterone system (RAAS) increases blood volume. Cardiac output and heart rate are increased. This causes an increased oxygen demand in the myocardium. If this is not compensated for, the cardiac muscle strength is reduced, which in turn leads to a reduced cardiogenic output. As a result, tissue perfusion and oxygen supply are reduced.

Another type of shock that leads to a relative reduction in perfusion is **neurogenic shock**. Here, vasodilation develops due to increased parasympathetic or decreased sympathetic activity. Causal factors are various abrupt neurogenic disturbances, such as spinal cord trauma or infarction. As a result of vasodilation, cardiac output is relatively reduced because blood volume is adequate but vascular volume is too high. A reduced perfusion is the further consequence.

Anaphylactic shock has a similar genesis. The primary event in this case is an allergic reaction, as a result of which vasoactive mediators are released on a massive scale. Different allergens, often inhalation allergens, cause a type I hypersensitivity reaction. As a result, IgE is released in high concentrations, which binds to inflammatory cells and induces the release of vasoactive mediators there. These lead to generalised vasodilation associated with increased vascular permeability. The latter leads to tissue oedema formation, which is responsible for numerous symptoms. Another mechanism is the increased release of mediators that lead to increased contraction of smooth muscle cells.

Textbook of Small Animal Pathophysiology, First Edition. Stephan Neumann.
© 2025 John Wiley & Sons Ltd. Published 2025 by John Wiley & Sons Ltd.

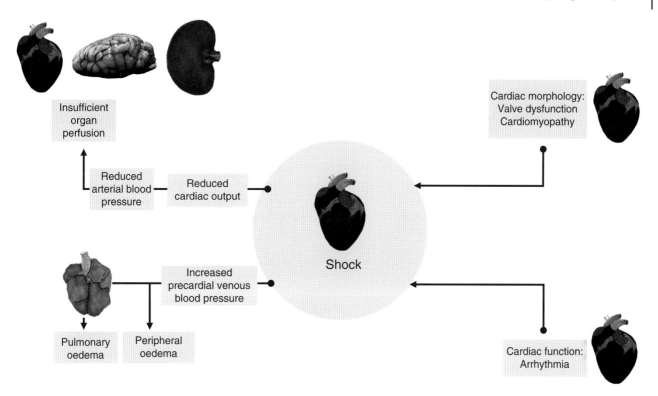

Figure 31.1   Pathomechanism of shock based on cardiogenic shock.

In **septic shock,** vasoactive mediators are increasingly released as a result of a bacterial infection. The causal factor is usually a systemic infection (bacteraemia). The release of bacterial toxins (PAMPS) stimulates surface receptors of the macrophages. These are often toll-like receptors. The macrophages in turn secrete various, mostly proinflammatory, cytokines, such as interleukin 1 (IL-1) and tumour necrosis factor (TNF-α). Under the influence of the cytokines, a systemic inflammatory response syndrome (SIRS) develops.

In contrast to the forms described so far, **hypovolaemic shock** is the result of an absolute volume deficiency. Causes are accordingly acute blood loss or acute loss of interstitial fluid in massive diarrhoea or diuresis. The volume deficiency reduces cardiac output (Figure 31.1).

Pathophysiologic Consequences

The consequences of a shock situation first develop on a cellular level. Due to the reduced oxygen supply, cellular energy production is reduced. The consequence is a reduced function of ATP-dependent transport mechanisms. If the Na^+/K^+ exchange is affected, the intracellular sodium and water concentration increases. This leads to cell swelling and possibly to cell rupture, but at least to an overall disturbed cell metabolism. Another consequence of the reduced oxygen supply is the change from aerobic to anaerobic energy production. The latter induces acidosis due to an increased accumulation of lactate. An altered pH value disrupts enzyme function and, thus, influences all cellular mechanisms.

In addition to the reduced supply of oxygen in the case of shock-induced reduced perfusion, other nutrients are also made available to the cells in a reduced form. The reduction in glucose supply leads to activated gluconeogenesis due to the effect of stress hormones, such as cortisol. Further consequences are an increased protein metabolism with an increase in protein breakdown products, such as ammonia and urea. Some metabolites, especially ammonia, are cytotoxic as they destroy the cell membrane.

Systemically, the different types of shock lead to **multi-organ failure**, which by definition is reached when two organ systems become insufficient. The mechanisms leading to multi-organ failure develop as a result of activation of stress hormones and pre-inflammatory cytokines. Vascular erosions activate blood coagulation, which leads to the formation of microthrombi with increased consumption of coagulation factors, and DIC develops.

Influenced organ systems	Clinical symptoms	Clinical pathological alterations
Systemic	Tachycardia	Polycythaemia
	Tachypnoea	Hypocoagulation
	Oliguria	Increased urea and creatinine
		Acidosis/alkalosis

Using septic shock as an example, the pathophysiological mechanisms will be presented.

The course of a septic shock is carried by the bacterially induced release of proinflammatory cytokines. TNF-α influences the activity of cardiac myocytes by inhibiting the β-receptors. Furthermore, it increases the expression of IL-1, IL-2, IL-6, platelet-activating factor (PAF) and the induction of the hepatic formation of acute phase proteins.

Further, bioactive mediators are formed under the initiation of the shock event. These include:

Kallikrein
Thrombin
Plasmin
Bradykinin
Fibrinogen and fibrin cleavage products
Complement C3a and C5a.

These mediators increase the inflammatory response and activate inflammatory cells, such as granulocytes, monocytes/macrophages and endothelial cells.

Cells activated in this way also release cytokines and mediators (TNF-α, IL-1β, IL-6, IL-8), which initiate a cascade of further cell activation and proteolytic reactions through paracrine mechanisms. The cleavage of cell-bound adhesion molecules, the secretion of oxidants, arachidonic acid molecules and, in particular, of lysosomal proteinases, such as elastase, leads to proteolysis of the vessel wall structures and to increased permeability. These processes can ultimately lead to organ failure. The process is intensified by hypercoagulation, which in turn is caused by proteolytic inactivation of antithrombin III (AT III), the most important inhibitor of the coagulation system, by PMN elastase. The same applies to protein C and other inhibitors of the blood coagulation cascade, such as α-2-plasmin inhibitor, C1-inactivator and α-2-macroglobulin (Figure 31.2).

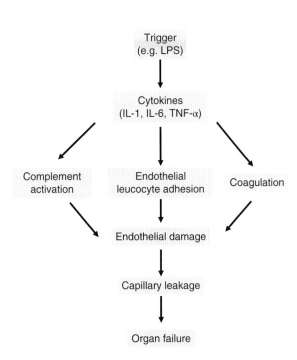

Figure 31.2 Septic shock process.

Further Reading

Bertini, P. and Guarracino, F. (2021). Pathophysiology of cardiogenic shock. *Current Opinion in Critical Care* 27 (4): 409–415. https://doi.org/10.1097/MCC.0000000000000853.

Blumlein, D. and Griffiths, I. (2022). Shock: aetiology, pathophysiology and management. *British Journal of Nursing (Mark Allen Publishing)* 31 (8): 422–428. https://doi.org/10.12968/bjon.2022.31.8.422.

Cannon, J.W. (2018). Hemorrhagic shock. *The New England Journal of Medicine* 378 (4): 370–379. https://doi.org/10.1056/NEJMra1705649.

Kuo, K. and Palmer, L. (2022). Pathophysiology of hemorrhagic shock. *Journal of Veterinary Emergency and Critical Care (San Antonio, Tex.: 2001)* 32 (S1): 22–31. https://doi.org/10.1111/vec.13126.

Russell, J.A., Rush, B., and Boyd, J. (2018). Pathophysiology of septic shock. *Critical Care Clinics* 34 (1): 43–61. https://doi.org/10.1016/j.ccc.2017.08.005.

32

Syncope

Definition

Syncope, also called 'circulatory collapse', is a short, spontaneously reversible loss of consciousness as a result of impaired blood flow to the brain.

Physiological Basics

The blood flow in the organism depends on cardiac output, arterial pressure, peripheral resistance and blood volume.

The resting blood flow to the brain in humans is 50–60 ml/min per 100 g. This corresponds to 12–15% of the cardiac output (Brignole et al. 2004).

Central blood flow to the brain is subject of an autoregulatory mechanism.

Autoregulation keeps the cerebral blood pressure stable at a peripheral blood pressure of approximately 60–160 mmHg. In this range, the cerebral blood pressure is kept constant by vascular contraction or dilatation (Bayliss effect). If the peripheral blood pressure drops sharply, the cerebral blood flow decreases. If the blood flow is no longer adequate, functional failures and loss of consciousness occur within a few seconds.

An important factor for cerebral blood flow is the interaction of the autonomic nervous system with the blood vessels and the heart.

Stretch receptors located in the high-pressure system at the bifurcation of the common carotid artery, the so-called 'carotid sinus', and at the aortic arch register the vessel width. The receptors are located as free nerve endings in the media and adventitia of the vessel wall. The excitation depends on the vessel wall dilatation. The impulses are transmitted via afferent nerves (C-fibres) to the vegetative core areas of the brain stem (nucleus tractus solitarii). In the event of a rise in blood pressure, the tonic sympathetic innervation of the blood vessels is inhibited in the vegetative core area. This results in vessel wall dilatation and a drop in blood pressure. If the receptors are less excited due to reduced arterial pressure or stroke volume, there is an increase in peripheral sympathetic tone and peripheral resistance increases. Similarly, sympathetic activity at the heart increases with an increase in frequency and there is an increase in stroke volume (Figure 32.1).

Aetiology

The causes of syncope can be differentiated into cardiogenic, neurogenic and metabolic causalities.

Neurogenic	Cardiogenic	Metabolic
Diffuse cerebral dysfunction (D/C)	Myocardial failure (D/C)	Hyper-, hypocalcaemia
Encephalopathy	Bradyarrhythmia (D)	Hyper-, hypokalaemia
Hydrocephalus	Tachyarrhythmia (D/C)	Hyper-, hyponatraemia
Brain tumour		Hypoglycaemia

D – Dog, C – Cat

Textbook of Small Animal Pathophysiology, First Edition. Stephan Neumann.
© 2025 John Wiley & Sons Ltd. Published 2025 by John Wiley & Sons Ltd.

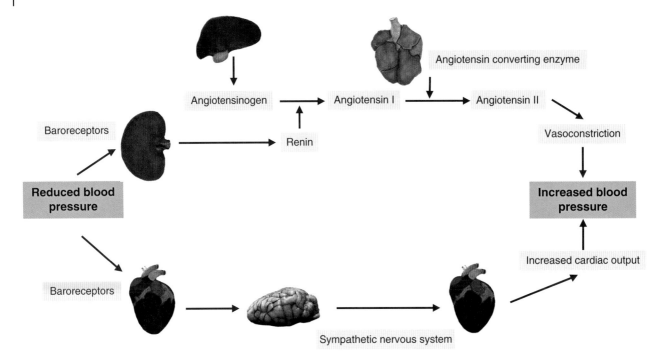

Figure 32.1 Mechanism of blood pressure regulation.

Pathogenesis

Neurogenic syncope can be caused causally by morphological changes in the brain. Lesions can stenose individual vessels and lead to a cerebral insufficiency. If intravascular stenosis occurs due to a thrombus, this leads to a similar mechanism.

Functional causes of neurogenic syncope are often based on dysfunction of the autonomic nervous system. Parasympathetic hyperactivity can lead to reduced cardiac output by influencing cardiac function; this causes blood pressure to fall below cerebral autoregulation and results in reduced blood flow with syncope. In the case of sympathetic underactivity, vascular dilatation develops with downstream reduced blood flow.

Cardiogenic syncope occurs as a result of morphological diseases of the heart or cardiac arrhythmias. In both cases, the consequence is a reduced cardiac output with reduced peripheral blood flow.

Metabolic syncope has no direct influence on cerebral blood flow, but is clinically comparable. Hypoglycaemia in particular has been described as a trigger of syncope. The pathogenetic mechanism begins after a drop in blood glucose with glucagon secretion within a few seconds. Glucagon leads to an increase in blood glucose concentration through activation of glucagon receptors in the liver. Receptor activation, in turn, causes glycogen breakdown and glucose release. This is followed within a few minutes by the release of cortisol, which causes increased gluconeogenesis and thus an increase in blood glucose concentration. In addition, cortisol can reduce peripheral glucose uptake via peripheral vasoconstriction, making more glucose available for cerebral function. At the same time, the expression of glucose transporters on the nerve cells increases. If the compensatory mechanisms are not sufficient and the glucose concentration remains low, an energy deficit of the nerve cells develops with their function being restricted, which can present itself clinically as weakness or syncope (Figure 32.2).

Disturbances of the electrolytes, especially potassium, sodium and calcium, lead to syncope by affecting the formation and conduction of excitation in nerves and muscle cells. The individual functions of the electrolytes are summarised below:

Sodium (Na^+) is a positively charged ion that enters the cell during depolarisation.
Potassium (K^+) is also a positively charged ion that flows out of the cell during repolarisation.
Calcium (Ca^{2+}) is another positively charged ion that plays an important role in the contraction of muscles and the transmission of signals between nerve cells.

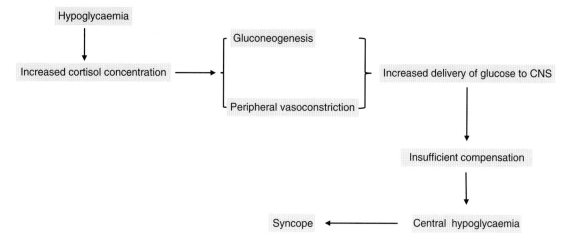

Figure 32.2 Pathomechanism of hypoglycaemia.

Sodium and potassium are both important for generating the action potential in nerve and muscle cells.

The resting potential of a cell is maintained by the function of potassium channels.

The potassium channels allow K^+ to flow out of the cell, which causes the cell membrane to remain negatively charged.

When an action potential is generated, the voltage-dependent sodium channels in the cell membrane open and Na^+ flows into the cell.

The incoming Na^+ ions cause a depolarisation of the cell as they change the charge of the cell from negative to positive.

This generates an electrical signal that is transmitted along the cell.

When the action potential has reached its peak, the voltage-dependent potassium channels, in the cell membrane, open and K^+ flows out of the cell.

The outflow of K^+ ions leads to a repolarisation of the cell, as the charge of the cell returns from positive to negative.

The ratio of sodium and potassium in the cell is important for the generation and regulation of action potentials.

A change in the ratio of Na^+ and K^+ can influence the action potentials and lead to problems.

Calcium is important for muscle contraction as it stimulates the release of calcium ions from the sarcoplasmic reticulum (SR).

Calcium ions then bind to troponin on the thin filaments of the muscle cells and initiate contraction.

Calcium also plays an important role in signal transmission between nerve cells. When an action potential arrives at the synapse, the voltage-dependent calcium channels open and Ca^{2+} flows into the cell.

The increase in Ca^{2+} stimulates the release of neurotransmitters from the synaptic vesicles.

The released neurotransmitters bind to receptors on the postsynaptic membrane and initiate a new action potential (Figure 32.3).

Regardless of the cause, syncope is essentially the pathogenetic consequence of an oxygen deficiency in the nerve cells. Hypoxia leads to a reduced formation of ATP, since in the case of hypoxia aerobic glycolysis is reduced and the anaerobic form can synthesise ATP less effectively. The critical oxygen tension for the synthesis of ATP is given as 25–40 mmHg, below which a reduction in ATP concentration of about 90% develops within a few minutes (Erecińska and Silver 2001). The consequence of this deficiency is a dysfunction of the ion channels. This can cause Na^+-influx. Water enters the nerve cells with the sodium, causing cell swelling and dysfunction. The breakdown of the sodium concentration gradient also results in an outflow of glutamate from the nerve cells via the sodium-glutamate cotransporter. The consequence is the increased expression of glutamate receptors on the nerve cells. These, in turn, increase Ca^{2+} influx into the nerve cells. Increased Ca^{2+} concentrations can initiate necrotic or apoptotic mechanisms.

There are various protective mechanisms to protect nerve cells from hypoxia. For example, a switch to anaerobic glycolysis or a reduction in cellular metabolism. However, these mechanisms are not sufficient to compensate for a pronounced hypoxia, especially, if it occurs abruptly (Table 32.1).

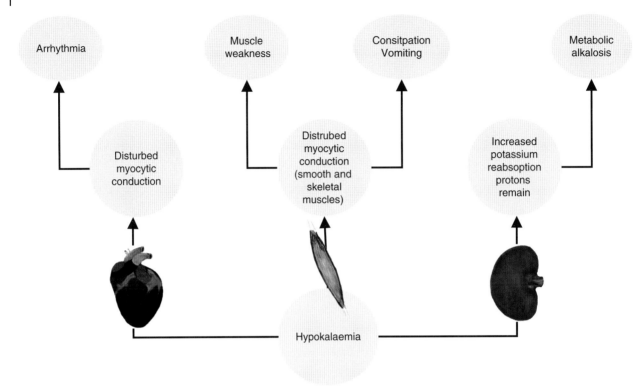

Figure 32.3 Pathomechanism of hypokalaemic syncope.

Table 32.1 Consequences of hypoxia on different ion channels.

Channel	Effect of hypoxia	Mechanism
Potassium	Inhibition	Influencing the channel proteins
Sodium	Activation/inhibition	Influence on channel protein expression
Calcium	Inhibition	

Source: Adapted from Bickler and Donohoe (2002).

Pathophysiologic Consequences

The main consequence of syncope is loss of consciousness. Since syncope is mainly triggered by habitual causes, there are often no further symptoms after the crisis has passed. Permanent syncope in the sense of a reduction in the cerebral oxygen supply can lead to permanent cognitive impairment and death.

Influenced organ systems	Clinical symptoms
Cardiovascular system	Loss of consciousness
Central nervous system	

References

Bickler, P.E. and Donohoe, P.H. (2002). Adaptive responses of vertebrate neurons to hypoxia. *The Journal of Experimental Biology* 205 (Pt 23): 3579–3586. https://doi.org/10.1242/jeb.205.23.3579.

Brignole, M., Alboni, P., Benditt, D.G. et al. (2004). Guidelines on management (diagnosis and treatment) of syncope-update 2004. *Journal of the Working Groups on Cardiac Pacing, Arrhythmias, and Cardiac Cellular Electrophysiology of the European Society of Cardiology* 6 (6): 467–537. PMID: 15519256.

Erecińska, M. and Silver, I.A. (2001). Tissue oxygen tension and brain sensitivity to hypoxia. *Respiration Physiology* 128 (3): 263–276. https://doi.org/10.1016/s0034-5687(01)00306-1.

Further Reading

Borgeat, K., Pack, M., Harris, J. et al. (2021). Prevalence of sudden cardiac death in dogs with atrial fibrillation. *Journal of Veterinary Internal Medicine* 35 (6): 2588–2595. https://doi.org/10.1111/jvim.16297.

He, W., Wang, X., Liu, S. et al. (2018). Sympathetic mechanisms in an animal model of vasovagal syncope. *Clinical Autonomic Research: Official Journal of the Clinical Autonomic Research Society* 28 (3): 333–340. https://doi.org/10.1007/s10286-018-0503-5.

Rossi, D.J., Oshima, T., and Attwell, D. (2000). Glutamate release in severe brain ischaemia is mainly by reversed uptake. *Nature* 403 (6767): 316–321. https://doi.org/10.1038/35002090.

33

Urinary Disorders

Definition

Difficulties in urination are defined as micturition disorders. *Dysuria* describes disturbed urination in general, which is often accompanied by painful urination (stranguria) and higher frequency urination (pollakisuria). Other changes in urine output are uncontrolled urination (incontinence) and the absence of urine output (anuria/oliguria) or increased urine output (polyuria).

Physiological Basics

The physiological basics are described in Chapter 41.

Aetiology

The causes for the different micturition disorders are manifold. They consist of diseases that lead to disorders in urine production, such as anuria and oliguria, as well as polyuria. On the other hand, they are the consequence of disturbed urination, such as stranguria or incontinence, and are caused by diseases that directly or indirectly affect bladder function.

Anuria/oliguria	Polyuria	Dysuria, stranguria, pollakisuria	Incontinence
Pre-renal	Endocrine diseases (D/C)	Behavioural alterations	Urethral sphincter incompetence (D)
Shock (D/C)	Hepatobiliary diseases	Feline lower urinary tract diseases (C)	Detrusor hypocontractility (D)
Hypoadrenocorticism (D)	Electrolyte disorders (D/C)	Infection (D/C)	Reflex dyssynergia (D/C)
Dehydration (D/C)	Renal disorders (D/C)	Urolithiasis (D/C)	
Renal		Neoplasia (D/C)	
Acute and chronic kidney diseases (D/C)		Reflex dyssynergia (D/C)	
Post-renal			
Urethra obstruction (D/C)			

D – Dog, C – Cat

Pathogenesis

Anuria or oliguria: Normal urine production depends essentially on glomerular filtration, which in turn depends on renal blood flow. Accordingly, the main causes of a lack of urine output are diseases that lead to reduced glomerular filtration. These include diseases associated with reduced blood pressure, such as shock or hypoadrenocorticism. The reduction

Textbook of Small Animal Pathophysiology, First Edition. Stephan Neumann.
© 2025 John Wiley & Sons Ltd. Published 2025 by John Wiley & Sons Ltd.

of glomerular filtration reduces the volume of primary urine. Reabsorption of water in the tubule and collecting tube further reduces the amount of water to be excreted.

Physiological urine production associated with urine outflow obstruction due to urethral obstruction is the cause of postrenal anuria.

Polyuria is often associated with polydipsia. In the vast majority of cases, the polyuria is in the foreground, and the polydipsia is a compensatory mechanism.

The feeling of thirst develops through an increase in plasma osmolarity or a reduction in blood pressure. Both are detected by receptors in the vascular walls. Osmosensors develop impulses, when plasma osmolarity increases, and induce a feeling of thirst via the hypothalamus, which leads to increased drinking and a reduction in osmolarity. Hypovolaemia can be perceived via baroreceptors at different locations. Activation of the renin-angiotensin-aldosterone system and an increase in the feeling of thirst induce increased water intake, which increases extracellular volume and blood pressure.

In polyuria, the water-conserving function of the kidneys is disturbed. This is primarily achieved by water reabsorption in the area of the proximal tubules and loops of Henle, with an osmotic gradient to the renal medulla being the driving force. This is generated by Na-K-Cl transporters, which increase the concentration of Na and Cl in the interstitial fluid. In addition, antidiuretic hormone (ADH) increases the reabsorption of urea in the collecting tubules. Both mechanisms together increase the interstitial osmolarity in the parenchyma of the renal medulla to >1000 mosm/l. Diseases that lower the medullary osmolarity can lead to reduced water reabsorption via the reduction of the osmotic gradient and thus trigger polyuria.

In **chronic renal failure,** functional nephrons are lost due to fibrotic remodelling in the renal parenchyma. As a result, hyperfiltration develops in the remaining nephrons, but this is not sufficient to adequately maintain medullary osmolarity. This is followed by a reduction in the osmotic gradient and thus reduced water reabsorption. **Liver diseases** leading to hepatic insufficiency may be associated with reduced urea synthesis. In such a case, less urea would be available to maintain medullary osmolarity. A different mechanism in the medullary area is suspected in hyperthyroidism. Here, increased medullary blood flow could lead to increased removal of osmotically active molecules and thereby reduce the medullary osmotic gradient.

Another mechanism through which the preservative function of the kidney can be disturbed in polyuria concerns the reabsorption of water in the area of the collecting tubes. Here, ADH acts on aquaporins. ADH is secreted from the neurohypophysis after its synthesis has been induced by impulses from the hypothalamus. ADH is transported via the blood to the epithelial cells of the collecting duct in the kidney. These cells are normally not permeable to water. The binding of ADH to membrane receptors increases the cytoplasmic calcium concentration, which in turn initiates the incorporation of aquaporins into the cell membrane. The aquaporins allow water to be reabsorbed from the collecting tube following an osmotic gradient.

Diseases that act on the ADH receptors via toxins can reduce the formation and incorporation of aquaporins and thus cause polyuria. The polyuria associated with pyometra is explained in this way because infection with toxin-producing *Escherichia coli* is often present in pyometra. A deficiency of ADH can also reduce the formation of aquaporins and thus cause polyuria. This is present in diabetes insipidus.

Another mechanism that leads to polyuria is based on a tubular osmotic gradient. This is the result of increased glomerular filtration of osmotically active molecules. Glucose is the most important osmotically active molecule. Diseases that lead to increased glucosuria primarily induce hyperglycaemia. From a serum glucose concentration of >180 mg/dl, glucosuria occurs. Primary glucosuria, which develops independently of hyperglycaemia, must be distinguished from this. These include tubular insufficiencies, as in Fanconi syndrome (see Chapter 41.3).

Finally, polyuria can be caused by a deficiency of ADH, which is present in central diabetes mellitus (Figure 33.1, Table 33.1).

Micturition is a reflex that is essentially triggered by an increase in bladder filling. When the bladder fills, the smooth musculature of the bladder wall is first stretched. If the degree of stretching increases, impulses are sent from stretch receptors in the bladder wall via afferents first to the sacral medulla and from there upwards to the formatio reticularis in the central nervous system (CNS). From there, impulses travel via the spinal cord and the hypogastric nerve to the smooth bladder wall muscles (detrusor). There, the nervous impulses produce a coordinated, sustained contraction of the detrusor muscles. At the same time, the tone of the external sphincter muscle is reduced via the pudendal nerve. The result is urine output. When the bladder is emptied, the sensory impulses decrease and the micturition reflex is terminated.

Micturition disorders can lead to difficult urination or to more frequent micturition of small amounts of urine or to incontinence. Micturition disorders are often the consequence of neurogenic diseases.

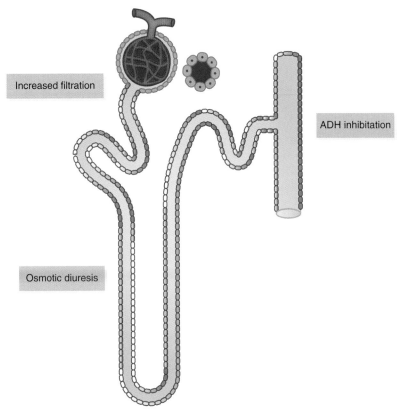

Figure 33.1 Mechanisms of polyuria.

Increased filtration

ADH inhibitation

Osmotic diuresis

Table 33.1 Causes for polyuria and polydipsia in dogs and cats.

Dog	Cat
Endocrine	**Endocrine**
Diabetes mellitus	Diabetes mellitus
Hyperadrenocorticism	Hyperthyroidism
Hypoadrencorticism	Central diabetes insipidus
Diabetes insipidus (central, peripheral)	Acromegaly
Acromegaly	Hyperadrenocorticism
Renal	**Renal**
Chronic kidney disease	Chronic kidney disease
Fanconi syndrome	Pyelonephritis
Electrolytes	**Electrolytes**
Hypercalcaemia	Hypercalcaemia
Hypokalaemia	Hypokalaemia
Miscellaneous	**Miscellaneous**
Liver diseases	Liver disease
Pyometra	

The following micturition disorders can develop.

Reduced Detrusor Reflex with Simultaneous Sphincter Hypertonus

The cause is a lesion between the brainstem and the spinal lumbar swelling. The consequence is a lack of micturition with an overflow bladder as a result of increasing internal bladder pressure that overcomes the sphincter tone. In these cases, the bladder is not actively and completely emptied.

A similar picture arises when the detrusor is areflectoric but the sphincter tone is normal.

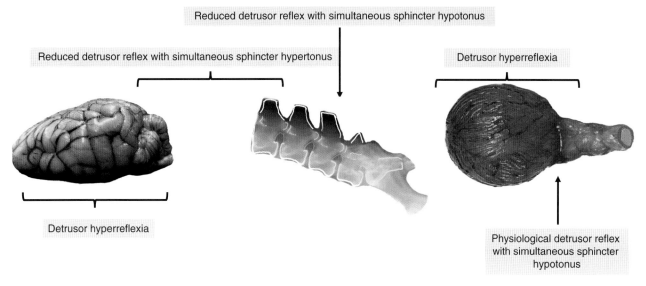

Figure 33.2 Causes and localisation of dysfunctional micturition.

Reduced Detrusor Reflex with Simultaneous Sphincter Hypotonus

The cause is usually a lesion in the sacral medulla. The consequence is leakage of urine as the bladder fills up.

Detrusor Hyperreflexia

Causes include cerebral diseases. The consequence is frequent micturation of small amounts of urine. Cystitis can produce a similar clinical picture.

Reflex Dyssynergy

The cause is a lesion in the upper motor neuron. This leads to a lack of coordination between the detrusor and the sphincter. Affected animals, mostly male dogs, initially pass urine physiologically, but after a short time urination is interrupted.

Physiological Detrusor Reflex with Simultaneous Sphincter Hypotonus

The cause is reduced pudendal nerve activity or reduced sympathetic activity at the urethra. Disturbances in the area of the sphincter musculature are also possible. This clinical picture appears more frequently in connection with the castration of bitches. The result is leakage of urine even with small urinary bladder volumes (Figure 33.2).

Further Reading

Acierno, M.J. and Labato, M.A. (2019). Canine incontinence. *The Veterinary Clinics of North America. Small Animal Practice* 49 (2): 125–140. https://doi.org/10.1016/j.cvsm.2018.11.003.

Byron, J.K. (2015). Micturition disorders. *The Veterinary Clinics of North America. Small Animal Practice* 45 (4): 769–782. https://doi.org/10.1016/j.cvsm.2015.02.006.

Feldman, E.C. and Nelson, R.W. (1989). Diagnostic approach to polydipsia and polyuria. *The Veterinary Clinics of North America. Small Animal Practice* 19 (2): 327–341. https://doi.org/10.1016/s0195-5616(89)50033-0.

Gouvêa, F.N., Pennacchi, C.S., Assaf, N.D. et al. (2021). Acromegaly in dogs and cats. *Annales d'Endocrinologie* 82 (2): 107–111. https://doi.org/10.1016/j.ando.2021.03.002.

Hagman, R. (2018). Pyometra in small animals. *The Veterinary Clinics of North America. Small Animal Practice* 48 (4): 639–661. https://doi.org/10.1016/j.cvsm.2018.03.001.

Ramírez-Guerrero, G., Müller-Ortiz, H., and Pedreros-Rosales, C. (2022). Polyuria in adults. A diagnostic approach based on pathophysiology. *Revista clinica espanola* 222 (5): 301–308. https://doi.org/10.1016/j.rceng.2021.03.003.

Wang, S., Mitu, G.M., and Hirschberg, R. (2008). Osmotic polyuria: an overlooked mechanism in diabetic nephropathy. *Nephrology, Dialysis, Transplantation: Official Publication of the European Dialysis and Transplant Association – European Renal Association* 23 (7): 2167–2172. https://doi.org/10.1093/ndt/gfn115.

34

Vomiting

Definition

Vomiting is a reflex controlled by the vomiting centre, which leads to emptying the stomach or parts of the intestine. The sensation that precedes vomiting is called 'nausea'.

Aetiology

The causes that lead to vomiting can be divided into gastrointestinal and extra-gastrointestinal causes.

Gastrointestinal	Extra-gastrointestinal	Endocrine	CNS
Dietary intolerance (D)	Pancreatitis (D/C)	Hyperthyroidism (C)	Vestibular diseases (D)
Food allergy (D)	Renal failure (D/C)	Hypoadrenocorticism (D)	Hydrocephalus (D/C)
Gastritis (D/C)	Liver failure (D/C)	Ketoacidosis (D/C)	
Gastroenteritis (D/C)			
Gastrointestinal obstruction(D/C)			

D – Dog, C – Cat

Pathogenesis

Vomiting is a protective reflex that is intended to protect the organism from potentially or actually toxic substances. This reflex is controlled by the vomiting centre, which is located in the brain stem in the area of the fourth ventricle. Vomiting is often accompanied by a preparatory mechanism of nausea. Rarely, vomiting is not accompanied by nausea. Triggering factors are described in the aetiologies.

To trigger the vomiting stimulus, the various causalities can either irritate receptors in the stomach and intestinal wall or stimulate the vomiting centre via nervous afferents, mostly of the vagus nerve. In addition, toxins or mediators can directly stimulate the vomiting centre. Direct vagal irritation originating from visceral structures can also induce vomiting.

Numerous emetic triggers act on chromaffin cells in the gastric and intestinal mucosa. The consequence is an increased synthesis and release of serotonin or substance P. Both substances stimulate compatible receptors in the mucosa, which act on the vomiting centre via vagal afferents. A direct effect on the vomiting centre is assumed for substance P (Chappa et al. 2006) (Figure 34.1).

Bacterial infections can be accompanied by vomiting. The pathogens act via receptor-associated emesis. Bacterial toxins (enterotoxin, endotoxin) stimulate chromaffin cells to synthesise serotonin and thus cause vomiting. Viruses can also induce serotonin synthesis in chromaffin cells. Another mechanism described is the virus-induced disruption of cellular calcium homeostasis. Certain viruses (e.g. rotaviruses) can induce a calcium release from the endoplasmic reticulum via

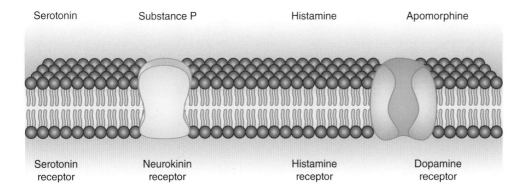

Figure 34.1 Representation of emetic receptors and triggers. *Source:* Adapted from Zhong et al. (2021).

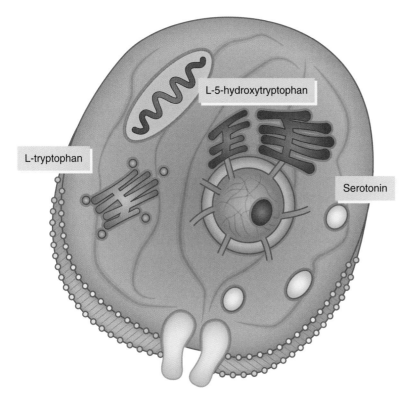

Figure 34.2 Function of the chromaffin cells. *Source:* Adapted from Rezzani et al. (2022).

so-called 'viroporins' and thus increase the cytoplasmic calcium concentration. At the same time, the reduction of the calcium concentration in the endoplasmic reticulum can stimulate calcium influx across the cell membrane. Both increase the intracellular calcium concentration, which causes the release of serotonin in the corresponding cells (Figure 34.2).

Stimulation of the vomiting centre results in the initiation of vomiting. This is essentially initiated by vagal efferents. This is followed by inspiration and closure of the epiglottis. At the same time, contractions of the stomach wall muscles develop from the pylorus towards the cardia. The onset of salivation and relaxation of the oesophagus and the proximal gastric sphincter allow the food pulp to enter the oesophagus. The onset of expiratory muscle contraction results in increased pressure in the thorax and oesophagus, accompanied by contractions of the oesophageal muscles, and the food pulp is vomited via the relaxed proximal oesophageal sphincter.

Pathophysiologic Consequences

The main consequences of vomiting occur in the chronic course. These include a reduced supply of nutrients and the loss of fluids and electrolytes.

Influenced organ systems	Clinical symptoms	Clinical pathological alterations
Systemic	Dehydration	Alkalosis
		Hypokalaemia
		Hyponatraemia

Dehydration occurs when large amounts of fluid are lost through vomiting, or when no more water is taken in due to nausea.

Different types of dehydration can be distinguished.

In isotonic dehydration, there is a balance between the loss of water and sodium. Clinical symptoms are characterised by hypovolaemia, hypotension and tachycardia. Laboratory diagnostics show an increase in serum protein and the PCV.

In hypotonic dehydration, the sodium loss is more marked than the water loss. As a result, the osmotic gradient between the inside and outside of the cell decreases. Water penetrates the cells and leads to intracellular oedema formation.

Clinically, the symptoms are similar to isotonic dehydration, but neurological symptoms up to fighting seizures may be more likely.

Hypertonic dehydration results from a high loss of free water. The increased osmolarity in the extracellular space causes a shift of water from intracellular to extracellular.

Isotonic or hypertonic dehydration usually develops during vomiting.

The consequences can be increased thirst. This is ADH controlled and is caused by the decrease in blood volume and the resulting lowered blood pressure. Dry mucous membranes are also a consequence of dehydration, which is also used for the clinical assessment of the disease. Neurological consequences, such as fatigue, weakness and disorientation are due to the effects of blood pressure and shifts in electrolyte concentrations.

The loss of protons through vomiting can also trigger **metabolic alkalosis**. Some symptoms may develop as a result of this. Alkalosis can temporarily reduce the oxygen release of haemoglobin. Furthermore, alkalosis increases the dissociation of proteins with the consequence of increased calcium binding to the free valences of the proteins. This can result in a reduction of ionised calcium, which can lead to muscle weakness. Cardially, metabolic alkalosis can cause arrhythmias and reduced cardiac output, and neurologically, neuronal excitability can be affected by alkalosis.

Further effects of alkalosis are often caused by hypokalaemia. This can be exacerbated in addition to potassium loss through vomiting, as in the case of alkalosis, cells secrete protons in exchange for potassium ions to compensate for the alkalosis.

Vomiting can cause hypovolaemic **hyponatraemia**. In advanced cases (Na < 135 mEq/l), this reduces plasma osmolarity. This causes a water shift from extra- to intracellular. The result is cell swelling. In the brain, swelling of the nerve cells causes symptoms, such as nausea, lethargy and coma.

The consequence of **hypokalaemia** develops due to hypokalaemic hyperpolarisation of the cell membrane. This prolongs the action potential and the refractory phase. In the various organ systems, this produces weakness, paralysis or tetany in the muscles, cardiac arrhythmia and gastrointestinal ileus can develop due to impaired intestinal motility (Figure 34.3).

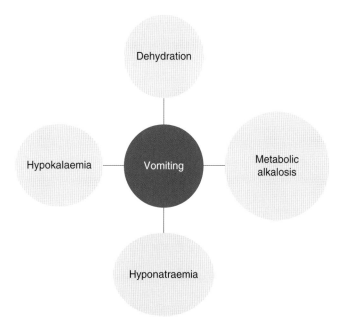

Figure 34.3 Consequences of chronic vomiting.

References

Chappa, A.K., Audus, K.L., and Lunte, S.M. (2006). Characteristics of substance P transport across the blood-brain barrier. *Pharmaceutical Research* 23 (6): 1201–1208. https://doi.org/10.1007/s11095-006-0068-1.

Rezzani, R., Franco, C., Franceschetti, L. et al. (2022). A focus on Enterochromaffin cells among the Enteroendocrine cells: localization, morphology, and role. *International Journal of Molecular Sciences* 23 (7): 3758. https://doi.org/10.3390/ijms23073758.

Zhong, W., Shahbaz, O., Teskey, G. et al. (2021). Mechanisms of nausea and vomiting: current knowledge and recent advances in intracellular emetic signaling systems. *International Journal of Molecular Sciences* 22 (11): 5797. https://doi.org/10.3390/ijms22115797.

35

Weight Loss

Definition

Weight loss is the reduction in body weight.

Aetiology

The causes of weight loss are inadequate food intake, inadequate absorption of food components or loss of nutrients.

Insufficient food intake	Malabsorption	Loss
Diseases of the teeth	Pancreatic insufficiency (D)	Protein-losing enteropathy (D/C)
the chewing muscles	Inflammatory bowel disease (IBD) (D/C)	Protein-losing nephropathy (D/C)
the oesophagus (D/C)	Cholangiectasia (D)	Tumour cachexia (D/C)

D – Dog, C – Cat

Pathogenesis

Regardless of causality, the reduced absorption of nutrients leads to an increased breakdown of the body's own substance.

An essential biochemical mechanism leading to the breakdown of body substance and weight loss is the ubiquitin-mediated proteolytic system.

The 26S proteasome is the proteolytically active part of the ubiquitin-proteasome system (UPS), through which the majority of intracellular proteins are highly selectively degraded. Triggers of this system include glucocorticoids and cytokines.

Weight loss associated with heart failure and chronic renal failure is often triggered by increased expression of proinflammatory cytokines. These cause an increase in metabolism and a reduction in food intake by influencing the satiety centre (Figure 35.1).

Cachexia is a frequent accompanying symptom in the severe course of cancer. This is triggered by different mechanisms through which the neoplasia influences the metabolism.

Inflammatory reactions: In many cancers, there is a systemic inflammatory response that can reduce appetite and food intake.

Some tumours can produce hormones that affect metabolism and can lead to weight loss.

Examples from humans are lung carcinomas, which can produce adrenocorticotropin (ACTH). ACTH in turn leads to increased cortisol synthesis, which can lead to an increase in blood glucose levels, a reduction in muscle tissue and an increase in fat loss, which in turn leads to weight loss. Another example is somatostatin synthesis by pancreatic

Textbook of Small Animal Pathophysiology, First Edition. Stephan Neumann.
© 2025 John Wiley & Sons Ltd. Published 2025 by John Wiley & Sons Ltd.

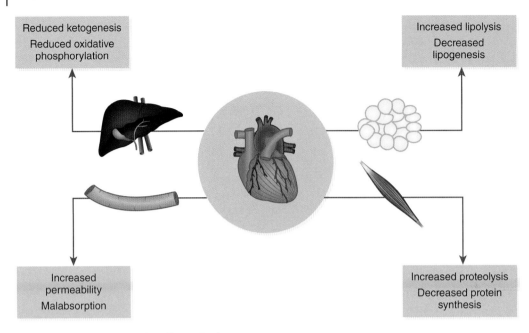

Figure 35.1 Mechanism of cardiac cachexia.

carcinomas. Somatostatin is a hormone, normally, produced by the pituitary gland and the intestine that regulates the metabolism of hormones, such as insulin, glucagon and growth hormone. When a pancreatic cancer produces somatostatin, it can affect the metabolism of these hormones in the body, which in turn can lead to weight loss.

Changes in fat metabolism: Cancer cells can affect the body's fat metabolism and lead to increased breakdown of fat tissue.

Lack of nutrients: Some tumours can affect the body's absorption of food, which can lead to a lack of important nutrients, such as proteins and vitamins.

Overproduction of cytokines: Certain tumours can trigger an overproduction of cytokines, which can increase inflammatory reactions in the body and reduce appetite.

Changes in insulin metabolism: Some tumours can impair insulin sensitivity and lead to increased insulin resistance, which in turn affects metabolism.

Changes in protein metabolism: Some tumours can affect the body's protein metabolism and lead to an increased loss of muscle mass.

Toxins: Some cancers can produce toxins that can reduce appetite and lead to nutritional deficiencies (Figure 35.2).

Pathophysiologic Consequences

The morphological and functional consequences of cachexia affect numerous organs and functions.

Influenced organ systems	Clinical symptoms
Systemic	Anorexia or increased appetite
	Weight loss
	Cachexia
	Sarcopenia

At the cellular level, cachexia is associated with mitochondrial dysfunction. This results in reduced protein synthesis associated with activation of the ubiquitin-26-S proteasome pathway, which leads to degradation of muscle proteins (Brown et al. 2017).

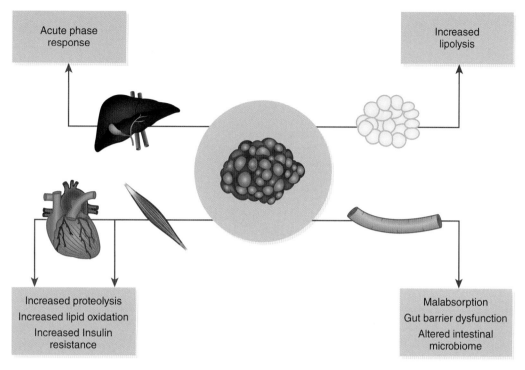

Figure 35.2 Influence of tumour diseases on food intake and weight loss. *Source:* Adapted from Morley et al. (2006).

The consequences of cachexia are a breakdown of **striated muscle** due to mitochondrial dysfunction, increased autophagy or apoptosis. Cachexia also has an effect on the **heart muscle**. Here, too, autophagy plays a role, and increased protein catabolism and oxidative stress also occur due to mitochondrial dysfunction. The consequences for the heart are an increasing fibrosis of the heart muscle and, functionally, a reduced contractility.

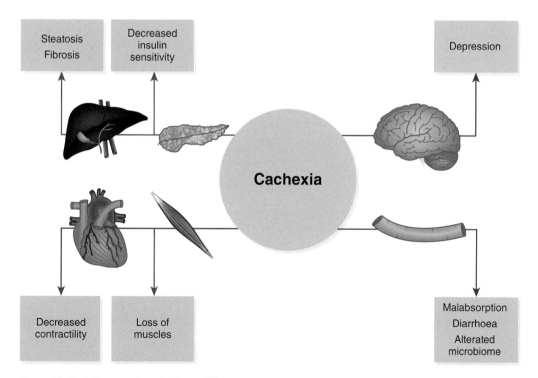

Figure 35.3 Influence of cachexia on different organ systems.

The influence of cachexia on **adipose tissue** is an increase in lipolysis with a simultaneous reduction in lipogenesis. In addition, glucose uptake by fat cells is reduced in cachexia. This is also a consequence of insulin resistance associated with cachexia. Since insulin is a potent anabolic hormone, the anabolic effect is lost in insulin resistance. This promotes protein breakdown. In the **liver**, ketogenesis is reduced and acute phase protein formation is increased, both triggered by IL-6. Ketone bodies are formed from fatty acids and are used for the energy supply of skeletal muscles, cardiac muscles and the nervous system. Reduction increases the generation of energy by protein breakdown, which is further enhanced by increased proteolysis to provide acute phase proteins. In the liver, metabolic conversion in cachexia leads to fibrosis and hepatic lipidosis.

A direct influence of cachexia on the **central nervous system** is a reduced supply of energy-providing molecules (e.g. ketone bodies) or through direct action of the proinflammatory cytokines active in cachexia. Functionally, this produces a reduction in appetite, which further increases catabolism.

Due to alteration of the tight-junctions between the enterocytes and reduced formation of antimicrobial peptides (AMP), **enteric consequences** also develop in cachexia. These are associated with malabsorption and lead to a disturbance of the intestinal microbiota.

Finally, cachexia also leads to a loss of **bone substance**, which negatively affects bone stability. The mechanism could be an activation of the transcription factor NF-kB.

Since many organ changes in cachexia are accompanied by local inflammatory reactions, an influence of cachexia on the **immune system** can also be suspected (Di Girolamo and Tajbakhsh 2022; Wyart et al. 2020) (Figure 35.3).

References

Brown, J.L., Rosa-Caldwell, M.E., Lee, D.E. et al. (2017). Mitochondrial degeneration precedes the development of muscle atrophy in progression of cancer cachexia in tumour-bearing mice. *Journal of Cachexia, Sarcopenia and Muscle* 8 (6): 926–938. https://doi.org/10.1002/jcsm.12232.

Di Girolamo, D. and Tajbakhsh, S. (2022). Pathological features of tissues and cell populations during cancer cachexia. *Cell Regeneration (London, England)* 11 (1): 15. https://doi.org/10.1186/s13619-022-00108-9.

Morley, J.E., Thomas, D.R., and Wilson, M.M. (2006). Cachexia: pathophysiology and clinical relevance. *The American Journal of Clinical Nutrition* 83 (4): 735–743. https://doi.org/10.1093/ajcn/83.4.735.

Wyart, E., Bindels, L.B., Mina, E. et al. (2020). Cachexia, a systemic disease beyond muscle atrophy. *International Journal of Molecular Sciences* 21 (22): 8592. https://doi.org/10.3390/ijms21228592.

Part III

Pathophysiology of Organ Systems

36

Cardiac System, Hypertension

36.1

Physiological Functions and General Pathophysiology of Organ Insufficiency

The essential function of the heart is to maintain the transport of blood. It is integrated into the circulatory system as a muscular pump and works more or less autonomously to maintain blood pressure and blood flow.

In order to be able to fulfil this function, some anatomical prerequisites and regulatory mechanisms are required, which will be explained in the following text.

Anatomy of the Heart

The mammalian heart is a hollow muscle that can be divided into two halves, each consisting of a ventricle and an atrium separated by the cardiac septum. The left half of the heart, which in dogs and cats is located caudally on the left side of the thorax due to a rotation of the heart axis, is responsible for transporting oxygen-rich blood into the body. The right half of the heart, on the other hand, which lies cranially on the right, transports deoxygenated blood to the lungs. The functions have an influence on the wall thickness of the half of the heart. The left half of the heart has a thicker wall than the right half, because the former has to build up a blood pressure of about 100 mmHg to transport the blood to the distant capillary networks of the organism. The right half of the heart is thin-walled, as blood only has to be transported from it to the lungs located in the immediate region, for which the right half of the heart has to build up an arterial blood pressure of approximately 20–30 mmHg.

To control the flow of blood, valves are created in the heart muscle that allow the blood to flow in one direction after heart contraction. In the left side of the heart, the mitral valve is located between the atrium and the ventricle, and the aortic valve is located between the ventricle and the aorta. In the right side of the heart, the tricuspid valve lies between the atrium and the ventricle and the pulmonary valve lies between the ventricle and the pulmonary artery. The heart valves are structures that are connected to the endocardium, the inner layer of the heart wall, which is followed on the outside by the myocardium, then the epicardium, and finally the heart lies in a pericardium (Figure 36.1.1).

Electrophysiological Automatism

In order to maintain its function, the heart muscles must contract in an orderly fashion to allow the flow of blood. The contracture of the heart muscles is primarily controlled autonomously. A hierarchically organised excitation formation and conduction system serves this purpose. This begins with the sinus node in the right atrium, after whose depolarisation the impulse can spread through the atrial musculature in the form of an action potential. Since the basic structures of the heart between the atrium and the ventricle do not transmit the electrical impulse, a connecting structure between the atrium and the ventricle is required, which is provided by the atrioventricular (AV) node. From here, the electrical impulse spreads via the septum in His's bundle and is distributed via Tawara legs and branched Purkinje fibres within the heart musculature.

The sinus node is composed of specialised cardiac muscle cells. These can be differentiated into P cells (pacemakers) and T cells (transition). The P cells are roundish and closely connected to each other via desmosomes. They lie together in small

Textbook of Small Animal Pathophysiology, First Edition. Stephan Neumann.
© 2025 John Wiley & Sons Ltd. Published 2025 by John Wiley & Sons Ltd.

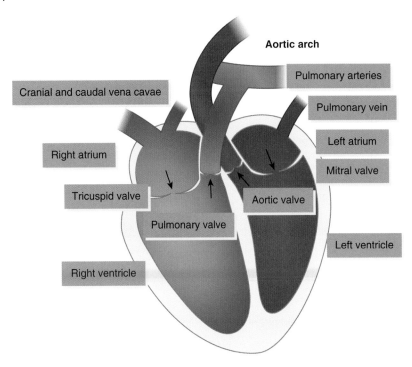

Figure 36.1.1 Anatomical overview of the heart structure.

groups. The T cells show an elongated structure, they surround the P-cell groups and connect them with the heart muscles. The excitation originates from the P cells. These are capable of independent depolarisation. This takes place because a low, unstable resting membrane potential prevails due to numerous ion channels in the cell membrane. Depolarisation is initiated by a sodium influx into the P cells due to the prevailing concentration difference between the cell exterior and interior. This is followed by a calcium influx. Then an action potential is formed due to the charge reversal in the cell interior. Repolarisation is initiated by an increased efflux of potassium ions along the concentration gradient from the inside to the outside. The frequency of depolarisations is 60–80/min in adult humans (Figure 36.1.2).

From the sinus node, the impulse spreads in the form of action potentials across the atrial myocardium at a speed of 1–2 m/s. For this purpose, the impulse is transmitted between the myocytes via existing gap junctions. These are channels that connect the cytoplasm of neighbouring cells. The gap junctions are formed by protein complexes called 'connexons'.

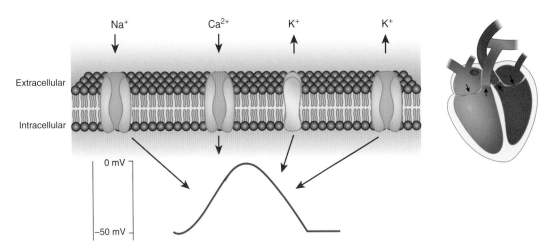

Figure 36.1.2 Ion fluxes and action potential structure in the P cells of the sinus node.

At the AV node, which is a secondary excitation centre with a lower frequency than the sinus node, the impulse is conducted from the atrial muscles into the septum of the ventricles. From there, the impulse propagates at a speed of about 2 m/s via His's bundle, Tawara's limb, Purkinje fibres and ventricular muscles.

Electromechanical Coupling

The conversion of an action potential into a muscle cell contraction is called 'electromechanical coupling'. When an impulse reaches the heart muscle cells (myocytes), an action potential is established there. First, the incoming action potential causes a change in the membrane resting potential. When a threshold value is reached, voltage-controlled Na channels open and a rapid influx of Na^+ ions follows along the concentration gradient. In this way, the membrane potential changes from −90 to 30 mV. This is followed by the so-called 'plateau phase', in which Ca influx and K outflow occur through channels along the cell membrane. In the subsequent repolarisation, the Ca channels close while the K channels remain open. In this way, the action potential returns to the resting potential. Subsequently, the original distribution of ions is restored by active mechanisms of the Na^+-K^+ pump (Figure 36.1.3).

During the Ca influx in the plateau phase of the action potential, the intracellular calcium concentration in the myocyte increases. This leads to a further release of calcium from the intracellular calcium store, the sarcoplasmic reticulum. The calcium binds to the myofibrils and causes contraction. The myofibrils are composed of the myofilaments actin and myosin. In the inactive, non-contracted, state, myosin and actin are separated from each other by the molecule tropomyosin. When calcium binds to the regulatory protein troponin, tropomyosin shifts and myosin can join with actin. This connection results in a conformational change at the myosin and a sliding into each other of the myosin and actin filaments is possible, and contraction takes place (Figure 36.1.4).

Physiological Heart Action

The task of the heart is the directed flow of blood. The following sequence of the heart's action serves this purpose. First, the heart fills with blood in what is called 'diastole'. To do this, the ventricular muscles relax and the pressure in the ventricle falls below the pressure in the atrium. The valves between the ventricles and the atria (mitral and tricuspid) open and blood flows from the atria into the ventricles. Initially, this happens as the base of the heart with the valves pushes over the blood in the atria. Only towards the end of diastole is more blood forced into the ventricles by an atrial contraction. This causes the pressure in the ventricles to rise above that of the atria, and the mitral and tricuspid valves close. Systole follows, in which the contraction of the ventricular muscles increases the intraventricular pressure. In the left ventricle from about 8 to about 80 mmHg and in the right ventricle from about 5 to about 25 mmHg. As a result, the ventricular pressure is higher than that of the aorta and pulmonary trunk. The aortic and pulmonary valves open and blood is ejected. During systole, the contracture of the heart muscles from the apex to the base of the heart causes a further increase in pressure to a peak in the left ventricle of 120 mmHg (Figure 36.1.5).

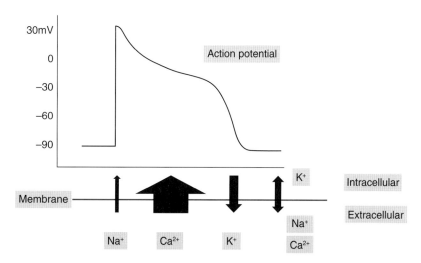

Figure 36.1.3 Ion fluxes in the generation of the action potential in the myocyte.

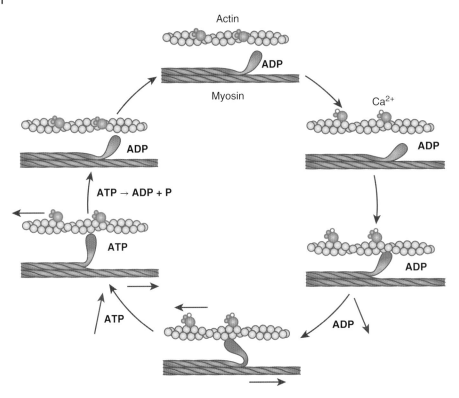

Figure 36.1.4 Sequence of muscle contraction. *Source:* Der Bewegungsapparat / https://bewegungsapparatjasmintamara.wordpress.com/das-skelett/die-muskelkontraktion-2/.

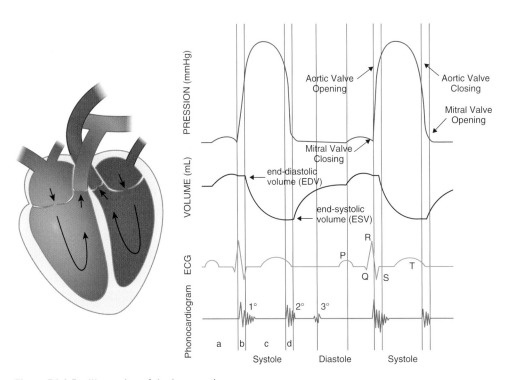

Figure 36.1.5 Illustration of the heart action.

Factors Influencing Heart Action

Although the heart works autonomously in principle, a situation-adapted cardiac output is important in order to always supply the organism with sufficient blood. An essential intracardiac mechanism of the adapted heart action is the 'Frank-Starling mechanism'. Here, the contractility of the heart muscle fibres increases when the volume in the ventricle increases. The reason for this mechanism is an increase in the sliding phase of myosin and actin filaments when they overlapped from 1.9 to 2.2 μm through pre-stretching.

A further adaptation of the cardiac action is given by the influence of the autonomic nervous system and its transmitters. The sympathetic nervous system acts via the transmitter noradrenaline on β receptors of the myocytes. These are coupled to G-protein and synthesise the second messenger cAMP. This increases the activity of protein kinase A, which increases the calcium influx into the cell. As a result, the contractile force of the myocyte increases. Overall, the sympathetic nervous system has an increasing effect on cardiac action.

The parasympathetic nervous system is connected to the heart via the vagus nerve. The transmitter is acetylcholine, which has a stabilising effect on the resting potential by opening K channels. In this way, the parasympathetic nervous system has an overall inhibitory effect on the heart's action (Table 36.1.1).

Basic Disorders of Cardiac Function

Cardiac function may be primarily disturbed by intracardiac pathomechanisms. Secondary dysfunction is when the trigger is extracardiac.

Primary disorders of cardiac function include congenital heart diseases. These include morphological defects of the heart muscle or the heart valves, as well as the blood vessels connected to the heart. This is discussed in Chapter 36.2.

Diseases of stimulus formation and conduction can arise primarily in the heart or be the result of an extracardiac disease. They are divided into supraventricular and ventricular according to their place of origin or effect (Table 36.1.2).

Among the **electrolyte changes**, changes in the potassium serum concentration have a particular effect on the heart. Depending on the concentration, these can influence the formation and transmission of excitation.

Hyperkalaemia leads to a lower resting membrane potential. This slows down depolarisation because fewer sodium channels are opened at the beginning of the action potential. At very high concentrations, the sodium channels are

Table 36.1.1   Effects of the sympathetic and parasympathetic nervous system on the heart.

Function	Sympathetic effect	Parasympathetic effect
Heart rate	Increase	Reduction
Contraction force	Increase	Reduction
Excitation conduction	Increase	Reduction
Blood pressure	Increase	Reduction

Table 36.1.2   Examples of intracardiac and extracardiac arrhythmias.

Supraventricular intracardiac	Ventricular intracardiac	Extracardiac
Mitral or tricuspid insufficiency	Congestive heart failure	Electrolyte imbalances
Dilated cardiomyopathy	Cardiomyopathy	Acid-base imbalances
Hypertrophic cardiomyopathy	Myocarditis	Hypoxia
	Pericarditis	

Source: Adapted from Ware, W.A. (2011).

inactivated so that an action potential can no longer develop, leading to cardiac arrest. **Hypokalaemia** leads to the active Na$^+$/K$^+$ ion transporter not being saturated. The consequence is a lower sodium level extracellularly, which impedes depolarisation.

Since the plateau phase of the action potential is carried by the calcium ion influx, changes in the serum calcium concentration also affect the cardiac action. **Hypercalcaemia** shortens the plateau phase because the concentration gradient supports accelerated calcium influx, which also shortens the action potential. The opposite occurs with **hypocalcaemia**, where the calcium influx slows down and the action potential lengthens.

Another factor that affects cardiac function is the **oxygen supply** to the myocytes. A reduction in the oxygen concentration due to disturbances of the pulmonary gas exchange or a reduced transport capacity due to anaemia leads to reduced ATP synthesis in the heart muscle cells. This affects the function of the Na$^+$/K$^+$-ATPase. This has the task of transporting sodium ions to the extracellular and potassium ions to the intracellular by means of active transport. The restriction of function reduces the sodium efflux, which means that no sufficient sodium concentration gradient can build up between the inside and outside of the cell. This affects depolarisation and reduces the contractile force of the myocytes. In extreme cases, cardiac arrest occurs.

General Consequences of Impaired Cardiac Function

Disturbances of cardiac function are differentiated according to their localisation in left- or right-sided disturbances.

Left-sided cardiac dysfunction leads to reduced ventricular output. Blood pressure and blood volume in the arterial system are reduced. This leads to a general undersupply of the organs in the capillary region of the arteries and to hypoxia. This induces a switch from aerobic to anaerobic glycolysis in the cells, resulting in lactate formation and acidosis. Due to the reduced organ perfusion, the acidosis is difficult to compensate for, as pulmonary and renal function is necessary for this, but this is reduced due to the reduced perfusion.

Acidosis induces vasodilation, which increases vascular permeability and can lead to the formation of oedema. At the same time, renal underperfusion due to water accumulation increases the effect of oedema formation. Chronic hypoxia also promotes the formation of erythropoietin, which leads to polycythaemia. This in turn affects the flow properties of the blood and can induce thrombus formation, which can cause emboli.

In the lungs, left-sided cardiac dysfunction causes blood stasis in the pulmonary veins; this in turn leads to increased pulmonary blood pressure and pulmonary oedema. The pulmonary oedema reduces the oxygen supply and worsens the hypoxia (Figure 36.1.6).

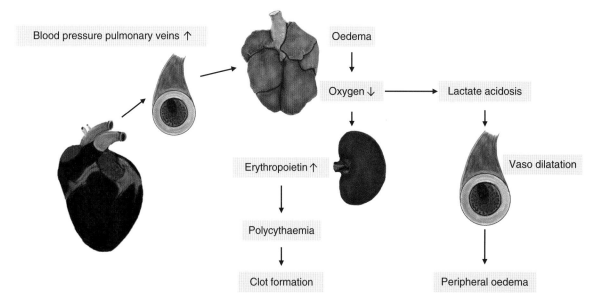

Figure 36.1.6　Mechanism of impaired left-sided cardiac function.

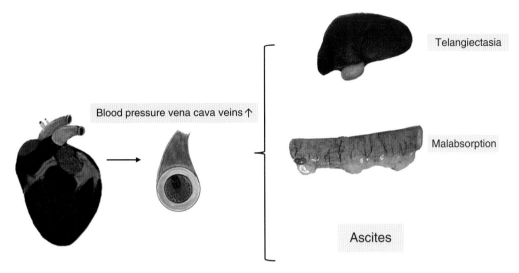

Figure 36.1.7   Mechanism of impaired right-sided heart function.

Right-sided cardiac dysfunction reduces blood flow in the peripheral veins, which results in blood stasis and vascular dilatation with an increase in vascular permeability and, as a result, oedema formation in the parenchymatous abdominal organs or ascites (Figure 36.1.7).

Compensation Mechanisms

Cardiac diseases induce different compensatory mechanisms to reduce the consequences for the organism. These can be divided into cardiac and peripheral mechanisms.

An increase in postcardiac peripheral resistance induces myocardial hypertrophy because myocardial cells are not capable of hyperplasia. As a result, hypertrophy can overcome the increased peripheral resistance and provide adequate peripheral perfusion. However, hypertrophy can only be increased within limits; in addition, there is a reduced supply of contraction force to the cardiac muscles, which limits compensation.

Peripheral Compensation Mechanisms

These occur as a result of a reduction in the cardiac output volume or with a lowered blood pressure. For compensation, the heart rate, contractility and peripheral resistance can be influenced via the sympathetic nervous system.

A second mechanism is based on the activation of the RAAS in the presence of reduced renal blood pressure. This results in an increase in blood pressure based on vasoconstriction and an increase in blood volume. The activation and consequences of the RAAS are as follows:

- It starts with the release of renin from kidney cells that are stimulated due to low blood pressure or low blood volume.
- Renin cleaves angiotensinogen, which is produced in the liver, into angiotensin I.
- Angiotensin I is converted into angiotensin II by the angiotensin-converting enzyme (ACE).
- Angiotensin II acts on blood vessels to constrict them and increase blood pressure.
- It also stimulates the release of aldosterone from the adrenal cortex.
- Aldosterone promotes the reabsorption of sodium and water in the kidneys, which leads to an increase in blood volume and blood pressure.
- Angiotensin II also stimulates the release of antidiuretic hormone (ADH), which increases water reabsorption in the kidneys.
- Angiotensin II can also act directly on the brain to increase thirst and reduce food intake to increase blood volume.
- Negative feedback of the RAAS system occurs when sufficient blood pressure and blood volume are achieved, which inhibits the release of renin.

Reference

Ware, W.A. (2011). *Cardiovascular Diseases in Small Animal Medicine*. Manson Publishing.

Further Reading

Binah, O. and Rosen, M.R. (1992). Mechanisms of ventricular arrhythmias. *Circulation* 85 (1 Suppl): I25–I31.

Nerbonne, J.M. and Kass, R.S. (2005). Molecular physiology of cardiac repolarization. *Physiological Reviews* 85 (4): 1205–1253. https://doi.org/10.1152/physrev.00002.2005.

Weidmann, S. (1974). Heart: electrophysiology. *Annual Review of Physiology* 36: 155–169. https://doi.org/10.1146/annurev.ph.36.030174.001103.

36.2

Congenital Cardiac Diseases

Definition

A heart disease is considered congenital if it is present at the time of birth and detectable in young animals. In many of these diseases, a breed disposition is recognisable, and dogs are more likely than cats to be affected by congenital heart disease.

Aetiology

Congenital heart disease occurs in dogs and cats. The prevalence is less than 1% for both species (Tidholm et al. 2015). The most common congenital changes involve morphological changes in the heart valves, followed by shunts between the atria or ventricles.

Shunts are direct connections between two fluid-filled structures with different pressures. The pressure gradient causes a flow from high pressure to low pressure.

Functionally, congenital heart diseases are differentiated into acyanotic and cyanotic. In acyanotic diseases, there is no shunt, a left-right shunt or an obstruction. Whereas in cyanotic heart diseases, a right-left shunt is found.

Most congenital heart diseases in dogs and cats are considered acyanotic because there is no blood flow from the venous low-pressure system to the arterial high-pressure system. An exception is tetralogy of Fallot, for example (Table 36.2.1).

Pathogenesis

The main congenital heart diseases in dogs and cats are explained below.

Valvular dysplasias are congenital malformations of the heart valve, the chordae tendineae or the papillary muscles. They occur in the mitral and tricuspid valves.

Mitral valve dysplasia develops due to shortened or elongated chordae tendineae, thickening or shortening of the leaflets or malposition of the papillary muscles. The result is valve insufficiency with valvular regurgitation and ventricular and atrial volume overload. This leads to left ventricular and left atrial dilatation.

The morphological changes in **tricuspid dysplasia** are comparable to those in mitral valve dysplasia. A described causality is an apical displacement of the valve attachment (Ebstein's syndrome) (Eyster et al. 1977). The functional consequence of tricuspid valve dysplasia is valve insufficiency with regurgitation and right atrial and ventricular dilatation.

Aortic stenosis leads to left ventricular outflow tract obstruction. Depending on the location of the narrowing, a distinction can be made between subvalvular, valvular and supravalvular aortic stenosis. Subvalvular aortic stenosis is the most common form of aortic stenosis in dogs; in this form, the narrowing of the outflow tract lies below the valve. The constricting structure can be fibrotic, muscular or fibromuscular in origin and can lead to static or dynamic stenosis. In the dynamic form, for example, a protrusion of the ventricular septum shifts systolically into the outflow tract. The consequences of aortic stenosis are increased left ventricular pressure, which can lead to enlargement and hypertrophy of the left ventricle. The poststenotic aorta is usually dilated.

Textbook of Small Animal Pathophysiology, First Edition. Stephan Neumann.
© 2025 John Wiley & Sons Ltd. Published 2025 by John Wiley & Sons Ltd.

Table 36.2.1 Common congenital heart diseases in dogs and cats.

Defect	Some affected breeds
Mitral valve dysplasia	Bull Terrier, German Shepherd Dog, Golden Retriever, Cats
Tricuspid valve dysplasia	Retriever, Boxer, Great Dane
Aortic stenosis	Newfoundland Dog, Rottweiler, Boxer, Cats
Pulmonic stenosis	English Bulldog, Miniature Schnauzer, West Highland White Terrier
Atrial septal defect	Boxer, Doberman Pinscher
Ventricular septal defect	English, Bulldog, Springer Spaniel, Cats
Patent ductus arteriosus	Maltese, Miniature Poodle, Yorkshire Terrier, Chihuahua

Pulmonary stenosis develops from a dysplastic pulmonary valve or a fusion of the valve parts. Supravalvular or subvalvular forms are rarely found. The consequence of pulmonary valve stenosis is right ventricular hypertrophy and poststenotic dilatation of the pulmonary arteries.

Atrial and **ventricular connections** are based on the special nature of the foetal blood circulation. In which the blood flowing into the right side of the heart has already been enriched with oxygen in the placenta. Since the lungs are not yet ventilated at this stage, only a small amount of blood needs to flow through the pulmonary artery. Most of the blood from the right side of the heart bypasses the lungs through the **foramen ovale** and the ductus arteriosus.

After the first breath, fundamental changes occur in this system, due to the expansion of the lungs, the pulmonary arterial resistance decreases acutely. This leads to increased blood flow to the lungs and increased venous return from the lungs to the left atrium. There, the blood pressure rises, reducing the pressure difference between the left and right atrium. As a result, the septa of the foramen ovale overlap and lead to its closure. If closure does not occur or does not develop completely, there is an **atrial septal defect**. The consequence of the septal defect is an atrial left-right shunt with increased blood filling and dilatation of the right atrium. As a consequence of the increased atrial blood filling, right ventricular dilatation may also develop.

Another congenital heart disease is a connection between the two ventricles of the heart, called a **ventricular septal defect**. Different localisations are possible, but the most common is the perimembranous type with a defect below the tricuspid valve. The consequences are a left-right shunt, which can be restrictive or non-restrictive.

In a restrictive ventricular septal defect, only small defects are present with minimal left-to-right shunt and sligthly elevated pulmonary artery pressure.

In a non-restrictive ventricular septal defect, blood flows through a large defect. This causes a marked left-right shunt to develop and subsequently an increase in right ventricular pressure with the development of right ventricular hypertrophy and pulmonary hypertension. In the case of pronounced pulmonary hypertension, a right-to-left shunt can develop due to the increased pulmonary vascular resistance; this is known as 'Eisenmenger's syndrome'. The consequence of a right-to-left shunt is an increase in the proportion of oxygen-depleted blood in the systemic circulation with the consequences of hypoxia and the clinical picture of cyanosis, whereby this clinical picture is classified as a cyanotic congenital heart disease.

The **persistent ductus arteriosus** is a connection between the pulmonary artery and the aorta that has persisted from foetal development. Since the lungs do not yet have a respiratory function during the foetal period, the blood coming from the right heart, oxygenated by the placenta, is conducted via the pulmonary artery and the ductus directly into the aorta, bypassing the lungs. Birth interrupts the maternal vascular supply, and the onset of respiration occurs due to the resulting hypoxia. The pulmonary arteries fill with blood and there is a drop in pulmonary vascular resistance. This reduces the volume of blood flowing from right to left in the first hours of life. As a result, the vascular intima of the duct proliferates. Another effect that leads to occlusion is caused by a postpartum drop in prostaglandin.

During the foetal phase, prostaglandin synthesis takes place in the placenta, which is why the prostaglandin serum concentration in the foetal blood is high overall.

The prostaglandin PGE2 has a vasodilatory effect on the ductus arteriosus via the prostaglandin EP4 receptor. Postpartum, there is a decrease in the PGE2 concentration and thus a vascular contraction of the ductus arteriosus. This mechanism is

Figure 36.2.1 Illustration of the different heart malformations.

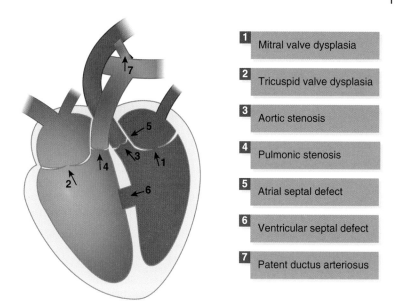

1	Mitral valve dysplasia
2	Tricuspid valve dysplasia
3	Aortic stenosis
4	Pulmonic stenosis
5	Atrial septal defect
6	Ventricular septal defect
7	Patent ductus arteriosus

supported by the inhibition of voltage-dependent potassium channels and the increase in the influx of calcium into the vascular wall muscle cells due to the increased oxygen tension in the blood, which leads to vasoconstriction (Michelakis et al. 2000).

An unclosed or partially closed ductus arteriosus leads to a left-right shunt, which can lead to dilatation of the left side of the heart and pulmonary artery hypertension.

Tetralogy of Fallot is characterised by four congenital changes in the heart, the ventricular septal defect, pulmonary stenosis, right-sided aorta and right ventricular hypertrophy. This leads to a left-right shunt, which, however, can develop into a right-left shunt in the sense of a shunt reversal in the case of pronounced pulmonary stenosis and right ventricular hypertrophy. Thus, it belongs to the cyanotic congenital heart diseases (Figure 36.2.1).

Diagnostics

Clinical signs	Clinical pathology	Imaging	Histopathology	Microbiology
Weakness	Non-specific	**Ultrasonography**	Not necessary	Not necessary
Cyanosis		Representation of the heart change		

Pathophysiologic Consequences

The congenital heart diseases have a pathophysiologic effect through

Increased afterload (aortic stenosis, pulmonary valve stenosis)
Increased preload (mitral valve dysplasia, tricuspid valve dysplasia)
a left-right shunt (atrial closure defect, septal closure defect)
a right-left shunt (tetralogy of Fallot)

as well as by acyanotic or cyanotic symptoms.

Complex diseases can also cause multiple pathophysiologic consequences. In general, congenital heart diseases become pathophysiologically and clinically manifest depending on the degree of alteration.

Influenced organ systems	Clinical symptoms	Clinical pathological alterations
Cardiovascular system	Exercise intolerance	Polycythaemia
Respiratory system	Syncope	Increased liver enzymes
Gastrointestinal system	Dyspnoea	
Hepatobiliary system	Liver congestion	
Haematological system	Abdominal effusion	
Systemic	Cyanosis	

Regardless of its location, **aortic stenosis** leads to decreased aortic pressure and reduced ejection. This can lead to reduced perfusion in the periphery. Cerebral underperfusion can lead to hypoxia, which causes **syncope**. Aortic stenosis increases the end-systolic blood volume in the left ventricle. As a consequence, this increases end-diastolic pressure, leading to enlargement of the left atrium and backpressure into the pulmonary arteries. This increases the hydrostatic pressure in the pulmonary capillaries and promotes extravasation into the interstitium and alveoli. The result is alveolar pulmonary oedema with clinically recognisable **dyspnoea**.

Compensatory changes in filling and pressure lead to a mostly concentric left ventricular hypertrophy. This reduces the coronary blood flow but at the same time increases the oxygen demand due to the hypertrophy. The ischaemia induces hypoxia in the myocytes and thus a switch to anaerobic glycolysis with intracellular acidosis. As a result, there is increased H^+ efflux through the Na^+/H^+ exchanger. This increases the intracellular Na^+ concentration, which eventually increases intracellular Ca^{2+} via Na^+/Ca^{2+} exchange. The increase of Ca^{2+} causes a mitochondrial Ca^{2+}- accumulation. This influences mitochondrial activity and reduces ATP synthesis. As a result, cellular ion homeostasis is disturbed, permeability of the cell membrane increases and cell death occurs. This can be necrotic or apoptotic (Murphy and Steenbergen 2008; Zhang et al. 2019).

At the same time, mitochondrial dysfunction can trigger arrhythmias. Mitochondrial dysfunction can cause a further increase in Ca^{2+} from the sarcoplasmic reticulum through oxidative stress (Gambardella et al. 2017).

The pathophysiologic consequences of **pulmonary stenosis** are increased volume and pressure in the right ventricle with the consequence of right heart hypertrophy and right heart failure with the described consequences of coronary underperfusion. Reflux via the right atrium into the caudal vena cava leads via **liver congestion** to hepatomegaly, portal hypertension with **ascites** and hepatocellular consequences of congestion, such as **liver enzyme elevations**. A hypertrophied right ventricle can reduce the volume of the left ventricle and thus the ejection volume by displacement of the septum. The consequences are a peripheral reduced perfusion as in aortic stenosis and thus possible triggering of a cerebral reduced supply and **syncope** (Figure 36.2.2).

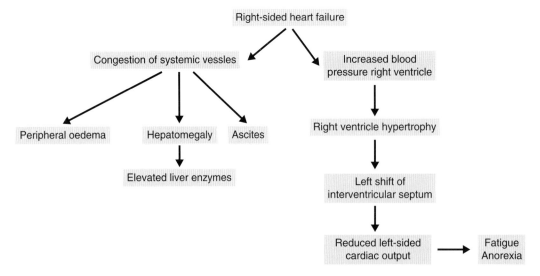

Figure 36.2.2 Pathophysiologic consequences of right heart failure.

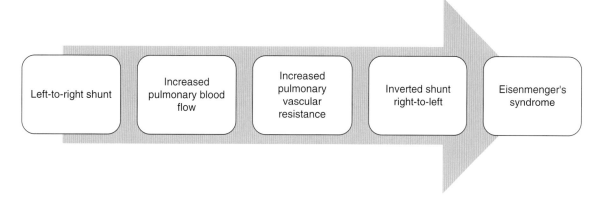

Figure 36.2.3 Pathophysiologic consequences of the left-right shunt.

Dysplasia of mitral and tricuspid valves causes regurgitation of blood volume into the left and right atrium, respectively. From there, blood backs up into the respective venous systems, causing pulmonary oedema in the left heart and ascites as a haemodynamic consequence in the right heart. The consequences are similar to those of valve insufficiencies and are described in Chapter 36.3.

The pathophysiologic consequences of atrial or septal occlusion defect or persistent ductus arteriosus vary according to severity and cause **left-right shunt**. This results in blood flow along the pressure gradient from the left to the right side of the heart. As a result, there is dilatation of the left ventricle and left atrium with left heart failure. Hypervolaemia also develops in the pulmonary vessels, leading to their vasoconstriction and pulmonary hypertension. **Pulmonary oedema** with **dyspnoea** and cough may be clinical sequelae. In addition, pulmonary hypertension causes right-sided cardiac wall hypertrophy and, in severe cases, right-to-left shunt (shunt reversal) resulting in an Eisenmenger's reaction (Figure 36.2.3).

Fallot's tetralogy is associated with the most severe pathophysiologic consequences. Due to the right-left shunt, consequences of systemic hypoxia develop. These are clinically recognisable by **weakness**, **syncope**, **dyspnoea** and **cyanosis**. Haematologically, the reduced oxygen concentration leads to **erythrocytosis** via the release of **erythropoietin**. This in turn can influence the flow properties of the blood and lead to blood stasis with thrombus formation and emboli or post-thrombotic ischaemia. An obstruction of capillary end-flow areas can negatively affect the function of the lungs, liver and kidneys, as well as the CNS.

Therapy

The therapy of congenital heart diseases is complex and therefore cannot be summarised in a table. Reference is made here to textbooks on cardiology. In principle, causal therapies for most diseases are only possible through surgical intervention or cardiac catheterisation. Therapeutic options for some secondary disease mechanisms are summarised below.

Symptom	Therapy
Pulmonary hypertension	Phosphodiesterase (PDE) type 5 inhibitor
Polycythaemia	Infusion, phlebotomy, hydroxyurea

References

Eyster, G.E., Anderson, L., Evans, A.T. et al. (1977). Ebstein's anomaly: a report of 3 cases in the dog. *Journal of the American Veterinary Medical Association* 170 (7): 709–713.

Gambardella, J., Sorriento, D., Ciccarelli, M. et al. (2017). Functional role of mitochondria in arrhythmogenesis. *Advances in Experimental Medicine and Biology* 982: 191–202. https://doi.org/10.1007/978-3-319-55330-6_10.

Michelakis, E., Rebeyka, I., Bateson, J. et al. (2000). Voltage-gated potassium channels in human ductus arteriosus. *Lancet (London, England)* 356 (9224): 134–137. https://doi.org/10.1016/S0140-6736(00)02452-1.

Murphy, E. and Steenbergen, C. (2008). Mechanisms underlying acute protection from cardiac ischemia-reperfusion injury. *Physiological Reviews* 88 (2): 581–609. https://doi.org/10.1152/physrev.00024.2007.

Tidholm, A., Ljungvall, I., Michal, J. et al. (2015). Congenital heart defects in cats: a retrospective study of 162 cats (1996–2013). *Journal of Veterinary Cardiology: The Official Journal of the European Society of Veterinary Cardiology* 17 (Suppl 1): S215–S219.

Zhang, J., Liu, D., Zhang, M., and Zhang, Y. (2019). Programmed necrosis in cardiomyocytes: mitochondria, death receptors and beyond. *British Journal of Pharmacology* 176 (22): 4319–4339. https://doi.org/10.1111/bph.14363.

Further Reading

Oliveira, P., Domenech, O., Silva, J. et al. (2011). Retrospective review of congenital heart disease in 976 dogs. *Journal of Veterinary Internal Medicine* 25 (3): 477–483.

Saunders, A.B. (2021). Key considerations in the approach to congenital heart disease in dogs and cats. *The Journal of Small Animal Practice* 62 (8): 613–623. https://doi.org/10.1111/jsap.13360.

Schrope, D.P. (2015). Prevalence of congenital heart disease in 76,301 mixed-breed dogs and 57,025 mixed-breed cats. *Journal of Veterinary Cardiology: The Official Journal of the European Society of Veterinary Cardiology* 17 (3): 192–202.

36.3

Atrioventricular Valvular Diseases

Definition

Atrioventricular valve disease is more common as an insufficiency than a stenosis and is a disorder of the valvular mechanism with inadequate closure of the valve.

Aetiology

Atrioventricular heart disease is more common in dogs than cats and more often affects the mitral valve than the tricuspid valve.

The causes can be differentiated into primary congenital or secondary forms and can be morphologically either degenerative or inflammatory.

Endocardiosis of the mitral valve is a degenerative heart valve disease. The disease occurs more frequently in certain breeds of dogs, for example, the dachshund. Accordingly, a genetic predisposition is suspected. Comparative studies on humans show homologies to Barlow's syndrome, which describes a mitral valve prolapse associated with a genetic disease called 'Marfan's syndrome'. In this disease, there is a mutation in the gene that codes for the protein fibrillin. This in turn is a component of the extracellular matrix (Oyama et al. 2020).

Another causality for valve insufficiency is infective endocarditis. This is usually triggered by streptococci (Table 36.3.1).

Pathogenesis

The morphological alterations to the valves in endocardiosis are degenerative in nature and are characterised by an increase in the extracellular matrix in the valve parenchyma. This leads to a thickening of the valve; the chordae tendinae are often also thickened and partially ruptured.

Endothelial lesions are possible triggers. There structures of the valve interstitium are exposed, which cause platelet aggregation. The result is a repair of the damaged valve apparatus with the consequences of scarring, connective tissue formation and contracture. The hypothesis does not explain all the circumstances of valve degeneration, but it helps to get an idea of the pathogenesis. The altered heart valve shows a lack of valve closure due to the apical thickening, so that an insufficiency develops. Furthermore, the morphological valve changes can cause the chordae tendinae to rupture and thus further negatively influence valve closure by allowing prolapse of the valve apex.

The pathogenesis of infective endocarditis depends on predisposing factors, such as pre-existing valve lesions, hypercoagulability or the virulence of the pathogen. If the bacteraemic pathogens settle, an inflammatory reaction develops, which is carried by platelet aggregation, fibrin formation and thickening of the heart valve. This in turn facilitates the colonisation of further pathogens (Figure 36.3.1).

Table 36.3.1 Causalities of mitral valve regurgitation.

Congenital	Infectious pathogen
	Streptococcus spp.

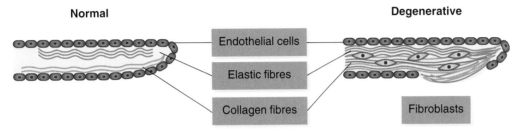

Figure 36.3.1 Morphological changes in mitral valve degeneration.

Diagnostics

Clinical signs	Clinical pathology	Imaging	Histopathology	Microbiology
Weakness Cough Abdominal distension	Non-specific	**Ultrasonography** Visualisation of the lesion and cardiac remodelling processes	Not necessary	Blood culture for suspected infective endocarditis

Pathophysiologic Consequences

The consequences of valve insufficiencies vary depending on whether the mitral or tricuspid valve is affected. The consequences of mitral valve insufficiency will be presented first.

Mitral Valve Insufficiency

Influenced organ systems	Clinical symptoms
Cardiovascular system	Cough
Respiratory system	Weakness
Urinary tract	Pre-renal failure

Systolic blood return from the left ventricle to the left atrium increases blood volume in the left atrium. This leads to backflow into the pulmonary alveolar area. The alveolar tissue consists of the alveolus, with closely connected alveolar cells, the interstitium and the alveolar capillaries. Here, the alveolus is largely free of fluid, apart from a low-grade fluid film that exerts no influence on resorption. There is hydrostatic and opposing oncotic pressure in the alveolar capillaries, both of which hold fluid as blood plasma in the capillary. A small outflow of fluid occurs into the interstitium, which is drained by peribronchial lymphatic vessels.

Cardiogenic pulmonary oedema is characterised by increased pulmonary venous pressure due to increased left atrial end-diastolic pressure. If the left atrial venous pressure exceeds 25 mmHg, the hydrostatic alveolar capillary pressure exceeds the opposing oncotic pressure and fluid can leak into the interstitium and alveolus. As a compensatory mechanism, interstitial lymphatic drainage is increased and the precapillary arteries are constricted. If the compensatory mechanisms are overwhelmed, cardiogenic pulmonary oedema develops. This affects the alveoli and the interstitium. The clinical symptom is **cough**.

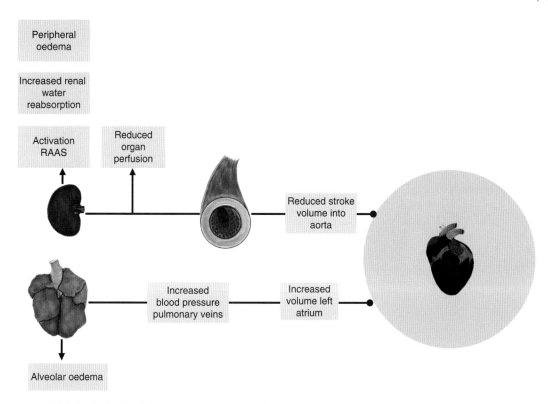

Figure 36.3.2 Pathophysiologic consequences of mitral valve regurgitation.

Systemic consequences can arise if the reduced systolic ejection from the left heart leads to peripheral underperfusion. This has different consequences.

Reduced renal perfusion leads to **pre-renal renal failure** by decreasing glomerular filtration due to reduced blood pressure in the precapillary arterioles. Accordingly, there is reduced formation of primary filtrate and eventually azotaemia. Reduced perfusion of the central nervous system (CNS) leads to hypoxia of the neurons, which reduces the formation of ATP due to reduced aerobic glycolysis. Clinical symptoms may include **weakness** and **fatigue** (Figure 36.3.2).

The consequences of mitral valve regurgitation following bacterial endocarditis are similar to those of endocardiosis. During acute endocarditis, however, further symptoms are added due to the infection. Due to the formation of inflammatory thrombi, which can be detached from the heart valves, an embolism of the coronary arteries is possible with the danger of an infarction. If the bacterial infection spreads to the myocardium, this causes a secondary myocarditis, which significantly worsens the clinical picture. Pericarditis due to invasion of the pericardium by the bacteria is also possible.

Extracardiac consequences of bacterial endocarditis usually result from bacteraemia of the pathogens, which can lead to metastatic inflammation. Or immune-mediated diseases develop due to the strong immune response to the infection. Metastatic inflammation may present as septic arthritis, osteomyelitis or myositis. Immune-mediated glomerulonephritis with proteinuria, and vasculitides with thrombus formation are also possible.

Laboratory diagnosis focuses on leucocytosis with nuclear left shift, and elevation of acute phase proteins. Mild non-regenerative anaemia due to chronic infection is also seen.

Tricuspid Valve Insufficiency

Influenced organ systems	Clinical symptoms
Cardiovascular system	Liver cirrhosis
Respiratory system	Ascites
Gastrointestinal system	Anorexia
Hepatobiliary system	Cachexia
	Dyspnoea

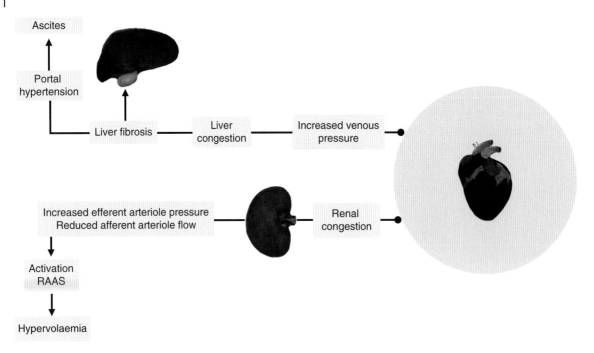

Figure 36.3.3 Pathophysiologic consequences of tricuspid regurgitation.

Due to the insufficiency of the tricuspid valve, blood congestion develops in the right atrium. This continues into the vessels of the splanchnic vascular system and initially leads to congestion in the liver. Chronic blood stasis in the liver leads to thrombosis in the vessels and sinusoids. The consequence is ischaemia of the hepatocytes. This causes a chronic inflammatory reaction with fibrotic remodelling of the liver parenchyma and **liver cirrhosis**. As a result, intrahepatic resistance increases and portal hypertension occurs. At the same time, albumin synthesis in the liver is reduced. Both lead to **ascites** with a modified transudate. At the same time, portal hypertension causes congestion of the intestinal vessels. The congestion causes ischaemia and hypoxia of the enterocytes. A cytokine-mediated reaction leads to the destruction of the tight-junctions between the enterocytes. The result is reduced absorption of food components and translocation of intestinal bacteria. The resorption disorders lead to reduced nutrition and cachexia. The process is worsened by associated anorexia. This is caused by absorbed active molecules that act directly on the satiety centre in the brain; these include short-chain fatty acids (Chen et al. 2021).

Increasing ascites leads to pressure on the diaphragm and can thus constrict the lung field and lead to **dyspnoea** (Figure 36.3.3).

Therapy

Symptom	Therapy
Reduction of the afterload	ACE inhibitor
Reduction of the afterload and increase of the contraction force	Pimobendan
Pulmonary oedema	Diuretics (e.g. Furosemide, Spironolactone)
Endocarditis, infection	Antibiotics

References

Chen, Y., Pu, W., Maswikiti, E.P. et al. (2021). Intestinal congestion and reperfusion injury: damage caused to the intestinal tract and distal organs. *Bioscience Reports* 41 (9): BSR20211560. https://doi.org/10.1042/BSR20211560.

Oyama, M.A., Elliott, C., Loughran, K.A. et al. (2020). Comparative pathology of human and canine myxomatous mitral valve degeneration: 5HT and TGF-β mechanisms. *Cardiovascular Pathology: The Official Journal of the Society for Cardiovascular Pathology* 46: 107196. https://doi.org/10.1016/j.carpath.2019.107196.

Further Reading

O'Brien, M.J., Beijerink, N.J., and Wade, C.M. (2021). Genetics of canine myxomatous mitral valve disease. *Animal Genetics* 52 (4): 409–421. https://doi.org/10.1111/age.13082.

Fox, P.R. (2012). Pathology of myxomatous mitral valve disease in the dog. *Journal of Veterinary Cardiology: The Official Journal of the European Society of Veterinary Cardiology* 14 (1): 103–126. https://doi.org/10.1016/j.jvc.2012.02.001.

Keene, B.W., Atkins, C.E., Bonagura, J.D. et al. (2019). ACVIM consensus guidelines for the diagnosis and treatment of myxomatous mitral valve disease in dogs. *Journal of Veterinary Internal Medicine* 33 (3): 1127–1140. https://doi.org/10.1111/jvim.15488.

Murray, J.F. (2011). Pulmonary edema: pathophysiology and diagnosis. *The International Journal of Tuberculosis and Lung Disease: The Official Journal of the International Union Against Tuberculosis and Lung Disease* 15 (2): 155. i.

36.4

Cardiomyopathy, Hypertrophic

Definition

Hypertrophic cardiomyopathies are defined as hypertrophy of the heart wall. They can be primary, idiopathic or secondary, and they are more often seen in cats than in dogs.

Aetiology

Genetically determined diseases are possible causes of primary idiopathic hypertrophic cardiomyopathy. A mutation in the gene encoding myosin-binding protein C has been described in Main Coon cats (Meurs et al. 2005; Fries et al. 2008). Other genetically determined diseases associated with hypertrophic cardiomyopathy are Duchenne-like muscular dystrophy in cats (Gaschen et al. 1999).

Secondary hypertrophies of the cardiac musculature are caused by diseases of the cardiac musculature; these can be consequences of inflammatory diseases or infiltrative processes such as lymphoma. Hypertrophies due to increased resistance, as in the case of obstruction of the outflow tracts (e.g. aortic stenosis), are to be distinguished from this. Finally, systemic diseases, such as endocrinopathies can lead to myocardial hypertrophy (Ferasin 2009) (Table 36.4.1).

Pathogenesis

The hypertrophy of the heart muscle in genetically determined diseases will be explained using the example of Duchenne-like muscular dystrophy.

The force generated during muscle contraction is transmitted via a membrane-bound complex that is connected intracellularly to the actin filaments and extracellularly to the basement membrane.

Dystrophin, a structural protein located on the inner cell membrane, binds to actin. While the N-terminus binds to actin, the C-terminus is connected to the so-called 'DAGPK' via dystroglycan. This complex includes $\alpha + \beta$ dystroglycan, as well as α, β, $\gamma + \delta$ sarcoglycan. The complex is membrane-bound and binds to the extracellular matrix via laminin. In addition to pure force transmission, DAGPK is also thought to play a role in stabilising the cell membrane, maintaining cell shape, Ca-shift and other metabolic processes. Dysfunctions of the DAGPK proteins lead, among other things, to the clinical picture of muscular dystrophy. In cats with Duchenne-like muscular dystrophy, reduced expression of dystrophin was found in the cardiac muscle cells (Gaschen et al. 1999). Hypertrophies of the muscles in muscular dystrophies are associated with increased remodelling of the dystrophic muscle cells and secondary fat storage and fibrosis and loss of contractile function. Compensatory hypertrophy occurs in the still intact myocytes (Cros et al. 1989) (Figure 36.4.1).

The secondary hypertrophies of the cardiac musculature develop, for example, in intra- or postcardiac obstructions. Hypertrophy of the cardiac musculature as a result of aortic stenosis is caused by increased systolic myocardial work.

The mechanism could be comparable to muscle hypertrophy through training. This is possibly mediated via the DAGPK. Repeated stretching of the complex can initiate the expression of structural proteins that lead to hypertrophy of the cell (Schiaffino et al. 2021).

The secondary endocrine cardiac hypertrophies are initiated by different mediators. In acromegaly, increased growth hormone is produced in the pituitary gland, which induces the formation of insulin like growth factor I (IGF I) in the

Textbook of Small Animal Pathophysiology, First Edition. Stephan Neumann.

Table 36.4.1 Causes of cardiac hypertrophy.

Primary	Secondary
Mutations	Vascular (D/C)
Myosin-binding protein C (C)	Stenoses
Dystrophin (C)	Systemic hypertension
	Cardiac (D/C)
	Myocarditis
	Systemic
	Hyperthyroidism (C)
	Acromegaly (C)

D – Dog, C – Cat.

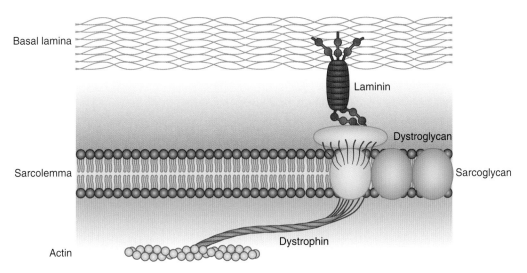

Figure 36.4.1 Dystrophin associated glycoprotein complex.

liver. This is an important anabolic hormone. It causes hypertrophy by binding to a membrane receptor. Secondary signal transduction initiates protein expression and thus the formation of structural components that lead to hypertrophy.

The influence of thyroid hormones on cardiac muscle cells takes place, on the one hand, via functional and, on the other hand, via morphological changes. Functionally, the influence takes place through an increased expression of Na^+-K^+ channel proteins, which promotes electromechanical coupling. Morphological changes are based on a binding of triiodothyronine (T3) to nuclear receptors and the initiation of protein expression (Barreto-Chaves et al. 2020).

Muscle hypertrophy in cats with hypertrophic cardiomyopathy is usually asymmetrical. The consequences of myocardial hypertrophy are disturbances in muscle relaxation associated with muscle stiffness. This in turn can reduce coronary blood flow and lead to ischaemia and fibrotic remodelling of the muscles. The remodelling processes lead to reduced ventricular filling or increased pressure is required for ventricular filling. Disturbances in the formation and transmission of excitation in the remodelled musculature can trigger arrhythmias.

Diagnostics

Clinical signs	Clinical pathology	Imaging	Histopathology	Microbiology
Weakness	Natriuretic peptides	**Ultrasonography** Visualisation of heart wall thickness and morphological remodelling processes	Not necessary	Not necessary

Pathophysiologic Consequences

Influenced organ systems	Clinical symptoms
Cardiovascular system	Abnormal heart sounds
Respiratory system	Dyspnoea
Urinary tract	Pleural effusion
Haematological system	Ascites
	Pre-renal failure
	Limb paresis or paralysis

Source: Adapted from Ferasin et al. (2003).

The pathophysiologic consequences of hypertrophic remodelling processes are based on cardiac dysfunction. These are due to disturbances in cardiac blood flow and the formation of turbulence. In cats with hypertrophic cardiomyopathy, diastolic dysfunction is manifested by reduced left ventricular filling capacity. This results in increased left atrial pressure and atrial enlargement. Consequently, increased pulmonary vein pressure develops. The altered blood flows lead to turbulence associated with the formation of thrombi.

The turbulence of the blood flow produces audible **heart murmurs**. Reduced blood flow or stagnation in the pulmonary veins causes pulmonary congestion with the formation of pulmonary oedema; this causes **dyspnoea**. Unlike dogs with pulmonary oedema, cats rarely show cough as a symptom. Reflux into the pulmonary veins increases hydrostatic pressure there and causes transudative **pleural effusion**. Less commonly, cats with hypertrophic cardiomyopathy may also have **ascites** due to reflux into the abdomen. As hypertrophic cardiomyopathy also causes reduced cardiac output, reduced renal blood flow may occur with the development of **pre-renal renal failure**.

Paresis or **paralysis** in cats with hypertrophic cardiomyopathy is caused by thrombus formation due to turbulent blood flow, particularly in the left atrium. Thrombus formation is probably mediated by von Willebrand factor (vWF). This is activated by shear forces acting on the endothelial cells during turbulent blood flow, binds to platelets and initiates thrombus formation. The process of platelet activation begins with the binding of vWF to glycoprotein Ib (GPIb) on the surface of platelets. The binding of vWF to GPIb leads to a conformational change of the GPIb complex, which activates other proteins on the platelet surface, including integrin, which promotes platelet aggregation. In addition, granules are released from the platelets. These granules contain, among other things, ADP and serotonin, which contribute to further platelet activation and platelet aggregation (Hathcock 2006).

The thrombus can be carried from the left atrium via the ventricle into the systemic circulation and cause an embolus. In cats with hypertrophic cardiomyopathy, the emboli usually occur in the bifurcation of the aorta and thus affect the supply to the hind limbs. In the postobstructive region, ischaemia leads to hypoxia and cell necrosis. The consequences are paralysis of the hind limbs (Figure 36.4.2).

Therapy

Symptom	Therapy
Relief of the heart through volume reduction and reduction of afterload	Diuretic (e.g. Furosemide, Torasemide, Spironolactone), ACE inhibitor
Pulmonary oedema, pleural effusion	Diuretic
Tachyarrhythmias	β-blockers (e.g. Atenolol), Ca-channel blockers (e.g. Diltiazem), K-channel blockers (e.g. Sotalol)
Thrombotic prophylaxis	Acetylsalicylic acid, Clopidogrel

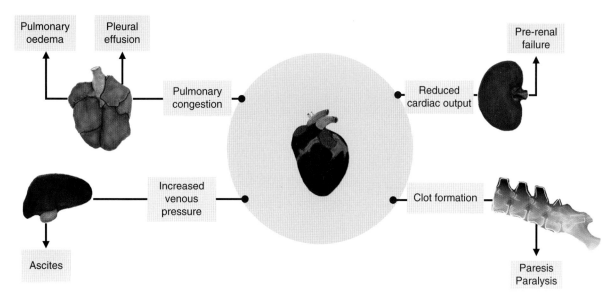

Figure 36.4.2 Pathophysiologic consequences of hypertrophic cardiomyopathy.

References

Barreto-Chaves, M.L., Senger, N., Fevereiro, M. et al. (2020). Impact of hyperthyroidism on cardiac hypertrophy. *Endocrine Connections* 9 (3): R59–R69. Advance online publication. https://doi.org/10.1530/EC-19-0543.

Cros, D., Harnden, P., Pellissier, J.F., and Serratrice, G. (1989). Muscle hypertrophy in Duchenne muscular dystrophy. A pathological and morphometric study. *Journal of Neurology* 236 (1): 43–47. https://doi.org/10.1007/BF00314217.

Ferasin, L. (2009). Feline myocardial disease. 1: Classification, pathophysiology and clinical presentation. *Journal of Feline Medicine and Surgery* 11 (1): 3–13. https://doi.org/10.1016/j.jfms.2008.11.008.

Ferasin, L., Sturgess, C.P., Cannon, M.J. et al. (2003). Feline idiopathic cardiomyopathy: a retrospective study of 106 cats (1994–2001). *Journal of Feline Medicine and Surgery* 5 (3): 151–159. https://doi.org/10.1016/S1098-612X(02)00133-X.

Fries, R., Heaney, A.M., and Meurs, K.M. (2008). Prevalence of the myosin-binding protein C mutation in Maine Coon cats. *Journal of Veterinary Internal Medicine* 22 (4): 893–896. https://doi.org/10.1111/j.1939-1676.2008.0113.x.

Gaschen, L., Lang, J., Lin, S. et al. (1999). Cardiomyopathy in dystrophin-deficient hypertrophic feline muscular dystrophy. *Journal of Veterinary Internal Medicine* 13 (4): 346–356. https://doi.org/10.1892/0891-6640(1999)013<0346:ciddhf>2.3.co;2.

Hathcock, J.J. (2006). Flow effects on coagulation and thrombosis. *Arteriosclerosis, Thrombosis, and Vascular Biology* 26 (8): 1729–1737. https://doi.org/10.1161/01.ATV.0000229658.76797.30.

Meurs, K.M., Sanchez, X., David, R.M. et al. (2005). A cardiac myosin binding protein C mutation in the Maine Coon cat with familial hypertrophic cardiomyopathy. *Human Molecular Genetics* 14 (23): 3587–3593. https://doi.org/10.1093/hmg/ddi386.

Schiaffino, S., Reggiani, C., Akimoto, T., and Blaauw, B. (2021). Molecular mechanisms of skeletal muscle hypertrophy. *Journal of Neuromuscular Diseases* 8 (2): 169–183. https://doi.org/10.3233/JND-200568.

Further Reading

Luis Fuentes, V., Abbott, J., Chetboul, V. et al. (2020). ACVIM consensus statement guidelines for the classification, diagnosis, and management of cardiomyopathies in cats. *Journal of Veterinary Internal Medicine* 34 (3): 1062–1077.

Kittleson, M.D. and Côté, E. (2021). The feline cardiomyopathies: 2. Hypertrophic cardiomyopathy. *Journal of Feline Medicine and Surgery* 23 (11): 1028–1051.

Maron, B.J. and Fox, P.R. (2015). Hypertrophic cardiomyopathy in man and cats. *Journal of Veterinary Cardiology: The Official Journal of the European Society of Veterinary Cardiology* 17 (Suppl 1): S6–S9.

Stern, J.A. and Ueda, Y. (2019). Inherited cardiomyopathies in veterinary medicine. *Pflugers Archiv: European Journal of Physiology* 471 (5): 745–753.

36.5

Cardiomyopathy, Dilated

Definition

Dilated cardiomyopathy (DCM) is characterised by impaired myocardial contractility of the left ventricle or both ventricles. The consequence is dilatation of the ventricles and reduced cardiac output.

Aetiology

Dilated cardiomyopathy is genetically induced in most cases. A familial accumulation is present in some dog breeds, such as Boxer and Doberman. Secondary dilated cardiomyopathies are described as a result of taurine and carnitine deficiency, chronic tachyarrhythmia and infectious myocarditis, as after parvovirus infections. Dogs are more often affected than cats.

Genetic	Metabolic	Cardiovascular
	Taurine deficiency (C)	Chronic tachyarrhythmia (D/C)
	Carnitine deficiency (D)	Myocarditis (D/C)

D – Dog, C – Cat

Pathogenesis

Primary DCM in dogs is generally considered idiopathic due to its unexplained pathogenesis. Numerous studies on genetic variations are available, in which different candidate molecules were investigated. Since the process is probably polygenetic, the possible pathogenesis is presented here as an example using a genetic variation of the endothelin (Matsa et al. 2014).

Endothelin is a peptide consisting of 21 amino acids, which is released by vascular endothelial cells under the influence of angiotensin, antidiuretic hormone, reactive oxygen species (ROS) and various cytokines as an inactive precursor. Under the influence of endothelin-converting enzymes, the biologically active 21-amino acid endothelin is released from the 39 amino acid precursor. Endothelin acts on different cell types, including the heart muscle cells, where it acts via a G-protein. G-proteins are connected to an enzyme, adenylate cyclase, which forms cyclic AMP (cAMP) from ATP. This acts as a second messenger in intracellular signal transduction. cAMP activates a protein kinase and induces Ca^+ influx from the sarcoplasmic reticulum. This results in increased myocardial contractility, an increase in heart rate and an increase in electrical conductivity.

In addition, endothelin has a stimulating effect on aldosterone secretion, reduces renal blood flow and thus the glomerular filtration rate and releases atrial natriuretic peptide (ANP). In the case of a gene mutation, the endothelin structure and effect are altered. This is a possible pathogenetic mechanism of canine DCM (Leary et al. 2020).

Other possible causes of DCM are disturbances in the energy production of the myocytes. This can be due to a disturbed expression of mitochondrial proteins of complexes I and V, which are involved in the synthesis of ATP (Lopes et al. 2006).

The consequences of both patterns of dysfunction are a reduced cardiac output, which activates the RAAS, leading to increased Na^+ and water retention. The result is a volume overload of the heart, which can be compensated. If the maximum compensation is exceeded, congestive heart failure develops, which is responsible for the pathophysiologic consequences (Figure 36.5.1).

Textbook of Small Animal Pathophysiology, First Edition. Stephan Neumann.
© 2025 John Wiley & Sons Ltd. Published 2025 by John Wiley & Sons Ltd.

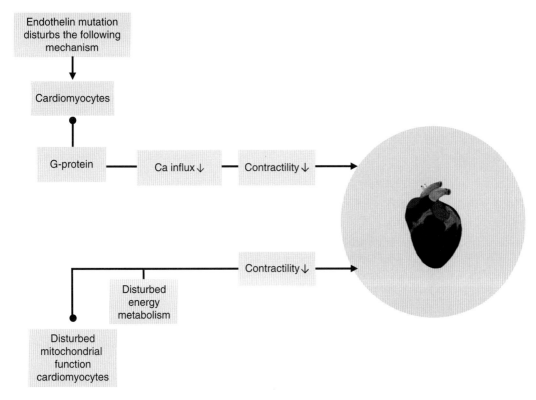

Figure 36.5.1 Pathogenesis of dilated cardiomyopathy.

Diagnostics

Clinical signs	Clinical pathology	Imaging	Histopathology	Microbiology
Weakness Syncope Cough	Mainly non-specific, Natriuretic peptides	**Ultrasonography** Visualisation of ventricular wall thickness and contractility	Not necessary	Not necessary

Pathophysiologic Consequences

Influenced organ systems	Clinical symptoms	Clinical pathology
Cardiovascular system	Weakness	Natriuretic peptides increased
Respiratory system	Weight loss	ALT, AST, GLDH increased
Urinary tract	Abdominal effusion	ALP increased
	Dyspnoea	Urea, creatinine Phosphorus increased
	Syncope	

The pathophysiologic consequences of DCM usually develop in the advanced stage of the disease and manifest as congestive heart failure, which is pronounced on the left and right sides. This results in organ damage due to congestion, and at the same time the ejection capacity is reduced, leading to organ diminished perfusion.

In **right-sided** congestive heart failure, at the end of the compensatory phase, the myocardium is unable to ensure adequate cardiac ejection. Reflux develops into the right atrium. From there, blood stasis continues via the vena cavae. Abdominal organs develop congestion-induced insufficiency.

Liver congestion is characterised by congested hepatic veins, an increase in transaminases indicating impaired hepatocellular integrity and congestion in the portal vessels. This indicates portal hypertension and **ascites**. The effect is intensified by reduced liver function as a result of liver congestion, which causes reduced albumin synthesis. This reduces oncotic pressure and may increase abdominal effusion.

The renal consequences of congestive heart failure are based, on the one hand, on reduced cardiac output and the resulting reduced renal perfusion, and on the other hand, on reduced venous outflow from the kidneys. The consequences are renal hypoxia, increased interstitial pressure and, as a result, interstitial fibrosis. This, combined with a reduction in glomerular filtration, leads to renal failure (Figure 36.5.2).

Intestinal morphology, permeability and absorption are also altered in heart failure. Systemic/venous congestion, sympathetic vasoconstriction and low cardiac output contribute to reduced splanchnic microcirculation and increase the risk of intestinal ischaemia. Resorption disorders resulting in **weight loss** and **weakness** are the consequences. In addition, ischaemia causes epithelial cell dysfunction and loss of gut barrier function, allowing lipopolysaccharide or endotoxin produced by gram-negative gut bacteria to enter the circulatory system and trigger systemic inflammation (Harjola et al. 2017).

Left-sided congestive heart failure primarily affects the lungs through congestion and the brain through reduced peripheral perfusion.

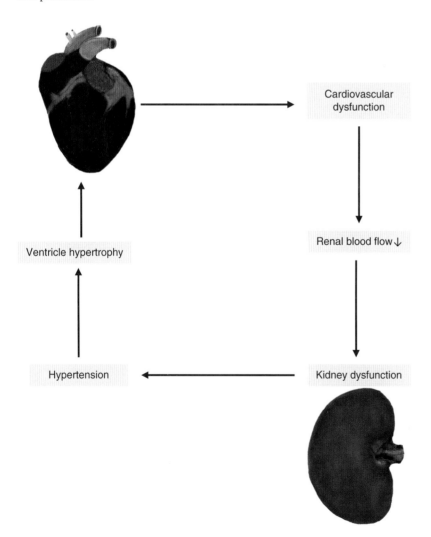

Figure 36.5.2 Relationship between cardiac dysfunction and renal failure. *Source:* Pouchelon et al. (2015) / John Wiley & Sons.

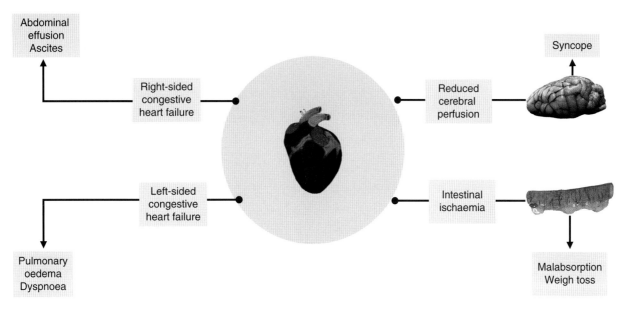

Figure 36.5.3 Pathophysiologic consequences of dilated cardiomyopathy.

Reduced blood flow from the left ventricle causes increased hydrostatic blood pressure in the pulmonary capillaries, which exaggerates the oncotic pressure, therefore leading to extravasation into the pulmonary interstitium and alveoli, with alveolar pulmonary oedema and **dyspnoea**.

The reduced perfusion in the brain leads to cerebral deficits and even syncope (Harjola et al. 2017) (Figure 36.5.3).

Therapy

Symptom	Therapy
Reduced cardiac output	ACE inhibitor, Pimobendan
Tachyarrhythmia	β-blockers (e.g. Atenolol), Ca-channel blockers (e.g. Diltiazem),
Effusion	Diuretics (e.g. Furosemide)

References

Harjola, V.P., Mullens, W., Banaszewski, M. et al. (2017). Organ dysfunction, injury and failure in acute heart failure: from pathophysiology to diagnosis and management. A review on behalf of the Acute Heart Failure Committee of the Heart Failure Association (HFA) of the European Society of Cardiology (ESC). *European Journal of Heart Failure* 19 (7): 821–836. https://doi.org/10.1002/ejhf.872.

Leary, P.J., Jenny, N.S., Bluemke, D.A. et al. (2020). Endothelin-1, cardiac morphology, and heart failure: the MESA angiogenesis study. *The Journal of Heart and Lung Transplantation: The Official Publication of the International Society for Heart Transplantation* 39 (1): 45–52. https://doi.org/10.1016/j.healun.2019.07.007.

Lopes, R., Solter, P.F., Sisson, D.D. et al. (2006). Correlation of mitochondrial protein expression in complexes I to V with natural and induced forms of canine idiopathic dilated cardiomyopathy. *American Journal of Veterinary Research* 67 (6): 971–977. https://doi.org/10.2460/ajvr.67.6.971.

Matsa, L.S., Sagurthi, S.R., Ananthapur, V. et al. (2014). Endothelin 1 gene as a modifier in dilated cardiomyopathy. *Genes* 548 (2): 256–262. https://doi.org/10.1016/j.gene.2014.07.043.

Pouchelon, J.L., Atkins, C.E., Bussadori, C. et al. (2015). Cardiovascular-renal axis disorders in the domestic dog and cat: a veterinary consensus statement. *The Journal of Small Animal Practice* 56 (9): 537–552. https://doi.org/10.1111/jsap.12387.

Further Reading

Freid, K.J., Freeman, L.M., Rush, J.E. et al. (2021). Retrospective study of dilated cardiomyopathy in dogs. *Journal of Veterinary Internal Medicine* 35 (1): 58–67.

Kittleson, M.D. and Côté, E. (2021). The feline cardiomyopathies: 3. Cardiomyopathies other than HCM. *Journal of Feline Medicine and Surgery* 23 (11): 1053–1067.

Pion, P.D., Kittleson, M.D., Rogers, Q.R., and Morris, J.G. (1987). Myocardial failure in cats associated with low plasma taurine: a reversible cardiomyopathy. *Science (New York, N.Y.)* 237 (4816): 764–768.

Stern, J.A. and Ueda, Y. (2019). Inherited cardiomyopathies in veterinary medicine. *Pflugers Archiv: European Journal of Physiology* 471 (5): 745–753.

Wright, K.N., Gompf, R.E., and DeNovo, R.C. (1999). Peritoneal effusion in cats: 65 cases (1981–1997). *Journal American Veterinary Medical Association* 214: 375–381.

36.6

Heart Arrhythmia

Definition

Cardiac arrhythmias are disturbances in the heart rhythm resulting in irregular heart activity.

Aetiology

Cardiac arrhythmias can be the cause or consequence of heart disease and can develop due to systemic diseases. They are principally differentiated into increased activity, tachyarrhythmia, and reduced activity, bradyarrhythmia. Cardiac arrhythmias are more common in dogs than in cats (Tables 36.6.1 and 36.6.2).

Bradyarrhythmias occur when excitation or conduction are disturbed; this can affect all elements of the conduction system. Causes are, for example inflammations, which induce tissue destruction in the acute phase and can thus impede impulse conduction. In the chronic phase, a connective tissue substitute develops in the form of a scar, which can also impede impulse conduction. However, many clinically manifest bradycardias in dogs and cats are idiopathic or the consequence of an extracardiac disease.

These include diseases that are localised outside the heart and affect cardiac function. Metabolic diseases, such as hypothyroidism are among them. Cardiological consequences of hypothyroidism are disturbances in lipid metabolism, which increase oxidative stress in the cardiocytes and can lead to apoptosis, which triggers a local inflammatory reaction with an influence on impulse transmission. Another mechanism that occurs in hypothyroidism is a reduction in energy metabolism. A reduction in ATP concentration interferes with energy-dependent ion channels and, by interfering with repolarisation, also interferes with depolarisation (Abdel-Moneim et al. 2020).

Further, extracardiac factors influencing conduction develop from electrolyte changes. In particular, hyperkalaemia has a significant influence on the formation of excitation in the heart. Depending on the serum concentration, hyperkalaemia leads to an increased influx of potassium ions into excitable cells. This leads to a lower resting membrane potential. As a result, depolarisation is slowed down because fewer sodium channels are opened at the beginning of the action potential. In the late plateau phase of the action potential, the conductivity for potassium increases, which shortens repolarisation. The result is extrasystoles. At very high concentrations, the sodium channels are inactivated.

Tachyarrhythmias are also cardiogenic, but more often due to the influence of sympathetic nerve fibres on the heart's action. The influence of the sympathetic nervous system on the excitable cells of the sinus node takes place via so-called 'pacemaker channels'. These enable an immediate sodium influx after repolarisation. The channels are activated when an impulse reaches the presynaptic membrane of the sympathetic nervous system. This results in the release of noradrenaline as a transmitter, which acts on β-adrenergic receptors in the postsynaptic membrane. This leads to a release of cAMP as a second messenger, which acts on the pacemaker channels and influences the ion flux by conformational change (Vedantham and Scheinman 2017).

Table 36.6.1 Causes of bradyarrhythmia.

Cardiac	Electrolytes	Metabolic
Sick sinus syndrome (D)	Hypercalcaemia (D/C)	Hypothyroidism (D)
Third degree AV-block (D)	Hypocalcaemia (D/C)	Hypoadrenocorticism (D)

Table 36.6.2 Causes of tachyarrhythmia.

Cardiac	Metabolic	Sympathicus
Atrial fibrillation (D/C)	Hyperthyroidism (C)	Fever (D/C)
Ventricular fibrillation (D/C)		Pain (D/C)

D – Dog, C – Cat

The influence of hyperthyroidism on the heart is manifold. An influence on the heart rhythm with the formation of a tachycardia is probably triggered via the autonomic nervous system, an increased sympathetic tone or probably more likely a parasympatholytic increase the heart rate. Another mechanism could result from an influence of the thyroid hormones on the potassium channels with the consequence of a shortening of the action potential (Hu et al. 2005; Ahmad et al. 2022).

Diagnostics

Clinical signs	Clinical pathology	Imaging	Histopathology	Microbiology
Weakness	Non-specific	**ECG**	Not necessary	Not necessary
Syncope		Diagnosis and differentiation of arrhythmias		

Pathophysiologic Consequences

The pathophysiologic consequences of arrhythmias result primarily from disturbed cardiac functions and can be divided into right-heart and left-heart dysfunction.

The individual consequences have already been explained in the other chapters of this section. Therefore, here is a general overview:

Influenced organ systems	Clinical symptoms
Cardiovascular system	Weakness
Respiratory system	Anorexia
Gastrointestinal system	Dyspnoea
Hepatobiliary system	Abdominal distension
Pancreas	
Urinary tract	

Cardiac arrhythmias lead to an impairment of the heart muscle contraction and thus reduce the pumping function of the heart.

An irregular heart rate can lead to the heart not being supplied with sufficient blood and oxygen, which can lead to hypoxia and impaired organ function. This also relates to other organs, such as the central nervous system. Decreased renal perfusion can lead to renal failure.

In addition, cardiac arrhythmias can lead to an increased release of stress hormones such as adrenaline. Finally, due to turbulence in the blood flow, thrombi can be formed, leading to emboli (Figure 36.6.1).

Figure 36.6.1 Summary of right and left-heart failure.

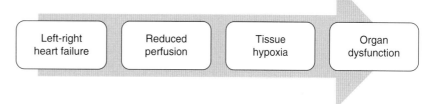

Figure 36.6.2 Mode of action of the antiarrhythmic drugs.

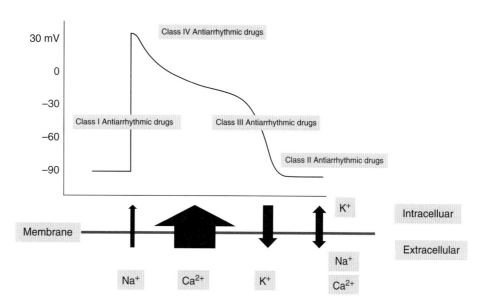

Therapy

Symptom	Therapy
Tachycardia	Class I-IV antiarrhythmics (Class Ia e.g. Procainamide; Class Ib e.g. Lidocaine, Mexilitin; Class II beta-blockers; Class III e.g. Sotalol; Class IV e.g. Diltiazem, Verapamil)
Bradycardia	Atropine, pacemaker implantation (Figure 36.6.2)

References

Abdel-Moneim, A., Gaber, A.M., Gouda, S. et al. (2020). Relationship of thyroid dysfunction with cardiovascular diseases: updated review on heart failure progression. *Hormones (Athens, Greece)* 19 (3): 301–309. https://doi.org/10.1007/s42000-020-00208-8.

Ahmad, M., Reddy, S., Barkhane, Z. et al. (2022). Hyperthyroidism and the risk of cardiac arrhythmias: anarrative review. *Cureus* 14 (4): e24378. https://doi.org/10.7759/cureus.24378.

Hu, L.W., Liberti, E.A., and Barreto-Chaves, M.L. (2005). Myocardial ultrastructure in cardiac hypertrophy induced by thyroid hormone–an acute study in rats. *Virchows Archiv* 446 (3): 265–269. https://doi.org/10.1007/s00428-004-1175-1.

Vedantham, V. and Scheinman, M.M. (2017). Familial inappropriate sinus tachycardia: a new chapter in the story of HCN4 channelopathies. *European Heart Journal* 38 (4): 289–291. https://doi.org/10.1093/eurheartj/ehv635.

36.7

Pericardial Disease

Definition

Pericardial diseases are diseases of the pericardium of varying aetiology.

Aetiology

The different aetiologies most often cause effusion in the pericardium. Neoplastic diseases are particularly frequent. Inflammations leading to pericarditis are rare and often associated with FIP in the cat. Finally, pericardial effusion can also be a consequence of coagulopathy. Overall, pericardial disease is more common in dogs than in cats.

Neoplasms	Inflammation	Coagulopathy
Heart base tumour (D)	FIP (C)	Extrinsic (D)
Mesothelioma (D/C)		Intrinsic (D)
Metastasis e.g. haemangiosarcoma (D)		
Lymphoma (C)		

D – Dog, C – Cat

Pathogenesis

Most of the causal diseases lead to pericardial effusion due to vascular coagulopathy, tumour haemorrhage due to vascular erosion or inflammatory secretion from the pericardium.

The pericardium surrounds the heart and forms the pericardium; it is composed of a visceral serosa and a parietal serosa. The innermost cell layer in the pericardium is composed of flat to cubic mesothelial cells, which carry numerous microvilli lumenward for secretion and absorption of the pericardial fluid. Below the mesothelial cells follows a subserosal layer with connective tissue cells and blood vessels, nerves and sessile macrophages (Figure 36.7.1).

Pericardial tumours have an impact on the heart through a direct impression due to expansive growth. The connective tissue structure of the pericardium promotes expansion towards the myocardium. Furthermore, tumour growth can cause vascular compression of the subserosal vessels in the parietal pericardium. This increases hydrostatic pressure in the vessels and leads to increased fluid secretion into the pericardium. Finally, the tumour may invasively grow into or originate from a blood vessel (haemangiosarcoma); in either case, bleeding develops into the pericardium (Refaat and Katz 2011).

Tumour growth is often associated with angiogenesis, which can be induced by angiogenic growth factors of the tumour cells (e.g. vascular endothelial growth factor (VEGF)). Local haemorrhages as a result of tumour diseases can arise through different mechanisms. On the one hand, erosion of the blood vessels by ingrowing tumour tissue leads to

Figure 36.7.1 Histology of the pericardium.

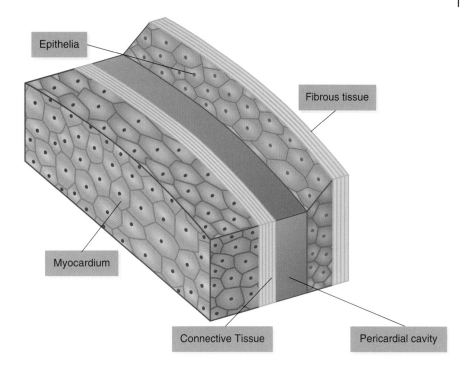

destruction of the vessel wall structure and leakage of blood, and on the other hand, increased tumour growth leads to an insufficient oxygen supply with the consequence of hypoxia and final cell necrosis. This destroys parts of the internal structure of the tumour, including vessels, whose destruction leads to bleeding (Figure 36.7.2).

Inflammatory pericardial diseases induce the formation of an exudate. This is a protein- and cell-rich inflammatory secretion that is formed due to the inflammatory process. On the one hand, the inflammation-induced increase in blood flow leads to an increased hydrostatic vascular pressure and consequently to a higher movement of fluid into the surrounding tissue. At the same time, however, the vascular permeability is also increased during inflammation, which leads to a displacement of proteins into the interstitium. This increases the colloid osmotic pressure there, which leads to further fluid movement out of the vessels.

In coagulopathy, the lack of blood clotting causes leakage from the pericardial blood vessels into the pericardium (Figure 36.7.3).

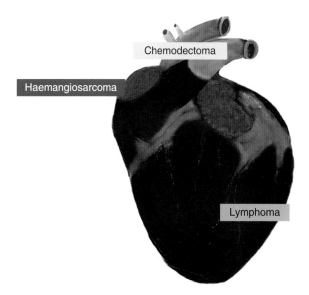

Figure 36.7.2 Typical localisations of cardiac neoplasms.

A highly haemodynamically relevant filling of the pericardial sac with fluid is called 'pericardial tamponade'. This can be caused by accumulation of secretions due to inflammation or as transudate due to a high reduction in oncotic pressure. The most frequent cause, however, is bleeding into the pericardium. If the fluid accumulation occurs slowly, limited distension of the pericardium may develop. If it fills rapidly, the pericardium hardly stretches at all and compression of the heart and cardiac vessels occurs. This is often due to haemorrhage into the pericardium and is more common in dogs than cats.

The compression of the heart muscle as a result of the tamponade causes a reduced filling of the heart chambers, which reduces the cardiac output. This leads to reduced perfusion of peripheral organs with the development of corresponding organ insufficiencies. At the same time, the coronary blood flow to the heart muscle is reduced. This leads to reduced perfusion and ischaemia with hypoxia. This has an additional influence on the heart function.

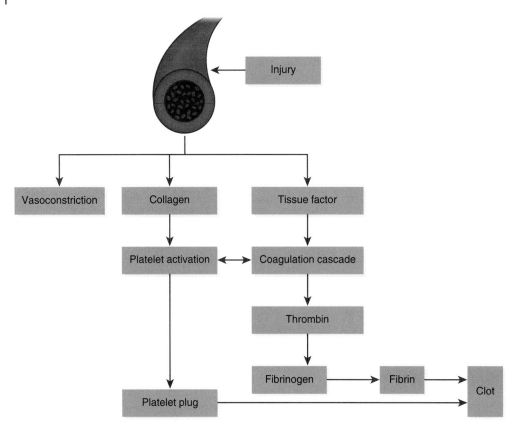

Figure 36.7.3 Mechanism of blood clotting.

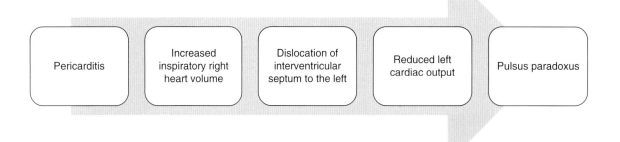

Figure 36.7.4 Mechanism of the 'Pulsus paradoxus'.

One consequence of pericardial tamponade is increased respiratory-influenced variation in blood pressure. Under physiological conditions, the intrapericardial pressure is reduced during inspiration, which increases the filling of the right side of the heart. This results in a leftward shift of the intraventricular septum intracardially. This leads to a reduced left ventricular filling compared to expiration. This reduces inspiratory left ventricular ejection and thus arterial blood pressure. In the case of an effusion in the pericardium, the inspiratory pressure reduction is increased, resulting in an increased drop in arterial pressure of ≥10 mmHg during inspiration. This also reduces coronary blood flow and increases inferior perfusion of the myocardium (Savitt et al. 1993) (Figure 36.7.4).

Diagnostics

Clinical signs	Clinical pathology	Imaging	Histopathology	Microbiology
Weakness Syncope	Non-specific	**Ultrasonography** Visualisation of pericardial effusion and possible pericardial thickening	**Cytology** Identification of tumour cells	Mostly not necessary

Pathophysiologic Consequences

The main consequences of pericardial diseases result from a mass in the pericardium. The total amount of pericardial fluid, whose composition is similar to blood plasma, is a few millilitres under physiological conditions. If the amount of fluid increases, the pressure in the pericardium increases. This acts in all directions, including on the pericardium, which can yield to the pressure and expand due to elastic fibres in the subserosa. However, this only happens gradually as the volume slowly increases. If the volume in the pericardium increases rapidly before the fibres can yield to the pressure increase by stretching, or if the chronic pericardial filling reaches a point at which stretching is no longer possible, the pressure causes an impairment of cardiac action. The intrapericardial pressure is between 0 and 4 mmHg, depending on breathing. If the pressure reaches the pressure in the right atrium (4–8 mmHg), venous blood flow to the heart and cardiac filling is impaired. As the pressure rises, the function of the left heart is also affected.

Influenced organs	Clinical symptoms	Clinical pathological alterations
Cardiovascular system	Lethargy	Azotaemia
Respiratory system	Anorexia	Increased liver enzymes
Hepatobiliary system	Syncope	
Urinary tract	Abdominal distension	

The pathophysiologic consequences of pericardial disease are due to congestive heart failure. This develops due to compression of the myocardium and compression of the venous and arterial blood supply. The resulting peripheral underperfusion reduces the central nervous oxygen supply. In acute cases, compensatory mechanisms fail and **lethargy** and **syncope** occurs. This is due to a disturbance of the central energy metabolism. The brain is a metabolically highly active organ with a high demand for oxygen. Even short-term interruptions of the oxygen supply lead to a disturbance of the cellular energy supply. As a result, ATP-dependent ion transporters and ion homeostasis at the nervous cell membrane are disturbed. This causes a reduction in nervous impulse activity and can clinically cause a syncope (Markus 2004).

Systemic reduced perfusion can lead to a reduction in preglomerular blood pressure. As a result, the filtration pressure in the glomerulum is reduced because the hydrostatic vascular pressure decreases. This leads to retention of substances physiologically excreted via urine. The reduced perfusion also reduces the oxygen supply to the renal parenchyma, especially the tubular epithelia. This reduces renal reabsorption processes and disrupts systemic homeostasis. The reduced perfusion also initiates damage to the tubular epithelial cells with the formation of apoptosis and necrosis. The latter induces an inflammatory reaction, which in turn can have a further unfavourable influence on the course of the disease, as the inflammatory infiltration additionally hinders the reabsorption processes at the epithelium. This is followed by renal failure with **azotaemia**.

The increasing pressure in the pericardium leads to ventricular compression resulting in decreased ventricular filling, which can cause right ventricular congestion leading to right heart failure with congestion of the abdominal vessels, with **abdominal effusion**. Vascular congestion in the liver leads to reduced perfusion and hypoxia of the hepatocytes. This initially induces damage to the cell membrane integrity and thus a release of hepatic enzymes. The result is a moderate hepatopathy with elevation of **liver** enzymes (Ramasamy et al. 2018; Prabhakar et al. 2019).

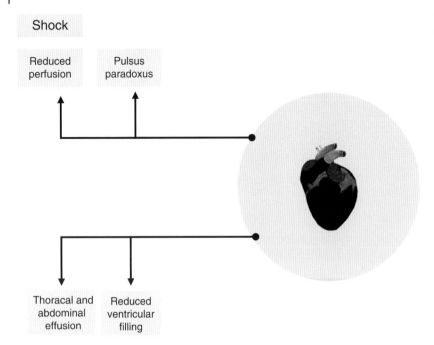

Figure 36.7.5 Pathophysiologic consequences of pericardial disease.

A special pericardial disease with severe clinical consequences is the congenital peritoneal-pericardial diaphragmatic hernia. The cause is assumed to be an embryonic developmental disorder of the septum transversum. Due to the displacement of abdominal organs into the pericardium, cardiological, respiratory and abdominal symptoms may develop. These include syncope, which may result from reduced cardiac output due to compression on the pericardium by abdominal organs. Respiratory symptoms, such as dyspnoea and cough result from thoracic space-occupying herniation and dilatation of the pericardium with restriction of the lung field. Finally, abdominal symptoms, such as vomiting and diarrhoea develop due to interference with the peristalsis of the stomach and intestines and due to altered vascularisation. The former can lead to vomiting; the latter can reduce intestinal absorption, leading to osmotic diarrhoea. All factors together affect nutrient absorption and the oxygen supply for nutrient metabolism, which can lead to weakness and emaciation (Figure 36.7.5).

Therapy

Symptom	Therapy
Chronic recurrent pericardial effusion	Fenestration of the pericardium
Coagulopathy	e.g. Vitamin K in case of intoxication with Vitamin K antagonists

References

Markus, H.S. (2004). Cerebral perfusion and stroke. *Journal of Neurology, Neurosurgery, and Psychiatry* 75 (3): 353–361. https://doi.org/10.1136/jnnp.2003.025825.

Prabhakar, Y., Goyal, A., Khalid, N. et al. (2019). Pericardial decompression syndrome: a comprehensive review. *World Journal of Cardiology* 11 (12): 282–291. https://doi.org/10.4330/wjc.v11.i12.282.

Ramasamy, V., Mayosi, B.M., Sturrock, E.D., and Ntsekhe, M. (2018). Established and novel pathophysiological mechanisms of pericardial injury and constrictive pericarditis. *World Journal of Cardiology* 10 (9): 87–96. https://doi.org/10.4330/wjc.v10.i9.87.

Refaat, M.M. and Katz, W.E. (2011). Neoplastic pericardial effusion. *Clinical Cardiology* 34 (10): 593–598. https://doi.org/10.1002/clc.20936.

Savitt, M.A., Tyson, G.S., Elbeery, J.R. et al. (1993). Physiology of cardiac tamponade and paradoxical pulse in conscious dogs. *The American Journal of Physiology* 265 (6 Pt 2): H1996–H2008. https://doi.org/10.1152/ajpheart.1993.265.6.H1996.

Further Reading

Aupperle, H., März, I., Ellenberger, C. et al. (2007). Primary and secondary heart tumours in dogs and cats. *Journal of Comparative Pathology* 136 (1): 18–26.

Lombard, C.W. (1983). Pericardial disease. *The Veterinary Clinics of North America. Small Animal Practice* 13 (2): 337–353.

Treggiari, E., Pedro, B., Dukes-McEwan, J. et al. (2017). A descriptive review of cardiac tumours in dogs and cats. *Veterinary and Comparative Oncology* 15 (2): 273–288.

36.8

Hypertension

Definition

Hypertension is defined as sustained, elevated arterial blood pressure. A systolic blood pressure of 160 mmHg is seen as the threshold value.

Aetiology

Elevated blood pressure can be a consequence of various organ dysfunctions. In many cases, the hypertension is idiopathic. The regulation of blood pressure is principally influenced by cardiac output and peripheral vascular resistance.

The regulation of blood pressure can be divided into short-term regulation, which is activated within a few seconds. This takes place through vascular baroreceptors in the aorta and carotid artery, which transmit information about blood pressure via afferent nerve pathways of the IX and X cranial nerves to the central nervous system. Sympathetic efferents adjust cardiac output and vascular tone accordingly.

Medium-term regulation (minutes to hours) of blood pressure is controlled by the RAAS. The trigger for the blood pressure adjustment is the perfusion of the renal glomeruli. In case of reduced perfusion, the ultrafiltrate in the proximal renal tubule is reduced. The resulting reduced Na^+ concentration is detected by specialised cells of the macula densa and renin is released. Renin acts as a protease and cleaves angiotensin I from angiotensinogen, which is produced in the liver. Under the catalysis of the angiotensin converting enzyme, which is predominantly expressed in the endothelial cells of the pulmonary vessels, angiotensin II is cleaved from angiotensin I. Angiotensin II has a direct vasoconstrictor effect via a G-protein-mediated intracellular Ca^{2+} release. Furthermore, a vasoconstrictor effect takes place via noradrenalin. The long-term regulation of blood pressure (hours to days) is controlled by the adjustment of fluid balance via ADH, aldosterone and natriuretic peptides. A blood pressure-increasing effect takes place through an increase in blood volume. This is achieved through increased water reabsorption. Aldosterone causes increased Na^+ and water reabsorption in the distal tubule. ADH can induce the increased synthesis of aquaporins in the collecting tube in a receptor-controlled manner and thereby increase water reabsorption. The antagonists are natriuretic peptides. These are formed in the atria when the volume load increases there. The result is reduced Na^+ and water reabsorption in the proximal tubule (Figure 36.8.1).

The aetiologies for hypertension are diverse according to the regulatory mechanisms. Besides the frequently occurring idiopathic hypertension, renal and hormonal diseases are in the foreground. Dogs and cats are equally affected by hypertension.

Idiopathic	Renal	Endocrine
Primary Hypertension (D/C)	Acute kidney disease (D/C)	Hyperadrenocorticism (D)
	Chronic kidney disease (D/C)	Hyperthyroidism (C)
		Diabetes mellitus (D/C)
		Hyperaldosteronism (D/C)
		Pheochromocytoma (D/C)

D – Dog, C – Cat

Textbook of Small Animal Pathophysiology, First Edition. Stephan Neumann.
© 2025 John Wiley & Sons Ltd. Published 2025 by John Wiley & Sons Ltd.

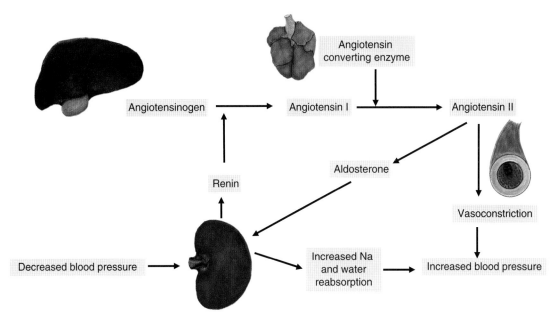

Figure 36.8.1 Physiology of blood pressure.

Pathogenesis

Primary idiopathic hypertension can cause an increase in blood pressure due to increased cardiac output and increased peripheral vascular resistance. Possible triggers are an increased sympathetic effect on the heart muscle and local vasoconstrictor factors. The latter can be based on an increased synthesis of vasoactive mediators, such as endothelins. These are a group of peptide hormones which are expressed, in particular, by the endothelial cells of the vessels. Endothelins act via G-protein-coupled receptors of the vascular smooth muscle cells and cause contraction there through increased Ca^+ influx.

The secondary diseases leading to hypertension can be divided into renal and endocrine dysfunctions. In **acute renal failure**, the increase in blood pressure is mainly due to compensatory mechanisms of reduced renal blood flow. Regardless of the localisation (pre- or intra-renal), glomerular filtration is reduced, this causes reduced Na^+ reabsorption in the proximal tubule and thereby activates the RAAS. The result is an increase in blood pressure.

In **chronic renal failure**, reduced glomerular filtration also plays an essential role in the pathogenesis of secondary hypertension. The reduced glomerular filtration rate (GFR) in this case is due to a loss of nephrons resulting from renal glomerulosclerosis. The reduced GFR increases the blood volume through a reduction in Na^+ and water excretion, which in turn increases the blood pressure.

Hyperadrenocorticism causes hypertension through different mechanisms. The extent of hypertension is related to the duration and extent of corticosteroid excess. Glucocorticoids develop mineralocorticoid effects by binding to the corresponding receptors. The binding activity is significantly lower than that of mineral corticoids, but in Cushing's disease there is a glucocorticoid excess, so there is a recognisable mineralocorticoid effect.

In addition, glucocorticoids lead to increased angiotensinogen release and increased sensitivity of angiotensin II receptors, thereby mimicking RAAS activation.

Furthermore, they increase the sensitivity of the ß-adrenergic receptors to catecholamines, which show a direct vasoconstrictor effect.

Finally, glucocorticoids inhibit NO synthetase, an enzyme that causes the synthesis of NO, an important vasodilator (Cicala and Mantero 2010) (Table 36.8.1).

Animals with **hyperthyroidism** show increased heart rate and cardiac output. This occurs through different mechanisms. Thyroid hormones can stimulate the activity of the sympathetic nervous system, which plays an important role in regulating heart rate and blood pressure. Increased sympathetic activity leads to an increase in heart rate and blood pressure.

In addition, thyroid hormones increase the sensitivity of the heart muscle cells to catecholamines, such as adrenaline and noradrenaline. These neurotransmitters stimulate the heart and increase the heartbeat and blood pressure.

Table 36.8.1 Mechanisms of hypertension in Cushing's disease.

Mineralocorticoid activity of cortisol
Activation of RAAS
Enhancement of cardiovascular sensitivity to vasoconstrictors
Increased β-adrenergic receptor sensitivity to catecholamines
Suppression of the vasodilatory system

Excessive production of thyroid hormones can lead to an increase in renin levels and an increase in aldosterone production, resulting in an increase in blood pressure. In addition, the increased thyroid hormone levels cause an increased release of endothelin. As a consequence, blood pressure increases (Berta et al. 2019).

Hypertension and **diabetes mellitus** are related, especially in type II diabetes mellitus. In this form of the disease, a structure of inflammation develops due to the release of proinflammatory cytokines and insulin resistance, which leads to a disturbance in the balance between vasoconstrictors (endothelin, angiotensin II) and vasodilators (nitric oxide, prostacyclin). In addition, the chronic inflammation attributed to obesity leads to dysfunction of endothelial cells and vascular smooth muscle, which leads to a cascade of proliferation, hypertrophy, remodelling and apoptosis.

This interferes with the balance between the arterial wall scaffolding proteins, elastin and collagen, which determine vascular compliance, a form of 'vascular ageing', that is a characteristic phenotype in hypertension (Petrie et al. 2018).

Other endocrine diseases associated with **hypertension** are **hyperaldosteronism** and **pheochromocytoma**. In both cases, the associated hypertension can be explained by an increase in blood volume and a direct catecholamine effect.

Diagnostics

Clinical signs	Clinical pathology	Imaging	Histopathology	Microbiology
Mostly non-specific	Non-specific	**Blood pressure measurement**	Not necessary	Not necessary

Pathophysiologic Consequences

The pathophysiologic consequences of hypertension are often masked by the underlying disease and are described, in detail, in the corresponding organ diseases. Some symptoms, however, can be traced back to lesions caused by the hypertension itself.

Influenced organ systems	Clinical symptoms
Cardiovascular system	Lethargy
Urinary tract	Headache
Central nervous system	Blindness
Ophthalmic system	Epistaxis

Central nervous and **ophthalmological** changes due to hypertension are particularly prominent. One of the primary effects of hypertension on the central nervous system is the disruption of the blood-brain barrier. The blood-brain barrier is a specialised membrane that separates the circulating blood from the brain tissue, and it regulates the exchange of substances between the two compartments. When hypertension occurs, it can cause damage to the blood-brain barrier, leading to the leakage of blood components into the brain tissue. This can trigger a cascade of inflammatory responses, including the activation of microglia, the brain's immune cells, which can produce proinflammatory cytokines and reactive oxygen species that further damage brain cells. Another consequence of hypertension on the central nervous system

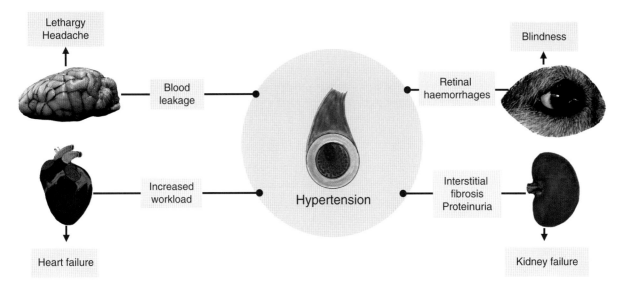

Figure 36.8.2 Pathophysiologic consequences of hypertension.

is the impairment of cerebral blood flow. Hypertension can lead to the constriction of blood vessels in the brain, reducing cerebral blood flow and depriving the brain of oxygen and nutrients. Clinical consequences can include **lethargy** and **headaches**.

The ophthalmological changes are mainly due to haemorrhages or exudation in the retinal area. Acute **blindness** is described as a major symptom, which occurs when the receptor function and nervous transmission are interrupted by haemorrhages in the retina.

Epistaxis in hypertension is a consequence of the rupture of blood vessels in the nasal cavity due to high blood pressure. The force of the blood flow can cause the weakened vessel walls to rupture, leading to bleeding. Another potential mechanism is the formation of microaneurysms, which weaken blood vessels. These microaneurysms can eventually rupture, causing bleeding and epistaxis (Figure 36.8.2).

Therapy

Therapy
ACE inhibitors
Calcium channel blocker
β-adrenergic blockers
Diuretics

References

Berta, E., Lengyel, I., Halmi, S. et al. (2019). Hypertension in thyroid disorders. *Frontiers in Endocrinology* 10: 482. https://doi.org/10.3389/fendo.2019.00482.

Cicala, M.V. and Mantero, F. (2010). Hypertension in Cushing's syndrome: from pathogenesis to treatment. *Neuroendocrinology* 92 (Suppl 1): 44–49. https://doi.org/10.1159/000314315.

Petrie, J.R., Guzik, T.J., and Touyz, R.M. (2018). Diabetes, hypertension, and cardiovascular disease: clinical insights and vascular mechanisms. *The Canadian Journal of Cardiology* 34 (5): 575–584. https://doi.org/10.1016/j.cjca.2017.12.005.

Further Reading

Acierno, M.J., Brown, S., Coleman, A.E. et al. (2018). ACVIM consensus statement: guidelines for the identification, evaluation, and management of systemic hypertension in dogs and cats. *Journal of Veterinary Internal Medicine* 32 (6): 1803–1822.

Brown, S., Atkins, C., Bagley, R. et al. (2007). Guidelines for the identification, evaluation, and management of systemic hypertension in dogs and cats. *Journal of Veterinary Internal Medicine* 21 (3): 542–558.

Henik, R.A. (1997). Systemic hypertension and its management. *The Veterinary Clinics of North America. Small Animal Practice* 27 (6): 1355–1372.

37

Respiratory System

37.1

Physiological Functions and General Pathophysiology of Organ Insufficiency

Functions

The essential functions of respiration are to supply the organism with oxygen in order to effectively maintain the body's internal energy supply. At the same time, respiration serves to eliminate CO_2, which is produced as a degradation product during glycolysis.

In addition, respiration is actively involved in the regulation of the acid-base balance via CO_2 elimination. Other functions include involvement in the regulation of blood pressure via the formation of angiotensin II from angiotensin I.

The intake and release of respiratory gases, as well as the exchange of gases in the lungs, is called 'external respiration', while the exchange of gases at the cellular level is called 'internal respiration'. The processes of gas exchange consist of:

Ventilation, Diffusion and Perfusion

The term **ventilation** describes the exchange of air between the atmosphere and the alveoli. Alveolar pressure differences serve as driving forces for air exchange. A lower alveolar pressure leads to inspiration and an increased alveolar pressure to expiration.

The air is moved in the upper and lower airways. Since there is no gas exchange in the upper airways (nose, larynx, trachea), the air there is called 'dead space volume' and accounts for about one-third of the total inhaled air.

The driving force for alveolar negative pressure and thus inspiration is considered to be the inspiratory negative pressure that occurs in the lungs when the chest expands. In the chest, visceral and parietal serosa lie on top of each other and are separated by a capillary gap. There is a small amount of 'pleural fluid' in this gap that allows the serosa surfaces to move smoothly. There is a negative pressure (about −4 mmHg) in the pleural gap, which causes the lungs to expand as the chest expands. Expansion of the rib cage is made possible by the contracting of the intercostal muscles and the additional flattening of the diaphragm. Both cause an enlargement of the rib cage, which the lungs passively follow (Figure 37.1.1).

In this way, the air reaches the terminal bronchioles and the alveoli via the trachea and bronchi. The air-carrying upper airways have the task of warming and humidifying the air and removing particles from it.

The connection of the respiratory apparatus with the outside world leads to an exposure of the respiratory mucosa to particles and pathogens. Accordingly, the respiratory apparatus has non-specific and specific forms of defence (Table 37.1.1).

Non-specific forms of defence include mechanisms that transport material out of the respiratory system, such as: cough, sneezing, mucociliary transport and bronchoconstriction.

The specific forms include: innate immune defence (lysozyme, complement, macrophages) and acquired defence (Ig A, T lymphocytes, B lymphocytes).

For defence based on mucociliary transport, there are cilia on the mucosal surface that rest in a mucus produced by mucosa cells. The top layer of mucus is more viscous than the layer below. Particles adhere to the top layer and can be transported by cilia movement on the less viscous bottom layer towards the larynx to be coughed up or swallowed (Figure 37.1.2).

Textbook of Small Animal Pathophysiology, First Edition. Stephan Neumann.
© 2025 John Wiley & Sons Ltd. Published 2025 by John Wiley & Sons Ltd.

Inspiration   Expiration

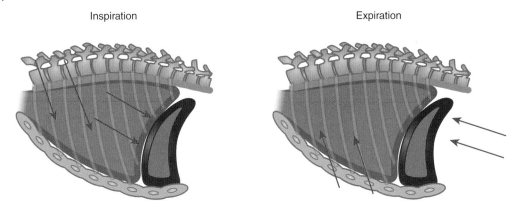

Figure 37.1.1 Movement of the chest during breathing.

Table 37.1.1 Defence systems in the airways.

Innate defence mechanisms	Adaptive defence mechanisms	Antimicrobial peptides
Mucociliary clearance	T-, B lymphocytes	Lysozyme
Epithelial cells	Antibody	Defensin
Alveolar macrophages		Lactoferrin
Neutrophilic granulocytes		
Surfactant		

Source: Adapted from Pilette et al. (2001).

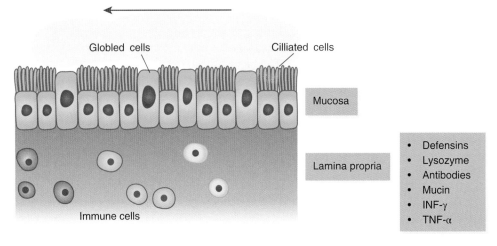

Figure 37.1.2 Illustration of mucociliary transport.

Diffusion is the second process in gas exchange. In this process, the respiratory gases are exchanged between the alveolar space and the alveolar-capillary blood. The diffusion distance is approximately 0.6 μm and includes the alveolar lipoprotein film, the alveolar epithelium, the basement membrane and the capillary endothelium. Diffusion is influenced by the diffusion distance, but also by the concentration gradient between the alveolar space and the capillary and the solubility of the gas. While the latter influencing factor is constant, the previous factors can be influenced by disease processes (Figure 37.1.3).

The third process of gas exchange is **perfusion**. The perfusion time is described as the period of time that the capillary blood is in alveolar contact, which is 0.7 seconds under normal conditions and 0.3 seconds under stress. Perfusion is controlled by respiratory gas concentrations. Hypoxaemia and hypercapnia lead to a constriction of pulmonary vessels and increase perfusion.

Connected to the gas exchange is the **gas transport**. This connects the lungs with the peripheral tissue. Oxygen transport mainly takes place via binding to haemoglobin. In the blood, haemoglobin is predominantly present in a form that allows oxygen binding. A small amount of haemoglobin is not available as CO-haemoglobin or met-haemoglobin. A very small amount of oxygen is present dissolved in the blood (1/70). The binding of oxygen to haemoglobin can be shown by the O_2-binding curve. This shows that effective binding to haemoglobin is possible especially at medium oxygen partial pressure.

At the cellular level, **oxygen exchange** is also driven by the pressure gradient. In the peripheral arterial blood, the partial pressure of oxygen is 100 mmHg and intercellularly the pressure is 39 mmHg. Diffusion of oxygen across the capillary endothelium, interstitium and cell membrane follows this pressure gradient. CO_2 is produced as the end product of energetic cellular metabolism. This is transported to the lungs dissolved in the blood or bound to haemoglobin. There, diffusion occurs from the capillary blood to the alveolus along the diffusion path described for oxygen and driven by a concentration gradient between capillary blood and alveolus (Figure 37.1.4).

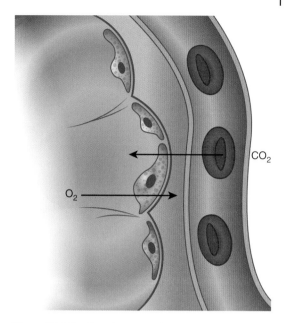

Figure 37.1.3 Alveolar gas exchange.

Pathological Mechanisms

Pathological mechanisms in respiratory diseases often involve the alveoli. The processes of ventilation, diffusion and perfusion are adversely affected. Regardless of the aetiology, some pathomechanisms can be summarised that show an influence on respiratory insufficiency:

Pulmonary oedema
Lung emphysema
Lung atelectasis

Pulmonary oedema impacts the respiratory mechanisms of ventilation, diffusion and perfusion, uniformly. It denotes an excessive accumulation of fluid within the lung parenchyma, situated beyond the vascular confines. The localisation of this condition allows differentiation between interstitial and alveolar types of pulmonary oedema.

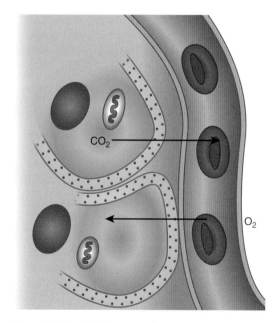

Figure 37.1.4 Cellular gas exchange.

The underlying pathophysiology involves an imbalance between the generation of interstitial fluid and its clearance through the pulmonary lymphatic system. Transvascular fluid movement is intrinsically linked to factors such as hydrostatic pressure, oncotic pressure and permeability.

Elevations in hydrostatic pressure, reductions in oncotic pressure or enhancements in transvascular permeability result in the ingress of plasma from the vasculature into the pulmonary interstitium or alveoli. Concurrently, hindered fluid removal occurs due to compromised lymphatic drainage (Figure 37.1.5). Numerous diseases are associated with the occurrence of pulmonary oedema (Table 37.1.2).

Hydrostatic pulmonary oedema predominantly arises from left-sided heart failure. The consequential elevation in ventricular filling pressure precipitates a decline in blood outflow from the pulmonary veins. Consequently, there is a marked escalation in pulmonary venous and capillary pressures. Once capillary pressure surpasses the threshold of 20–25 mmHg, it triggers the extravasation of fluid from the capillaries into the surrounding tissues.

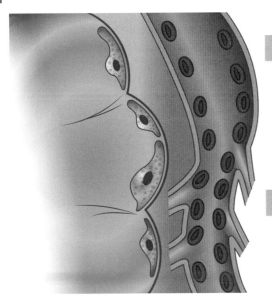

Increased capillary volume

Increased capillary permeability

Figure 37.1.5 Mechanisms of pulmonary oedema formation.

Table 37.1.2 Causes for the development of pulmonary oedema.

Aetiology	Increased hydrostatic pressure	Increased permeability
Left heart failure	+	−
Overinfusion (iatrogenic)	+	−
Sepsis	+	+
Uraemia	+	+
Pulmonary emboli	+	+

Source: Adapted from Hartmann, H. (1994).

The occurrence of increased vascular permeability manifests as '**permeability oedema**', constituting the second most prevalent condition. Primarily driven by inflammatory processes, augmented permeability contributes to the leakage of blood plasma, proteins and inflammatory cells, fostering the formation of oedema within the pulmonary interstitium (Assaad et al. 2018; Herrero et al. 2018).

Emphysema, a significant contributor to pulmonary dysfunction, is characterised by an abnormal and excessive accumulation of air distal to the terminal bronchi, resulting in the over-inflation of alveoli and subsequent rupture. This pathological condition leads to an increase in alveolar surface area but concomitantly diminishes the surface available for gas exchange through the alveoli.

Emphysema can manifest either as alveolar or interstitial expansion. The fundamental mechanism underlying its development involves the action of elastase released by neutrophilic granulocytes or macrophages during an inflammatory process. Elastase, an enzyme, targets and damages the elastic fibres within the alveolar walls and interstitium. The impairment of these elastic fibres results in their inability to recoil after being stretched, leading to a progressive and irreversible accumulation of air within the alveoli.

This persistent air accumulation predisposes the alveoli to structural damage and subsequent rupture, thereby contributing to the development and progression of emphysema (Bagdonas et al. 2015; Liang and He 2019) (Figure 37.1.6).

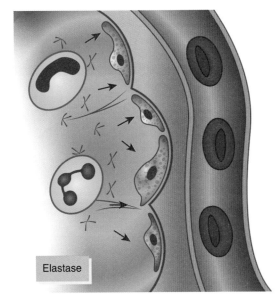

Elastase

Figure 37.1.6 Mechanisms of emphysema formation.

Atelectasis, characterised by the collapse or airlessness of a lung area, represents a significant factor contributing to respiratory failure. While foetal lung atelectasis is normal due to the timing of lung development occurring predominantly intra-post-partum, disturbances during this developmental phase may result in partial or persistent atelectasis.

In acquired cases, atelectasis arises as a consequence of processes involving alveolar remodeling, often linked to inflammatory responses and the accumulation of inflammatory secretions within the alveoli. This accumulation initiates an inflammatory cascade, potentially leading to fibrosis within the alveoli and subsequent filling of the alveolar lumen (Peroni and Boner 2000) (Figure 37.1.7).

The main principle consequences of respiratory diseases result from a reduced oxygen supply to the organism and are reflected in hypoxaemia and hypoxia. At the same time, respiratory insufficiency leads to an increased CO_2 concentration (hypercapnia) and can thus influence the acid-base balance (Roussos and Koutsoukou 2003; Lamba et al. 2016).

In case of respiratory insufficiency, the body develops compensatory mechanisms. Alveolar hyperventilation of healthy lung segments increases CO_2 expiration and decreases hypercapnia. (Epstein and Singh 2001).

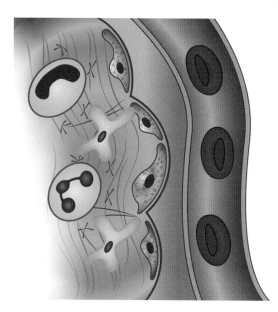

Figure 37.1.7 Mechanisms of lung atelectasis.

The hypoxaemia is partially compensated by a change in oxygen binding to haemoglobin.

If the compensation mechanisms are exceeded, cellular and tissue-based disorders follow as a result of the hypoxia (see Chapter 6).

Initially, the cellular consequence of hypoxia may include a change in energy metabolism towards anaerobic glycolysis, with increased production of lactic acid and lactic acidosis could be the consequence. Lactic acidosis affects muscle contraction, the vasoconstrictor effects of catecholamines are reduced, and vasoactive substances are released that cause vascular dilatation.

References

Assaad, S., Kratzert, W.B., Shelley, B. et al. (2018). Assessment of pulmonary edema: principles and practice. *Journal of Cardiothoracic and Vascular Anesthesia* 32 (2): 901–914. https://doi.org/10.1053/j.jvca.2017.08.028.

Bagdonas, E., Raudoniute, J., Bruzauskaite, I., and Aldonyte, R. (2015). Novel aspects of pathogenesis and regeneration mechanisms in COPD. *International Journal of Chronic Obstructive Pulmonary Disease* 10: 995–1013. https://doi.org/10.2147/COPD.S82518.

Epstein, S.K. and Singh, N. (2001). Respiratory acidosis. *Respiratory Care* 46 (4): 366–383.

Hartmann, H. (1994). *Clinical Pathology of Domestic Animals*. Jena: Gustav Fischer Verlag.

Herrero, R., Sanchez, G., and Lorente, J.A. (2018). New insights into the mechanisms of pulmonary edema in acute lung injury. *Annals of Translational Medicine* 6 (2): 32. https://doi.org/10.21037/atm.2017.12.18.

Lamba, T.S., Sharara, R.S., Singh, A.C., and Balaan, M. (2016). Pathophysiology and classification of respiratory failure. *Critical Care Nursing Quarterly* 39 (2): 85–93. https://doi.org/10.1097/CNQ.0000000000000102.

Liang, G.B. and He, Z.H. (2019). Animal models of emphysema. *Chinese Medical Journal* 132 (20): 2465–2475. https://doi.org/10.1097/CM9.0000000000000469.

Peroni, D.G. and Boner, A.L. (2000). Atelectasis: mechanisms, diagnosis and management. *Paediatric Respiratory Reviews* 1 (3): 274–278. https://doi.org/10.1053/prrv.2000.0059.

Pilette, C., Godding, V., Kiss, R. et al. (2001). Reduced epithelial expression of secretory component in small airways correlates with airflow obstruction in chronic obstructive pulmonary disease. *American Journal of Respiratory and Critical Care Medicine* 163 (1): 185–194. https://doi.org/10.1164/ajrccm.163.1.9912137.

Roussos, C. and Koutsoukou, A. (2003). Respiratory failure. *The European Respiratory Journal. Supplement* 47: 3s–14s. https://doi.org/10.1183/09031936.03.00038503.

37.2

Brachiocephalic Syndrome

Definition

The disease is defined as a limitation of the respiratory function of brachiocephalic breeds.

Aetiology

Brachiocephalic breeds occur in the dog and cat species. The clinical relevance of the syndrome described here is found more often in the dog. The syndrome is composed of several anatomical variations, which include:

Constricted nostrils
Deformation of the choans
Thickened and lengthened soft palate
Laryngeal collapse
Evert tuning pockets
Hypoplasia of the trachea

The changes do not occur all at the same time and can also vary in severity.

Pathogenesis

The anatomical variations lead to the clinically manifest syndrome via various mechanisms. Increased breathing resistance due to the various stenoses in the respiratory system is a possible causality for the syndrome. The nostrils, the choanae, the larynx and the trachea are seen as stenoses. The increased breathing resistance requires increased activity of the respiratory muscles. Nevertheless, the oxygen demand cannot always be completely provided, which can lead to hypoxia with resulting symptoms. (Oechtering et al. 2007; Ginn et al. 2008; Piroth 2020) (Figure 37.2.1).

Diagnostics

Clinical signs	Clinical pathology	Imaging	Histopathology	Microbiology
Exercise and heat intolerance	Non-specific	**Endoscopy**	Not necessary	Not necessary
Snoring				

Textbook of Small Animal Pathophysiology, First Edition. Stephan Neumann.
© 2025 John Wiley & Sons Ltd. Published 2025 by John Wiley & Sons Ltd.

Figure 37.2.1 Localisation of stenoses in the respiratory system of brachiocephalic dogs.

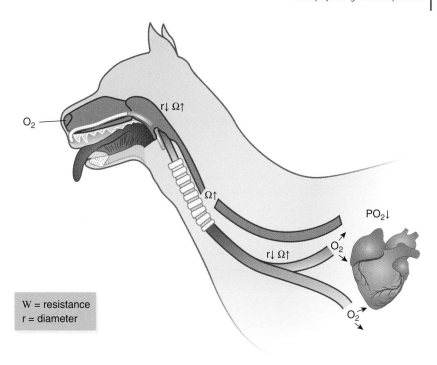

Pathophysiologic Consequences

The pathophysiologic consequences result from the impaired function of the respiratory system.

Influenced organ systems	Clinical symptoms	Clinical pathological alterations
Cardiovascular system	Exercise intolerance	Increased liver enzymes
Respiratory system	Snoring	
Gastrointestinal system	Cough	
Central nervous system	Vomiting	
	Dyspnoea	
	Disturbed thermoregulation	
	Syncope	

Heat intolerance is caused by the reduced mucosal surface area in the area of the nasal cavity and the stenotic airways, which are involved in the regulation of body temperature through evaporative cooling.

Exercise intolerance is caused by a reduced oxygen supply in the body. This is a consequence of anatomical changes. According to Hagen-Poiseuille's law, the airflow depends on pressure differences between the beginning and the end of the respiratory system, which in turn depends on the local resistance. Furthermore, the airflow depends on the diameter of the air-conducting pathways and finally on its length. In brachiocephalic animals, resistance is increased in the area of the nasal cavity due to deformed choans, in the area of the laryngopharynx due to an elongated and hyperplastic soft palate, and in the area of the trachea due to hypoplasia resulting from tracheal cartilage dysplasia. This results in a reduced partial pressure of oxygen in the arteries, which in turn stimulates the respiratory mechanics, which become hypertrophic due to an increased work capacity caused by the high air resistance.

Snoring, caused by turbulence of the airflow in the hyperplastic nasal passages and in the area of the elongated soft palate.

Coughing may result from a mechanical stimulus resulting from the frequent air movement of the hypoplastic trachea. Hyperplastic mucosa in the area of the trachea and bronchi can also trigger the cough stimulus by increased air movement irritating the mucosa.

In particular, the elongated soft palate can lead to pharyngo-laryngeal irritation, which stimulates the vomiting centre via vagal afferents and induces vomiting. Another mechanism may arise due to aerophagia, which can occur with increased breathing resistance. This leads to irritation of the gastric mucosa with **vomiting** as a symptom.

The increased breathing resistance implies increased activity of the respiratory muscles, making inspiration more difficult. Swelling in the airways due to hyperplastic mucosa may also impede expiration, resulting in **dyspnoea**.

Due to the reduced or stenotic mucosal surface area, the surface area for heat dissipation during panting is reduced. This means that affected dogs are unable to dissipate sufficient body heat when the outside temperature is high. It is due to **hyperthermia**.

In pronounced cases with clearly restricted respiratory function or with an increased demand for oxygen, for example during physical activity, a short-term oxygen deficiency may occur. This can cause a loss of consciousness in brachiocephalic dogs in the sense of **syncope**.

Finally, in brachiocephalic dogs, due to hypoxia, there is also a damage of hepatocytes associated with a release of **cytosolic enzymes**, resulting in their increased activity in the serum.

Therapy

Symptom	Therapy
Stenoses in the air-carrying airways	Surgery
Swelling of the mucous membranes of the respiratory system	Corticoids

References

Ginn, J.A., Kumar, M.S., McKiernan, B.C., and Powers, B.E. (2008). Nasopharyngeal turbinates in brachycephalic dogs and cats. *Journal of the American Animal Hospital Association* 44 (5): 243–249. https://doi.org/10.5326/0440243.

Oechtering, T.H., Oechtering, G.U., and Nöller, C. (2007). Structural characteristics of the nose in brachycephalic dog breeds analysed by computed tomography. Structural characteristics of the nose in brachycephalic dog breeds analysed by computed tomography. *Veterinary Practice. Issue K, Small Animals/Pets* 35 (3): 177–187. https://doi.org/10.1055/s-0038-1622615.

Piroth, A.C. (2020) The role of thermoregulation in the development of canine brachycephalic respiratory distress syndrome. Diss University of Zurich.

37.3

Acute Respiratory Distress Syndrome (ARDS)

Definition

Acute respiratory distress syndrome (ARDS) is a respiratory insufficiency due to alveolar damage and can be triggered by a variety of processes, mostly inflammatory in nature.

Aetiology

The causes of ARDS are divided into pulmonary and systemic causalities. In the foreground of the local causes are different forms of pneumonia, such as aspiration pneumonia, but also infectious pneumonia caused by viruses, bacteria and fungi. Pulmonary contusion or lobe torsion are also possible local causalities. In the case of systemic causes, strong inflammatory reactions, such as pancreatitis are promoted, in addition, all forms of sepsis and shock. The disease occurs equally in dogs and cats (Table 37.3.1).

Pathogenesis

The course of ARDS can be divided into an exudative, a proliferative and a fibrotic phase according to the general course of an inflammatory event (Table 37.3.2).

The **first phase** of the pathomechanism of ARDS is the recruitment of neutrophilic granulocytes due to an inflammatory stimulus. Recruitment is a complex process that is illustrated using the example of a bacterial infection.

Invading bacteria act by producing bacterial toxins, for example, lipopolysaccharides (LPS). These are compounds composed of a lipid and a saccharide, which are connected to each other via a core region. The LPS are components of the outer bacterial membrane. During bacterial decay, the molecules are released from the membrane. Free LPS react with membrane receptors, such as cluster of differentiation 14 (CD 14) or toll-like receptor 4 (TLR4), which are expressed on numerous cells, for example macrophages. The binding induces the synthesis of proinflammatory cytokines, such as TNF-α or IL-1 via the transcription factor NF-κB as a second messenger.

Such reactive cells are localised as alveolar macrophages or dendritic cells in the area of the alveolus (Table 37.3.3).

Activation of the local macrophages activates alveolar endothelial cells via the paracrine-acting cytokines. These express different surface molecules, such as selectins. Circulating defence cells can form a connection with the activated endothelial cells via expressed selectin ligands. In this way, the leukocytes are 'captured'. First, the leukocytes roll on the endothelial cell surfaces. In the next step, the leukocytes adhere to the endothelial cell surface and eventually transmigrate into the environment (Phillipson and Kubes 2011; Weckbach et al. 2014; Wessel et al. 2014).

Through transmigration, proteolytic enzymes released by granulocytes, together with activated macrophages, lead to further destruction of the periendothelial area. This leads to destruction of the alveolar-capillary barrier with infiltration of plasma and further neutrophilic granulocytes and macrophages into the interstitium and alveoli. Fibrin is formed from the fibrinogen dissolved in the plasma, causing microscopically visible hyaline membranes. The fibrin inhibits the synthesis of surfactant by type 2 alveolar cells.

Surfactant consists of phospholipids, cholesterol esters and proteins and reduces the surface tension in the alveolus. As a result, even the low alveolar air pressure makes it possible to expand the alveolus with the consequence of an increase in

Table 37.3.1 Aetiologies of ARDS.

Local	Systemic
Different forms of pneumonia (D/C)	Sepsis (D/C)
Pulmonary contusion (D)	Pancreatitis (D/C)
	Shock (D/C)

D – Dog, C – Cat

Table 37.3.2 Phases of ARDS.

Phase	Start (days)	Microscopic change
Exudative phase	1–7	Infiltration of neutrophilic granulocytes, microthrombi, alveolar cell necrosis, loss of basement membrane
Proliferative phase	3	Proliferation of alveolar cells, myofibroblasts and fibroblasts
Fibrotic phase	7	Connective tissue remodelling of the alveoli and alveolar septa

Table 37.3.3 Alveolar cells.

Cell	Function
Alveolar cell type 1	Alveolar surface cell
Alveolar cell type 2	Alveolar stem cell, for alveolar regeneration, surfactant formation
Alveolar macrophages	Non-specific defence, antigen presentation, phagocytosis
Alveolar dendritic cell	Antigen presentation
Fibroblasts	Remodelling
Alveolar endothelial cells	Conversion of angiotensin I to angiotensin II

lung expandability (compliance). This in turn leads to less work for the respiratory muscles, which are necessary for inspiration.

The lack of surfactant causes the alveoli to collapse.

After granulocyte recruitment and the onset of alveolar destruction, the **second phase** of ARDS, the proliferation phase, follows. Due to the increasing destruction in the alveolar area, type 2 alveolar cells attempt to repair destroyed tissue. In parallel or, in the case of massive damage, resident fibroblasts are activated. The mechanisms of fibroblast activation are controlled by proinflammatory cytokines and growth factors (e.g. TGF) that are active in the inflammatory area. Another mechanism of fibroblast activation is the mechanical stretching of the tissue. This has an influence on the cellular structures of the cytoskeleton and can trigger signal transduction (Liu et al. 1995).

If the alveolar and perialveolar fibrosis processes continue, the **third phase** of ARDS is fibrosis. This is characterised by the increased formation of collagen by the fibroblasts. The mechanism of fibroblast activation begins with the receptor binding of activating growth factors, for example TGF. Cellular signal transduction via the SMAD pathway leads to the transcription and secretion of profibrotic proteins (Inui et al. 2021).

The remodelling process increases local vascular resistance; this induces pulmonary hypertension, which in turn increases hydrostatic pressure, which increases permeability and increases alveolar oedema (Figure 37.3.1).

Diagnostics

Clinical signs	Clinical pathology	Imaging	Histopathology	Microbiology
Weakness	Non-specific	**Radiology**	Necessary for final diagnosis, seldom performed	Not necessary
Dyspnoea		Interstitial and alveolar pattern		
Cough				

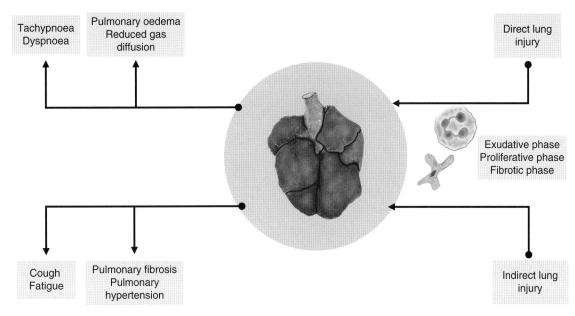

Figure 37.3.1 Mechanisms in ARDS.

Pathophysiologic Consequences

The main pathophysiologic consequences of ARDS are due to impaired lung function (hypoxia and hypercapnia).

Influenced organs	Clinical symptoms	Clinical pathological alterations
Respiratory system Cardiovascular system	Fatigue	Hypoxaemia
	Cyanosis	Hypercapnia
	Tachypnoea	Respiratory acidosis
	Cough	Increased liver enzymes

Source: Greensmith and Cortellini (2018) and DeClue and Cohn (2007).

The pathophysiologic consequences of ARDS are essentially based on the consequences of **hypoxaemia** and **hypercapnia**. The lack of oxygen causes a metabolic change in the energy metabolism in different organs. Aerobic glycolysis develops into anaerobic glycolysis, which is possible under oxygen reduction. The result is a reduced synthesis of ATP and thus a lower energy reserve for cellular processes. The mechanisms of ion transport at the cell membrane are particularly affected. Under the influence of reduced ion fluxes, more sodium remains in the cells; this binds water and leads to 'over-hydration' of the cell, which impairs cell function. The brain is particularly sensitive to hypoxaemia, which explains the symptoms of **fatigue** in ARDS.

The reduced oxygen concentration in the blood causes the visible **cyanosis**. This can be central or peripheral. Peripheral cyanosis is mainly related to reduced perfusion in the periphery, for example, due to shock or cold. Central cyanosis, on the other hand, is the consequence of haemoglobin colour in the presence of reduced arterial oxygen saturation from >95% to <85%. It is thus a consequence of respiratory hypoventilation and is associated with ARDS (Pahal and Goyal 2023).

Tachypnoea develops as a compensatory symptom following reduced oxygen saturation. It is defined as an increased respiratory rate with a constant depth of breath. The respiratory rate is controlled by the respiratory centre in the medulla oblongata. In the context of ARDS, hypoxaemia and especially hypercapnia lead to stimulation of arterial chemoreceptors in the aorta or the carotid artery of the central chemoreceptors in the area of the IV ventricle of the brain. These register the concentrations of O_2 and CO_2 in the blood. When O_2 is reduced or CO_2 is increased, transmembrane Ca^{2+} channels open in the glomus cells of the chemoreceptors. Ca^{2+}-influx increases transmitter release at the glomus cells and a frequency increase of action potentials at the postsynaptic membrane is conducted via the vagus nerve to the respiratory centre. There, the increase in frequency of the action potentials induces the increase in respiratory frequency (Ortega-Sáenz et al. 2020).

Cough develops due to inflammation and impaired lung function with accumulation of inflammatory detritus in the bronchial membrane area and its clearance.

The increase in CO_2 concentration leads to **respiratory acidosis**. This is compensated for renally. The pathophysiologic consequences are mostly central nervous symptoms, such as depression.

Finally, the increase in pulmonary resistance leads to right-heart dysfunction. This can cause liver congestion with **elevated liver enzymes** and ascites due to stagnation in the splanchnic system.

Therapy

Symptom	Therapy
Hypoxia	Oxygen therapy
Respiratory acidosis	Infusion buffered saline

References

DeClue, A.E. and Cohn, L.A. (2007). Acute respiratory distress syndrome in dogs and cats: a review of clinical findings and pathophysiology. *Journal of Veterinary Emergency and Critical Care* 17 (4): 340–347.

Greensmith, T.D. and Cortellini, S. (2018). Successful treatment of canine acute respiratory distress syndrome secondary to inhalant toxin exposure. *Journal of Veterinary Emergency and Critical Care (San Antonio, Tex.)* 28 (5): 469–475.

Inui, N., Sakai, S., and Kitagawa, M. (2021). Molecular pathogenesis of pulmonary fibrosis, with focus on pathways related to TGF-β and the ubiquitin-proteasome pathway. *International Journal of Molecular Sciences* 22 (11): 6107. https://doi.org/10.3390/ijms22116107.

Liu, M., Xu, J., Souza, P. et al. (1995). The effect of mechanical strain on fetal rat lung cell proliferation: comparison of two- and three-dimensional culture systems. In vitro cellular & developmental biology. *Animal* 31 (11): 858–866. https://doi.org/10.1007/BF02634570.

Ortega-Sáenz, P., Moreno-Domínguez, A., Gao, L., and López-Barneo, J. (2020). Molecular mechanisms of acute oxygen sensing by arterial chemoreceptor cells. Role of Hif2α. *Frontiers in Physiology* 11: 614893. https://doi.org/10.3389/fphys.2020.614893.

Pahal, P. and Goyal. A. (2023). Central and Peripheral Cyanosis. [Updated 2022 Oct 3]. StatPearls [Internet]. Treasure Island (FL): StatPearls Publishing. https://www.ncbi.nlm.nih.gov/books/NBK559167/.

Phillipson, M. and Kubes, P. (2011). The neutrophil in vascular inflammation. *Nature Medicine* 17 (11): 1381–1390. https://doi.org/10.1038/nm.2514.

Weckbach, L.T., Gola, A., Winkelmann, M. et al. (2014). The cytokine midkine supports neutrophil trafficking during acute inflammation by promoting adhesion via β2 integrins (CD11/CD18). *Blood* 123 (12): 1887–1896. https://doi.org/10.1182/blood-2013-06-510875.

Wessel, F., Winderlich, M., Holm, M. et al. (2014). Leukocyte extravasation and vascular permeability are each controlled in vivo by different tyrosine residues of VE-cadherin. *Nature Immunology* 15 (3): 223–230. https://doi.org/10.1038/ni.2824.

Further Reading

Boiron, L., Hopper, K., and Borchers, A. (2019). Risk factors, characteristics, and outcomes of acute respiratory distress syndrome in dogs and cats: 54 cases. *Journal of Veterinary Emergency and Critical Care (San Antonio, Tex.: 2001)* 29 (2): 173–179.

37.4

Asthma (Feline Lower Respiratory Tract Disease)

Definition

Asthma is defined as a reversible obstructive airway disease due to a hypersensitivity reaction. The clinical picture is described in cats.

Aetiology

The exact cause of feline asthma is unknown.

Pathogenesis

The causal allergic reaction of type I begins with a reaction to an allergen. This is taken up by dendritic cells in the respiratory system and presented to T lymphocytes. Subsequently, plasma cells produce IgE, which binds to mast cells and sensitises them. Upon renewed allergen contact, the sensitised mast cells react by secreting mediators, such as histamine. These induce a constriction of the smooth airway muscles, increased mucus production and vasodilation. At the same time, capillary permeability increases and there is a secretion of blood plasma into the airways.

The increase in permeability with the extravasation of leukocytes and proteins is discussed as a consequence of a down-regulation of cadherin. Cadherins are transmembrane glycoproteins. They are part of the desmosomes and connect cell membranes to each other to stabilise a cell association. Intracellularly, cadherins are connected to the cytoskeleton. Inflammatory mediators, such as histamine, which increase vascular permeability, can structurally alter cadherins via the phosphorylation of tyrosine residues, inducing a loosening of the cell association with the formation of gaps between endothelial cells through which leukocytes or proteins can enter the surrounding tissue (Wessel et al. 2014).

The leakage of plasma proteins leads to swelling and oedema of the bronchial walls and thus to a narrowing of the airway lumen. Activation of T cells releases cytokines thought to play a role in the late reaction, including IL-2 and IL-5. Chronic exposure leads to epithelial changes, hypertrophy of the bronchial wall muscles and bronchoconstriction in the peripheral airways.

Bronchoconstriction is caused by the contraction of peribronchial smooth muscle cells. Under physiological conditions, smooth muscle cells contract by release of Ca^{2+} from the sarcoplasmic reticulum and interaction of actin and myosin filaments. This is described, in detail, in Chapter 36. In the case of chronic obstructive bronchitis, such as feline asthma, the peribronchial smooth muscle cells change. The proportion of proliferating muscle cells increases compared to contracting forms. Furthermore, the muscle cells are capable of synthesising proinflammatory cytokines, such as IL-1, IL-6 or IL-8, and can thus increase the inflammatory process. In addition, the contraction behaviour of the cells changes. All changes together lead to clinically relevant bronchoconstriction (Yan et al. 2018).

Diagnostics

Clinical signs	Clinical pathology	Imaging	Histopathology	Microbiology
Cough	Non-specific	**Radiology**	Not necessary	Not necessary
Tachypnoea		Bronchial or bronchointerstitial pattern		

Pathophysiologic Consequences

All clinical symptoms of feline asthma result from the pathomorphological changes in the terminal lung area. Especially in chronic cases, cough and dyspnoea are in the foreground of the clinical symptoms.

Influenced organ systems	Clinical symptoms	Clinical pathological consequences
Respiratory system	Cough	Hypoxia
	Dyspnoea	Hypercapnia

Cough is the consequence of bronchial changes in feline asthma. Chemical and physical triggers of the asthmatic inflammatory process, such as prostaglandins, protease or hyperthermia, cause an irritation of transient receptor potential vanilloid 1 (TRPV) receptors. These are expressed more frequently in asthma patients and thus increase sensitivity. The impulse goes from the receptors via afferent vagus nerves to the cough centre (Lee and Gu 2009).

Other consequences include impaired respiratory function, which can manifest clinically as **dyspnoea**. This can lead to hypoxaemia and hypercapnia. Both cause disruption of peripheral organs, such as the central nervous system or liver, by altering energy metabolism, resulting in a reduced amount of energy for transmembrane ion transport. Their disruption in turn causes water accumulation, cell swelling and dysfunction (Figure 37.4.1).

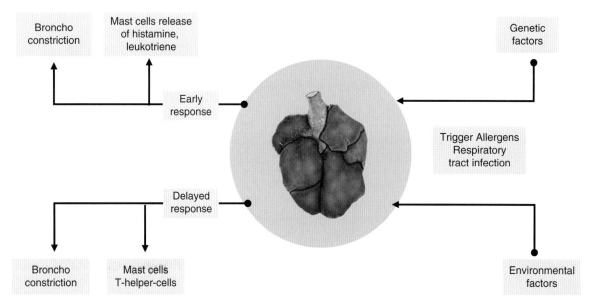

Figure 37.4.1 Pathomechanisms in asthma.

Therapy

Symptom	Therapy
Inflammatory response	Anti-inflammatory drugs (e.g. Corticoids)
Bronchoconstriction	Bronchodilators (e.g. Methylxanthine, β-2 agonists)
Dyspnoea	Oxygen therapy

References

Lee, L.Y. and Gu, Q. (2009). Role of TRPV1 in inflammation-induced airway hypersensitivity. *Current Opinion in Pharmacology* 9 (3): 243–249. https://doi.org/10.1016/j.coph.2009.02.002.

Wessel, F., Winderlich, M., Holm, M. et al. (2014). Leukocyte extravasation and vascular permeability are each controlled in vivo by different tyrosine residues of VE-cadherin. *Nature Immunology* 15 (3): 223–230. https://doi.org/10.1038/ni.2824.

Yan, F., Gao, H., Zhao, H. et al. (2018). Roles of airway smooth muscle dysfunction in chronic obstructive pulmonary disease. *Journal of Translational Medicine* 16 (1): 262. https://doi.org/10.1186/s12967-018-1635-z.

Further Reading

Grotheer, M. and Schulz, B. (2019). Feline asthma and chronic bronchitis – an overview of diagnostics and therapy. *Veterinary Practice. Issue K, Small Animals/Pets* 47 (3): 175–187. https://doi.org/10.1055/a-0917-6245.

Reinero, C.R. (2011). Advances in the understanding of pathogenesis, and diagnostics and therapeutics for feline allergic asthma. *Veterinary journal (London, England: 1997)* 190 (1): 28–33. https://doi.org/10.1016/j.tvjl.2010.09.022.

37.5

Chronic Obstructive Bronchitis

Definition

Chronic obstructive bronchitis (COB) is a non-reversible disease of the bronchial tract that leads to a narrowing of the bronchial lumen due to inflammation or remodelling processes.

Aetiology

Chronic obstructive bronchitis is a consequence of a chronic inflammatory process, so potentially any inflammatory bronchitis can develop into a chronic obstructive form. The disease occurs equally in dogs and cats (Table 37.5.1).

Pathogenesis

The chronic inflammatory process that is responsible for COB causes bronchiolar obstruction by different mechanisms. In the final stage, there is a mixture of morphological stenosis due to oedema, inflammation and fibrosis, as well as reflex bronchoconstriction. Chronic inflammation activates alveolar macrophages to phagocytose the triggering agents. The alveolar macrophages have the following tasks:

1) Initiation of inflammation through the release of IL-1 and TNF-α.
2) Control of inflammation through the release of inhibitors, such as the IL-1 receptor antagonists or soluble TNF-α receptors and the production of the anti-inflammatory interleukin 10 (IL-10).
3) Secretion of bactericidal molecules, such as lysozymes and defensins. Defensins are cationic proteins capable of killing bacteria and fungi.
4) Reconstruction of the lung by the secretion of metalloelastases, collagenases and metalloproteases. These enzymes are able to dissolve fibrin and release a growth factor for fibroblasts.
5) Support of opsonisation by production of components of the complement system. This releases proteases that lead to tissue irritation.

At the same time, the inflammatory process, mediated by the activation of epithelial cells, chemotactically attracts neutrophilic granulocytes via epithelial release of IL-8 and TNF-α. The neutrophilic granulocytes support the activity of the macrophages. In this process, neutrophilic granulocytes produce various proteases, including secretory and membrane-bound metalloproteases, serine proteases, cysteine proteases and other lysosomal enzymes. Serine proteases, such as proteinase 3 (PRTN3), neutrophil elastase (ELA2) and cathepsin G (CathG) are produced in high concentrations during myelogenesis and stored in the azurophilic granules of neutrophilic granulocytes. Under the influence of the combined effects of the inflammatory cells, degradation of the bronchus-associated connective tissue occurs. This also disrupts the pulmonary defence mechanism of mucociliary clearance by hypertrophying the bronchus-associated smooth muscle cells, destroying the cilia-bearing epithelial cells and inducing hyperplasia of the mucus-producing goblet cells to form more mucus.

Table 37.5.1 Causes of bronchitis.

Infection	Inflammatory	Other
Viral	Asthma (C)	Aspiration (D/C)
e.g. Canine adenovirus	Eosinophilic bronchopneumonia (D)	
Canine reovirus		
Feline herpesvirus		
Feline calicivirus		
Bacterial (D/C)		
Bordetella bronchiseptica		
Pasteurella		
Mycoplasma		
Streptococci		
Parasitic		
e.g. *Aelurostrongylus* (C)		
Angiostrongylus (D)		

D – Dog, C – Cat

In combination, the following morphological remodelling process develops. The alveolus is atelectatic or emphysematous, the walls of the bronchioli are thickened, there is increased mucus production, reflex constriction is increased and the morphology of the bronchial tree is disturbed by remodelling of the connective tissue.

Diagnostics

Clinical signs	Clinical pathology	Imaging	Histopathology	Microbiology
Dyspnoea	Non-specific	Radiology	Cytology	Bronchoalveolar lavage
		Bronchial or bronchointerstitial pattern		
		Endoscopy		

Pathophysiologic Consequences

The pathophysiologic consequences of COB primarily affect the respiratory system, but the remodelling processes increase the lung pressure, which leads to a right-heart failure. At the same time, hypoxia promotes erythropoietin synthesis resulting in polycythaemia.

Influenced organ systems	Clinical symptoms	Clinical pathological alterations
Cardiovascular system	Weakness	Respiratory acidosis
Respiratory system	Dyspnoea	Polycythaemia
Hepatobiliary system	Cough	Increased liver enzymes

In particular, the right-heart failure is causative for the clinically manifest **weakness**. Pulmonary hypertension develops from the pulmonary remodelling processes. This increases right ventricular afterload, thereby increasing right ventricular systolic blood pressure and causing wall hypertrophy. This can lead to tricuspid and pulmonary insufficiency. At the same time, the septum shifts to the left ventricle, reducing left ventricular volume and thus left ventricular ejection. If the right heart is no longer able to increase ejection, blood flows back into the right atrium and systemic venous system. A developing liver congestion leads to an increase in **liver enzymes**. Late consequences can also be ascites as a result of the congestion.

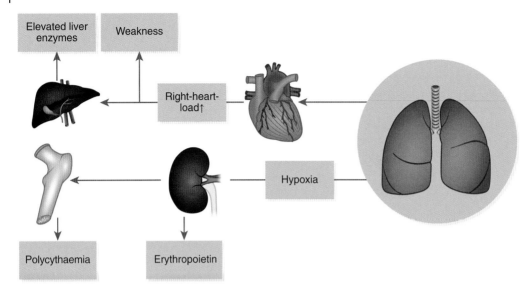

Figure 37.5.1 Pathophysiologic consequences of chronic bronchitis.

In addition to the cardiological consequences, the remodelling process in the lungs leads to **dyspnoea** and **cough** as a consequence of the restricted diffusion field and the permanent irritation of the cough reflex arc.

Respiratory insufficiency causes **polycythaemia** via hypoxia. Erythropoietin is produced by oxygen-sensitive cells of the renal cortex. These cells register the oxygen tension via membrane receptors. In the case of hypoxia, a transcription factor is formed, which induces the expression of erythropoietin in the nucleus. Produced erythropoietin reaches the bone marrow via the blood. There, erythropoietin binds to a receptor and induces erythropoiesis.

Finally, the reduced CO_2 exhalation leads to respiratory acidosis (Figure 37.5.1).

Therapy

Symptom	Therapy
Cough	Antitussives (e.g. Hydrocodone)
Bronchospasm	Bronchodilators (e.g. Sympathomimetics, Salbutamol; Theophylline)
Chronic inflammation	Corticosteroids

Further Reading

Bagdonas, E., Raudoniute, J., Bruzauskaite, I., and Aldonyte, R. (2015). Novel aspects of pathogenesis and regeneration mechanisms in COPD. *International Journal of Chronic Obstructive Pulmonary Disease* 10: 995–1013. https://doi.org/10.2147/COPD.S82518.

Barnes, P.J. (2017). Cellular and molecular mechanisms of asthma and COPD. *Clinical science (London, England: 1979)* 131 (13): 1541–1558. https://doi.org/10.1042/CS20160487.

37.6

Pneumonia

Definition

Pneumonia refers to an inflammation of the alveolar space and/or the interstitial lung tissue, which is mainly caused by infections.

Aetiology

The following causes of pneumonia in dogs and cats are described.

Aspiration pneumonia arises when food is inhaled from the oral cavity, this can occur as a result of regurgitation, vomiting and laryngeal dysfunction. Infection-related pneumonia is viral, bacterial, parasitic or fungal. Here, the pathogen spectrum differs between dog and cat. Virus-related pneumonia in dogs is associated with canine influenza virus, canine distemper virus, adenovirus, parainfluenza virus and herpes virus. *Bordetella bronchiseptica*, *Staphylococcus* spp., *Streptococcus* spp., *Escherichia coli*, *Klebsiella* spp., *Pseudomonas* spp. and *Pasteurella* spp. have been described as bacterial infectious agents in dogs with pneumonia.

In cats, the viral spectrum of pneumonia is often associated with caliciviruses. Bacterial pathogens are *Pasteurella* spp., *E. coli*, *Staphylococcus* spp., *Streptococcus* spp., *Pseudomonas* spp., *B. bronchiseptica* and *Mycoplasma* spp. (Dear 2014).

Parasitic pneumonia is often associated with lungworm infestation, such as feline aelurostrongylosis and canine angiostrongylosis (Traversa and Guglielmini 2008). Finally, cryptococcosis and histoplasmosis are described as fungal. The disease occurs equally in dogs and cats.

Virus	Bacteria	Parasite	Fungi
Influenza virus (D)	*Bordetella bronchiseptica* (D/C)	*Aelurostrongylus* (C)	Blastomycosis (D)
Distemper virus (D)	*Staphylococcus* spp. (D/C)	*Angiostrongylus* (D)	Cryptococcosis (C)
Adenovirus (D)	*Streptococcus* spp. (D/C)	Crenosoma (D)	Histoplasmosis (C)
Parainfluenza virus (D)	*Pasteurella* spp. (D/C)	*Capillaria* (D/C)	
Herpes virus (D/C)	*Escherichia coli* (D/C)		
Calicivirus (C)	*Pseudomonas* spp. (D/C)		
	Mycoplasma spp. (D/C)		

D – Dog, C – Cat

A special form of pneumonia is the eosinophilic bronchopneumonia described in dogs.

Textbook of Small Animal Pathophysiology, First Edition. Stephan Neumann.
© 2025 John Wiley & Sons Ltd. Published 2025 by John Wiley & Sons Ltd.

Pathogenesis

Due to the localisation of the lungs to the outside world, the body protects itself from infection in the lungs by numerous defence mechanisms. These include mucociliary transport and cough, by which foreign material is transported out of the respiratory system. When foreign particles reach the terminal bronchi and alveoli, there is a defence consisting of alveolar macrophages, immunoglobulins, complement and surfactant. In addition to the inflammatory reaction, the process is influenced by vegetative reflexes. Cholinergic stimulation leads to glandular secretion, bronchoconstriction, increased mucus production and vasodilation (Randall 2010).

If the defence systems are overcome, pneumonia develops. This is often associated with the terminal bronchi as bronchopneumonia. Furthermore, it can occur alveolar and/or interstitial. Alveolar pneumonia develops more frequently after aerogenic transmission and begins in the terminal bronchi. According to the course of an inflammatory event, infiltration with inflammatory cells and cytokine-initiated permeability increase of the pulmonary capillaries with exudation into the alvcoli and interstitium develops. In interstitial pneumonia, the inflammatory response is more likely to occur in the interstitium and is carried by macrophages and mononuclear inflammatory cells (Figure 37.6.1).

Diagnostics

Clinical signs	Clinical pathology	Imaging	Histopathology	Microbiology
Dyspnoea	Non-specific	**Radiology** Bronchial or bronchointerstitial pattern	Not necessary	Bronchoalveolar lavage

Pathophysiologic Consequences

The pathophysiologic consequences of pneumonia are initially concentrated on the respiratory system and can eventually have systemic effects.

Influenced organ systems	Clinical symptoms
Respiratory system	Weakness
Systemic	Fatigue
	Dyspnoea
	Cough

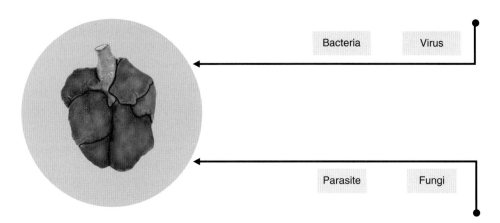

Figure 37.6.1 Mechanism of pneumonia.

In particular, the increased inflammation-related infiltration and exudation in the area of the alveoli and bronchi reduces the diffusion surface for gas exchange. This leads to hypoxia and hypercapnia. As a result, respiratory activity is increased in a compensatory manner, which can lead to tachypnoea and **dyspnoea**.

The consequences of hypoxia are particularly noticeable at the cellular level. Here, hypoxia causes an energy deficiency. This is due to reduced intracellular ATP synthesis as a result of the switch to anaerobic glycolysis. A lack of ATP affects, among other things, the ATP-dependent Na^+/K^+ pump, with the result of reduced sodium efflux and potassium influx. This causes water accumulation in the cell, as well as disturbances of the membrane balance. This opens calcium channels and leads to increased calcium influx.

The consequences of an increased cellular calcium concentration are multiple. Intra-mitochondrially, the complexes of the respiratory chain are affected, resulting in an increased synthesis of reactive oxygen species (ROS). At the same time, intra-mitochondrial glutathione is lost, which reduces oxidative stress as a 'radical scavenger'. As a result, mitochondrial membrane damage and organelle dysfunction occur.

Further consequences of an increased cellular calcium concentration are the increases in activity of lipases, protease and endonucleases. All of these lead to progressive cellular dysfunction.

Hypercapnia due to reduced alveolar gas exchange causes respiratory acidosis. Due to compensatory mechanisms by the buffering effect of haemoglobin and increased H^+ excretion via the kidneys, clinical consequences of hypercapnia are not very noticeable.

In pronounced, chronic cases, cardiovascular, neurological and metabolic consequences are possible. Acidosis has a direct negative inotropic effect on the heart muscles. At the same time, sensitivity to catecholamines decreases and peripheral vasodilation develops. As a consequence, cardiac function and blood pressure are reduced. This in turn can cause hypoxia, as discussed earlier. Neurologically, respiratory acidosis causes a disturbance of the Na^+-K^+ transport mechanism with the consequence of water accumulation in the nervous tissue and thus a restriction of nervous function (Staub et al. 1994). As a consequence, **weakness** and **fatigue** may develop.

The clinically prominent symptom of cough is due to bronchioalveolar remodelling processes. Dry cough develops due to interstitial infiltration with inflammatory cells. This can lead to permanent irritation of the cough receptors by mediators of the inflammatory cells. A wet cough develops when there has been an exudation of inflammatory secretions in the alveolar and bronchial areas due to inflammation. This, combined with existing bronchial mucus, forms a viscous fluid that is no longer transported by mucocilliary clearance. Remaining secretions irritate the receptors of the bronchial wall and induce the cough reflex (Figure 37.6.2).

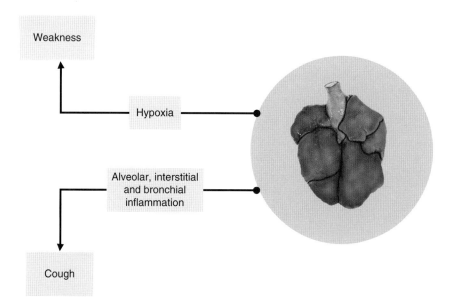

Figure 37.6.2 Pathophysiologic consequences of pneumonia.

Therapy

Symptom	Therapy
Infection	Antibiotics
Cough	Secretolytics (e.g. Bromhexine, Acetylcysteine)
Dry cough	Antitussives (e.g. Hydrocodone)

References

Dear, J.D. (2014). Bacterial pneumonia in dogs and cats. *The Veterinary Clinics of North America. Small Animal Practice* 44 (1): 143–159. https://doi.org/10.1016/j.cvsm.2013.09.003.

Randall, T.D. (2010). Bronchus-associated lymphoid tissue (BALT) structure and function. *Advances in Immunology* 107: 187–241. https://doi.org/10.1016/B978-0-12-381300-8.00007-1.

Staub, F., Mackert, B., Kempski, O. et al. (1994). Swelling and damage to nerves and glial cells by acidosis. *Anasthesiology, Intensive Care, Emergency Medicine, Pain Therapy: AINS* 29 (4): 203–209. https://doi.org/10.1055/s-2007-996719.

Traversa, D. and Guglielmini, C. (2008). Feline aelurostrongylosis and canine angiostrongylosis: a challenging diagnosis for two emerging verminous pneumonia infections. *Veterinary Parasitology* 157 (3–4): 163–174.

Further Reading

Reinero, C. (2019). Interstitial lung diseases in dogs and cats part I: the idiopathic interstitial pneumonias. *Veterinary Journal (London, England: 1997)* 243: 48–54.

Reinero, C. (2019). Interstitial lung diseases in dogs and cats part II: known cause and other discrete forms. *Veterinary Journal (London, England: 1997)* 243: 55–64.

37.7

Idiopathic Lung Fibrosis

Definition

Idiopathic pulmonary fibrosis is a fibrotic remodelling of the lung parenchyma of unknown origin.

Aetiology

The disease occurs primarily in West Highland White Terriers.

Pathogenesis

The main histopathological finding in affected animals is interstitial fibrosis in the alveolar wall and bronchioles. This is accompanied by proliferation of resident myofibroblasts and smooth muscle cell hyperplasia. Inflammatory cells in the form of lymphocytes and plasma cells are hardly present. As a consequence of fibrosis, stenosis of the air-conducting pathways occurs (Corcoran et al. 1999; Syrjä et al. 2013).

According to current knowledge, the pathogenesis is based on the destruction of the alveolar cells sine causa. This leads to a compensatory proliferation of type 2 alveolar cells. Profibrotic cytokines, such as TGF-β are secreted by these cells. This binds to membrane receptors of fibroblasts. Via signal transduction through the SMAD pathway, TGF-β affects gene expression in the nucleus. As a result, a differentiation from fibroblasts via promyofibroblasts to myofibroblasts develops. This differentiation is accompanied by an increased synthesis of actin filaments. The process can be positively influenced by mechanical stimulation. Finally, myofibroblasts are capable of synthesising collagens, thus implicating tissue fibrosis (King et al. 2011; Tai et al. 2021) (Figure 37.7.1).

Diagnostics

Clinical signs	Clinical pathology	Imaging	Histopathology	Microbiology
Dyspnoea	Non-specific	**Radiology**	Not necessary	Not necessary
Cough		Interstitial lung pattern		

Pathophysiologic Consequences

The pathophysiologic consequences focus on the respiratory system and the clinical consequences of its insufficiency.

Textbook of Small Animal Pathophysiology, First Edition. Stephan Neumann.

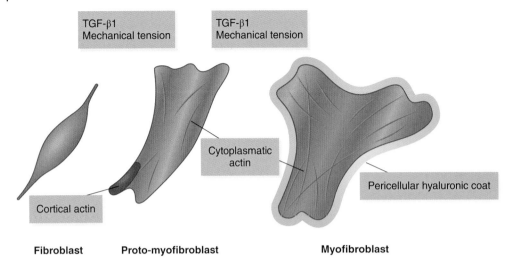

Figure 37.7.1 Differentiation of fibroblasts into myofibroblasts.

Influenced organ systems	Clinical symptoms	Clinical pathological alterations
Respiratory system	Exercise intolerance	Polycythaemia
Systemic	Dyspnoea	
	Cough	

The **exercise intolerance** develops from the restricted gas exchange area and the wider resorption pathway due to fibrosis; this also causes the dyspnoea.

In addition, fibrosis disturbs the overall organ architecture, with blood vessels being displaced. This leads to thrombosis of the vessels with the need for the formation of collateral vessels. This can lead to a reduced supply of oxygen to the tissue. In addition, the reduced removal of CO_2 can contribute to an accumulation in the tissue and formation of acidosis. This in turn also leads to cellular dysfunction.

The remodelling processes of the lungs also influence the bronchial transport mechanisms and additionally irritate the bronchial mucosa. As a consequence of the reduced mucociliary clearance and the receptor irritation, cough develops.

In some advanced cases, systemic hypoxia leads to reactive polycythaemia by inducing renal erythropoietin secretion due to arterial oxygen deficiency.

Therapy

Symptom	Therapy
Fibrosis reduction	Corticoids
Bronchodilation	Methylxanthine derivatives, e.g. theophylline

References

Corcoran, B.M., Cobb, M., Martin, M.W. et al. (1999). Chronic pulmonary disease in West Highland white terriers. *The Veterinary Record* 144 (22): 611–616. https://doi.org/10.1136/vr.144.22.611.

King, T.E. Jr., Pardo, A., and Selman, M. (2011). Idiopathic pulmonary fibrosis. *Lancet (London, England)* 378 (9807): 1949–1961. https://doi.org/10.1016/S0140-6736(11)60052-4.

Syrjä, P., Heikkilä, H.P., Lilja-Maula, L. et al. (2013). The histopathology of idiopathic pulmonary fibrosis in West Highland white terriers shares features of both non-specific interstitial pneumonia and usual interstitial pneumonia in man. *Journal of Comparative Pathology* 149 (2–3): 303–313. https://doi.org/10.1016/j.jcpa.2013.03.006.

Tai, Y., Woods, E.L., Dally, J. et al. (2021). Myofibroblasts: function, formation, and scope of molecular therapies for skin fibrosis. *Biomolecules* 11 (8): 1095. https://doi.org/10.3390/biom11081095.

Further Reading

Laurila, H.P. and Rajamäki, M.M. (2020). Update on canine idiopathic pulmonary fibrosis in West Highland white terriers. *The Veterinary Clinics of North America. Small Animal Practice* 50 (2): 431–446. https://doi.org/10.1016/j.cvsm.2019.11.004.

38

Gastrointestinal System

38.1

Physiological Functions and General Pathophysiology of Organ Insufficiency

Digestion

The gastrointestinal tract has the essential task of supplying an organism with nutrients. Functionally, the organ system can be divided into the following areas:

Food intake
Food transport
Food digestion
Nutrient intake

The sections belonging to the gastrointestinal tract can perform these functions due to their anatomical structure.

Food intake takes place via the mouth cavity. There, the food is taken in, chopped into swallowable bites and swallowed. The presence of saliva is important for the function of the swallowing process. This is produced by three pairs of salivary glands, the Glandula parotis, Glandula mandibularis and Glandula sublingualis, as well as numerous smaller salivary glands in the buccal mucosa. The different glands secrete secretions of different compositions, which, in their sum, essentially contain mucin, electrolytes and water. Mucin is a glycoprotein and gives saliva its viscosity. Electrolytes are present in saliva in more or less identical concentrations to those in blood plasma, and their secretion is associated with the secretion of water, another essential component of saliva. Water can dissolve nutrients to be better identified by the taste receptors. This is an essential prerequisite for the nervous and hormonal control of digestion (Table 38.1.1).

The digestive process is controlled by nervous reflexes and hormones and begins with the production of saliva in the oral cavity. Saliva production is controlled by the nerves of the autonomic nervous system, with the parasympathetic nervous system developing and facilitating reflexes and the sympathetic nervous system inhibiting reflexes. Salivary secretion is promoted by olfactory and gustatory stimuli.

After the bite has been swallowed, the digestion process of the food begins in the stomach. The control takes place both neurologically and hormonally. Already the intake of food promotes gastric juice secretion via the parasympathetic nervous system. In addition, gastric juice secretion is promoted by the formation of gastrin. This is secreted by G-cells of the gastric mucosa, the pancreas and the duodenum. The secretion is controlled by the parasympathetic nervous system and by food in the pyloric region. Via the bloodstream, gastrin reaches the parietal cells of the stomach wall and promotes the formation of hydrochloric acid. The secretion of hydrochloric acid by the parietal cells is an essential function of the stomach. The secretion initiates the digestion of proteins. Hydrochloric acid production is controlled by gastrin, but also by histamine, as well as by parasympathetic nerve fibres of the vagus nerve.

The molecular mechanisms of hydrochloric acid secretion are explained here. In this process, protons are secreted into the gastric lumen against potassium ions via an ATPase-controlled exchange. The protons are the product of the dissociation of carbonic acid under the influence of carbonic anhydrase. The chloride ions originate from NaCl, which is channelled through the parietal cell.

Another important function of digestion is the secretion of pepsin. Pepsin is formed by the gastric chief cells of the stomach wall and secreted as an inactive precursor (pepsinogen). The formation takes place under the influence of the parasympathetic nervous system. Pepsinogen is degraded to pepsin by cleavage of a peptide at a pH value below 6 up to an optimum

Textbook of Small Animal Pathophysiology, First Edition. Stephan Neumann.

Table 38.1.1 Functions of the saliva.

Component	Food	Teeth	Oral microbiome
Mucin	Bolus formation		
Water	Taste		
Bicarbonate		Buffer	
Calcium phosphate		Remineralisation	
Immunoglobulins			Antiviral, antibacterial and antifungal, defence
Lysozyme			
Defensin			

Table 38.1.2 Stomach function.

	Function
Temporary feed storage	Dosed release of food pulp into the small intestine
Non-specific defence	Reduction of the bacterial flora of the feed
Iron and vitamin B12	Mechanisms preparing for resorption

at a pH value of 3–4. In addition to activation by acidic environments, pepsin itself can also initiate a smaller part of the activation by autocatalysis. Pepsin is able to divide proteins by hydrolytic cleavage. Pepsin cleaves bonds with phenylalanine, tyrosine and leucine most easily, but can hydrolyse almost all other peptide bonds as well.

Other stomach functions are summarised in Table 38.1.2.

Gastric motility is important for the portioning of the chyme and its further transport into the small intestine. The movements of the stomach are controlled by the autonomic nervous system. The parasympathetic nervous system shows stimulatory activity and the sympathetic nervous system shows inhibitory activity. After food pulp has reached the stomach and the stomach wall is stretched, this initiates contraction waves of the stomach wall muscles that mix the chyme. The release of chyme into the small intestine is reached by peristaltic contraction waves from the cardia to the pyloric sphincter. Through transport via the pylorus, acidic chyme reaches the small intestine.

There, further digestion and later the resorption of the food components is located. Digestion is initially ensured by the influence of pancreatic and bile secretions and later by enterocyte enzymes. It is controlled vegetatively and via enteric hormones. Table 38.1.3 lists hormones of the digestive tract.

Table 38.1.3 Important hormones of the digestive system with essential functions.

Hormone	Function
Gastrin	Secretion of H^+ by parietal cells
	Regeneration of gastrointestinal mucosa
Cholecystokinin	Gall bladder emptying
	Secretion of the pancreatic juice
Secretin	Inhibition of gastric acid secretion
	Stimulation of bicarbonate secretion (bile, pancreatic juice)
Gastric inhibitory polypeptide (GIP)	Stimulation of insulin secretion
	Stimulation of lipase activity
	Inhibition of gastric juice secretion
	Inhibition of gastric emptying
Motilin	Stimulation of intestinal motility

Table 38.1.4 Overview of intestinal enzymes.

Enzyme	Substrate	Product
Lactase	Lactose	Glucose-galactose
Enterokinase	Trypsinogen	Trypsin
Aminopeptidase	Terminal amino acids	Peptide cleavage

Source: Adapted from Kanecko et al. (2008).

After the acidic chyme has reached the small intestine, secretin is formed by the intestinal mucosa cells. This secretin reaches the pancreas via the blood and initiates the release of pancreatic juice. Due to its bicarbonate concentration, this initially buffers the acidic chyme. At the same time, the secretion of pancreatic enzymes initiates the digestion of the food components.

The continued digestion of the food components is carried out by enzymes of the mucosal cells of the intestine. The final processes of digestion can take place through intestinal peristalsis, which, like gastric wall peristalsis, mixes, transports and presents the chyme to the mucosal surface. These processes are also controlled vegetatively and hormonally (Table 38.1.4).

After the digestion process is complete, the individual food components are absorbed. The mechanisms during this process vary.

The absorption processes is located in the small intestine, and accordingly the surface area of the small intestine is significantly enlarged.

Carbohydrates are absorbed as monosaccharides. Pentoses are absorbed faster than hexoses. They are transported via carriers on the luminal epithelial cell membrane. Glucose is used as an example to illustrate the transport. Glucose is transported into the cell together with sodium via an epithelial carrier. The intracellular concentration gradient of Na^+ is the driving force. Inside the cell, glucose and sodium dissociate from the carrier. Sodium is transported back to the luminal membrane surface via an ATP-consuming process.

Proteins are absorbed in the form of amino acids. The transport mechanism is similar to that of glucose in that cotransport with sodium takes place.

Fats are absorbed as tri-, di- and monoglycerides, as well as fatty acids, glycerol and cholesterol. In the process, the bile acids act as detergents and bring the fats into contact with the mucosal surface. Absorption usually happens via pinocytosis. The onward transport of the fats is special. Long-chain triglycerides form chylomicrons with proteins, which are released by the mucosal cells into the lymphatic system. They then enter the venous system via the milk duct. Short-chain fatty acids are released to the portal venous system after absorption and go directly to the liver.

The absorption of electrolytes is an active absorption processes. Water can be absorbed in cotransport with electrolytes or glucose and other absorbed food components. Another form of water absorption is located in the large intestine. Here, water is absorbed via Na cotransport through the mucosa. The expression of aquaporins in the colonic epithelium also enables water absorption.

The further transport of the food pulp into the large intestine via the ileocaecal valve is to prevent a backflow of the chyme from the large intestine into the small intestine. The mixing would be suboptimal in that the intestinal flora differs in quality and quantity between the small and large intestine. However, an adapted physiological intestinal flora is essential for digestive processes. In the large intestine, water is extracted from the chyme. However, this is only one task. Bacterial fermentation is also located in the large intestine, which supplies nutrients (Figure 38.1.1).

Gut-associated Lymphoid Tissue (GALT)

The gastrointestinal tract represents a large interface of the organism with the outside world. Accordingly, a pronounced confrontation with antigen from the environment, as microbiological antigen or dietary antigen, is located here. Accordingly, the intestinal barrier assumes an important defence function. The defence function of the intestinal wall is based on various mechanisms:

1) Tight-junctions between the enterocytes
2) Lymphatic tissues as Peyer's plates, mesenteric lymph nodes and lymph follicles in the intestinal wall

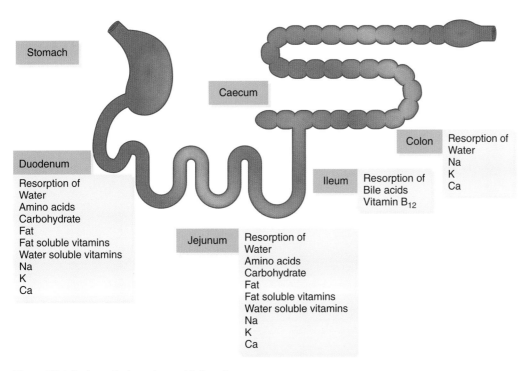

Figure 38.1.1 Intestinal sections with function.

3) IgA secretion
4) Paneth cells
5) Gastric juice pH
6) Intestinal peristalsis

1. The tight-junctions establish a firm impermeable connection between the enterocytes. This prevents direct contact between the intestine-associated antigen and the defence cells of the lamina propria in the intestinal wall. The tight-junctions are mainly formed by the proteins claudin and occludin. If there is a leakage through the tight-junctions, this implies the secretion of proinflammatory cytokines (TNF-α, interferon-γ) by the enterocytes.

2. If enteric antigens pass through this first protective barrier, there is a second defence by cells of the non-specific defence, the dendritic cells. These can bind antigenic components (PAMPS) via toll-like receptors and present the antigen to the cells of the specific defence through the expression of major histocompatibility complex (MHC). These are localised in the intestine-associated lymphatic system. After antigen presentation, the native lymphocytes differentiate into TH1 and TH2 lymphocytes. The former secretes various proinflammatory cytokines and initiates the inflammatory response, while the latter regulates the inflammatory process through the secretion of anti-inflammatory cytokines (IL-10).

In addition to the dendritic cells in the lamina propria, so-called 'M-cells' are localised in the epithelium between the enterocytes, which function as non-specific antigen-presenting defence cells. The enterocytes are largely protected from direct contact with the microbiota by a layer of mucus. M-cells lack this covering, so that direct antigen contact can occur. M-cells can take up antigen via endocytosis and also present it to native lymphocytes.

3. Another defence function of the intestinal wall is the secretion of IgA. This is secreted by plasma cells in the lamina propria and reaches the intestinal lumen via transcytosis through the enterocytes.

4. Another cell type that represents the intestinal defence function are the paneth cells. These are localised in the Lieberkühn's crypts and can secrete antimicrobial proteins (AMP) after antigen contact.

In the physiological pH environment, the majority of AMPs are positively charged. In contrast, the surface of microorganisms expresses many negatively charged molecules, e.g. lipopolysaccharides. Due to this, a charge-dependent interaction with components of the bacterial cell wall occurs. This leads to the formation of pores in the bacterial cell wall. Electrolyte balance can occur via these and the existing membrane potential collapses. The result is lysis of the bacterial cell.

Since the proportion of negatively charged molecules on the prokaryotic cell surface is higher than in eukaryotic cells, the AMPs show a certain specificity.

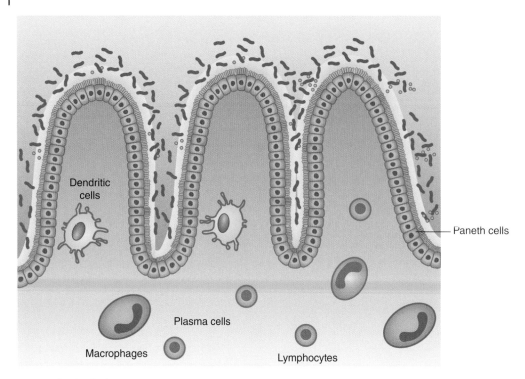

Figure 38.1.2 Defence system in the intestinal wall.

5. and 6. Two other non-specific defence mechanisms of the intestinal tract are the inactivation of ingested bacteria by gastric acid and the prevention of colonisation of bacteria due to intestinal peristalsis (Figure 38.1.2).

In recent decades, knowledge and awareness of and for the intestinal **microbiome** has grown considerably. The term 'intestinal microbiome' refers to the total amount of intestinal flora, which includes bacteria, viruses, fungi, archaea and protozoa. Colonisation of the intestine takes place around and after birth and is species-specific but also varies from individual to individual. Changes in the microbiome also happens during life. Several hundred species of bacteria alone have been described. In principle, the number of microorganisms increases in the course of the intestine from the stomach to the large intestine, and there is also a shift from aerobically growing germs to anaerobes in the large intestine.

The number of different bacterial species in the intestinal microbiome belongs to 14 phyla, 27 classes, 56 orders, 106 families, 286 genera and 533 species (Table 38.1.5).

Physiological functions in the gastrointestinal tract are attributed to the microbiome. The metabolic function of the bacteria is based on the fermentation of carbohydrates. These are predominantly fermented in the colon to short-chain fatty acids (acetate, propionate, butyrate). In addition, endogenous peptides of the enterocytes, mucins, enzymes or undigested food protein are also degraded by bacteria in the colon. The degradation products are branched-chain fatty acids. At the same time, ammonia, amines, phenols, indoles and thiols are formed. Certain bacteria can synthesise vitamins, such as vitamin K, folic acid, biotin and thiamine.

In addition to the metabolic function, the microbiome takes on a trophic function by feeding the epithelial cells of the intestinal wall. Short-chain fatty acids, which are an important source of energy for the enterocytes, serve this purpose. In addition, the microbiome serves the development and maturation of the resident immune system.

Another function of the microbiome is the generation of colonisation resistance. This prevents ingested pathogens from colonising and later infecting by occupying the biotope.

A functional insufficiency of the gastrointestinal tract leads to an undersupply of nutrients and other ingredients of the food. The insufficiency can be divided into a digestive insufficiency and an absorption insufficiency.

Table 38.1.5 List of quantitatively important bacterial strains in the microbiome of 96 healthy dogs.

Actinobacter
Bacteroides
Cyanobacteria
Deferribacteria
Firmicutes
Fusobacteria
Proteobacteria
Spirochaeta
Tenericutes
Verrucomicrobia

Source: Adapted from You and Kim (2021).

Table 38.1.6 Consequences of malassimilation.

Deficiency	Consequence
Protein deficiency	Cachexia, oedema formation
Carbohydrate deficiency	Reduced supply of the energy source glucose
Vitamin deficiency	
Vitamin A	Night blindness, reduced tear secretion, dry skin, hyperkeratosis
Vitamin K	Increased bleeding tendency (reduced activity of factor II, factor VII, factor IX, factor X)
Vitamin B12	Macrocytic anaemia
Potassium deficiency	Weakness, cardiac arrhythmia
Calcium deficiency	Secondary hyperparathyroidism
Iron deficiency	Hypochromic anaemia

Consequences of this malassimilation are disturbances in the absorption of nutrients. These can lead to the following changes listed in Table 38.1.6.

References

Kanecko, J.J., Harvey, J.W., and Bruss, M.L. (ed.) (2008). *Clinical Biochemistry of Domestic Animals*, 425. Academic Press.

You, I. and Kim, M.J. (2021). Comparison of gut microbiota of 96 healthy dogs by individual traits: breed, age, and body condition score. *Animals: an Open Access Journal from MDPI* 11 (8): 2432. https://doi.org/10.3390/ani11082432.

Further Reading

Cheng, L.K., O'Grady, G., Du, P. et al. (2010). Gastrointestinal system. *Wiley Interdisciplinary Reviews. Systems Biology and Medicine* 2 (1): 65–79. https://doi.org/10.1002/wsbm.19.

Granger, D.N., Holm, L., and Kvietys, P. (2015). The gastrointestinal circulation: physiology and pathophysiology. *Comprehensive Physiology* 5 (3): 1541–1583. https://doi.org/10.1002/cphy.c150007.

Greenwood-Van Meerveld, B., Johnson, A.C., and Grundy, D. (2017). Gastrointestinal physiology and function. *Handbook of Experimental Pharmacology* 239: 1–16. https://doi.org/10.1007/164_2016_118.

Hunt, R.H., Camilleri, M., Crowe, S.E. et al. (2014). The mucus and mucins of the goblet cells and enterocytes provide the first defense line of the gastrointestinal tract and interact with the immune system. *Immunological Reviews* 260 (1): 8–20. https://doi.org/10.1111/imr.12182.

Lidbury, J.A., Cook, A.K., and Steiner, J.M. (2016). Hepatic encephalopathy in dogs and cats. *Journal of Veterinary Emergency and Critical Care (San Antonio, Tex.: 2001)* 26 (4): 471–487.

Mason, K.L., Huffnagle, G.B., Noverr, M.C., and Kao, J.Y. (2008). Overview of gut immunology. *Advances in Experimental Medicine and Biology* 635: 1–14. https://doi.org/10.1007/978-0-387-09550-9_1.

Parikh, A. and Thevenin, C. (2022). Physiology, gastrointestinal hormonal control. In: *StatPearls [Internet]*. Treasure Island (FL): StatPearls Publishing.

Pelaseyed, T., Bergström, J.H., Gustafsson, J.K. et al. (2018). Intestinal microbiota and the immune system in metabolic diseases. *Journal of Microbiology (Seoul, Korea)* 56 (3): 154–162. https://doi.org/10.1007/s12275-018-7548-y.

Soenen, S., Rayner, C.K., Jones, K.L., and Horowitz, M. (2016). The ageing gastrointestinal tract. *Current Opinion in Clinical Nutrition and Metabolic Care* 19 (1): 12–18. https://doi.org/10.1097/MCO.0000000000000238.

Stokes, C. and Waly, N. (2006). Mucosal defence along the gastrointestinal tract of cats and dogs. *Veterinary Research* 37 (3): 281–293. https://doi.org/10.1051/vetres:2006015.

Suchodolski, J.S. (2011). Companion animals symposium: microbes and gastrointestinal health of dogs and cats. *Journal of Animal Science* 89 (5): 1520–1530. https://doi.org/10.2527/jas.2010-3377.

Tack, J. (2015). The stomach in health and disease. *Gut* 64 (10): 1650–1668. https://doi.org/10.1136/gutjnl-2014-307595.

38.2

Megaoesophagus

Definition

The *megaoesophagus* is defined as a local or generalised dilation of the oesophageal lumen.

Aetiology

The causes of oesophageal dilatation are usually neurogenic or myogenic. Numerous causes are idiopathic. Megaoesophagus occurs regularly in dogs but is rare in cats.

Idiopathic	Genetic	Neurological	Myogenic
(D)	Congenital myasthenia gravis (D)	Myasthenia gravis (D)	Systemic lupus erythematosus (D)
		Polyneuropathy (D)	Myositis (D)
		Hypoadrenocorticism (D)	
		Hypothyroidism (D)	

D-dog C-cat

Pathogenesis

For a better understanding, the physiology of the swallowing process should be briefly explained.

This can be divided into an oral, a pharyngeal and an oesophageal phase. The first phase involves the preparation of the food bolus for the act of swallowing and can be influenced voluntarily. The bolus is transported to the base of the tongue by the activity of the oral cavity muscles and the tongue. Subsequently, the tongue rises under the hard and soft palate, transporting the bolus towards the oesophagus. In the pharyngeal phase, which is subject to nervous control by the 'swallowing centre' in the medulla oblongata, the proximal oesophageal sphincter relaxes and the food bolus can be moved into the oesophagus. At the same time, the soft palate closes the nasal cavity and the epiglottis closes the larynx. Once the food bolus has passed the sphincter, the oesophageal phase begins by contraction of the proximal oesophageal sphincter. The oesophageal transport is performed based on the peristalsis of the oesophageal muscles. The main trigger for the initiation of oesophageal peristalsis is the stretching of the oesophageal wall. Peristalsis is involuntary. It is controlled by vagal reflex arcs. When the food bolus reaches the distal oesophageal sphincter, it relaxes and the food can enter the cardia of the stomach.

The musculature and the autonomic nervous supply of the oesophagus are responsible for its peristalsis. Accordingly, primary diseases of the nerves, neuromuscular transmission or musculature can lead to a disturbance of peristalsis with subsequent lumen dilatation and megaoesophagus.

A common disease associated with megaoesophagus is myasthenia gravis. In this case, there is a receptor blockade at the postsynaptic membrane, which leads to reduced impulse formation in the oesophageal musculature, with the consequence of hypomotility with subsequent dilatation. Polymyopathies lead to megaoesophagus via similar mechanisms.

Textbook of Small Animal Pathophysiology, First Edition. Stephan Neumann.

The significance of hypothyroidism as a cause of megaoesophagus is controversial. It is possible that the autoimmune thyroiditis causally involved in primary hypothyroidism leads to the formation of autoantibodies that become active at the neuromuscular end plate of the oesophageal muscles. There, a disturbance of neuromuscular impulse transmission develops (Emami et al. 2007).

The occurrence of transient megaoesophagus in Addison's disease is observed more frequently. The electrolyte changes that occur in the disease, especially hyperkalaemia, are held responsible for the symptoms. If the extracellular potassium concentration increases, this causes a reduction in the chemical potassium gradient between the intracellular and extracellular space. As a result, the resting membrane potential decreases. Initially, this leads to easier formation of an action potential. However, chronic membrane depolarisation causes a reduction in the sensitivity of Na^+ channels and thus a reduced generation of an action potential and overall excitability of the cell membrane. The involvement of potassium channels in the contraction of oesophageal striated and smooth muscle has been investigated (Horii et al. 2019). In addition autoimmune mechanisms may also play a role in hypoadrenocorticism.

Diagnostics

Clinical signs	Clinical pathology	Imaging	Histopathology	Microbiology
Regurgitation	Non-specific	**Radiology**	Not necessary	Not necessary
Dyspnoea	If applicable, myasthenia gravis AK	Contrast, cave aspiration		
		Endoscopy		

Pathophysiologic Consequences

The pathophysiologic consequences of megaoesophagus are essentially due to a reduced supply of food to the organism and to disturbances caused by inhalation of food.

Influenced organ systems	Clinical symptoms
Gastrointestinal system	Regurgitation
Respiratory system	Weight loss
Neuromuscular system	Weakness
	Dyspnoea

The impaired oesophageal function impedes the act of swallowing, which can lead to a stasis of food pulp in the oesophagus, accompanied by **regurgitation**. This is a mechanism in which chyme flows from the oesophagus into the oral cavity without the mechanisms of abdominal pressure increase typical of vomiting. However, due to the distension of food within the oesophagus, there is an activation of muscle contraction of the striated and smooth oesophageal muscles (Lang et al. 2019).

Regurgitation results in reduced feed intake, which can lead to **cachexia** and **weakness**. A reduction in oesophageal motility can also cause increased salivation as saliva produced does not reach the stomach.

Finally, the disturbance of the swallowing act can cause food components to enter the trachea and lungs via the larynx, leading to aspiration pneumonia. This is caused by different components of the aspirate: If gastric acid is present in the aspirate, the epithelial cells in the airways are destroyed. The mechanism is similar to that of an inflammatory reaction and is carried by neutrophilic granulocytes and macrophages and their secretion of mediators, such as proinflammatory cytokines or eicosanoids. Bacterial colonisation takes place through microorganisms of the oral cavity flora, which are still active in the aspirate, as the bactericidal gastric acid is not or only partially effective. A major clinical symptom of aspiration pneumonia is **dyspnoea** (Son et al. 2017) (Figure 38.2.1).

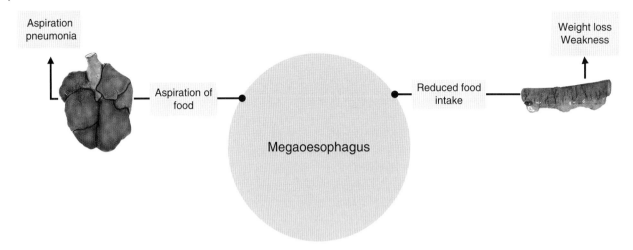

Figure 38.2.1 Pathophysiologic consequences in megaoesophagus.

Therapy

Symptom	Therapy
Regurgitation	Elevated oral feeding
Aspiration pneumonia	Antibiotics
If myasthenia gravis	Anticholinesterase inhibitors (e.g. Pyridostigmine)

References

Emami, M.H., Raisi, M., Amini, J., and Daghaghzadeh, H. (2007). Achalasia and thyroid disease. *World Journal of Gastroenterology* 13 (4): 594–599. https://doi.org/10.3748/wjg.v13.i4.594.

Horii, K., Suzuki, Y., Shiina, T. et al. (2019). ATP-dependent potassium channels contribute to motor regulation of esophageal striated muscle in rats. *The Journal of Veterinary Medical Science* 81 (9): 1266–1272. https://doi.org/10.1292/jvms.19-0197.

Lang, I.M., Medda, B.K., and Shaker, R. (2019). Characterization and mechanism of the esophago-esophageal contractile reflex of the striated muscle esophagus. *American Journal of Physiology. Gastrointestinal and Liver Physiology* 317 (3): G304–G313. https://doi.org/10.1152/ajpgi.00138.2019.

Son, Y.G., Shin, J., and Ryu, H.G. (2017). Pneumonitis and pneumonia after aspiration. *Journal of Dental Anesthesia and Pain Medicine* 17 (1): 1–12. https://doi.org/10.17245/jdapm.2017.17.1.1.

Further Reading

Guilford, W.G. (1990). Megaesophagus in the dog and cat. *Seminars in Veterinary Medicine and Surgery (Small Animal)* 5 (1): 37–45.

Mace, S., Shelton, G.D., and Eddlestone, S. (2013). Megaesophagus in the dog and cat. *Veterinary Practice. Issue K, Small Animals/Pets* 41 (2): 123–132.

38.3

Gastritis/Ulceration

Definition

Gastritis is, by definition, an inflammation of the gastric mucosa, which can be acute or chronic. If the inflammatory process extends beyond the mucosa, there is an ulceration.

Aetiology

Gastritis can occur primarily as a result of ingestion of intolerable food or drugs. Secondarily, gastritis is associated with diseases of the intestine, hormonal diseases, liver and pancreatic diseases. Gastritis occurs regularly in dogs and cats.

Gastral	Endocrine	Metabolic
Food sensitivity (D)	Hypoadrenocorticism (D)	Pancreatitis (D,C)
Drugs (D,C)	Hyperthyroidism (C)	Liver diseases (D,C)
NSAID		Kidney diseases (D,C)
Infection (D)		
Helicobacter spp.		

D – Dog, C – Cat

Pathogenesis

The various triggers of gastritis produce damage to the gastric mucosa via different mechanisms. This can be caused by reduced blood flow (hypoadrenocorticism), inflammatory reactions (food sensitivity) or toxic metabolites (liver disease).

As a result, an imbalance develops between protective and aggressive factors with the consequence of further damage to the mucous membrane by the gastric juice. The protection of the gastric mucosa is disturbed.

The protection of the gastric mucosa is based on the formation of mucus. The mucus that protects the gastric mucosa is secreted by goblet cells of the gastric mucosa. It is composed of water and mucins, the latter are glycoproteins with a special swelling behaviour. Through secretion, the gastric mucosa is covered with a viscous mucus of approximately 0.1–0.5 mm. The production of mucus is promoted by the influence of prostaglandins.

In addition, prostaglandins induce bicarbonate secretion in gastric muscle cells, which buffer protons.

For the formation of mucus and bicarbonate, as well as the transport of protons, the blood circulation of the gastric mucosa is essential.

Helicobacter-associated gastritis and the NSAID-induced form are used to illustrate the pathogenesis of gastritis.

The development of gastritis by infection with *Helicobacter* spp. in dogs and cats is controversially discussed. Although the pathogen is found in the stomach of both species, its role in the genesis of gastritis is not fully understood (Neiger and Simpson 2000; Taillieu et al. 2022).

Textbook of Small Animal Pathophysiology, First Edition. Stephan Neumann.
© 2025 John Wiley & Sons Ltd. Published 2025 by John Wiley & Sons Ltd.

However, since the pathogenesis of infection in humans is largely understood, this mechanism is presented here as an example. Due to the principally antibacterial milieu in the stomach, bacterial infective pathogens must be resistant to the acidic gastric environment. They must overcome the mucus barrier to colonise the gastric mucosa. Furthermore, they must adhere to the mucosal cells and finally produce a pathological effect, for example, through the synthesis of toxins.

It is possible for *Helicobacter* spp. to overcome the acidic gastric milieu because urease is formed in the cytoplasm of the bacteria. This can convert urea into ammonia and ammonium ions, which can penetrate the bacterial plasma membrane and bind protons periplasmically, i.e. between the bacterial membrane and the bacterial wall. In this way, the bacteria protect themselves from gastric acid. The influx of urea takes place via pH-dependent channels, so it is only activated when the pH in the stomach drops. In the second step of the infection, the *Helicobacter* bacteria move towards the mucosal cells by means of flagella. There they adhere to receptors of the epithelial cells via various binding proteins (adhesins). The cytotoxicity of *Helicobacter* is mediated by cytotoxin-associated gene A and vacuolating cytotoxin A. The former can influence cell signalling by binding to phosphatases, manipulate the cytoskeleton, inhibit cell proliferation and influence the secretion of IL-8. This is an important chemotactic factor to migrate neutrophilic granulocytes. Vacuolating cytotoxin A is able to induce anion channels in epithelial cells of the gastric mucosa. This allows efflux of cellular components, possibly to feed the bacterium. In addition, the toxin induces the formation of intracellular vacuoles. These can expand due to water influx and thus disturb cellular metabolism (Szabò et al. 1999; Kao et al. 2016; Cheok et al. 2021).

The induction of gastritis by the application of NSAIDs is known in dogs and cats. The mechanism of mucosal damage is based on the inhibition of cyclooxygenase 1, an enzyme involved in prostaglandin synthesis, which protects the gastric mucosa from gastric acid by increasing blood flow and initiating the synthesis of bicarbonate. Secondly, NSAIDs show a direct cytotoxic effect against epithelial cells. They increase membrane permeability and thus alter the transport mechanisms at the cell membrane resulting in cell apoptosis or necrosis. In addition, they can activate caspases. Caspases are intracellular proteases that can induce apoptosis. After prolonged use, NSAIDs induce the formation of leukotrienes, as the inhibition of cyclooxygenase makes increased arachidonic acid concentrations available for leukotriene synthesis. Leukotrienes induce the synthesis of proinflammatory cytokines and cause an inflammatory response. At the same time, they reduce blood flow and can promote the formation of radicals via ischaemia and hypoxia. Both mechanisms can damage epithelial cells (Lichtenberger 1995; Tomisato et al. 2001; Gudis and Sakamoto 2005).

Permanent overcoming of the defence mechanisms and disturbance of the repair mechanisms can lead to profound mucosal changes, the gastric ulcer.

Diagnostics

Clinical signs	Clinical pathology	Imaging	Histopathology	Microbiology
Vomiting Inappetence	Non-specific	**Endoscopy** Biopsy or visual ulcer diagnosis Possibly **ultrasonography** for ulcer diagnosis	Histopathological diagnosis	Mostly not necessary

Pathophysiologic Consequences

The pathophysiologic consequences of gastritis and gastric ulcer are similar, but can be more serious in the case of ulcer. They predominantly affect the gastrointestinal tract.

Influenced organ systems	Clinical symptoms	Clinical pathological alterations
Gastrointestinal system	Vomiting Nausea Pain Inappetence Weight loss Dehydration	Haemoconcentration Anaemia Metabolic alkalosis

The symptoms are closely related to the changes in the gastric mucosa. These cause **vomiting** via two main mechanisms. Firstly, receptors in the stomach wall are irritated and act on the vomiting centre via nervous afferents, mostly of the vagus nerve. Another emetic factor is the increased synthesis and release of serotonin or substance P by chromaffin cells of the gastric wall. Both substances stimulate compatible receptors in the mucosa, which act on the vomiting centre via vagal afferents. A direct effect on the vomiting centre is also suspected for substance P. Nausea is associated with this effect. **Nausea** is to be seen as an associated symptom of vomiting. Nausea is triggered by a variety of stimuli from the gastrointestinal tract, but also from the vestibular apparatus and the central nervous system. Metabolic diseases, such as uraemia are also accompanied by nausea. The target organ is the central vomiting centre. Dopamine and serotonin, among others, are seen as mediators that lead to the triggering of symptoms via corresponding receptors.

Pain in gastritis and ulcers results from the irritation of nociceptors in the stomach and peritoneal cavity. These are activated by stimulus modalities, such as stretching or chemical stimuli. Inflammation causes a lowering of the stimulus threshold. This is achieved by the inflammatory mediators binding to receptors of the nociceptors and facilitating the generation of an action potential through a sodium influx. Afferents reach the pain centre in the reticular formation and the limbic system via the spinal cord.

As a result of nausea, vomiting and visceral pain, **inappetence** occurs, which in turn can lead to **weight loss** in the chronic course. Reduction of water intake can lead to **dehydration** and **haemoconcentration**. In case of ulcer bleeding, blood is released into the gastrointestinal tract. Due to the influence of gastric acid, haemoglobin is oxidised to haematin, which is reduced during intestinal passage, and becomes visible as **melena**. The bleeding can also lead to **anaemia**. This is regenerative as bleeding anaemia. However, non-bleeding chronic gastritis can also cause non-regenerative anaemia of chronic disease. This is caused by depression of erythropoietin synthesis mediated by proinflammatory cytokines. Due to the loss of gastric juice, vomiting can also lead to disturbances of the acid-base balance, especially in the case of chronic disease. During the formation of gastric acid in the parietal cells of the gastric wall, protons are discharged into the gastric lumen. These originate from a synthesis of carbonic acid from CO_2 and H_2O catalysed by carbonic anhydrase. After dissociation, bicarbonate is exchanged for chloride at the basement membrane. This slightly increases the bicarbonate concentration in the serum. In chronic vomiting, however, chloride ions and protons have to be constantly re-synthesised, and the bicarbonate concentration in the serum rises accordingly, resulting in metabolic alkalosis. This in turn can lead to hypokalaemia. The increased bicarbonate concentration in the serum during metabolic alkalosis leads to increased filtration in the kidneys. Accordingly, the bicarbonate concentration in the primary urine increases. Tubularly, this leads to the synthesis of CO_2 and OH^-, catalysed by carbonic anhydrase. Due to a proton efflux from the tubular epithelia, $OH^- + H^+ > H_2O$ is formed. For this, however, sodium must be exchanged for protons at the luminal membrane. In the basal membrane, sodium is exchanged for potassium. As a result, hypokalaemia can develop (Figure 38.3.1).

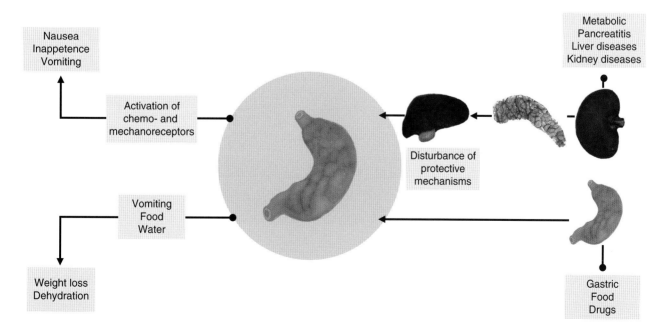

Figure 38.3.1 Pathogenesis and pathophysiologic consequences of gastritis.

Therapy

Symptom	Therapy
Vomiting	Antiemetic drugs (e.g. Maropitant, Metoclopramide, Ondansetron)
Nausea	Antiemetic drugs
Pain	Painkiller (e.g. Morphine)
Mucosa alteration	Protective drugs
Dehydration	Infusion

References

Cheok, Y.Y., Lee, C.Y.Q., Cheong, H.C. et al. (2021). An overview of Helicobacter pylori survival tactics in the hostile human stomach environment. *Microorganisms* 9 (12): 2502. https://doi.org/10.3390/microorganisms9122502.

Gudis, K. and Sakamoto, C. (2005). The role of cyclooxygenase in gastric mucosal protection. *Digestive Diseases and Sciences* 50 (Suppl 1): S16–S23. https://doi.org/10.1007/s10620-005-2802-7.

Kao, C.Y., Sheu, B.S., and Wu, J.J. (2016). Helicobacter pylori infection: an overview of bacterial virulence factors and pathogenesis. *Biomedical Journal* 39 (1): 14–23. https://doi.org/10.1016/j.bj.2015.06.002.

Lichtenberger, L.M. (1995). The hydrophobic barrier properties of gastrointestinal mucus. *Annual Review of Physiology* 57: 565–583. https://doi.org/10.1146/annurev.ph.57.030195.003025.

Neiger, R. and Simpson, K.W. (2000). Helicobacter infection in dogs and cats: facts and fiction. *Journal of Veterinary Internal Medicine* 14 (2): 125–133. https://doi.org/10.1892/0891-6640(2000)014<0125:iidacf>2.3.co;2.

Szabò, I., Brutsche, S., Tombola, F. et al. (1999). Formation of anion-selective channels in the cell plasma membrane by the toxin VacA of Helicobacter pylori is required for its biological activity. *The EMBO Journal* 18 (20): 5517–5527. https://doi.org/10.1093/emboj/18.20.5517.

Taillieu, E., Chiers, K., Amorim, I. et al. (2022). Gastric Helicobacter species associated with dogs, cats and pigs: significance for public and animal health. *Veterinary Research* 53 (1): 42. https://doi.org/10.1186/s13567-022-01059-4.

Tomisato, W., Tsutsumi, S., Rokutan, K. et al. (2001). NSAIDs induce both necrosis and apoptosis in guinea pig gastric mucosal cells in primary culture. *American Journal of Physiology. Gastrointestinal and Liver Physiology* 281 (4): G1092–G1100. https://doi.org/10.1152/ajpgi.2001.281.4.G1092.

Further Reading

Amorim, I., Taulescu, M.A., Day, M.J. et al. (2016). Canine gastric pathology: areview. *Journal of Comparative Pathology* 154 (1): 9–37. https://doi.org/10.1016/j.jcpa.2015.10.181.

Davis, M.S. and Williamson, K.K. (2016). Gastritis and gastric ulcers in working dogs. *Frontiers in Veterinary Science* 3: 30. https://doi.org/10.3389/fvets.2016.00030.

Sinha, M., Gautam, L., Shukla, P.K. et al. (2013). Current perspectives in NSAID-induced gastropathy. *Mediators of Inflammation* 2013: 258209. https://doi.org/10.1155/2013/258209.

Sullivan, M. and Yool, D.A. (1998). Gastric disease in the dog and cat. *Veterinary Journal (London, England: 1997)* 156 (2): 91–106. https://doi.org/10.1016/s1090-0233(05)80035-8.

38.4

Gastric Dilatation–Volvulus Syndrome

Definition

Gastric dilatation–volvulus is defined as dilation of the stomach and torsion of the gastric axis clockwise.

Aetiology

The cause of the disease is not fully understood, but a variety of risk factors have been described. The disease is specific to the dog. Large-breed dogs with a deep rib cage are preferentially affected. A correlation with food quantity, type of food and feeding frequency has been described. A previous splenectomy is also considered a risk factor, as are elevated gastrin concentrations.

The importance of the microbiome in the development of gastric distortion is also discussed. Alteration of the microbiome is suspected, for example, due to congenital gene variations of the immune system (Harkey et al. 2017; Hullar et al. 2018).

Genetic	Feeding
Large breeds	Large amount of feed
Large thoracic depth	Rapid feed intake
	Stress

Pathogenesis

The disease is composed of its dilatation of the stomach and its torsion. It is not finally clear whether the stomach dilates first and then turns or vice versa. In the case of primary torsion, digestive activity in the stomach would be impeded. Dilation would develop secondarily through bacterial fermentation of carbohydrates in the stomach or the formation of CO_2 from bicarbonate and hydrochloric acid (Brockman et al. 1995). The consequence would be the further clockwise rotation of the stomach around its own axis. In the process, the pylorus first moves from the right side to the left side and dorsally. The consequence is the torsion of the oesophagus and duodenum and thus the interruption of the gastric transport function (Figure 38.4.1).

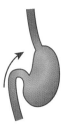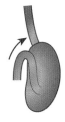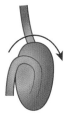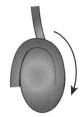

Figure 38.4.1 Mechanism of gastric torsion.

Diagnostics

Clinical signs	Clinical pathology	Imaging	Histopathology	Microbiology
Disturbed general condition	Non-specific	**Radiology**	Not necessary	Not necessary
Distended abdomen		Distended and twisted stomach		

Pathophysiologic Consequences

The pathophysiologic consequences of gastric torsion are based to a considerable extent on the consequences of the disturbed blood flow. The dilated and turned stomach first affects the venous blood flow in the caudal vena cava and in the portal vein. This results in 'blood stasis' in the stomach wall. It leads to ischaemia of the gastric wall cells, which become necrotic if 'blood stasis' persists for a long time.

The death of cells in the stomach wall releases vasoactive metabolites. These can lead to pathophysiologic consequences. Reperfusion after retorsion can be equally serious. This follows the mechanisms of the ischaemia-reperfusion syndrome.

Influenced organ systems	Clinical symptoms	Clinical pathological alterations
Cardiovascular system	Shock	Azotaemia
Respiratory system	Heart arrhythmia	Increased liver enzymes
Gastrointestinal system	Dyspnoea	DIC
Hepatobiliary system	Lethargy	Prolonged PT and apTT
Urinary tract	Pre-renal failure	Thrombocytopenia
Systemic		Acidosis/alkalosis

Gastric dilatation increases intra-abdominal pressure in the sense of a compartment syndrome. This affects the venous flow in the abdomen and later the arterial supply to the organs. The consequence of the reduced blood flow in the caudal vena cava and the portal vein is a reduced venous return to the right side of the heart, which continues via the pulmonary circulation to the left side of the heart. This causes reduced cardiac output and leads to **hypovolaemic shock**. Even after retorsion with reperfusion, increased vascular permeability in the necrotic stomach wall can lead to fluid leakage into the parenchyma, resulting in a volume deficiency.

The consequence of hypovolaemic shock is reduced perfusion of numerous organs.

This also affects the heart itself, so that hypoxia of the myocytes occurs as a result of the reduced perfusion. This can disrupt cell integrity and is discussed as the cause of the **arrhythmias** that occur. These regularly occur as ventricular premature complexes and ventricular tachycardia (Miller et al. 2000).

Another factor that affects cardiac function in dogs with gastric torsion is myocardial depressant factor (MDF). This is released when pancreatic perfusion is reduced and leads to decreased contractility of the cardiac muscle cells (Greene et al. 1977).

The situation of cardiac and systemic underperfusion is aggravated by compensatory mechanisms. Both the reduced perfusion and the release of MDFs lead to vasoconstriction via the renin-angiotensin-aldosterone system (RAAS), resulting in an increased oxygen demand of the myocardial cells.

At the same time, gastric dilatation causes **dyspnoea** due to a diaphragmatic elevation and consequently reduces the lung breathing volume. Alveolar gas exchange is reduced. Hypoxia and hypercapnia are the result. As a compensatory mechanism, the organism tries to improve lung ventilation by means of increased ventilation pressure, but this is accompanied by increased lung resistance, which increases the right cardiac load.

The reduced organ perfusion causes a reduction in glomerular filtration in the kidneys, leading to **pre-renal renal failure**. Hypoxia also damages the oxygen-sensitive tubular cells, limiting renal tubular function.

An increase in **liver enzymes**, ALT, AST and GLDH, as cytosolic and mitochondrial enzymes, is the consequence of liver congestion due to a reduction in caval reflux or the consequence of reduced arterial perfusion of the liver as a result of hypovolaemic shock. Both lead to hypoxia, which in turn disturbs cellular energy production, thus affecting transport processes at the cell membrane, which loses its integrity and leads to the release of cytosolic enzymes. In the liver, the pericentral hepatocytes in particular, which are sensitive to hypoxia, react.

The impaired perfusion of the intestine leads to alterations of the mucosal barrier resulting in translocation of bacteria to mesenteric lymph nodes, liver and spleen. The translocation activates proinflammatory cytokines (IL-1, IL-6 and IL-8, TNF-α). The consequence can be sepsis. This can also develop into **septic shock**. The development of sepsis is also possible if a gastric rupture with subsequent peritonitis develops as a result of the gastric wall necrosis. However, this rarely occurs.

Numerous causalities of gastric torsion lead to a loss of factors of the coagulation and fibrinolytic system. These include cell necrosis, reperfusion and sepsis. The consequence is **DIC** with prolonged coagulation (PT, apTT) and thrombocytopenia. DIC in turn can lead to thrombosis of vessels resulting in ischaemia, hypoxia and cell necrosis.

Gastric torsion can affect the **acid-base balance** in different ways. The consequence of ischaemia in the stomach wall is a cellular change from aerobic to anaerobic glycolysis with increased lactate formation. This can lead to metabolic acidosis. However, metabolic alkalosis is also possible through the sequestration of gastric acid, or if the animals can still vomit, through the loss of gastric acid. This in turn can lead to hypokalaemia.

Another pathophysiologic consequence also arises after gastric decompression and retorsion have occurred. Here, there is a risk of cell damage due to the reversal of ischaemia to reperfusion.

The cellular consequence of ischaemia is a change in energy production from aerobic to anaerobic glycolysis, which on the one hand reduces ATP formation and on the other develops an intracellular acidosis. The consequence is intracellular water accumulation, with destruction of cell organelles and later followed by cell death.

The reduction of ATP is accompanied by a conversion via AMP to hypoxanthine. In the case of reperfusion, the increasing oxygen concentration converts hypoxanthine to xanthine by means of xanthine oxidase. Uric acid and superoxide are formed from xanthine. The consequence of the increased superoxide formation is an increase in free radicals, which in turn can destroy the cells through lipid peroxidation (Figure 38.4.2).

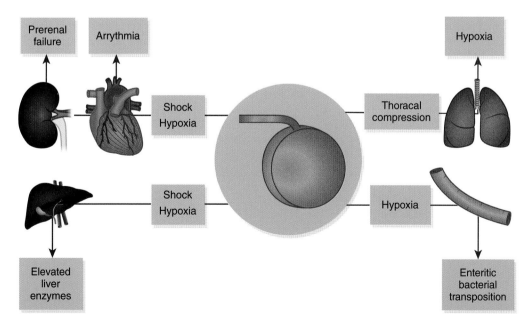

Figure 38.4.2 Pathophysiologic consequences of gastric torsion.

Therapy

Symptom	Therapy
Dilation and torsion	Decompression, surgery
Shock	Infusion
DIC	Heparin
Heart arrhythmia	Antiarrhythmic therapy (e.g. Lidocaine)
Bacterial translocation	Antibiotics

References

Brockman, D.J., Washabau, R.J., and Drobatz, K.J. (1995). Canine gastric dilatation/volvulus syndrome in a veterinary critical care unit: 295 cases (1986–1992). *Journal of the American Veterinary Medical Association* 207 (4): 460–464.

Greene, L.J., Shapanka, R., Glenn, T.M., and Lefer, A.M. (1977). Isolation of myocardial depressant factor from plasma of dogs in hemorrhagic shock. *Biochimica et Biophysica Acta* 491 (1): 275–285. https://doi.org/10.1016/0005-2795(77)90063-0.

Harkey, M.A., Villagran, A.M., Venkataraman, G.M. et al. (2017). Associations between gastric dilatation-volvulus in Great Danes and specific alleles of the canine immune-system genes DLA88, DRB1, and TLR5. *American Journal of Veterinary Research* 78 (8): 934–945. https://doi.org/10.2460/ajvr.78.8.934.

Hullar, M.A.J., Lampe, J.W., Torok-Storb, B.J., and Harkey, M.A. (2018). The canine gut microbiome is associated with higher risk of gastric dilatation-volvulus and high risk genetic variants of the immune system. *PLoS One* 13 (6): e0197686. https://doi.org/10.1371/journal.pone.0197686.

Miller, T.L., Schwartz, D.S., Nakayama, T., and Hamlin, R.L. (2000). Effects of acute gastric distention and recovery on tendency for ventricular arrhythmia in dogs. *Journal of Veterinary Internal Medicine* 14 (4): 436–444. https://doi.org/10.1892/0891-6640(2000)014<0436:eoagda>2.3.co;2.

Further Reading

Gazzola, K.M. and Nelson, L.L. (2014). The relationship between gastrointestinal motility and gastric dilatation-volvulus in dogs. *Topics in Companion Animal Medicine* 29 (3): 64–66. https://doi.org/10.1053/j.tcam.2014.09.006.

Glickman, L.T., Glickman, N.W., Schellenberg, D.B. et al. (2000). Incidence of and breed-related risk factors for gastric dilatation-volvulus in dogs. *Journal of the American Veterinary Medical Association* 216 (1): 40–45. https://doi.org/10.2460/javma.2000.216.40.

Peycke, L.E., Hosgood, G., Davidson, J.R. et al. (2005). The effect of experimental gastric dilatation-volvulus on adenosine triphosphate content and conductance of the canine gastric and jejunal mucosa. *Canadian Journal of Veterinary Research = Revue canadienne de recherche veterinaire* 69 (3): 170–179.

Sharp, C.R. and Rozanski, E.A. (2014). Cardiovascular and systemic effects of gastric dilatation and volvulus in dogs. *Topics in Companion Animal Medicine* 29 (3): 67–70. https://doi.org/10.1053/j.tcam.2014.09.007.

Song, K.K., Goldsmid, S.E., Lee, J., and Simpson, D.J. (2020). Retrospective analysis of 736 cases of canine gastric dilatation volvulus. *Australian Veterinary Journal* 98 (6): 232–238. https://doi.org/10.1111/avj.12942.

38.5

Enteritis/Inflammatory Bowel Disease

Definition

Enteritis is an inflammation of the intestine; usually of the small intestine. It can take acute and chronic forms. The chronic inflammatory bowel disease (IBD) is a form of chronic intestinal wall inflammation.

Aetiology

The causes can be divided into local and systemic factors. In the local forms, feed intolerances or allergies are more common than infections. As systemic diseases, kidney and pancreas diseases can lead to secondary intestinal inflammation. Enteritis occurs equally in dogs and cats.

Food	Infection	Inflammation	Systemic
Intolerance (D/C)	Viral infection	Inflammatory bowel disease (D,C)	Pancreatitis (D,C)
Allergy (D/C)	Parvovirus (D)	Haemorrhagic gastroenteritis (D)	Pancreas insufficiency (D)
	Corona virus (D,C)		Kidney failure (D,C)
	FIV (C)		
	FeLv (C)		
	Bacterial infection		
	Campylobacter (D)		
	Salmonella (D)		
	Clostridia (D)		
	Yersinia (D)		
	Parasites		
	Giardia (D,C)		
	Trichomonas (C)		
	Worms (e.g. hookworm, tapeworm) (D/C)		

D – Dog, C – Cat

Pathogenesis

The different causalities influence intestinal function through various mechanisms. In principle, influences on mucosal permeability, secretion and motility can arise.

Textbook of Small Animal Pathophysiology, First Edition. Stephan Neumann.
© 2025 John Wiley & Sons Ltd. Published 2025 by John Wiley & Sons Ltd.

The transport of nutrients and water takes place via the enterocytes. Water, in particular, is absorbed from the intestinal lumen in cotransport with sodium. Permeability can change due to different causalities; it can decrease or increase. A decrease in permeability occurs when the carrier systems fail due to pathological changes in the enterocytes (e.g. swelling) or when the resorption surface is reduced due to a reduction of the brush border or the villi. The consequence is reduced fluid absorption from the intestine. This leads to a negative fluid balance and water remaining in the intestinal lumen can change the ingesta consistency and cause diarrhoea.

Increased permeability increases the permeability towards the intestinal lumen, for example, when the tight-junctions become permeable to sodium ions, which are transported intestinally and can carry water in the cotransport. At the same time, when the tight-junctions are disrupted, higher molecular weight molecules are also lost from the propria, creating an osmotic gradient towards the lumen. In extreme cases, this process can lead to protein loss into the intestine, which is the hallmark of 'protein-losing enteropathy'.

In addition to the change in permeability, increased secretions can occur in intestinal diseases. Secretory epithelial cells are mostly located in the crypts. Under the influence of mostly bacterial endotoxins, increased cAMP is formed in the enterocytes. This causes an opening of the luminal chloride channels and thus a luminal chloride secretion. To maintain electroneutrality, chloride is transported basally at the enterocytes in symport with sodium. The increased chloride secretion also leads to increased sodium secretion, which takes water with it in the cotransport, resulting in a significant shift of water into the intestinal lumen (Figure 38.5.1).

Many intestinal inflammations are associated with changes in intestinal motility. Intestinal movements originate from smooth muscle cells in the tunica muscularis. These are subject to the control of the enteric nervous system, which acts independently of the central nervous system. An important neurotransmitter is serotonin, which is localised in high concentrations in the intestinal wall, especially in enterochromaffin cells of the crypts. Under the influence of, for example, bacterial toxins, a Ca-influx into the enterochromaffin cells can occur. This increases its intracellular concentration, which increases serotonin secretion and contracts the smooth muscle cells (Guttman and Finlay 2008).

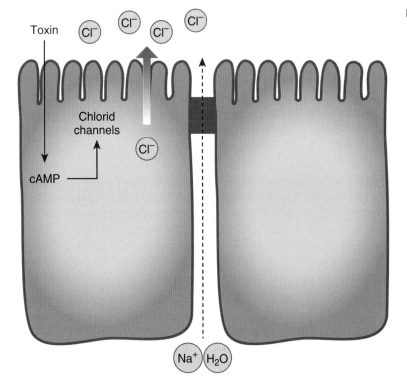

Figure 38.5.1 Mechanism of secretory diarrhoea.

In addition, motility changes are seen as a protective mechanism of the body to eliminate the 'damaging causalities' by shortening the transit time. In any case, increased motility is the functional consequence. This reduces the residence time of the ingesta, which leads to malabsorption and at the same time keeps osmotically active molecules in the intestine.

The causalities described cause the clinical picture of enteropathy via the mechanisms described. The term is more appropriate than that of enteritis, as not all processes are inflammatory.

Inflammatory bowel disease is a common chronic bowel disease. This is an inflammatory process in the intestinal wall. The cause and pathogenesis of the disease are not fully understood. Histologically, the disease ends with a diffuse inflammation in the intestinal wall. Infiltrates of different inflammatory cells, mostly lymphocytes and plasma cells, can be found in different layers of the intestinal wall, mostly in the submucosa. According to current findings, the pathogenesis is composed of genetic variations of the sessile immune cells and an altered immune response to different triggers as a result.

Physiologically, the immune system distinguishes between pathogenic and non-pathogenic commensals in the intestinal wall. When pathogens come into contact with antigen-presenting cells in the intestinal wall, the antigen is presented to naïve T cells. These proliferate into different T cells depending on the antigen. Parasites induce a proliferation of Th2 cells, while viruses induce a Th1 cell response and bacteria induce a Th17 cell response. The proliferated T cells induce the further immune response by which the pathogenic agent is eliminated. In contrast, commensals do not induce a corresponding immune response.

In the case of IBD, an altered immune response develops. One hypothesis is based on mutations of the surface receptors of the antigen-presenting cells. In such a case, contact with a non-pathogenic commensal would also trigger an immune response. After antigen presentation, Th17 cells would proliferate from naïve T cells in such a case, which would then lead to an inflammatory response.

The process is maintained by an inflammatory response that is sustained by numerous cytokines (Table 38.5.1).

The mechanism by which IBD leads to the main symptom of diarrhoea involves several of the primary diarrhoeal causalities. These include increased secretion, decreased absorption, increased permeability and increased motility. Mediated by proinflammatory cytokines, the inflammatory response leads to swelling of enterocytes, reducing their absorption properties. Furthermore, the inflammatory response leads to an intracellular increase in second messengers, cAMP and Ca^{2+}. These messengers activate Cl channels, leading to hypersecretion. Due to alterations of the cytoskeleton, intercellular tight-junctions are lost and paracellular permeability is increased (Michelangeli and Ruiz 2003) (Figure 38.5.2).

Table 38.5.1 Cytokines, with their respective changes in IBD.

Cytokines	Increased	Decreased	Unchanged
IL-1	X		
INF-γ	X		
IL-2			X
TNF	X		
IL-4			X
IL-5	X		
IL-6	X		
IL-7	X		
IL-8	X		
IL-9	X		
Il-10		X	

Source: Toutounji (2017).

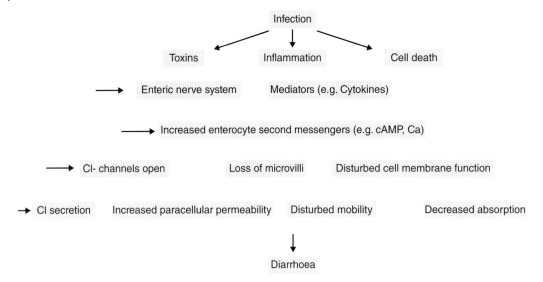

Figure 38.5.2 Molecular mechanisms of diarrhoea.

Diagnostics

Clinical signs	Clinical pathology	Imaging	Histopathology	Microbiology
Vomiting Diarrhoea	Non-specific	**Endoscopy** Taking biopsies	For diagnosis of IBD	Pathogenic agents if applicable Microbiome

Pathophysiologic Consequences

The main consequence of bowel diseases is diarrhoea. As a result, weight loss develops due to reduced absorption and loss of nutrients.

Influenced organ systems	Clinical symptoms	Clinical pathological alterations
Gastrointestinal System Systemic	Diarrhoea Weight loss Dehydration	Hypoalbuminaemia

Especially in the acute stage of the disease, water loss occurs. The disruption of tight-junctions allows interstitial fluid to escape into the intestinal lumen. In addition, various aquaporins are involved in water reabsorption from the intestine. Their number is reduced in bowel diseases, resulting in a reduction of water reabsorption (Guttman and Finlay 2008).

Water loss can be isotonic or hypotonic. In isotonic water loss, interstitial fluid is lost, with little change in plasma osmolarity and no osmotic gradient. In hypotonic water loss, hypertonic **dehydration develops**. This means that the plasma osmolarity increases, which leads to a water shift from the cells into the extracellular space.

Severe cases of diarrhoea with increased permeability are associated with a loss of protein, which can lead to hypoalbuminaemia due to protein-losing enteropathy. This mechanism is described in Chapter 38.6 (Figure 38.5.3).

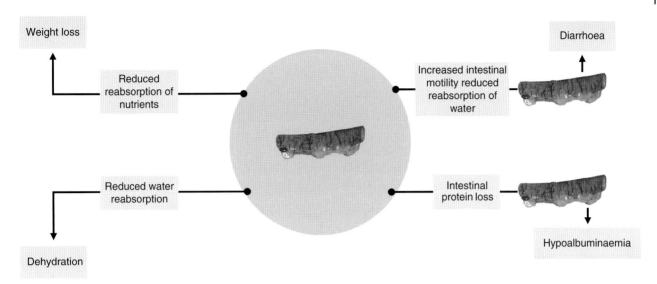

Figure 38.5.3 Pathophysiologic consequences of IBD.

Therapy

Symptom	Therapy
Food intolerance	Diet
Diarrhoea	Spasmolytics (e.g. Metamizole, Butylscopolamine bromide)
Dehydration	Infusion
Pathogenic bacterial infection	Antibiotics

References

Guttman, J.A. and Finlay, B.B. (2008). Subcellular alterations that lead to diarrhea during bacterial pathogenesis. *Trends in Microbiology* 16 (11): 535–542. https://doi.org/10.1016/j.tim.2008.08.004.

Michelangeli, F. and Ruiz, M. (2003). I, 2. Physiology and pathophysiology of the gut in relation to viral diarrhea. *Perspectives in Medical Virology* 9: 23–50. https://doi.org/10.1016/S0168-7069(03)09003-7.

Toutounji, M. (2017). Mimicking the pathogenesis of inflammatory bowel disease in an intestinal cell model: Role of ER stress and RhoA signalling in intestinal barrier dysfunction. Diss Hanover.

Further Reading

Allenspach, K. (2013). Diagnosis of small intestinal disorders in dogs and cats. *The Veterinary Clinics of North America. Small Animal Practice* 43 (6): 1227. v. https://doi.org/10.1016/j.cvsm.2013.07.001.

Dunowska, M. (2017). What is causing acute haemorrhagic diarrhoea syndrome in dogs? *The Veterinary Record* 180 (22): 539–541. https://doi.org/10.1136/vr.j2609.

Jergens, A.E. (1999). Inflammatory bowel disease. Current perspectives. *The Veterinary Clinics of North America. Small Animal Practice* 29 (2): 501–521.

Jergens, A.E. (2002). Feline inflammatory bowel disease--current perspectives on etiopathogenesis and therapy. *Journal of Feline Medicine and Surgery* 4 (3): 175–178. https://doi.org/10.1053/jfms.2002.0179.

Mandigers, P. and German, A.J. (2010). Dietary hypersensitivity in cats and dogs. *Tijdschrift voor Diergeneeskunde* 135 (19): 706–710.

Marks, S.L., Rankin, S.C., Byrne, B.A., and Weese, J.S. (2011). Enteropathogenic bacteria in dogs and cats: diagnosis, epidemiology, treatment, and control. *Journal of Veterinary Internal Medicine* 25 (6): 1195–1208. https://doi.org/ 10.1111/j.1939-1676.2011.00821.x.

Parrish, C.R. (1995). Pathogenesis of feline panleukopenia virus and canine parvovirus. *Bailliere's Clinical Haematology* 8 (1): 57–71. https://doi.org/10.1016/s0950-3536(05)80232-x.

Unterer, S. and Busch, K. (2021). Acute hemorrhagic diarrhea syndrome in dogs. *The Veterinary Clinics of North America. Small Animal Practice* 51 (1): 79–92. https://doi.org/10.1016/j.cvsm.2020.09.007.

Weese, J.S. (2011). Bacterial enteritis in dogs and cats: diagnosis, therapy, and zoonotic potential. *The Veterinary Clinics of North America. Small Animal Practice* 41 (2): 287–309. https://doi.org/10.1016/j.cvsm.2010.12.005.

38.6

Intestinal Lymphangiectasias

Definition

Intestinal lymphangiectasias are defined as dilation or rupture of lymphatic vessels in the intestinal wall. They occur primarily and secondarily. They induce protein-losing enteropathy.

Aetiology

The primary form is described as congenital lymphangiectasia, which occurs more frequently in certain dog breeds, such as Yorkshire terriers, and suggests a genetic cause. Secondary forms are caused by right heart disease or neoplastic alterations of the lymphatic ducts, as in lymphoma or mediastinal tumours. The disease complex is predominantly described in dogs.

Primary	Secondary
Congenital (D)	Right-sided-heart disease (D)
(Yorkshire Terrier, Basenji, Lundehund, Maltese)	Lymphoma (D/C)
	Mediastinal mass (D/C)

D-dog C-cat

Pathogenesis

First, the physiology of the lymphatic system will be explained.

The enteric lymphatic system is an important transport system for absorbed fats and fat-soluble molecules, such as vitamins A, D and E. The lymphatic capillaries of the system are part of the vascularisation of the villi and are surrounded by an arterio-venous plexus. In the submucosa, the lymphatic capillaries of several villi join and then run via tunica muscularis and serosa in the serous membranes of the mesentery to finally reach the venous blood system in front of the right atrium via the thoracic duct.

The flow of lymph fluid within the lymphatic system is maintained by different forces. Intrinsic contraction and smooth muscle cells along the lymphatic vessels maintain lymph flow; in addition, valves in the lymphatic ducts prevent lymph backflow. Finally, in the larger lymphatic vessels, lymph flow is influenced by movement of the diaphragm and variations in central venous pressure (Ohtani 1987; Bernier-Latmani et al. 2015).

Factors influencing lymph flow are vasoactive substances that can have a positive or negative influence. Cholecystokinin, glucagon, serotonin and bradykinin have a positive effect on lymph flow. The lymph flow is negatively influenced by nitric oxide (NO), prostaglandins and ADH.

In addition to transporting lipids absorbed in the intestine, the intestinal lymphatic system drains the extracellular intestinal fluid and is involved in the local defence of the intestine (Figure 38.6.1).

Textbook of Small Animal Pathophysiology, First Edition. Stephan Neumann.
© 2025 John Wiley & Sons Ltd. Published 2025 by John Wiley & Sons Ltd.

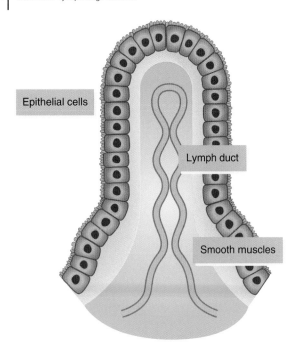

Figure 38.6.1 Structure of the intestinal lymphatic system.

Epithelial cells

Lymph duct

Smooth muscles

The absorption of lipids begins with the formation of micelles. These are formed when fats are cleaved by pancreatic lipase in the presence of emulsifying bile salts. Fatty acids and monoglycerides subsequently bind to binding proteins of the enterocyte membrane and, after endocytosis in the smooth endoplasmic reticulum, are combined with apoproteins to form chylomicrons. These reach the basolateral enterocyte membrane via Golgi apparatus. There, the chylomicron membrane fuses with the cell membrane and the chylomicrons are released. After absorption from the lymphatic capillaries, the fats are distributed systemically. The absorption of cholesterol also occurs after intestinal micelle formation by bile salts. A transmembrane carrier in the enterocyte membrane enables the influx of cholesterol into the enterocyte, where cholesterol is esterified by an acyltransferase and combined with apoproteins in the smooth endoplasmic reticulum to form a chylomicron. This is transported via the Golgi apparatus to the basolateral enterocyte membrane, where it passes out of the cell into the interstitium by exocytosis. The uptake of the chylomicrons by the lymph capillaries takes place paracellularly through a change in lymphatic vessel permeability. This is probably controlled by VEGF-A, which binds to a semaphorin receptor of the lymphatic capillary endothelial cells. Intracellular signal transduction controlled by a tyrosine kinase leads to a conformational change of the intercellular tight-junction, allowing the uptake of the chylomicrons (Soker et al. 1998; Becker et al. 2005).

The chemical composition of the lymph fluid in comparison to the serum shows that the former can be clearly variable depending on the food intake. Overall, however, the composition is comparable, although proteins are present in lymph fluid in somewhat lower concentrations than in serum (2.0–4.0 g/dl versus 5.5–7.5 g/dl). The opposite is true for fats, especially in the postprandial phase. Cellularly, a high number of lymphocytes are present in the lymph fluid (Friedel et al. 1976).

In addition to congenital causes of lymphangiectasia, secondary causes of intestinal lymphangiectasia are processes that increase central venous pressure. These include diseases of the right side of the heart and space-occupying processes in the thorax. These lead to lymphatic congestion in the thoracic duct, which continues into the periphery and into the intestinal lymphatic vessels. If the pressure increases, the vessels dilate and rupture and lymph fluid leaks into the intestinal lumen.

Another cause for the development of intestinal lymphangiectasia is chronic inflammatory reactions in the intestinal wall. Tumorous diseases, such as intestinal lymphoma or adenocarcinomas of the intestinal wall can also lead to increased pressure in the lymph duct system, the consequence of which is ultimately the rupture of the lymph capillaries and vessels (Figure 38.6.2).

Figure 38.6.2 Morphological changes in lymphangiectasia.

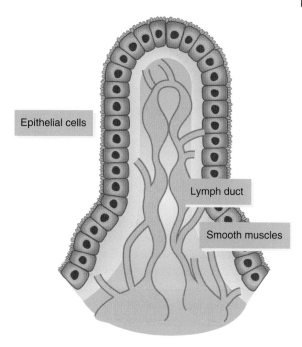

Epithelial cells

Lymph duct

Smooth muscles

Diagnostics

Clinical signs	Clinical pathology	Imaging	Histopathology	Microbiology
Diarrhoea	Hypoproteinaemia Hypocholesterolaemia	Endoscopy/laparotomy Taking a biopsy	Histopathology	Not necessary

Pathophysiologic Consequences

The pathophysiologic consequences primarily affect the gastrointestinal tract. However, increased protein loss also leads to systemic changes.

Influenced organ systems	Clinical symptoms	Clinical pathological alterations
Gastrointestinal system	Diarrhoea	Lymphopenia
Systemic	Ascites	Hypocholesterolaemia
	Oedema	Hypotriglyceridaemia
	Dyspnoea	Hypoproteinaemia

Rupture of the lymphatic vessels and intestinal lymphoedema can cause lymphatic fluid to enter the intestinal lumen. This is rich in osmotically active molecules, such as proteins. This increases the osmotic gradient between the interstitium of the intestinal wall and the intestinal lumen. This is followed by an efflux of water into the intestinal lumen. This also takes place to some extent during physiological digestion. There, after the breakdown of the food components with the formation of osmotically active molecules, an osmotic gradient initially develops in the direction of the intestinal lumen. Only when the osmotically active molecules are absorbed does the gradient reverse.

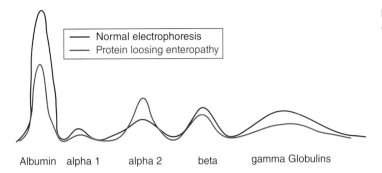

Figure 38.6.3 Protein electrophoresis in protein-losing enteropathy.

In the case of lymphangiectasia, due to lymph leakage into the intestinal lumen, the osmotic gradient towards the intestinal lumen remains high, which binds water in the intestine and leads to **diarrhoea.**

The loss of lymph into the intestinal lumen also results in the loss of components of the lymph, such as lymphocytes and fats. This leads to **lymphopenia** and **hypocholesterolaemia** or **hypotriglyceridaemia**.

The loss of protein leads to **hypoproteinaemia**. This usually leads to a decrease in serum albumin and serum gamma globulins, but an increase in serum α-2 macroglobulins, such as ceruloplasmin and haptoglobin (Figure 38.6.3).

The consequence of reduced albumin concentration affects all functions of albumin (Table 38.6.1).

Albumin is a transporter for numerous hydrophobic molecules. These are bound to albumin and transported in this way in the blood. The same applies to ions, which are also bound to albumin. Due to its ampholytic properties, albumin can bind and release protons, which also results in its buffering property.

By binding water, albumin prevents it from leaving the blood vessels.

A major clinical consequence of hypoalbuminaemia in protein-losing enteropathy is the reduction of oncotic pressure and the formation of **oedema** or **effusions** in the form of transudates in the body cavities.

The loss of water from the vascular system has a negative effect on blood pressure, which drops. As a result, ADH is increasingly released from the pituitary gland and increases renal water reabsorption through increased synthesis of aquaporins in the distal tubule and the collecting tube. At the same time, the activation of the RAAS attempts to stabilise blood pressure. This leads to aldosterone release from the adrenal cortex. This causes sodium reabsorption in the distal tubule and water in the cotransport to stabilise blood volume and blood pressure. The consequence of 'hyperaldosteronism' is a loss of potassium and alkalosis.

Another consequence of protein-losing enteropathy is the loss of antithrombin (Goodwin et al. 2011; Nagahara et al. 2021).

Antithrombin is a glycoprotein that is produced in the liver. It consists of 432 amino acids and has a molecular weight of 58 kDa, which is comparable to the number of amino acids and the molecular weight of albumin (584 amino acids and 66 kDa). For this reason, many albumin-loss diseases are accompanied by a simultaneous loss of antithrombin.

The functions of antithrombin are to inhibit the clotting factors thrombin, factor IXa, Xa, XIa, XIIa. This makes it an effective inhibitor of blood clotting. A deficiency of antithrombin increases the clotting tendency of the blood and leads to the formation of thrombi.

If thrombi move, an embolism develops. Emboli aggregate especially in organs with many vessels, such as the lungs, kidneys, heart or liver. There, an activation of the intrinsic coagulation system initiated by the embolus develops, whereby the embolus becomes a thrombus. In the lungs, the consequence of the emboli is a reduction in pulmonary

Table 38.6.1 Functions of albumin.

Function	Target molecules
Transport protein	Unconjugated bilirubin, fatty acids, hormones, vitamins, cations (Ca, Mg, Cu, Zn)
Colloid osmotic pressure	
Buffer	

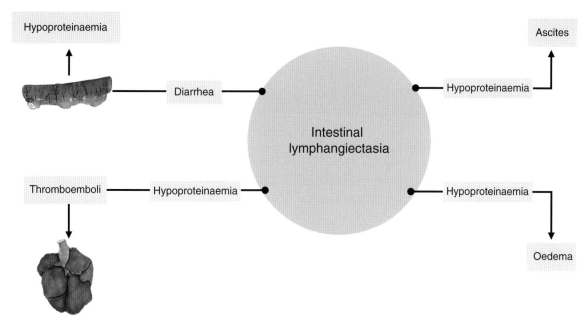

Figure 38.6.4 Pathophysiologic consequences of lymphangiectasia.

blood flow, which leads to a reduction in the lung parenchyma for gas exchange. The consequence can be arterial hypoxia. This in turn activates the respiratory centre via chemoreceptors with the consequence of tachypnoea. A possibly associated pleuritis due to the lung parenchymal changes leads to painful breathing movements and thus to **dyspnoea**. At the same time, pulmonary hypertension and right heart strain develops as pulmonary resistance increases due to the emboli (Figure 38.6.4).

Therapy

Symptom	Therapy
Protein loss	Diet
Hypercoagulability	Antiplatelet drugs (e.g. Clopidogrel)
Ascites severe	Diuretics (e.g. Furosemide)

References

Becker, P.M., Waltenberger, J., Yachechko, R. et al. (2005). Neuropilin-1 regulates vascular endothelial growth factor-mediated endothelial permeability. *Circulation Research* 96 (12): 1257–1265. https://doi.org/10.1161/01.RES.0000171756.13554.49.

Bernier-Latmani, J., Cisarovsky, C., Demir, C.S. et al. (2015). DLL4 promotes continuous adult intestinal lacteal regeneration and dietary fat transport. *The Journal of Clinical Investigation* 125 (12): 4572–4586. https://doi.org/10.1172/JCI82045.

Friedel, R., Bode, R., Trautschold, I., and Mattenheimer, H. (1976). Cell enzymes in lymph. Distribution and transport of cell enzymes within the extracellular space. *Journal of Clinical Chemistry and Clinical Biochemistry* 14 (3): 119–128.

Goodwin, L.V., Goggs, R., Chan, D.L., and Allenspach, K. (2011). Hypercoagulability in dogs with protein-losing enteropathy. *Journal of Veterinary Internal Medicine* 25 (2): 273–277. https://doi.org/10.1111/j.1939-1676.2011.0683.x.

Nagahara, T., Ohno, K., Nagao, I. et al. (2021). Changes in the coagulation parameters in dogs with protein-losing enteropathy between before and after treatment. *The Journal of Veterinary Medical Science* 83 (8): 1295–1302. https://doi.org/10.1292/jvms.21-0137.

Ohtani, O. (1987). Three-dimensional organization of lymphatics and its relationship to blood vessels in rat small intestine. *Cell and Tissue Research* 248 (2): 365–374. https://doi.org/10.1007/BF00218204.

Soker, S., Takashima, S., Miao, H.Q. et al. (1998). Neuropilin-1 is expressed by endothelial and tumor cells as an isoform-specific receptor for vascular endothelial growth factor. *Cell* 92 (6): 735–745. https://doi.org/10.1016/s0092-8674(00)81402-6.

Further Reading

Cifarelli, V. and Eichmann, A. (2019). The intestinal lymphatic system: functions and metabolic implications. *Cellular and Molecular Gastroenterology and Hepatology* 7 (3): 503–513. https://doi.org/10.1016/j.jcmgh.2018.12.002.

Craven, M.D. and Washabau, R.J. (2019). Comparative pathophysiology and management of protein-losing enteropathy. *Journal of Veterinary Internal Medicine* 33 (2): 383–402. https://doi.org/10.1111/jvim.15406.

Kull, P.A., Hess, R.S., Craig, L.E. et al. (2001). Clinical, clinicopathologic, radiographic, and ultrasonographic characteristics of intestinal lymphangiectasia in dogs: 17 cases (1996-1998). *Journal of the American Veterinary Medical Association* 219 (2): 197–202. https://doi.org/10.2460/javma.2001.219.197.

Okanishi, H., Yoshioka, R., Kagawa, Y., and Watari, T. (2014). The clinical efficacy of dietary fat restriction in treatment of dogs with intestinal lymphangiectasia. *Journal of Veterinary Internal Medicine* 28 (3): 809–817. https://doi.org/10.1111/jvim.12327.

38.7

Intestinal Obstruction

Definition

Intestinal obstruction is a partial or complete displacement of the intestinal lumen.

Aetiology

The causes can be divided into mechanical and functional forms. Intestinal obstruction occurs equally in dogs and cats.

Mechanical	Functional
Foreign bodies (D,C)	Hypomobility (D/C)
Neoplasia (D,C)	
Volvulus (D/C)	
Intussusception (D/C)	
Herniation (D/C)	

D – Dog, C – Cat

Pathogenesis

The mechanical causes can be divided into intestine-associated causes or foreign bodies. The latter are usually materials ingested with food that are not digested. During the intestinal passage, these can partially or completely obstruct the intestinal lumen and thus lead to an obstruction. Localisations for obstruction are natural constrictions in the course of the intestine, such as the area of the ileocaecal valve. Another location is the jejunum. This section of the intestine is particularly long and foreign bodies are initially transported by peristalsis. However, in the course of the jejunum, peristalsis can become insufficient because the contraction of the smooth muscle fibres is not sufficient to transport the foreign body. The consequence of the obstruction is first a spasm of the intestinal wall caused by the smooth muscle. This is followed by ischaemia of the intestinal wall at the obstruction, as well as pre-obstructive intestinal dilatation. This further complicates the transporting peristalsis. The ischaemia causes hypoxia of the intestinal wall. This leads to necrosis and eventually to rupture of the intestinal wall with translocation of intestinal bacteria into the peritoneal cavity. This leads to septic peritonitis.

In the section of the intestine before the obstruction, stasis of the ingesta leads to dilatation of the intestine. This causes an altered absorption of nutrients. The dilation reduces the contact between the ingesta and the mucosa, and accordingly, degradation and absorption processes are not completed. Osmotically active ingesta remains in the intestinal lumen and promotes secretion of water into the intestinal lumen, which worsens the process.

Textbook of Small Animal Pathophysiology, First Edition. Stephan Neumann.
© 2025 John Wiley & Sons Ltd. Published 2025 by John Wiley & Sons Ltd.

Table 38.7.1 Intestine-associated tumours in dogs and cats.

Organ	Adenocarcinoma	Leiomyosarcoma	Leiomyoma	Lymphoma
Stomach	+++	+	+	−
Small intestine	++	+	+	++
Colon	+	+	+	+

Intestine-associated causes of intestinal obstruction are dislocations of intestinal segments. These can push into each other, in which case there is intussusception, or they turn around the mesenteric blood supply (ileus). Both forms of intestinal dislocation are seen in the context of altered intestinal motility. For example, a partially increased intestinal motility, e.g. as a result of inflammation, can push the hypermotile intestine into the adjacent intestinal segment. The consequence of the dislocations is based on ischaemia and hypoxia of the affected intestinal segments. The resulting necrosis of the intestinal wall allows bacteria to dislocate and leads to septic peritonitis. Due to the good intestinal perfusion, inflammatory mediators and proinflammatory cytokines formed in the ischaemic-necrotic area can enter the systemic circulation and induce a systemic shock reaction.

Bowel-associated tumours are mostly adenocarcinomas or lymphomas. These can cause partial or complete intestinal obstruction. In addition, tumours damage the organism by metastasising. This takes place in the regional lymph nodes, in the liver or rarely in the lungs (Table 38.7.1).

Diagnostics

Clinical signs	Clinical pathology	Imaging	Histopathology	Microbiology
Vomiting	Non-specific	**Ultrasonography**/radiology (contrast)/laparotomy	Histopathology in cases of neoplasia	Not necessary

Pathophysiologic Consequences

The consequences of intestinal wall obstruction are based, on the one hand, on the altered absorption and, on the other hand, on the consequences of intestinal wall necrosis. They depend on the localisation and extent of the obstruction.

Symptom	Complete obstruction prox. small intestine	Complete obstruction dist. small intestine	Partial obstruction
Beginning	<24h	>24h	>24h
Vomiting	Yes, often	Yes, less often	Rare
Anorexia	Yes	Variable	Variable
Dehydration	Yes, hgr.	Yes, mgr.	Variable
Lethargy	Yes, hgr.	Yes, hgr.	Yes, mgr.
Shock	Yes	Variable	Rare
Abdominal pain	Yes, hgr.	Variable	Variable, mgr.

hgr = high grade; mgr = medium grade

Clinical pathological alterations
Haemoconcentration
Azotaemia
Hyponatraemia
Hypokalaemia

The systemic consequences of intestinal obstruction result from the alterations of the intestinal wall with necrosis and the disturbed intestinal function. In the pre-obstructive intestinal segment, intestinal dilatation develops. This is increased by fermentation processes of the bacterial intestinal flora and possibly aerophagy. The dilatation of the intestinal wall causes **abdominal pain** and **anorexia** via irritation of the autonomic nervous system and nerve receptors in the peritoneum. In addition, an osmotic gradient between the intestinal lumen and the intestinal wall develops pre-obstructive, since osmotically active molecules remain in the lumen due to the impaired resorption in the dilated intestine. The result is water influx into the intestinal lumen. This aggravates the process of dilatation and also leads to dehydration. **Dehydration**, in turn, can lead to hypovolaemia. This activates the ADH-RAAS to compensate for hypovolaemia and reduced blood pressure. If the compensation is insufficient, pre-renal renal failure with **azotaemia** can occur. In the further course, there is also hypovolaemic **shock**. The latter can also lead to septic shock due to bacterial translocation in the obstructive region as a result of intestinal wall necrosis and the associated systemic inflammation. The bacterial translocation already takes place before the actual intestinal wall necrosis. In addition to the mucus layer on the mucosa and the secretion of antibacterially active substances, the integrity of the enterocytes and their anchoring in the cell network primarily prevent the translocation of bacteria from the intestine. In the case of obstruction, an obstruction of the blood vessels and a local inflammatory process develops. Under the influence of vasoactive mediators in the area of inflammation, oedema develops in the intestinal wall. This disrupts the function of the intestinal wall cells, which can impair mucus secretion and anchorage of the enterocytes. Both facilitate bacterial translocation even before manifest necrosis develops.

Vomiting occurs in intestinal obstruction due to stasis of the ingesta and its distance from the stomach. If gastric emptying is impeded, the stomach and intestinal wall dilate. Irritation of the parasympathetic nervous system can induce vomiting. Bacterial overgrowth or translocation can also have a direct effect on the vomiting centre through bacterial toxin production.

The loss of protons through vomiting can trigger **metabolic alkalosis**. Alkalosis can temporarily reduce the oxygen release of haemoglobin. Furthermore, alkalosis increases the dissociation of proteins, with the consequence of increased calcium binding to the free proton valences of the proteins. This can result in a reduction of ionised calcium, which can lead to muscle weakness. Cardially, metabolic alkalosis can cause arrhythmias and reduced cardiac output, and neurologically, neuronal excitability can be affected by alkalosis.

Other effects of alkalosis are often caused by hypokalaemia. This can be made worse by vomiting, in addition to the loss of potassium, because in alkalosis, cells secrete protons in exchange for potassium ions to compensate for the alkalosis.

The consequence of **hypokalaemia** develops due to hypokalaemic hyperpolarisation of the cell membrane. This prolongs the action potential and the refractory phase. In the various organ systems, this produces weakness, paralysis or tetany in the muscles, cardiac arrhythmia and gastrointestinal ileus can develop due to impaired intestinal motility (Figure 38.7.1).

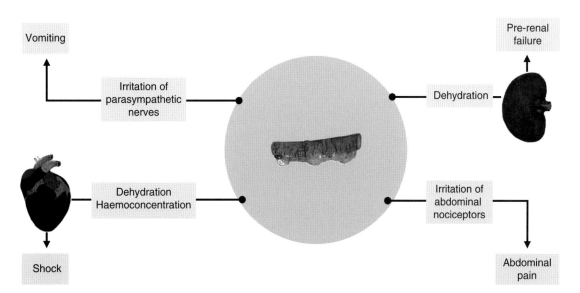

Figure 38.7.1 Pathophysiologic consequences of intestinal obstruction.

Vomiting can cause hypovolaemic **hyponatraemia**. In advanced cases (Na <135 mEq/l), this reduces plasma osmolality. This causes a water shift from extra- to intracellular. The result is cell swelling. In the brain, swelling of the nerve cells causes symptoms, such as nausea, lethargy and coma.

Therapy

Symptom	Therapy
Shock	Infusion
Acid-base balance	Buffering (e.g. Sodium bicarbonate)
Obstruction	Surgery

Further Reading

Bragg, D., El-Sharkawy, A.M., Psaltis, E. et al. (2015). Postoperative ileus: recent developments in pathophysiology and management. *Clinical Nutrition (Edinburgh, Scotland)* 34 (3): 367–376. https://doi.org/10.1016/j.clnu.2015.01.016.

Gieger, T. (2011). Alimentary lymphoma in cats and dogs. *The Veterinary Clinics of North America. Small Animal Practice* 41 (2): 419–432. https://doi.org/10.1016/j.cvsm.2011.02.001.

Hill, T.L. (2019). Gastrointestinal tract dysfunction with critical illness: clinical assessment and management. *Topics in Companion Animal Medicine* 35: 47–52. https://doi.org/10.1053/j.tcam.2019.04.002.

Willard, M.D. (2012). Alimentary neoplasia in geriatric dogs and cats. *The Veterinary Clinics of North America. Small Animal Practice* 42 (4): 693. vi. https://doi.org/10.1016/j.cvsm.2012.04.006.

Whitehead, K., Cortes, Y., and Eirmann, L. (2016). Gastrointestinal dysmotility disorders in critically ill dogs and cats. *Journal of Veterinary Emergency and Critical Care (San Antonio, Tex. 2001)* 26 (2): 234–253. https://doi.org/10.1111/vec.12449.

39

Hepatobiliary System

39.1

Physiological Functions and General Pathophysiology of Organ Insufficiency

Functions

The liver is at the centre of metabolism with anabolic and catabolic functions. It influences haemostasis, the synthesis of the body's own proteins and the storage of carbohydrates and fats. In addition, it is capable of detoxification by conjugation of lipophilic molecules and is an excretory organ through bile production. Liver function is influenced by the number of hepatocytes, the blood supply to the organ, its reserve capacity and regeneration capacity (Table 39.1.1).

The liver is composed of the hepatic parenchyma, consisting of hepatocytes, Kupffer's cells, Ito cells, Pit cells and vascular endothelia of the sinusoids, the bile duct tissue with the gallbladder, and the hepatic vascular system, consisting of arteries, portal veins and systemic veins. The largest part of the liver mass is made up of the parenchyma, whose smallest anatomical unit is the hepatic lobule (lobulus). This forms a polygonal body, at the corners of which vessels in the form of artery and portal vein as well as the bile duct are located and form the so-called 'Glisson's triangle'. In the centre of the liver lobule, as part of the systemic venous system, is the central vein. From the corners to the centre run the sinusoids, capillaries in which the exchange of substances with the hepatocytes takes place. Due to functionally different performances, the hepatocytes are divided into zones I–III along the sinusoid.

The sinusoids are large-lumen capillaries with a length of 350–500 μm and a variable diameter of 5–15 μm. Endothelial cells rest on a network of reticulin fibres of collagen type III, which have intercellular gaps of 0.1–0.5 μm as well as pores of 100 nm in their cytoplasm. A basement membrane is not formed. Between the endothelial cells, the Kupffer's stellate cells as well as the Ito cells of the sinusoid and the hepatocytes lies the space of Diss, in which the cell-free phase of the blood can come into direct contact with the apical membrane of the hepatocytes. This, together with the slow blood flow, due to the large diameter of the sinusoids, serves the optimal exchange of substances at the sinusoidal hepatocyte membrane. The hepatocytes are located along the sinusoid. According to the theory of the 'flowing liver', the regeneration of the hepatocytes takes place periportally, at the beginning of the sinusoid. The hepatocytes push further and further into the centre of the liver lobule through cell division and are eliminated perivenously through apoptosis. Through this cycle, the liver parenchyma is constantly renewed. As already briefly explained above, the liver cells are divided into three zones along the sinusoid.

Zone I of the hepatocytes lies periportally, zone III perivenously and zone II represents the intermediate zone between zone I and zone III. Different metabolic functions distinguish the hepatocytes in the three zones (Figure 39.1.1).

The cellular components of the liver parenchyma are differentiated as hepatocytes, Kupffer's stellate cells, Ito cells and Pit cells.

The hepatocytes are large, polygonal cells with a diameter of 20–30 μm, a weakly basophilic cytoplasm and a centrally located nucleus with one or two large nucleoli. The hepatocytes are connected to each other by 'gap junctions'. Between these, the intercellular space expands into a tubular gap space, the bile canaliculus. This tubular space is separated from the rest of the extracellular space by tight-junctions, so that no bile can enter the space of Diss and thus the blood. The high functional capacity of hepatocytes is morphologically expressed by the fact that about 25% of hepatocytes are binucleate and that hepatocytes are rich in mitochondria (up to 1700 mitochondria per hepatocyte in humans) and have a distinct smooth (detoxification and cholesterol metabolism) and rough (protein synthesis) endoplasmic reticulum. Extensive Golgi fields are located near the bile ductuli. The cells are rich in lysosomes and peroxisomes. Under physiological conditions, only single lipid droplets can be detected in the cytoplasm.

Textbook of Small Animal Pathophysiology, First Edition. Stephan Neumann.
© 2025 John Wiley & Sons Ltd. Published 2025 by John Wiley & Sons Ltd.

Table 39.1.1 Functions of the liver.

Storage	Synthesis	Detoxification	Excretion
Glycogen	Albumin	Lipophilic molecules	Bile
Fat	Coagulation factors		

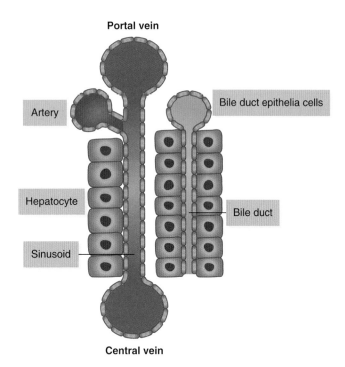

Figure 39.1.1 Illustration of the liver lobule with the sinusoid.

Kupffer cells are components of the mononuclear phagocyte system (MPS). They are located in the lumen of the sinusoids and the space of Diss and maintain contact with the endothelial cells and the hepatocytes. Their functions include phagocytosis and pinocytosis activity as part of the defence function. Furthermore, they release cytokines as signalling substances of the organised defence, are involved in the clearance of endotoxins from the portal blood and synthesise collagenases that influence the composition of the extracellular matrix.

The Ito cells are also called 'fat storage cells'. These 5–10 μm large cells are located in the space of Diss and store fats and vitamin A. They also contain many filaments as well as organelles for protein synthesis. They are capable of transformation into myofibroblasts. Under the influence of cytokines from damaged hepatocytes and Kupffer cells, the differentiation of the Ito cells into myofibroblasts takes place. These, in turn, are extensively involved in the formation of extracellular matrix and thus take on a central role in the pathogenesis of liver fibrosis and ultimately liver cirrhosis.

Finally, the pit cells are attached to endothelial cells in the sinusoids. They belong to the group of 'Large Granular Lymphocytes' and have a defence function as natural killer cells (McCuskey 2000; Kolios et al. 2006; Senoo 2004; Nakatani et al. 2004).

The activities of the liver begin in the **prepartum phase**. During foetal development, the liver is considered the centre of haematopoiesis for a certain period of time (9–24 weeks of gestation in humans). Under the influence of interleukin-3 (IL-3) and erythropoietin, erythrocytes are formed from hepatic stem cells. This mechanism stops after birth, but can be reactivated in the case of bone marrow aplasia. In adults, the liver indirectly influences haematopoiesis via iron, folic acid and vitamin B_{12} metabolism. Rudimentary erythropoietin synthesis in the liver is also maintained in the adult. The hepatogenic influence on iron metabolism and thus on haematopoiesis is based on the synthesis of apotransferrin, the transport protein for iron, and the storage of iron in the form of ferritin and haemosiderin. Iron bound to apotransferrin, a complex called 'transferrin', is taken up by hepatocytes for storage by endocytosis. Within the hepatocytes, iron is released from the transferrin complex and reversibly stored by binding to ferritin. When the ferritin store is full, further storage takes place in the form of haemosiderin. In addition to iron storage, the liver plays a role in haem synthesis and haem degradation. The latter takes place primarily in Kupffer cells and ends with the synthesis of indirect bilirubin, which is bound to albumin, taken up by the hepatocytes and glucuronidated to direct bilirubin.

The liver also has an influence on haematopoiesis via folic acid metabolism. Folic acid is involved in nucleic acid synthesis and is stored in the liver as folate polyglutamate after its absorption from the gastrointestinal tract (Yu et al. 1993; Donovan and Andrews 2004).

The liver plays a central role in **protein metabolism** through the synthesis and degradation of body proteins. The end products of protein biosynthesis in the liver are primarily plasma proteins, which, with the exception of albumin and pre-albumin, occur as glycoproteins. In addition to albumin, 100% of which is synthesised in the liver, alpha-globulins (80%), fibrinogen (100%) and prothrombin (100%) are produced in the liver. Of the plasma proteins, albumin is the most common (50–60%). It is synthesised exclusively in the liver. Its synthesis rate is positively influenced by hormones (cortisol and thyroxine), as well as by colloid osmotic pressure. Inflammatory mediators have a negative influence on albumin synthesis. For this reason, albumin is counted among the negative 'acute phase proteins' whose plasma concentration decreases in the acute inflammatory phase. The half-life of albumin in dogs is about eight days. The catabolism of the protein takes place not only in the liver but also in numerous other tissues (muscles, kidneys). The function of albumin is, primarily, to maintain the osmotic pressure (albumin is responsible for 75% of the osmotic activity in plasma). In addition, it is an important transport protein for numerous mediators (e.g. hormones such as thyroxine, elements such as calcium, vitamins such as tryptophan, metabolites such as bilirubin and bile acids). The central function of the liver in relation to haemostasis results from its synthesis function of coagulation factors. In addition, numerous factors of the fibrinolytic system, such as plasminogen, antithrombin III, α_2-macroglobulin are also produced in the liver. Another influence of the liver on blood coagulation results from the fact that factors II, VII, IX and X are activated by a vitamin K-dependent carboxylation reaction. Vitamin K, in turn, is absorbed in the small intestine in a bile acid-dependent manner (De Feo and Lucidi 2002; Lisman et al. 2002).

In the small intestine, carbohydrates from food are broken down into absorbable monosaccharides. These are partially absorbed actively (glucose and galactose) or passively (fructose, sorbitol and also glucose and galactose). The individual sugars are subject to considerable fluctuating concentrations in the portal venous system, which are balanced in the liver. The important metabolic activities of the liver in connection with carbohydrate metabolism are **glycogen storage, glycogenolysis, glycolysis** and **gluconeogenesis**.

The regulation of carbohydrate metabolism is influenced by hormones. Insulin promotes the uptake of glucose into the hepatocytes and the metabolism there. Glucagon, a functional antagonist of insulin, leads to an increase in blood glucose through increased formation and reduced breakdown of glucose. Furthermore, adrenaline and cortisone influence the carbohydrate metabolism of the liver. The former promotes the formation of glucose and its degradation to ATP; the latter, as a peripheral insulin antagonist, leads to an increase in the blood glucose concentration (Raddatz and Ramadori 2007).

Also **fat metabolism** takes place in the liver. Fatty acids are synthesised from acetyl-CoA and NADPH and are thus a product of glucose degradation. Fats serve the body as energy carriers and energy reserves and are released into the blood as lipoproteins. In addition to fatty acid synthesis, acetyl-CoA serves the synthesis of ketone bodies. These are formed in the liver and also serve as energy carriers. Finally, cholesterol metabolism as the basis of steroids and membrane cholesterols also takes place in the liver.

The initial substances for fat metabolism are supplied to the liver from the intestine via the portal vein or the lymphatic system. The fats are absorbed as fatty acids, monoglycerides, cholesterol and phospholipids. While short-chain fatty acids freely enter the blood vascular system, the long-chain fatty acids are built up into triglycerides in the enterocytes and transported away as chylomicrons together with lipoproteins via the lymphatic system.

The degradation of fatty acids in the citric acid cycle are an important part of the catabolic fat metabolism. The biochemical reactions of the citric acid cycle take place in the mitochondria, especially in the liver cell. The provision of acyl-CoA, as the starting product of β-oxidation, is a cytosolic reaction. Both reaction chains are connected via the carnitine shuttle.

For transport across the inner mitochondrial membrane, acyl-CoA molecules are bound to carnitine by carnitine acyltransferase (I). A carnitine-acylcarnitine translocase transports the carnitine fatty acid ester into the mitochondrial matrix in exchange for free mitochondrial carnitine. There, carnitine acyltransferase (II) transfers the acyl residue back to CoA. The free carnitine is transported back into the cytosol where it is available to take over another activated acyl residue (Jump 2011).

The excretory capacity of the liver is concentrated on **bile** with bile pigments and bile acids.

Bilirubin is a degradation product of haemoglobin metabolism. Its synthesis is a step in the degradation of the porphyrin ring (haem) from haemoglobin. Initially, biliverdin is formed during this degradation, which occurs under natural conditions as part of cell maturation in the MPS. Under the catalysis of biliverdin reductase, biliverdin is reduced to bilirubin. Since it is hydrophobic, it is bound to albumin and transported from the site of its formation to the liver. There, the conjugation of water-insoluble to water-soluble bilirubin takes place as glucuronisation. The latter reaches the intestine via the bile duct system, where it is further reduced to stercobilin and excreted. A small amount returns to the liver via the enterohepatic circulation. Most of the bilirubin formed in the liver comes from haemoglobin degradation; other sources include cytochromes.

Bile acids are steroids and are synthesised from cholesterol. In the hepatocytes, the so-called 'primary bile acids', 'cholic acid' and 'chenodeoxycholic acid', are formed first. These are excreted into the intestine via the bile. There, under the influence of bacterial enzymes, hydroxyl groups are removed, which leads to the formation of the so-called 'secondary bile acids', deoxycholic acid and litho acid. In the intestine, bile acids take on an important function in the digestion of lipids and fat-soluble vitamins. The bile acids are involved in the formation of micelles, through which the absorption of lipids is made possible. The bile acid pool is constantly renewed by synthesis of bile acids. Nevertheless, the organism behaves conservatively with regard to bile acids and tries to minimise enteral loss. This is done by returning 90 95% of the bile acids to the liver via the enterohepatic circulation. The bile acids contained in the portal blood are predominantly taken up in the liver by the hepatocytes on the sinusoidal membrane and secreted into the bile ducts at the basement membrane (Kullak-Ublick et al. 2004) (Table 39.1.2).

The functions of bile are to support the digestion of hydrophobic molecules. Due to the molecular structure, bile salts can form micelles with lipids and increase their water solubility and thus resorption capacity. The excretion of metabolic products, such as bile pigments, via the bile is a form of excretion by the organism. In addition to bile pigments as the end product of haemoglobin degradation, metals, cholesterol and lecithin are also excreted via the bile. Due to its content of buffering bicarbonate, bile is able to neutralise acid chyme that has entered the intestine. This is important for the protection of the intestinal epithelia, but also for the activation of digestive enzymes.

The following general pathophysiologic consequences are to be expected in hepatopathies of various causes with impairment of liver function.

Although the most common symptom, the **disturbance of general condition** is difficult to assign to a pathophysiologic mechanism. It is possible that this is a consequence of the disturbances of different metabolic processes. The influence of liver diseases on different neurotransmitters, such as serotonin or noradrenalin, is also discussed (Swain 2006). Antagonisation of the serotonin receptor, for example, led to an improvement in symptoms in people with hepatopathy due to a reduction in general well-being (Späth et al. 2000).

The development of **vomiting** and **diarrhoea** in dogs with hepatopathies is generally attributed to inflammation and ulceration of the gastrointestinal mucosa. In a study of 43 dogs with gastrointestinal ulcerations, 14 dogs had concomitant hepatopathy. Thus, liver disease was the most common single condition seen in association with ulceration in this study (Stanton and Bright 1989). Other reports describe vomiting associated with hepatoencephalopathy (HE) and hepatitis (Shih et al. 2007).

A reduced metabolism of gastrin and histamine in patients with hepatopathy is suspected as one mechanism. Increased serum gastrin and histamine concentrations have been demonstrated in people with hepatopathies, especially liver cirrhosis (Gittlen et al. 1990; Celinski et al. 2009). The consequences are increased gastric acid production with the consequence of mucosal irritation and ulceration (Maintz and Novak 2007). The results could not be fully confirmed for dogs. A study in dogs with hepatopathies did not show significantly increased gastrin concentrations compared to the healthy control

Table 39.1.2 Composition of bile.

Organic substances	Inorganic substances
Bile salts	Water
Bile pigments	Sodium
Cholesterol	Calcium
Fatty acids	Potassium
Mucin	Chloride
	Bicarbonate

group (Mazaki-Tovi et al. 2012). Histamine, however, was elevated in another study in dogs with liver failure (Zhang and Zhao 1998). Another mechanism considered to trigger gastro- or enteropathy is a disturbance of blood circulation in the gastrointestinal mucosa. This may develop as a result of portal hypertension, which has been described in canine hepatitis and hepatic fibrosis (James et al. 2008). Presumably, portal hypertension leads to blood stasis in the mucosa, which results in reduced mucin production, with the consequence of reduced protection of the mucosa from irritating gastric or intestinal contents.

In hepatoencephalopathy, neurotoxic substances that have not been metabolised in the liver and act on the central vomiting centre are also suspected as triggers (Tivers et al. 2015).

Polyuria and **polydipsia** are another clinical sign in dogs with hepatopathy. In one study, 21% of 100 dogs with various hepatopathies showed PU/PD (Neumann 2005). In another study, 89% of nine Labrador retrievers suffering from copper-associated hepatitis had PU/PD (Langlois et al. 2013).

Discussed mechanisms for PU/PD associated with hepatopathies include decreased urea synthesis in the insufficient liver resulting in a decreased urea gradient in the renal medulla and thus decreased water reabsorption. However, no studies have been found on this mechanism as a cause of PU/PD in dogs with liver disease. Also, in a study of eight dogs with hepatitis, only three dogs had a decreased urea concentration (Langlois et al. 2013), so this mechanism cannot explain all cases of PU/PD in dogs with hepatopathies.

Another mechanism could be due to secondary hyperaldosteronism, which occurs with reduced liver function. Aldosterone is predominantly metabolised in the liver (Kliman and Peterson 1958). A disturbance of this mechanism leads to an increase in the concentration of this hormone and thus to a reduced salt excretion via the kidney. The haematogenous salt increase causes polydipsia, which in turn is followed by compensatory polyuria (Warren et al. 1980; Jiménez et al. 1985). There are no studies on this mechanism in dogs either.

Finally, insufficient ADH secretion, which has been found in dogs with liver disease, could be a trigger of PU/PD (Kang and Park 2012).

The consequence of the reduced ADH concentration is increased diuresis, as ADH-induced water reabsorption in the collecting tube is reduced.

Pruritus is less commonly observed in association with hepatopathies. In a study of copper-associated hepatitis in Dalmatians, for example, two out of 10 dogs had pruritus as a clinical symptom (Webb et al. 2002). The mechanism is thought to be cholestasis and associated accumulation of bile acids in the skin. This hypothesis is supported by the observation that intracutaneous injections of bile acids cause itching. On the other hand, pruritus in liver patients is not related to the bile acid concentration in the serum (Weisshaar et al. 2003).

The improvement of pruritus in liver patients by the administration of morphine antagonists led to the hypothesis that endogenous opiates are involved in the development of hepatogenous pruritus (Jones and Bergasa 1990; Bergasa et al. 1994). It is assumed that the metabolism of endogenous opiates is disturbed in liver diseases and that an increased irritation of central opioid receptors leads to the symptom (Bergasa et al. 1994).

However, studies in dogs are lacking for the mechanisms described.

A **bleeding tendency** in dogs with hepatopathies is due to the fact that the liver is the site of synthesis of numerous factors involved in blood clotting and fibrinolysis. These include fibrinogen, as well as factors II, V, VII, VIII, IX, X and XI (Mischke and Nolte 2000). Disorders of coagulation or fibrinolysis have been described in dogs with various hepatopathies (Badylak et al. 1983; Toulza et al. 2006; Kummeling et al. 2006). The type of liver alteration seems to have an influence on the respective altered factors. In one study, factor IX, X and XI deficiency was observed in dogs with liver cirrhosis, while liver neoplasia was associated with factor VIII deficiency (Badylak et al. 1983). In dogs with chronic hepatitis and cirrhosis, activated partial thromboplastin time was prolonged and platelet count and antithrombin concentration were decreased in another study (Prins et al. 2010).

The underlying mechanisms for the lack of coagulation and fibrinolysis factors are seen in a reduced synthesis of these factors by the insufficient liver. Therefore, there also seems to be a correlation with the extent of liver disease (Prins et al. 2010). Thrombocytopenia in dogs with hepatopathies is thought to be caused by reduced production of thrombopoietin and increased consumption of platelets in cases of hepatogenic disseminated intravascular coagulopathy (Wigton et al. 1976).

Disturbances of consciousness in hepatopathies may occur as a result of HE, which is defined as a central nervous disorder caused by liver disease (Taboada and Dimski 1995). Symptoms have been described in dogs in association with portosystemic shunts and fulminant liver failure (Strombeck et al. 1975; Rothuizen 1993; Tivers et al. 2014).

The cause is discussed to be cytotoxic substances that are actually eliminated in the liver by means of biotransformation but enter the whole organism due to metabolic insufficiency or bypassing the liver (portosystemic collateral formation)

(Ferenci et al. 2002; Díaz-Gómez et al. 2011). In the brain, some of these substances can produce central nervous symptoms by occupying receptors and affecting excitation conduction. These substances include true (e.g. γ-aminobutyric acid, GABA) and false neurotransmitters (e.g. ammonia, octopamine, phenylethylamine) (Taboada and Dimski 1995).

Ascites is also described as a symptom in dogs with hepatopathies. The occurrence of ascites depends on the type of hepatopathy; in particular, marked morphological changes in the liver architecture lead to this symptom. Of 34 dogs with chronic hepatitis, 41% had ascites in one study (Raffan et al. 2009). The presence of ascites is evaluated as a negative prognostic factor in canine hepatopathies (Sevelius 1995; Raffan et al. 2009).

Currently, two mechanisms are being discussed that could be responsible for the development of ascites. The reduced albumin synthesis in the insufficient liver lowers the oncotic pressure in the vascular system and thus causes ascites formation. Albumin concentration below 15 g/l reduces the oncotic pressure markedly. However, even liver-diseased dogs with normal albumin concentrations can develop ascites (James et al. 2008; Rothuizen 2009). Another mechanism leading to ascites is portal hypertension, which occurs in chronic cirrhotic liver disease. This leads to disturbed blood flow in the liver parenchyma, which induces a backflow of blood into the splanchnic system (Buob et al. 2011).

References

Badylak, S.F., Dodds, W.J., and Van Vleet, J.F. (1983). Plasma coagulation factor abnormalities in dogs with naturally occurring hepatic disease. *American Journal of Veterinary Research* 44 (12): 2336–2340.

Bergasa, N.V., Alling, D.W., Vergalla, J., and Jones, E.A. (1994). Cholestasis in the male rat is associated with naloxone-reversible antinociception. *Journal of Hepatology* 20 (1): 85–90. https://doi.org/10.1016/s0168-8278(05)80471-4.

Buob, S., Johnston, A.N., and Webster, C.R. (2011). Portal hypertension: pathophysiology, diagnosis, and treatment. *Journal of Veterinary Internal Medicine* 25 (2): 169–186. https://doi.org/10.1111/j.1939-1676.2011.00691.x.

Celinski, K., Konturek, P.C., Slomka, M. et al. (2009). Altered basal and postprandial plasma melatonin, gastrin, ghrelin, leptin and insulin in patients with liver cirrhosis and portal hypertension without and with oral administration of melatonin or tryptophan. *Journal of Pineal Research* 46 (4): 408–414. https://doi.org/10.1111/j.1600-079X.2009.00677.x.

De Feo, P. and Lucidi, P. (2002). Liver protein synthesis in physiology and in disease states. *Current Opinion in Clinical Nutrition and Metabolic Care* 5 (1): 47–50. https://doi.org/10.1097/00075197-200201000-00009.

Díaz-Gómez, D., Jover, M., del Campo, J.A. et al. (2011). Experimental models for hepatic encephalopathy. *Revista espanola de enfermedades digestivas* 103 (10): 536–541. https://doi.org/10.4321/s1130-01082011001000006.

Donovan, A. and Andrews, N.C. (2004). The molecular regulation of iron metabolism. *The Hematology Journal: The Official Journal of the European Haematology Association* 5 (5): 373–380. https://doi.org/10.1038/sj.thj.6200540.

Ferenci, P., Lockwood, A., Mullen, K. et al. (2002). Hepatic encephalopathy – definition, nomenclature, diagnosis, and quantification: final report of the working party at the 11th World Congresses of Gastroenterology, Vienna. *Hepatology* 35 (3): 716–721.

Gittlen, S.D., Schulman, E.S., and Maddrey, W.C. (1990). Raised histamine concentrations in chronic cholestatic liver disease. *Gut* 31 (1): 96–99. https://doi.org/10.1136/gut.31.1.96.

James, F.E., Knowles, G.W., Mansfield, C.S., and Robertson, I.D. (2008). Ascites due to pre-sinusoidal portal hypertension in dogs: a retrospective analysis of 17 cases. *Australian Veterinary Journal* 86 (5): 180–186. https://doi.org/10.1111/j.1751-0813.2008.00284.x.

Jiménez, W., Martinez-Pardo, A., Arroyo, V. et al. (1985). Temporal relationship between hyperaldosteronism, sodium retention and ascites formation in rats with experimental cirrhosis. *Hepatology (Baltimore, Md.)* 5 (2): 245–250. https://doi.org/10.1002/hep.1840050215.

Jones, E.A. and Bergasa, N.V. (1990). The pruritus of cholestasis: from bile acids to opiate agonists. *Hepatology (Baltimore, Md.)* 11 (5): 884–887. https://doi.org/10.1002/hep.1840110526.

Jump, D.B. (2011). Fatty acid regulation of hepatic lipid metabolism. *Current Opinion in Clinical Nutrition and Metabolic Care* 14 (2): 115–120. https://doi.org/10.1097/MCO.0b013e328342991c.

Kang, M.H. and Park, H.M. (2012). Syndrome of inappropriate antidiuretic hormone secretion concurrent with liver disease in a dog. *The Journal of Veterinary Medical Science* 74 (5): 645–649. https://doi.org/10.1292/jvms.11-0483.

Kliman, B. and Peterson, R.E. (1958). The metabolism of titrated aldosterone in man. *40th Meeting Endocrine Society*.

Kolios, G., Valatas, V., and Kouroumalis, E. (2006). Role of Kupffer cells in the pathogenesis of liver disease. *World Journal of Gastroenterology* 12 (46): 7413–7420. https://doi.org/10.3748/wjg.v12.i46.7413.

Kullak-Ublick, G.A., Stieger, B., and Meier, P.J. (2004). Enterohepatic bile salt transporters in normal physiology and liver disease. *Gastroenterology* 126 (1): 322–342. https://doi.org/10.1053/j.gastro.2003.06.005.

Kummeling, A., Teske, E., Rothuizen, J., and Van Sluijs, F.J. (2006). Coagulation profiles in dogs with congenital portosystemic shunts before and after surgical attenuation. *Journal of Veterinary Internal Medicine* 20 (6): 1319–1326. https://doi.org/10.1892/0891-6640(2006)20[1319:cpidwc]2.0.co;2.

Langlois, D.K., Smedley, R.C., Schall, W.D., and Kruger, J.M. (2013). Acquired proximal renal tubular dysfunction in 9 Labrador Retrievers with copper-associated hepatitis (2006-2012). *Journal of Veterinary Internal Medicine* 27 (3): 491–499. https://doi.org/10.1111/jvim.12065.

Lisman, T., Leebeek, F.W., and de Groot, P.G. (2002). Haemostatic abnormalities in patients with liver disease. *Journal of Hepatology* 37 (2): 280–287. https://doi.org/10.1016/s0168-8278(02)00199-x.

Maintz, L. and Novak, N. (2007). Histamine and histamine intolerance. *The American Journal of Clinical Nutrition* 85 (5): 1185–1196. https://doi.org/10.1093/ajcn/85.5.1185.

Mazaki-Tovi, M., Segev, G., Yas-Natan, E., and Lavy, E. (2012). Serum gastrin concentrations in dogs with liver disorders. *The Veterinary Record* 171 (1): 19. https://doi.org/10.1136/vr.100627.

McCuskey, R.S. (2000). Morphological mechanisms for regulating blood flow through hepatic sinusoids. *Liver* 20 (1): 3–7. https://doi.org/10.1034/j.1600-0676.2000.020001003.x.

Mischke, R. and Nolte, I. (2000). Hemostasis: introduction, overview, laboratory techniques. In: *Schalm's Veterinary Hematology* (ed. B.F. Feldman, J.G. Zinkl, and N.C. Jain), 519–525. Philadelphia, PA: Lippincott Williams and Wilkins.

Nakatani, K., Kaneda, K., Seki, S., and Nakajima, Y. (2004). Pit cells as liver-associated natural killer cells: morphology and function. *Medical Electron Microscopy: Official Journal of the Clinical Electron Microscopy Society of Japan* 37 (1): 29–36. https://doi.org/10.1007/s00795-003-0229-9.

Neumann, S. (2005). Epidemiological, clinical and laboratory diagnostic findings in dogs with hepatopathies. *Kleintierpraxis* 50: 695–707.

Prins, M., Schellens, C.J., van Leeuwen, M.W. et al. (2010). Coagulation disorders in dogs with hepatic disease. *Veterinary Journal (London, England: 1997)* 185 (2): 163–168. https://doi.org/10.1016/j.tvjl.2009.05.009.

Raddatz, D. and Ramadori, G. (2007). Carbohydrate metabolism and the liver: actual aspects from physiology and disease. *Journal of Gastroenterology* 45 (1): 51–62. https://doi.org/10.1055/s-2006-927394.

Raffan, E., McCallum, A., Scase, T.J., and Watson, P.J. (2009). Ascites is a negative prognostic indicator in chronic hepatitis in dogs. *Journal of Veterinary Internal Medicine* 23 (1): 63–66. https://doi.org/10.1111/j.1939-1676.2008.0230.x.

Rothuizen, J. (1993). Portosystemic hepatic encephalopathy related with congenital and acquired hepatopathies in the dog. *Advances in Veterinary Science and Comparative Medicine* 37: 403–416.

Rothuizen, J. (2009). Important clinical syndromes associated with liver disease. *The Veterinary Clinics of North America. Small Animal Practice* 39 (3): 419–437. https://doi.org/10.1016/j.cvsm.2009.02.007.

Senoo, H. (2004). Structure and function of hepatic stellate cells. *Medical Electron Microscopy: Official Journal of the Clinical Electron Microscopy Society of Japan* 37 (1): 3–15. https://doi.org/10.1007/s00795-003-0230-3.

Sevelius, E. (1995). Diagnosis and prognosis of chronic hepatitis and cirrhosis in dogs. *The Journal of Small Animal Practice* 36 (12): 521–528. https://doi.org/10.1111/j.1748-5827.1995.tb02801.x.

Shih, J.L., Keating, J.H., Freeman, L.M., and Webster, C.R. (2007). Chronic hepatitis in Labrador retrievers: clinical presentation and prognostic factors. *Journal of Veterinary Internal Medicine* 21 (1): 33–39. https://doi.org/10.1892/0891-6640(2007)21[33:chilrc]2.0.co;2.

Späth, M., Welzel, D., and Färber, L. (2000). Treatment of chronic fatigue syndrome with 5-HT3 receptor antagonists–preliminary results. *Scandinavian Journal of Rheumatology. Supplement* 113: 72–77.

Stanton, M.E. and Bright, R.M. (1989). Gastroduodenal ulceration in dogs. Retrospective study of 43 cases and literature review. *Journal of Veterinary Internal Medicine* 3 (4): 238–244. https://doi.org/10.1111/j.1939-1676.1989.tb00863.x.

Strombeck, D.R., Meyer, D.J., and Freedland, R.A. (1975). Hyperammonemia due to a urea cycle enzyme deficiency in two dogs. *Journal of the American Veterinary Medical Association* 166 (11): 1109–1111.

Swain, M.G. (2006). Fatigue in liver disease: pathophysiology and clinical management. *Canadian journal of gastroenterology = Journal canadien de gastroenterologie* 20 (3): 181–188. https://doi.org/10.1155/2006/624832.

Taboada, J. and Dimski, D.S. (1995). Hepatic encephalopathy: clinical signs, pathogenesis, and treatment. *The Veterinary Clinics of North America. Small Animal Practice* 25 (2): 337–355.

Tivers, M.S., Handel, I., Gow, A.G. et al. (2014). Hyperammonemia and systemic inflammatory response syndrome predicts presence of hepatic encephalopathy in dogs with congenital portosystemic shunts. *PLoS One* 9 (1): e82303. https://doi.org/10.1371/journal.pone.0082303. eCollection 2014.

Tivers, M.S., Handel, I., Gow, A.G. et al. (2015). Attenuation of congenital portosystemic shunt reduces inflammation in dogs. *PLoS One* 10 (2): e0117557. https://doi.org/10.1371/journal.pone.0117557. eCollection 2015.

Toulza, O., Center, S.A., Brooks, M.B. et al. (2006). Evaluation of plasma protein C activity for detection of hepatobiliary disease and portosystemic shunting in dogs. *Journal of the American Veterinary Medical Association* 229 (11): 1761–1771. https://doi.org/10.2460/javma.229.11.1761.

Warren, S.E., Mitas, J.A. 2nd, and Swerdlin, A.H. (1980). Hypernatremia in hepatic failure. *JAMA* 243 (12): 1257–1260.

Webb, C.B., Twedt, D.C., and Meyer, D.J. (2002). Copper-associated liver disease in Dalmatians: a review of 10 dogs (1998-2001). *Journal of Veterinary Internal Medicine* 16 (6): 665–668. https://doi.org/10.1892/0891-6640(2002)016<0665:cldida>2.3.co;2.

Weisshaar, E., Kucenic, M.J., and Fleischer, A.B. Jr. (2003). Pruritus: a review. *Acta Dermato-Venereologica. Supplementum* 213: 5–32.

Wigton, D.H., Kociba, G.J., and Hoover, E.A. (1976). Infectious canine hepatitis: animal model for viral induced disseminated intravascular coagulation. *Blood* 47: 287–296.

Yu, H., Bauer, B., Lipke, G.K. et al. (1993). Apoptosis and hematopoiesis in murine fetal liver. *Blood* 81 (2): 373–384.

Zhang, L. and Zhao, Q. (1998). An experimental study on the disorders of hepatic hemodynamics and changes of plasma histamine in dogs with fulminant hepatic failure. *Journal of Tongji Medical University = Tong ji yi ke da xue xue bao* 18 (1): 33–36. https://doi.org/10.1007/BF02888276.

39.2

Acute Hepatic Failure

Definition

Acute hepatic failure is defined as the sudden onset of liver cell necrosis with loss of liver function.

Aetiology

Numerous drugs, environmental toxins or endotoxins have been described as causing acute liver failure. Dogs are more frequently affected by the disease. In cats, the disease is often associated with hepatolipidosis.

Drugs	Toxins	Infection
Tetracyclines, sulfonamides (D)	Arsenic (D/C)	Canine hepatitis virus (D)
Azathioprine, mitutane (D) Methimazole (C)	Mercury (D/C)	Canine herpes virus (D)
NSAID (D)	Lead (D/C)	Leptospirosis (D)
Phenobarbital (D)	Copper (D)	

D – Dog, C – Cat

Pathogenesis

Various causalities can trigger acute hepatocellular necrosis. Different mechanisms play a role, which also act in different regions of the liver lobule. Hypoxic causes often lead to cell necrosis in the pericentral region of the liver lobule. There, the oxygen supply of the cells is also physiologically reduced. Accordingly, these cells react sensitively to a further reduction in partial oxygen pressure. Shock can be a cause of pericentral liver failure. Drugs and toxins have a particularly toxic effect in the zone of the liver lobule where they are metabolised. Metabolites that cause cellular stress with the formation of reactive oxygen species (ROS) or a disturbance of mitochondrial function have a triggering effect here. If the cellular compensation mechanisms are exceeded, cell necrosis occurs.

The main point of attack of many causalities of acute liver failure in the cell is cellular respiration, which takes place in the mitochondria of the cell with the formation of ATP. ATP can no longer be provided in the cell if oxygen is lacking for the oxidative energy production of the cell. Chemical-toxic damage to the enzyme systems necessary for cellular respiration can also cause an ATP deficiency. ATP is produced in the mammalian cell either by oxidative phosphorylation or by the less efficient second pathway of anaerobic glycolysis. The liver, like skeletal muscle, the heart and the kidney, is able to store carbohydrates in the form of glycogen. In the absence of oxygen, the liver's glycogen supply is consumed to provide ATP via anaerobic glycolysis.

Since the Na^+-K^+ pump works under ATP consumption, its function is reduced during ATP depletion. Sodium is now no longer transported out of the cell and water follows the osmotic gradient into the cell. This disturbance of the water balance

Textbook of Small Animal Pathophysiology, First Edition. Stephan Neumann.

can be recognised microscopically by a cloudy swelling (mitochondria), after progressive water retention by vacuolar degeneration (mitochondria and endoplasmic reticulum) or as hydropic degeneration (cytoplasm).

In addition to disturbances of the cellular water balance in the case of energy deficiency, the change from aerobic to anaerobic glycolysis also leads to increased formation of lactate and thus lowers the intracellular pH value. This restricts the function of some pH-dependent enzymes. This leads to the deregulation of numerous metabolic processes in the cell, especially protein biosynthesis. Lack of structural proteins leads to a permeability disorder of the cell membrane and damage to cell organelles. Furthermore, important lipoproteins for the removal of neutral fats are no longer provided. Reduced removal and reduced fatty acid oxidation due to oxygen deficiency subsequently lead to fatty degeneration of the cell. In the further course of cell death, an increased calcium influx and the formation of cell-damaging radicals play a role. These mechanisms can also be at the beginning of cell damage. Thus, free radicals can damage DNA, cell organelles or the integrity of the cell membrane. A loss of calcium homeostasis due to ischaemic or toxic damage leads to an activation of cell-damaging enzymes.

Membrane integrity can also be disrupted by a number of other factors, such as toxins including endotoxins, radiation and the complement system. But an undersupply of vitamin E and selenium can also lead to membrane instability. Oxygen radicals oxidise polyunsaturated fatty acids to peroxides, among other things. Consequently, the function of the lipid bilayer of the biomembrane, the fluidity of the membrane and its transport and receptor function are impaired. The cell normally has various ways to protect itself against free oxygen radicals. Antioxidants, such as glutathione, s-adenosylmethionine, vitamin E, superoxide dismutase and ubiquinone Q10 serve as protection. In the case of massive ROS formation, however, the protective measures are overwhelmed. Lipid peroxidation by ROS is an important mechanism in liver cell damage in toxic hepatoses, biliary obstructions, chronic hepatitis and the iron and copper storage diseases. In some of these diseases, lipid peroxidation is the first pathological characteristic (Figure 39.2.1).

Diagnostics

Clinical signs	Clinical pathology	Imaging	Histopathology	Microbiology
Strongly disturbed general condition Coma	Severely increased liver enzymes	**Ultrasonography** Liver structure generalised hypoechogenic mainly	Mostly not necessary	Not necessary

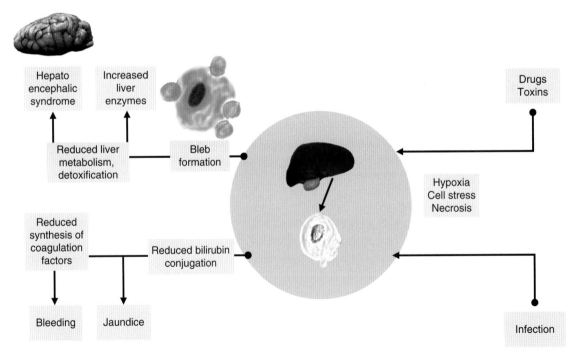

Figure 39.2.1 Pathogenesis and pathophysiologic consequences of acute liver failure.

Pathophysiologic Consequences

Due to the central metabolic function of the liver, acute liver failure is associated with a variety of organ symptoms.

Influenced organ systems	Clinical symptoms	Clinical pathological alterations
Cardiovascular system	Lethargy	Anaemia
Gastrointestinal system	Anorexia	Thrombocytopenia
Hepatobiliary system	Seizures	Increased ALT, AST, GLDH
Central nervous system	Vomiting	Increased ALP, bilirubin
Haematological system	Diarrhoea	Hypoglycaemia
Systemic	PU/PD	Hypoalbuminaemia
	Coagulopathy	

Although the most common symptoms, **lethargy** and **anorexia** are difficult to attribute to a pathophysiologic mechanism. It is possible that they are the consequence of disturbances in different metabolic processes.

Cytotoxic substances that are actually eliminated in the liver by means of biotransformation but enter the whole organism due to metabolic insufficiency are discussed as cause for lethargy and anorexia. In the brain, some of these substances can produce central nervous symptoms by occupying receptors and influencing neural conduction. These substances include true (e.g. γ-aminobutyric acid, GABA) and false neurotransmitters (e.g. ammonia, octopamine, phenylethylamine).

Seizures develop due to a hepato-encephalic syndrome, which can occur in acute liver dysfunction. The reduced liver output leads to inadequate detoxification of the ammonia in the urea cycle or glutamine synthesis, resulting in an increase in blood ammonia levels. Ammonia can cross the blood-brain barrier and is taken up by astrocytes, leading to complex functional impairment with changes in neurotransmitter concentrations. The mechanism is explained in detail in Chapter 39.4 (Figure 39.2.2).

The development of **vomiting and diarrhoea** in dogs with hepatopathies is generally attributed to inflammation and ulceration of the gastric and intestinal mucosa. A reduced metabolism of gastrin and histamine in patients with hepatopathy is thought to be one mechanism. The consequences are increased gastric acid production with the consequence of mucosal irritation and ulceration. Another mechanism considered to trigger gastro- or enteropathy is a disturbance of blood circulation in the gastrointestinal mucosa. In hepatoencephalopathy, neurotoxic substances that have not been metabolised in the liver and act on the central vomiting centre are also suspected as triggers.

Polyuria and polydipsia are another clinical symptom in dogs with hepatopathy. The discussed mechanisms for PU/PD associated with hepatopathies are decreased urea synthesis in the insufficient liver resulting in a decreased urea gradient in the renal medulla and thus decreased water reabsorption. However, no studies have been found on this mechanism as a cause of PU/PD in dogs with liver disease.

Another mechanism could be due to secondary hyperaldosteronism, which occurs with reduced liver function. Aldosterone is predominantly metabolised in the liver. A disturbance of this mechanism leads to an increase in the concentration of this hormone and thus to a reduced salt excretion via the kidney. The haematogenous salt increase causes polydipsia, which in turn is followed by compensatory polyuria. There are no studies on this mechanism in dogs either. Finally, insufficient ADH secretion, which has been found in dogs with liver disease, could be a trigger of PU/PD (Kang and Park 2012). The consequence of reduced ADH concentration is increased diuresis, as vasopressin-induced water reabsorption in the collecting duct is reduced.

A **bleeding tendency** in dogs with hepatopathies is likely due to the fact that the liver is the site of synthesis of numerous factors involved in blood clotting and fibrinolysis. These include fibrinogen, as well as factors II, V, VII, VIII, IX, X and XI. Disorders of coagulation or fibrinolysis have been described in dogs with various hepatopathies. The underlying mechanisms for the deficiency of coagulation and fibrinolysis factors are a reduced synthesis of these factors by the insufficient liver. Therefore, there also seems to be a correlation with the extent of liver disease. **Thrombocytopenia** in dogs with hepatopathies is thought to be caused by reduced production of thrombopoietin and increased consumption of platelets in cases of hepatogenic disseminated intravascular coagulopathy. The consequence of this bleeding tendency can be an initially non-regenerative **anaemia**.

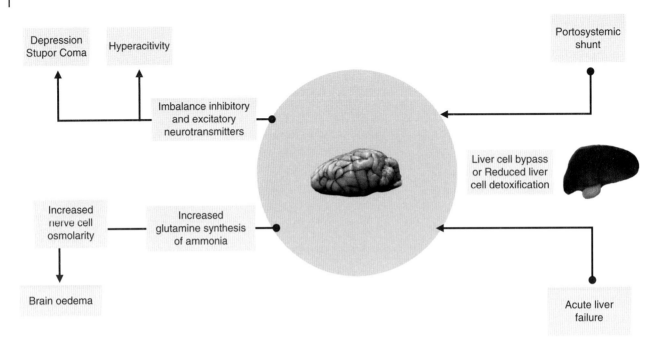

Figure 39.2.2 Mechanism of hepatoencephalopathy.

The massive hepatocellular destruction in acute liver failure is reflected in the usually very strongly increased activities of the liver enzymes **ALT**, **AST** and **GLDH**. The release of hepatocellular enzymes is usually the result of evagination and constriction of the cell membrane with enclosed cytoplasmic components. These so-called 'blebs' contain cytoplasmic enzymes of the hepatocytes and can cause increased activity in the blood when strangulated.

The bleb formation is due to a disturbance of the cytoskeleton. This in turn can result directly from toxin action or be the consequence of an energy deficiency due to ATP depletion. The lack of energy leads to actin depolarisation, which results in cellular structural loss with cellular blebs. These blebs can rupture intravascularly, releasing cellular enzymes (Gores et al. 1990). Alternatively, cellular structure may be directly affected by cellular necrosis, leading to leakage of cellular components.

Acute liver failure can also be accompanied by cholestasis, recognisable by increased **ALP activity** and **hyperbilirubinaemia**. Hyperbilirubinaemia in particular is also seen as a prognostic marker. The development of cholestasis in acute liver failure is intrahepatic. The cause of cholestasis is the disturbance of the synthesis or outflow of bile.

Bile is a mixture of organic and inorganic components that is synthesised by hepatocytes and then transported via the bile ducts.

The organic components cholesterol, phospholipids, bile salts and bilirubins are formed in the hepatocytes and then released via the hepatocyte membrane into the bile ducts. This transport is carrier-supported and ATP-dependent. Cholesterol and phospholipids are transported via the MDR 1 + 2 transporters. Bile salts have their own transporter. The secretion of organic components creates an osmotic gradient which is followed by water into the bile ducts.

In the case of liver failure, cholestasis may occur if the transport mechanisms at the hepatocyte membrane are disturbed and bile components accumulate in the hepatocytes. In addition, structural changes can destroy the tight-junctions between the hepatocytes, allowing leakage of bile into the sinusoids. The increase in ALP activity can be attributed to structural changes in the bile duct epithelia, which lead to an increased release of the enzyme.

Finally, the reduction of the liver's synthesis capacity can be seen in the reduced synthesis of, e.g. **albumin** or **glucose**.

The latter is the consequence of a more than 75% reduction in liver synthesis capacity. The liver is significantly involved in the synthesis of glucose from glycogen and in the form of gluconeogenesis from amino acids. With reduced liver function, glucose-forming mechanisms may be reduced, leading to hypoglycaemia (Grek and Arasi 2016; Riordan and Williams 2000; Gow 2017; Lidbury et al. 2016).

Therapy

Symptom	Therapy
Stabilisation of a lethargic patient	Infusion
Cerebral oedema	Diuresis Mannitol
Hepatic encephalopathy	Lactulose, antibiotics
Vomiting	Antiemetics (e.g. Ondansetron, Maropitant, Omeprazole)

References

Gores, G.J., Herman, B., and Lemasters, J.J. (1990). Plasma membrane bleb formation and rupture: a common feature of hepatocellular injury. *Hepatology (Baltimore, Md.)* 11 (4): 690–698. https://doi.org/10.1002/hep.1840110425.

Gow, A.G. (2017). Hepatic encephalopathy. *The Veterinary Clinics of North America. Small Animal Practice* 47 (3): 585–599. https://doi.org/10.1016/j.cvsm.2016.11.008.

Grek, A. and Arasi, L. (2016). Acute liver failure. *AACN Advanced Critical Care* 27 (4): 420–429. https://doi.org/10.4037/aacnacc2016324.

Kang, M.H. and Park, H.M. (2012). Syndrome of inappropriate antidiuretic hormone secretion concurrent with liver disease in a dog. *The Journal of Veterinary Medical Science* 74 (5): 645–649. https://doi.org/https:/doi.org/10.1292/jvms.11-0483.

Lidbury, J.A., Cook, A.K., and Steiner, J.M. (2016). Hepatic encephalopathy in dogs and cats. *Journal of Veterinary Emergency and Critical Care (San Antonio, Tex.: 2001) 26* (4): 471–487. https://doi.org/10.1111/vec.12473.

Riordan, S.M. and Williams, R. (2000). Fulminant hepatic failure. *Clinics in Liver Disease* 4 (1): 25–45. https://doi.org/10.1016/s1089-3261(05)70095-7.

Further Reading

Thawley, V. (2017). Acute liver injury and failure. *The Veterinary clinics of North America. Small Animal Practice* 47 (3): 617–630. https://doi.org/10.1016/j.cvsm.2016.11.010.

Weingarten, M.A. and Sande, A.A. (2015). Acute liver failure in dogs and cats. *Journal of Veterinary Emergency and Critical Care (San Antonio, Tex.:2001)* 25 (4): 455–473. https://doi.org/10.1111/vec.12304.

39.3

Chronic Hepatitis; Liver Fibrosis and Cirrhosis

Definition

Chronic hepatitis is a diffuse inflammation of the liver parenchyma. It is characterised by inflammatory cell infiltrates, as well as apoptosis and necrosis of hepatocytes. In the advanced stage, chronic hepatitis is the cause of the proliferation of fibroblasts and the increased formation of connective tissue, which leads to liver fibrosis and in the final stage to cirrhosis of the liver. Chronic hepatitis and liver cirrhosis are more prominent in dogs than in cats. In cats cholangiohepatitis is more common and discussed in Chapter 39.6.

Aetiology

Infectious agents play a minor role as etiological factors of chronic hepatitis in dogs and cats. Drugs and toxins have been described as causal agents. Autoimmune diseases are suspected and copper storage disease is the most common cause of chronic hepatitis in some breeds of dogs.

Drugs/toxins	Genetic	Autoimmune	Infection
Phenobarbital (D)	Copper storage disease (D)	Cholangiohepatitis, non-suppurative (C)	Hepatitis contagiosa canis (D)
NSAID (D)			Leptospirosis (D)

D – Dog, C – Cat

Pathogenesis

The mechanism by which toxins, in particular, trigger hepatitis begins with chemical-toxic hepatocyte damage and a subsequent immunological reaction. The hepatocyte damage is often the result of the biotransformation of the toxin, which produces intermediates that can trigger different reactions.

On the one hand, metabolites can induce the formation of reactive oxygen species (ROS). This generates oxidative stress when there is an imbalance between free radicals and radical scavengers. The ROS have an unbound electron, which makes them particularly reactive. The ROS can react with molecules in all cellular organelles and thus damage the hepatocyte. The damaged hepatocyte thereby releases molecules (e.g. heat shock proteins), which are recognised as so-called 'DAMPs' by non-parenchymatous cells, including the Kupffer cells, via pattern recognition receptors. These are activated by the reaction and induce the transcription of cytokines and the recruitment of further cytotoxic cells, e.g. neutrophilic granulocytes and monocytes (Martin-Murphy et al. 2010; Pessayre et al. 2012).

Bound to nucleic acids, proteins and fats, the metabolites can trigger an autoimmune reaction as haptens (Tailor et al. 2015). This is carried by autoantibodies and cytotoxic T lymphocytes. In dogs with hepatitis, autoantibodies against the nucleus (ANA, histones) and the hepatocyte membrane proteins have been found (Weiss et al. 1995; Dyggve et al. 2017).

Another mechanism that explains individual responses to hepatotoxins is a genetic polymorphism. Polymorphisms in genes coding for enzymes that metabolise toxins have been identified for humans. Such polymorphisms could lead to toxic consequences. Alternatively, a polymorphism in a gene encoding a cytoprotective factor could make individuals susceptible to therapeutic doses of drugs (Shaw et al. 2010).

For example, one paper demonstrated how ketoconazole develops a hepatotoxic effect. Different mechanisms were identified, including inhibition of sterol synthesis, activation of the CXCL8 pathway and the Nrf2-mediated oxidative stress response. These changes in turn led to activation of cytokine expression and secretion (Wewering 2017).

The hepatitis that develops from the mechanisms described can, in the case of chronicity, progress to liver fibrosis and later to liver cirrhosis.

While liver fibrosis initially represents an accumulation of connective tissue, cirrhosis changes the organ architecture and thus also has a considerable influence on organ function.

The mechanism of fibrosis involves not only hepatocytes but also other hepatogenic parenchymal cells, such as sessile macrophages (Kupffer cells), endothelial cells and fat-storing Ito cells.

First, damaged hepatocytes secrete various profibrotic and proinflammatory substances. The profibrotic factors include transforming growth factor-β (TGF-β) and platelet derived growth factor (PDGF). Among other things, these activate fat-storing Ito cells, which are localised in the space of Diss and store numerous vitamin A-containing fat droplets in the resting state. After activation, the Ito cells differentiate into contractile myofibroblasts. The transformation can be divided into two phases, the initiation phase and perpetuation.

During the initiation phase, changes occur in gene expression and in the phenotype of the Ito cells. On the one hand, the vitamin A storage function is lost; on the other hand, cytoskeletal proteins, such as α-smooth muscle actin (α-SMA) are increasingly expressed. In perpetuation, the cells proliferate and can also migrate to other liver areas through PDGF-mediated migration.

The activated Ito cells show an increased, TGF-β-mediated, synthesis of the extracellular matrix (ECM). The main components of the hepatic ECM are collagens. In the case of fibrosis, their quantity increases, the composition changes and other molecules, such as elastin, fibronectin, hyaluron, laminin and proteoglycans are formed. There is a loss of the balance between fibrogenesis and fibrolysis that exists in the physiological state.

In addition to Ito cells, other cell types, such as platelets or Kupffer cells are also involved in fibrogenesis (Ikeda et al. 1999; Bataller and Brenner 2005; Schuppan 2015).

Progressive fibrosis leads to a remodelling of the liver architecture. The consequence is the formation of connective tissue nodules (micro- and macronodullary) and alteration of the vascular supply, which eventually leads to delayed outflow from the portal vein system, causing portal hypertension (Figure 39.3.1).

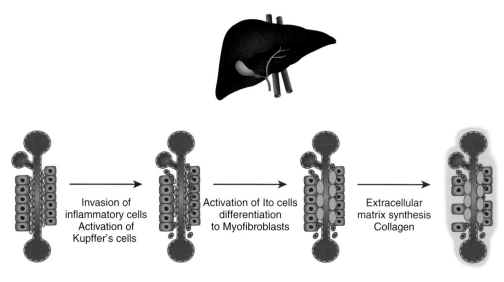

Figure 39.3.1 Mechanism of hepatogenic fibrogenesis.

Diagnostics

Clinical signs	Clinical pathology	Imaging	Histopathology	Microbiology
Non-specific	Elevated liver enzymes Decreased albumin Increased bile acids	**Ultrasonography** Mixed echogenicity	**Diagnostic**, evidence of connective tissue remodelling	Not necessary

Pathophysiologic Consequences

The pathophysiologic consequences are closely related to the extent of parenchymatous remodelling of the liver. While chronic hepatitis without fibrosis or cirrhosis essentially shows reactions of the white blood count and increases in markers of liver cell integrity (liver enzymes), fibrosis and cirrhosis are accompanied by a reduction in liver function (synthesis of albumin, coagulation factors, urea). Another consequence is the portal hypertension present in the cirrhotic remodelling process. This is involved in the development of ascites, as well as portosystemic collaterals and thus a hepatoencephalic syndrome.

Influenced organs	Clinical symptoms	Frequency (%)	Clinical pathological alterations
Hepatobiliary system	Lethargy	93	Leucocytosis
Gastrointestinal system	Inappetence	85	Anaemia
Central nervous system	Weight loss	45	Increased liver enzymes
Urinary tract	Vomiting	50	Hypoalbuminaemia
	Diarrhoea	30	Decreased urea
	Polydipsia	30	Increased bile acids
	Icterus	54	Coagulopathy
	Ascites	25	

Source: Bexfield et al. (2011).

As already shown in acute liver failure, **lethargy** and **inappetence** are difficult to assign to a pathophysiologic mechanism. It is possible that they are the consequence of disturbances of different metabolic processes.

Weight loss is partly the result of inappetence, but chronic liver diseases also show a lack of anabolically acting IGF I as well as an increased concentration of molecules of the ubiquitin-proteasome pathway, which is responsible for the degradation of the body's own proteins (Gerke et al. 2018).

Disturbances in digestion are held responsible for the gastrointestinal symptoms of **vomiting** and **diarrhoea**; this is also described in Chapter 39.4. The mechanisms are seen to be reduced liver function, which leads to reduced bile acid secretion. This reduces intestinal lipid absorption and triggers osmotic diarrhoea.

If portal hypertension is present, different mechanisms are described that lead to intestinal disorders. Essentially, motility disorders, dysbiosis and hyperpermeability are observed (Fukui and Wiest 2016).

The motility disorders observed in connection with portal hypertension are primarily prolonged transit times in the intestine due to reduced gastrointestinal motility. This in turn is probably due to a dysfunction of the autonomic nervous system in the sense of parasympathicolysis (Verne et al. 2004). The delayed motility in the intestine induces a 'bacterial overgrowth syndrome' which is associated with structural and functional changes in the intestinal mucosa that increase the intestinal permeability of bacteria and their products. Portal hypertensive gastro-enteropathy is associated with enlarged mucosal and submucosal vessels, as well as inflammatory infiltrates and epithelial erosion (Bellot et al. 2013; Fukui and West 2016).

Another reason for vomiting in connection with hepatitis is vagal stimulation by dislocation of the upper gastrointestinal tract when hepatomegaly is present (Rothuizen and Meyer 2000).

The presumed mechanisms for **PU/PD** have also already been presented in Chapter 39.4.

Another phenomenon that develops in fibrotic-cirrhotic liver remodelling is **icterus**. This is a consequence of mixed conjugated and unconjugated bilirubinaemia. The physiological serum bilirubin concentration in dogs is very low at 0–0.5 mg/dl.

A clear, clinically visible jaundice only occurs at serum bilirubin levels of 2–3 mg/dl. The yellowing of the blood plasma can already be perceived at 1.5–2.0 mg/dl. Causal factors are cholestatic changes due to the morphological remodelling of the liver, haemolytic changes and disturbances in renal bilirubin excretion caused by a hepato-renal syndrome.

The aetiology of haemolytic **anaemia** in patients with chronic hepatitis or liver cirrhosis is multifactorial and may be a consequence of red blood cell destruction by splenic sequestration, by disseminated intravascular coagulation (DIC) or by acanthocyte formation. The mechanism of acanthocyte formation is thought to be an alteration in lipid metabolism on the red cell membrane, resulting in the characteristic morphology that has a tendency to haemolysis. It has been observed that in liver disease the erythrocyte membrane has an increased ratio of cholesterol to phospholipid. This is partly due to the fact that in liver disease the activity of serum lecithin cholesterol acyltransferase, an enzyme that converts free cholesterol to cholesterol esters, is reduced and consequently free cholesterol is increased (Privitera and Meli 2016).

In hepato-renal syndrome, there is a reversible decrease in glomerular filtration rate due to renal vasoconstriction. The basis is formed by the compensatory mechanisms of cirrhotic ascites. Pathogenetically, portal hypertension, as well as hypoalbuminaemia, which is due to the reduced protein synthesis of the liver, with reduction of the colloid osmotic pressure, play a role in the development of ascites. Hypovolaemia leads to activation of the renin-angiotensin-aldosterone system, ADH (antidiuretic hormone) and catecholamines. Activation of these regulatory mechanisms leads to sodium and fluid reabsorption and renal vasoconstriction.

The formation of **ascites** as a sign of advanced liver cirrhosis is essentially based on two mechanisms. The morphological change in the cirrhotic liver increases the vascular resistance in the portal vessels. This increases the pressure in the splanchnic system, resulting in portal hypertension. Initially, portal hypertension develops as a consequence of increased intrahepatic vascular resistance caused by chronic liver disease leading to several pathological events in the sinusoidal circulation, such as stenosis due to fibrosis, microvascular thrombosis, dysfunction of sinusoidal endothelial cells and activation of hepatic Kupffer cells. In addition to hepatic vessels, mesenteric vessels are also involved in portal hypertension (McConnell and Iwakiri 2018).

Another trigger of ascites is the **hypoalbuminaemia** present in connection with the developing functional insufficiency of the liver. This, as well as the reduced **urea** concentration and **coagulopathy**, are consequences of the insufficiency. Hypoalbuminaemia reduces the oncotic pressure and, in cooperation with portal hypertension, leads to ascites.

Leukocytosis and elevated liver enzymes occur in chronic hepatitis and liver cirrhosis, particularly in the inflammatory form, and reflect the activity of the immune system and the disruption of liver cell integrity (Figure 39.3.2).

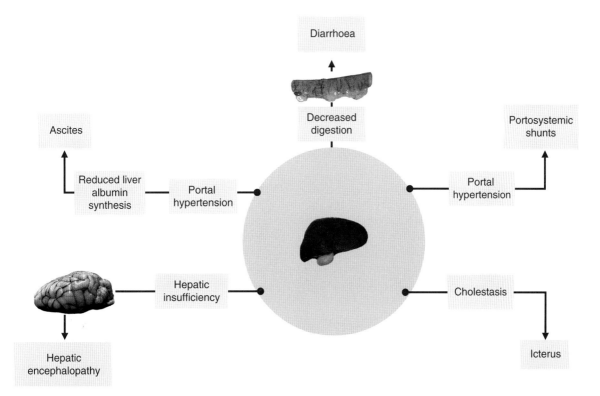

Figure 39.3.2 Pathophysiology of liver cirrhosis.

Therapy

Symptom	Therapy
Inflammation	Anti-inflammatory drugs (e.g. Corticoids)
Fibrosis	Anti-fibrotics (e.g. Corticoids)
Vomiting	Antiemetics (e.g. Maropitant)
Hepatopretectants	Ursodeoxycholic acid, SAM, Silimarien

References

Bataller, R. and Brenner, D.A. (2005). Liver fibrosis. *The Journal of Clinical Investigation* 115 (2): 209–218. https://doi.org/10.1172/JCI24282.

Bellot, P., Francés, R., and Such, J. (2013). Pathological bacterial translocation in cirrhosis: pathophysiology, diagnosis and clinical implications. *Liver International* 33 (1): 31–39. https://doi.org/10.1111/liv.12021.

Bexfield, N.H., Andres-Abdo, C., Scase, T.J. et al. (2011). Chronic hepatitis in the English Springer Spaniel: clinical presentation, histological description and outcome. *The Veterinary Record* 169 (16): 415. https://doi.org/10.1136/vr.d4665.

Dyggve, H., Meri, S., Spillmann, T. et al. (2017). Antihistone autoantibodies in Dobermans with hepatitis. *Journal of Veterinary Internal Medicine* 31 (6): 1717–1723. http://dx.doi.org/10.1111/jvim.14838.

Fukui, H. and Wiest, R. (2016). Changes of intestinal functions in liver cirrhosis. *Inflammatory Intestinal Diseases* 1 (1): 24–40. https://doi.org/10.1159/000444436.

Gerke, I., Kaup, F.J., and Neumann, S. (2018). Evaluation of serum insulin-like growth factor-1 and 26S proteasome concentrations in healthy dogs and dogs with chronic diseases depending on body condition score. *Research in Veterinary Science* 118: 484–490. https://doi.org/10.1016/j.rvsc.2018.04.009.

Ikeda, K., Wakahara, T., Wang, Y.Q. et al. (1999). In vitro migratory potential of rat quiescent hepatic stellate cells and its augmentation by cell activation. *Hepatology (Baltimore, Md.)* 29 (6): 1760–1767. https://doi.org/10.1002/hep.510290640.

Martin-Murphy, B.V., Holt, M.P., and Ju, C. (2010). The role of damage associated molecular pattern molecules in acetaminophen-induced liver injury in mice. *Toxicology Letters* 192 (3): 387–394. https://doi.org/10.1016/j.toxlet.2009.11.016.

McConnell, M. and Iwakiri, Y. (2018). Biology of portal hypertension. *Hepatology International* 12 (Suppl 1): 11–23. https://doi.org/10.1007/s12072-017-9826-x.

Pessayre, D., Fromenty, B., Berson, A. et al. (2012). Central role of mitochondria in drug-induced liver injury. *Drug Metabolism Reviews* 44 (1): 34–87. https://doi.org/10.3109/03602532.2011.604086.

Privitera, G. and Meli, G. (2016). An unusual cause of anemia in cirrhosis: spur cell anemia, a case report with review of literature. *Gastroenterology and Hepatology from Bed to Bench* 9 (4): 335–339.

Rothuizen, J. and Meyer, H.P. (2000). History, physical examination, and signs of liver diseases. In: *Textbook of Veterinary Internal Medicine (Hrsg)*, 5e (ed. S.J. Ettinger and E.C. Feldmann), 1272–1277. Philadelphia: Aufl., W.B. Saunders Company.

Schuppan, D. (2015). Liver fibrosis: common mechanisms and antifibrotic therapies. *Clinics and Research in Hepatology and Gastroenterology* 39 (Suppl 1): S51–S59. https://doi.org/10.1016/j.clinre.2015.05.005.

Shaw, P.J., Ganey, P.E., and Roth, R.A. (2010). Idiosyncratic drug-induced liver injury and the role of inflammatory stress with an emphasis on an animal model of trovafloxacin hepatotoxicity. *Toxicological Sciences: An Official Journal of the Society of Toxicology* 118 (1): 7–18. https://doi.org/10.1093/toxsci/kfq168.

Tailor, A., Faulkner, L., Naisbitt, D.J., and Park, B.K. (2015). The chemical, genetic and immunological basis of idiosyncratic drug-induced liver injury. *Human & Experimental Toxicology* 34 (12): 1310–1317. http://dx.doi.org/10.1177/0960327115606529.

Verne, G.N., Soldevia-Pico, C., Robinson, M.E. et al. (2004). Autonomic dysfunction and gastroparesis in cirrhosis. *Journal of Clinical Gastroenterology* 38 (1): 72–76. https://doi.org/10.1097/00004836-200401000-00015.

Weiss, D.J., Armstrong, P.J., and Mruthyunjaya, A. (1995). Anti-liver membrane protein antibodies in dogs with chronic hepatitis. *Journal of Veterinary Internal Medicine* 9 (4): 267–271. https://doi.org/10.1111/j.1939-1676.1995.tb01078.x.

Wewering, F. (2017). Characterisation of chemical-induced Drug-Induced Liver Injury (DILI). Diss Free University Berlin.

Further Reading

Dirksen, K., Spee, B., Penning, L.C. et al. (2017). Gene expression patterns in the progression of canine copper-associated chronic hepatitis. *PLoS One* 12 (5): e0176826.

Eulenberg, V.M. and Lidbury, J.A. (2018). Hepatic fibrosis in dogs. *Journal of Veterinary Internal Medicine* 32 (1): 26–41. https://doi.org/10.1111/jvim.14891.

Spee, B., Arends, B., van den Ingh, T.S. et al. (2006). Copper metabolism and oxidative stress in chronic inflammatory and cholestatic liver diseases in dogs. *Journal of Veterinary Internal Medicine* 20 (5): 1085–1092. https://doi.org/10.1892/0891-6640 (2006)20[1085,cmaosi]2.0.co;2.

Sterczer, A., Gaál, T., Perge, E., and Rothuizen, J. (2001). Chronic hepatitis in the dog—a review. *The Veterinary Quarterly* 23 (4): 148–152. https://doi.org/10.1080/01652176.2001.9695104.

Webster, C.R.L., Center, S.A., Cullen, J.M. et al. (2019). ACVIM consensus statement on the diagnosis and treatment of chronic hepatitis in dogs. *Journal of Veterinary Internal Medicine* 33 (3): 1173–1200. https://doi.org/10.1111/jvim.15467.

39.4

Portosystemic Shunts/Hepatoencephalopathy

Definition

Portosystemic shunts are direct links between the portal vein system and the systemic venous system, bypassing the liver. Hepatoencephalopathy is a central neurological syndrome that develops as a result of liver dysfunction, often due to a portosystemic shunt. Portosystemic shunts and hepatoencephalopathy are essentially described in dogs.

Aetiology

The exact causality of the congenital portosystemic shunt in dogs and cats is unknown. In humans, a developmental disorder between the fourth and tenth week of embryonic development, during which hepatic and systemic vessels develop, is suspected as the cause (Tang et al. 2020). Molecular genetic studies in dogs have identified some candidate genes for shunt development (van Steenbeek et al. 2013).

Morphologically, the majority of congenital portosystemic shunts in large breeds are intrahepatic as a persistent venous duct or as a central intrahepatic shunt or right lateral intrahepatic shunt. Small breeds, on the other hand, more often have a congenital extrahepatic shunt as a porto-caval, porto-azygos or porto-phrenic variant. The congenital forms differ from the acquired forms in that portal hypertension occurs in the latter. This can lead to the formation of collateral vessels between the portal vein system and the systemic venous system within two to three months. Causes of acquired portosystemic shunt are remodelling processes in the liver in chronic hepatitis, liver fibrosis/cirrhosis, neoplasia or portal vein occlusion as thrombosis. In contrast to dogs, shunt diseases are rare in cats and tend to occur extrahepatically (Figure 39.4.1).

Congenital	Acquired
Intrahepatic small breeds	Chronic hepatitis
Extrahepatic large breeds	Liver fibrosis
	Cirrhosis
	Liver neoplasms

Pathogenesis

The vascular bypass of the liver has several consequences. Firstly, the liver is supplied with a reduced amount of blood and growth factors. This leads to reduced development in the liver and thus to limited function. Furthermore, with a portosystemic bypass of the liver, metabolites that would be metabolised in the liver accumulate in the organism (Table 39.4.1).

Textbook of Small Animal Pathophysiology, First Edition. Stephan Neumann.
© 2025 John Wiley & Sons Ltd. Published 2025 by John Wiley & Sons Ltd.

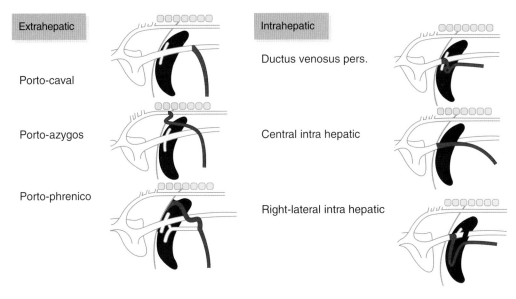

Figure 39.4.1 Types of portosystemic shunts.

Table 39.4.1 Metabolites with significance in hepatoencephalic syndrome.

Ammonia
Benzodiazepines
Aromatic amino acids
Mercaptans
Short-chain fatty acids
Phenols
Manganese

Diagnostics

Clinical signs	Clinical pathology	Imaging	Histopathology	Microbiology
Depressive behaviour Seizures	Significantly increased NH_3 and bile acids	**Ultrasonography** Visualisation of the shunt vessel intra- or extrahepatic	Not necessary	Not necessary

Pathophysiologic Consequences

The pathophysiologic consequences of a portosystemic shunt affect the organs of the gastrointestinal tract and, in the case of hepatoencephalopathy, also the central nervous system.

Influenced organ systems	Clinical symptoms	Clinical pathological alterations
Gastrointestinal system	Ataxia	Anaemia
Hepatobiliary system	Seizures	
Urinary tract	Circling	Hypoalbuminaemia
	Coma	Coagulopathy
Endocrine system		
	Hypersalivation	Hyperammonaemia
Central nervous system	Vomiting	Decreased urea
Haematological system	Diarrhoea	Hypoglycaemia
		Hypocholesterolaemia
	PU/PD	
	Dysuria	

Source: Hausmann (2017).

Many of the symptoms (**ataxia, seizures, circling, coma**) that occur as a result of a portosystemic shunt are due to a hepatoencephalic syndrome. Various mechanisms lead to the development of neurological symptoms. One mechanism is the accumulation of neurotoxic mediators, which are present in increased concentrations in the blood due to reduced liver function or bypassing of the liver. Ammonia seems to play a central role in this. It is formed in the intestine as a result of microbial protein degradation and amino acid deamination and reaches the liver in high concentrations (200–400 µmol/l) via the portal system. There, it is degraded via the urea cycle or glutamine synthesis. In the systemic blood, the ammonia concentration of approximately 40 µmol/l is clearly below the portal concentration. Under physiological conditions, ammonium ions predominate in the organism (98%) and only a small proportion consists of gaseous ammonia.

Ammonia can freely pass cell membranes and the ammonium ions use K^+-channels or transporters for transmembrane transport. As a result of a portosystemic shunt, ammonia and ammonium ions enter the brain in increased concentrations via the blood-brain barrier. At the astrocyte membrane, the Na^+-K^+-ATPase is activated as a result of the increased concentration of ammonium ions. Potassium and ammonium ions enter the cell and sodium ions are transported to the outside.

With the sodium, water molecules are discharged and shrinkage of the astrocytes occurs. At the same time, there is an excess of positive charges in the astrocytes, whereupon Cl^- is transported into the cells. The resulting depolarisation selectively impairs cortical inhibitory networks. Another mechanism is based on the intracellular excess of ammonium ions in the astrocytes. The consequence is increased glutamine synthesis (Hadjihambi et al. 2014, 2018).

Glutamine can accumulate intracellularly and induce osmotic swelling of astrocytes; at the same time extracellular glutamine acts as a neurotransmitter.

In this context, there is an increased release of proinflammatory cytokines from the astroglia (TNF-α, IL-1, IL-6). This has a supportive effect on the development of HE (Shawcross et al. 2010).

Depending on the extent of the clinical symptoms, four different degrees of HE are distinguished in human medicine:

1) Reduced behaviour, polyuria
2) Salivation, disorientation, blindness
3) Stupor, salivation, epileptic strokes
4) Coma

Disturbances in digestion are held responsible for the gastrointestinal symptoms of **vomiting** and **diarrhoea**. Due to the reduced liver function, fewer bile acids are secreted, which reduces intestinal lipid absorption and can thus trigger osmotic diarrhoea.

If the portosystemic shunt is a consequence of portal hypertension, different mechanisms are described that lead to intestinal disorders. Essentially, motility disorders, dysbiosis and hyperpermeability are observed (Fukui and Wiest 2016).

The motility disorders observed in connection with portal hypertension are primarily prolonged transit times in the intestine due to reduced gastrointestinal motility. This, in turn, is probably due to a dysfunction of the autonomic nervous system in the sense of parasympatholysis (Verne et al. 2004). The delayed motility in the intestine induces a 'bacterial overgrowth syndrome' which is associated with structural and functional changes in the intestinal mucosa that increase the intestinal permeability of bacteria and their products. Portal hypertensive gastroenteropathy is associated with enlarged mucosal and submucosal vessels, as well as inflammatory infiltrates and epithelial erosion (Bellot et al. 2013; Fukui and Wiest 2016).

The **PU/PD** observed in the context of a portosystemic shunt is explained by several mechanisms. First, the reduction of urea synthesis in the liver seems to lead to a lowered osmotic gradient in the renal medulla, which reduces the filtration pressure in Henle's loop. As a result, less water is reabsorbed and diuresis occurs. Polyuria is followed secondarily by polydipsia.

Another mechanism appears to trigger PU/PD via impaired neuroendocrine function. Dogs with portosystemic shunt and HE develop increased pituitary activity which may be caused by false neurotransmitters.

Chronic hypercortisolism which is seen in cases of portosystemic shunt and HE, in turn, is associated with impaired regulation of the release of ADH (Rothuizen et al. 1995).

Dysuria can be the result of urinary calculi, which are usually ammonium urates in the portosystemic shunt. Uric acid is formed when purine is broken down in the liver via various intermediates, such as xanthine.

This in turn is converted into the soluble allantoin.

In liver dysfunction, the formation of soluble allantoin is limited.

This leads to an excess of uric acid. With a corresponding partner, such as ammonia, crystals can be formed in the urine.

The most common haematological abnormality in dogs with congenital portosystemic shunts is microcytic hypochromic anaemia. The mechanism is not due to an absolute iron deficiency, as dogs with portosystemic shunts usually have high haemosiderin concentrations in the liver. However, since they have low serum iron concentrations, the cause is a reduced synthesis of transport proteins, such as transferrin (Bunch et al. 1995; Yiannikourides and Latunde-Dada 2019).

Reduced serum concentrations of **urea, albumin, glucose** and **cholesterol** are collectively explained by reduced liver synthesis in congenital portosystemic shunt. A similar explanation is given for the presence of blood coagulation disorders associated with liver disease. The liver is the site of synthesis for numerous coagulation factors, as well as factors in fibrinolysis. Accordingly, liver dysfunction can influence primary and secondary haemostasis as well as fibrinolysis.

Changes that have been described in connection with the congenital portosystemic shunt are a reduction in platelets, protein C and antithrombin III, while Willebrand factor and factor VIII are increased. Such patients also show hypercoagulability (Webster 2017).

The cause of thrombocytopenia in acquired portosystemic shunt with portal hypertension is thought to be sequestration of platelets into the spleen. In the congenital form, a deficiency of thrombopoietin is more likely to be observed. Thrombopoietin is produced in the liver, kidney, bone marrow and striated muscle, triggered by a deficiency of platelets. In bone marrow, it induces thrombocytopoiesis. The differentiation of megakaryocytes is controlled by thrombopoietin via a receptor in their cell membrane. Binding of thrombopoietin to platelet cell membrane terminates its action (Poordad 2007).

Changes in the coagulation factors, as well as those of fibrinolysis, are seen as a consequence of a reduced synthesis capacity of the liver.

Therapy

Symptom	Therapy
Hyperammonaemia	Reduction intestinal bacteria; (e.g. Amoxycillin, Metronidazole, Lactulose)
Shunt	Surgical closure (Ameroid constrictor, cellophane banding)

References

Bellot, P., Francés, R., and Such, J. (2013). Pathological bacterial translocation in cirrhosis: pathophysiology, diagnosis and clinical implications. *Liver International: Official Journal of the International Association for the Study of the Liver* 33 (1): 31–39. https://doi.org/10.1111/liv.12021.

Bunch, S.E., Jordan, H.L., Sellon, R.K. et al. (1995). Characterization of iron status in young dogs with portosystemic shunt. *American Journal of VeterinaryResearch* 56: 853–858.

Fukui, H. and Wiest, R. (2016). Changes of intestinal functions in liver cirrhosis. *Inflammatory Intestinal Diseases* 1 (1): 24–40. https://doi.org/10.1159/000444436.

Hadjihambi, A., Rose, C.F., and Jalan, R. (2014). Novel insights into ammonia-mediated neurotoxicity pointing to potential new therapeutic strategies. *Hepatology (Baltimore, Md.)* 60 (3): 1101–1103. https://doi.org/10.1002/hep.27282.

Hadjihambi, A., Arias, N., Sheikh, M., and Jalan, R. (2018). Hepatic encephalopathy: a critical current review. *Hepatology International* 12 (Suppl 1): 135–147. https://doi.org/10.1007/s12072-017-9812-3.

Hausmann, L. (2017). Transcutaneous fluorometric determination of indocyanine green elimination as a dynamic liver function test in dogs with congenital extrahepatic protosystemic shunt. Dissertation University of Giessen.

Poordad, F. (2007). Review article: thrombocytopenia in chronic liver disease. *Alimentary Pharmacology & Therapeutics* 26 (Suppl 1): 5–11. https://doi.org/10.1111/j.1365-2036.2007.03510.x.

Rothuizen, J., Biewenga, W.J., and Mol, J.A. (1995). Chronic glucocorticoid excess and impaired osmoregulation of vasopressin release in dogs with hepatic encephalopathy. *Domestic Animal Endocrinology* 12 (1): 13–24. https://doi.org/10.1016/0739-7240(94)00005-l.

Shawcross, D.L., Shabbir, S.S., Taylor, N.J., and Hughes, R.D. (2010). Ammonia and the neutrophil in the pathogenesis of hepatic encephalopathy in cirrhosis. *Hepatology (Baltimore, Md.)* 51 (3): 1062–1069. https://doi.org/10.1002/hep.23367.

van Steenbeek, F.G., Van den Bossche, L., Grinwis, G.C. et al. (2013). Aberrant gene expression in dogs with portosystemic shunts. *PLoS One* 8 (2): e57662. https://doi.org/10.1371/journal.pone.0057662.

Tang, H., Song, P., Wang, Z. et al. (2020). A basic understanding of congenital extrahepatic portosystemic shunt: incidence, mechanism, complications, diagnosis, and treatment. *Intractable & Rare Diseases Research* 9 (2): 64–70. https://doi.org/10.5582/irdr.2020.03005.

Verne, G.N., Soldevia-Pico, C., Robinson, M.E. et al. (2004). Autonomic dysfunction and gastroparesis in cirrhosis. *Journal of Clinical Gastroenterology* 38 (1): 72–76. https://doi.org/10.1097/00004836-200401000-00015.

Webster, C.R. (2017). Hemostatic disorders associated with hepatobiliary disease. *The Veterinary Clinics of North America. Small Animal Practice* 47 (3): 601–615. https://doi.org/10.1016/j.cvsm.2016.11.009.

Yiannikourides, A. and Latunde-Dada, G.O. (2019). A short review of iron metabolism and pathophysiology of iron disorders. *Medicines (Basel, Switzerland)* 6 (3): 85. https://doi.org/10.3390/medicines6030085.

Further Reading

Berent, A.C. and Tobias, K.M. (2009). Portosystemic vascular anomalies. *The Veterinary Clinics of North America. Small Animal Practice* 39 (3): 513–541. https://doi.org/10.1016/j.cvsm.2009.02.004.

Buob, S., Johnston, A.N., and Webster, C.R. (2011). Portal hypertension: pathophysiology, diagnosis, and treatment. *Journal of Veterinary Internal Medicine* 25 (2): 169–186. https://doi.org/10.1111/j.1939-1676.2011.00691.x.

Gow, A.G. (2017). Hepatic encephalopathy. *The Veterinary Clinics of North America. Small Animal Practice* 47 (3): 585–599. https://doi.org/10.1016/j.cvsm.2016.11.008.

Sakamoto, Y., Sakai, M., Sato, K., and Watari, T. (2020). Plasma renin activity and aldosterone concentration in dogs with acquired portosystemic collaterals. *Journal of Veterinary Internal Medicine* 34 (1): 139–144. https://doi.org/10.1111/jvim.15661.

39.5

Feline Hepatic Lipidosis

Definition

Hepatic lipidosis is the accumulation of triglycerides in the hepatocytes. It is assumed when more than 50–80% of hepatocytes show fatty vacuoles. The clinical picture is rare in dogs, but a common clinical picture in cats develops in connection with anorexia.

Aetiology

Anorexia is seen as a major aetiological factor, resulting in the development of a disorder in the mobilisation and metabolism of fatty acids. As anorexia is associated with numerous diseases, many severe disease complexes in the cat are also at risk of hepatic lipidosis.

Primary	Secondary
Idiopathic	Diabetes mellitus
	Pancreatitis
	Renal failure
	Gastrointestinal diseases
	Hepatobiliary diseases
	Neoplasia

Pathogenesis

Hepatic lipidosis is a complex metabolic dysfunction of the cat, which in principle results from an increased need for fatty acids in cases of anorexia. The period between reduced food intake and the development of lipidosis is between 2 and 14 days. The consequence of anorexia is an increased secretion of hormones that regulate energy metabolism, such as glucagon, cortisol or catecholamines. These increase the activity of a hormone-sensitive lipase, which releases fatty acids from the abdominal adipose tissue and transports them to the liver via the portal vein. At the same time, a de novo synthesis of fatty acids takes place in the liver. After uptake of the fatty acids by the hepatocytes, they can be transported into the mitochondria with the help of L-carnitine and contribute to energy production there via β-oxidation. Alternatively, the fatty acids can also be transported to other organs via VLDL. If the possibilities of ß-oxidation or transport via VLDL are exceeded

Textbook of Small Animal Pathophysiology, First Edition. Stephan Neumann.
© 2025 John Wiley & Sons Ltd. Published 2025 by John Wiley & Sons Ltd.

due to the increased supply of fatty acids, the fatty acids accumulate and are stored in fat vacuoles. In addition, anorectic cats also show a reduction in protein intake, leading to a deficiency of essential amino acids needed for VLDL formation (Verbrugghe and Bakovic 2013).

Diagnostics

Clinical signs	Clinical pathology	Imaging	Histopathology	Microbiology
Disturbed general condition	Moderate increased liver enzymes Severe increased ALP	**Ultrasonography** Mixed or hyperechogenic liver texture	**Diagnostic** Hepatocytes with pronounced vacuolisation	Not necessary

Pathophysiologic Consequences

In the case of hepatic lipidosis, it is not always clear which symptoms are the cause or consequence of the disease.

Influenced organ systems	Clinical symptoms	Clinical pathological alterations
Hepatobiliary system	Anorexia	Increased liver enzymes
Central nervous system	Lethargy	Increased ALP
	Vomiting	Bilirubinaemia
	Nausea	Decreased urea
	Icterus	Hyperammonaemia
	Dehydration	

The clinical symptoms of **anorexia** and **lethargy**, for example, can be both a cause and a consequence of hepatic lipidosis. The consequence is based on the developing liver insufficiency and can also be accompanied by a hepatoencephalic syndrome. However, in hepatic lipidosis, this appears to be a consequence of a reduced arginine concentration. Arginine is an essential component of the urea cycle. If arginine is missing, the metabolism of ammonia to **urea** is disturbed and **hyperammonaemia** develops. This could also be responsible for the **nausea** and **vomiting**. Vomiting in turn coupled with reduced general condition can cause **dehydration**. The elevated **liver enzymes** are signs of a disturbance of liver cell integrity and the **bilirubinaemia** is a sign of cholestasis. Cholestasis causes marked changes in the cytoskeleton of the hepatocytes. First, the cell structure is disturbed by destruction of the actin filament scaffold. This causes a change in cell structure and cellular transport processes. The latter are also disturbed when, due to cholestasis, the canalicular transport of molecules is disturbed because the transport proteins (e.g. MDR I + II) are expressed less. Furthermore, cholestasis can cause bile flow into the sinusoids via destruction of the tight-junctions (Zollner and Trauner 2008).

The increased activity of the liver enzymes, **ALT** and **AST,** results from increased oxidative stress. This leads to the increased formation of reactive oxygen molecules, which react with the lipids of the cell membrane, among other things and form peroxides. As a result, the membrane structure is lost, leading to increased leakage of initially cytoplasmic enzymes (Itri et al. 2014).

In hepatolipidosis, hepatic lipid metabolism is disturbed. This consists of the uptake of fatty acids across the cell membrane by certain carrier proteins, a de novo synthesis of fatty acids from acetyl-CoA and fatty acid oxidation and is regulated by different proteins and transcription factors. For example, Fatty Acid-Binding Protein 1 (FABP1) is involved in intracellular fatty acid transport.

Fatty acid oxidation is controlled by peroxisome proliferator-activated receptor-alpha (PPAR-α), which reduces intrahepatic lipid content by using lipids as an energy source. While the process occurs mainly in the mitochondria, lipid overload forces a higher degree of fatty acid oxidation in the peroxisomes and cytochromes, generating ROS (Ipsen et al. 2018).

In addition to the elevation of the hepatocellular enzymes ALT, AST, an increased serum activity of **alkaline phosphatase** is typical for feline hepatolipidosis. Alkaline phosphatase is a hydrolase and belongs to the metalloenzymes that cleave phosphoric acid esters in an alkaline environment. It is expressed in different tissues. Within the liver, the enzyme is produced in hepatocytes at the canalicular membrane and by bile duct epithelia. In the case of cholestasis, biliary excretion of ALP into the bile ducts may be reduced, leading to increased serum activities. Another mechanism would be through increased expression of the enzyme. In cholestasis, human hepatocytes show increased expression of ALP at the hepatocyte canalicular membrane. The process could be triggered by an increased activity of cAMP. Under the influence of bile acids, cholestasis may destroy the hepatocyte membrane with the increased ALP expression, releasing ALP (Levitt et al. 2022).

Therapy

Symptom	Therapy
Dehydration	Fluid therapy
Anorexia	Diet, feeding via oesophageal tube
Vomiting	Antiemetics (e.g. Ondansetron, Maropitant, Metoclopramide)
Metabolic disturbance	L-carnitine, arginine

References

Ipsen, D.H., Lykkesfeldt, J., and Tveden-Nyborg, P. (2018). Molecular mechanisms of hepatic lipid accumulation in non-alcoholic fatty liver disease. *Cellular and Molecular Life Sciences: CMLS* 75 (18): 3313–3327. https://doi.org/10.1007/s00018-018-2860-6.

Itri, R., Junqueira, H.C., Mertins, O., and Baptista, M.S. (2014). Membrane changes under oxidative stress: the impact of oxidized lipids. *Biophysical Reviews* 6 (1): 47–61. https://doi.org/10.1007/s12551-013-0128-9.

Levitt, M.D., Hapak, S.M., and Levitt, D.G. (2022). Alkaline phosphatase pathophysiology with emphasis on the seldom-discussed role of defective elimination in unexplained elevations of serum ALP – a case report and literature review. *Clinical and Experimental Gastroenterology* 15: 41–49. https://doi.org/10.2147/CEG.S345531.

Verbrugghe, A. and Bakovic, M. (2013). Peculiarities of one-carbon metabolism in the strict carnivorous cat and the role in feline hepatic lipidosis. *Nutrients* 5 (7): 2811–2835. https://doi.org/10.3390/nu5072811.

Zollner, G. and Trauner, M. (2008). Mechanisms of cholestasis. *Clinics in Liver Disease* 12 (1): 1–vii. https://doi.org/10.1016/j.cld.2007.11.010.

Further Reading

Biourge, V.C., Groff, J.M., Munn, R.J. et al. (1994). Experimental induction of hepatic lipidosis in cats. *American Journal of Veterinary Research* 55 (9): 1291–1302.

Dimski, D.S. (1997). Feline hepatic lipidosis. *Seminars in Veterinary Medicine and Surgery (Small Animal)* 12 (1): 28–33. https://doi.org/10.1016/s1096-2867(97)80041-2.

Mazaki-Tovi, M., Abood, S.K., Segev, G., and Schenck, P.A. (2013). Alterations in adipokines in feline hepatic lipidosis. *Journal of Veterinary Internal Medicine* 27 (2): 242–249. https://doi.org/10.1111/jvim.12055.

Valtolina, C. and Favier, R.P. (2017). Feline hepatic lipidosis. *The Veterinary Clinics of North America. Small Animal Practice* 47 (3): 683–702. https://doi.org/10.1016/j.cvsm.2016.11.014.

39.6

Cholangiohepatitis

Definition

Cholangiohepatitis are inflammations of the liver parenchyma involving the bile duct area. They can be neutrophilic or lymphoplasma cellular.

Aetiology

Two types of cholangiohepatitis are also differentiated aetiologically; in the neutrophilic-suppurative form, infections are seen as the causative factor. In contrast, the lymphoplasma cellular non-suppurative form often coexists with pancreatitis and inflammatory bowel disease (IBD). Cholangiohepatitis is more common in cats than in dogs.

Suppurative	Non-suppurative
E. coli (C,D)	Autoimmunity
Enterobacter (C,D)	
Streptococci (C,D)	
Klebsiella (C)	
Clostridia (C,D)	
Bacteroides (C)	
Toxoplasma (C)	
Campylobacter (D)	

D – Dog, C – Cat

Pathogenesis

Neutrophilic cholangiohepatitis can occur as an acute or chronic form and is characterised by an infiltration of neutrophilic granulocytes into the bile ducts and bile duct parenchyma. In the acute form, associated changes are increased blood flow and inflammatory oedema; whereas in the chronic form, fibrotic changes are present. The changes may be diffuse or local within the liver. The aetiopathogenesis of neutrophilic cholangiohepatitis in the cat is not fully understood but seems to be triggered by obstructive changes in the bile ducts leading to slow bile flow or even bile stasis. Ruptures of the tight-junction allow bile flow into the liver parenchyma and induce an inflammatory response. Causally or associated with neutrophilic cholangio-hepatitis is a bacterial infection. The bacterial pathogens are primarily intestine-associated bacteria. These can enter the liver parenchyma via the bile duct system or be spread haematogenously into the liver after overcoming the intestinal barrier.

Textbook of Small Animal Pathophysiology, First Edition. Stephan Neumann.
© 2025 John Wiley & Sons Ltd. Published 2025 by John Wiley & Sons Ltd.

Initially, one assumes a bacterial overgrowth syndrome. The consequence is that the intestinal barrier is overcome by the bacterial load. The tight-junctions as a structural connection between the mucosa cells are destroyed, which increases the permeability for bacteria. Also, a reduction of the mucus layer, as well as a reduced expression of antimicrobial peptides (AMPs) leads to a reduced defence situation on the intestinal wall. Bacterial invasion triggers a local inflammatory process. This is initiated by sessile dendritic cells and macrophages and leads to cytokine release. Subsequently, further inflammatory cells are recruited. The inflammatory process increases local blood flow, which facilitates bacterial flushing and leads to bacteraemia (Janeczko et al. 2008; Lidbury et al. 2020; Simbrunner et al. 2021).

The non-suppurative form is distinguished from the suppurative cholangiohepatitis. This is characterised by infiltration with lymphocytes and plasma cells periportally and in the area of the bile ducts. In addition, fibrotic remodelling takes place in the parenchyma. The course of the disease tends to be chronic. An immune-mediated process is seen as the causal factor. This is supported by the simultaneous occurrence of IBD. The disease process is similar to that of human sclerosing cholangitis. Here, too, an immune-mediated process is assumed (Day 1998). This is composed of a susceptibility and a corresponding trigger. The predisposition seems to be due to changes in the genes of the major histocompatibility complex and certain HLA haplotypes. The trigger is probably a bacterial translocation from the intestine, which is called 'leaky gut'. The developing inflammation is carried by proinflammatory cytokines, such as TNF-α, IL-1 and IL-6, as well as by TGF and CD^{4+} and CD^{8+} T cells (Spurkland et al. 1999; Folseraas et al. 2011; Gidwaney et al. 2017).

Diagnostics

Clinical signs	Clinical pathology	Imaging	Histopathology	Microbiology
Unspecific	Moderate elevated liver enzymes	**Ultrasonography** Mixed echogenicity of liver parenchyma	**Diagnostic**, evidence of infiltration of inflammatory cells into the liver parenchyma.	Mostly not necessary Maybe culture of bile

Pathophysiologic Consequences

The pathophysiologic consequences of both syndromes are strongly influenced by the associated remodelling processes, such as fibrosis and jaundice and are variable in the course of the disease.

Influenced organ systems	Clinical symptoms	Clinical pathological alterations
Gastrointestinal system	Anorexia	Leucocytosis (supp.)
Hepatobiliary system	Lethargy	Increased liver enzymes
Pancreas	Vomiting	Hyperglobulinaemia (non-supp.)
	Diarrhoea	Bilirubinaemia
	Abdominal pain	
	Icterus	

Source: Boland and Beatty (2017).

The clinical findings are similar in cats suffering from the suppurative and non-suppurative forms of cholangiohepatitis. The difference is in the laboratory parameters, primarily in the leucocytes, which are elevated in the suppurative form. In the non-suppurative form, on the other hand, hyperglobulinaemia is regularly found.

Anorexia and **lethargy** are frequently observed symptoms in liver diseases with different causes. They have already been described in acute liver failure and chronic hepatitis. They are possibly the consequence of disturbances in various metabolic processes.

The cause is thought to be cytotoxic substances that are supposed to be eliminated by biotransformation in the liver, but end up in the whole body due to metabolic insufficiency. In the brain, some of these substances can produce central nervous symptoms by occupying receptors and influencing nerve conduction. These substances include true (e.g. γ-aminobutyric acid, GABA) and false neurotransmitters (e.g. ammonia, octopamine, phenylethylamine). In the present case, the anorexia could have a further influence on the symptoms via a developing liver lipidosis.

Diarrhoea, vomiting and **abdominal pain** may be caused by associated IBD or pancreatitis. The mechanism by which IBD causes diarrhoea involves several of the primary diarrhoeal causalities. These include increased secretion, decreased absorption, increased permeability and increased motility. Mediated by proinflammatory cytokines, the inflammatory response leads to swelling of enterocytes, reducing their absorption properties. Furthermore, the inflammatory reaction leads to an intracellular increase in the second messengers cAMP and Ca^{2+}. These messengers activate Cl channels, leading to hypersecretion. Due to alterations of the cytoskeleton, intercellular tight-junctions are lost and paracellular permeability is increased (Michelangeli and Ruiz 2003). Abdominal pain is a common symptom in pancreatitis. The irritation of intra-pancreatic nociceptors is a mechanism that occurs when mediators, such as serotonin, bradykinin or calcium are released from destroyed acinar cells (Demir et al. 2011).

Icterus is the consequence of disease-associated cholestasis. **Bilirubinaemia** can also be seen in this context.

A disturbance of the hepatogenic excretion of the bile components is seen as an essential mechanism. This is reduced by the influence of proinflammatory cytokines, such as TNF-α or IL-1. The cytokines have a reducing effect on the expression of hepatocellular transport proteins. In addition, the cytokines cause a reduction of aquaporins at the canalicular hepatocyte membrane, which impedes bile flow and supports cholestasis (Chand and Sanyal 2007; Ghenu et al. 2022).

The increase in **liver enzymes** reflects the inflammatory process in the liver. Liver enzymes are released more frequently by 'surface blebs' than by necrotic cell death. The bleb formation is due to a disruption of the cytoskeleton. This, in turn, can result directly from the action of inflammatory mediators or be the consequence of an energy deficiency due to ATP depletion. The energy deficiency leads to actin depolarisation, resulting in cellular structural loss with cellular blebs. These blebs can rupture intravascularly, releasing cellular enzymes (Gores et al. 1990).

Finally, **hyperglobulinaemia** is particularly noticeable in the non-suppurative form. Liver diseases influence the globulins and their fractions. In serum electrophoresis, the β +γ globulins are often elevated. The former are often transferrin and complement; the latter are immunoglobulins. This reflects the immunological process that takes place in the liver (Figure 39.6.1).

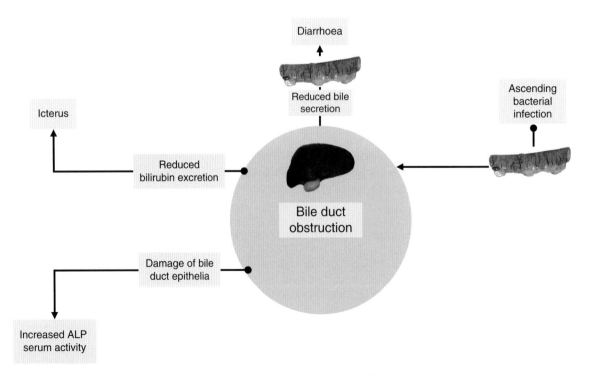

Figure 39.6.1 Pathogenesis and pathophysiologic consequences of cholangitis.

Therapy

Symptom	Therapy
Infection (suppurative)	Antibiotics (e.g. Amoxycillin, Metronidazole)
Inflammation (non-suppurative)	Corticosteroids
Hepatoprotection	S-adenosylmethionine (SAM), ursodeoxycholic acid

References

Chand, N. and Sanyal, A.J. (2007). Sepsis-induced cholestasis. *Hepatology (Baltimore, Md.)* 45 (1): 230–241. https://doi.org/10.1002/hep.21480.

Day, M.J. (1998). Immunohistochemical characterization of the lesions of feline progressive lymphocytic cholangitis/cholangiohepatitis. *Journal of Comparative Pathology* 119 (2): 135–147. https://doi.org/10.1016/s0021-9975(98)80058-3.

Demir, I.E., Tieftrunk, E., Maak, M. et al. (2011). Pain mechanisms in chronic pancreatitis: of a master and his fire. *Langenbeck's Archives of Surgery* 396 (2): 151–160. https://doi.org/10.1007/s00423-010-0731-1.

Folseraas, T., Melum, E., Franke, A., and Karlsen, T.H. (2011). Genetics in primary sclerosing cholangitis. *Best Practice & Research. Clinical Gastroenterology* 25 (6): 713–726. https://doi.org/10.1016/j.bpg.2011.09.010.

Ghenu, M.I., Dragoş, D., Manea, M.M. et al. (2022). Pathophysiology of sepsis-induced cholestasis: areview. *JGH Open: An Open Access Journal of Gastroenterology and Hepatology* 6 (6): 378–387. https://doi.org/10.1002/jgh3.12771.

Gidwaney, N.G., Pawa, S., and Das, K.M. (2017). Pathogenesis and clinical spectrum of primary sclerosing cholangitis. *World Journal of Gastroenterology* 23 (14): 2459–2469. https://doi.org/10.3748/wjg.v23.i14.2459.

Gores, G.J., Herman, B., and Lemasters, J.J. (1990). Plasma membrane bleb formation and rupture: a common feature of hepatocellular injury. *Hepatology (Baltimore, Md.)* 11 (4): 690–698. https://doi.org/10.1002/hep.1840110425.

Janeczko, S., Atwater, D., Bogel, E. et al. (2008). The relationship of mucosal bacteria to duodenal histopathology, cytokine mRNA, and clinical disease activity in cats with inflammatory bowel disease. *Veterinary Microbiology* 128 (1–2): 178–193. https://doi.org/10.1016/j.vetmic.2007.10.014.

Lidbury, J.A., Mooyottu, S., and Jergens, A.E. (2020). Triaditis: truth and consequences. *The Veterinary Clinics of North America. Small Animal Practice* 50 (5): 1135–1156. https://doi.org/10.1016/j.cvsm.2020.06.008.

Michelangeli, F. and Ruiz, M. (2003). I, 2. Physiology and pathophysiology of the gut in relation to viral diarrhea. *Perspectives in Medical Virology.* 9: 23–50. https://doi.org/10.1016/S0168-7069(03)09003-7.

Simbrunner, B., Trauner, M., and Reiberger, T. (2021). Review article: therapeutic aspects of bile acid signalling in the gut-liver axis. *Alimentary Pharmacology & Therapeutics* 54 (10): 1243–1262. https://doi.org/10.1111/apt.16602.

Spurkland, A., Saarinen, S., Boberg, K.M. et al. (1999). HLA class II haplotypes in primary sclerosing cholangitis patients from five European populations. *Tissue Antigens* 53 (5): 459–469. https://doi.org/10.1034/j.1399-0039.1999.530502.x.

Further Reading

Boland, L. and Beatty, J. (2017). Feline cholangitis. *The Veterinary Clinics of North America. Small Animal Practice* 47 (3): 703–724. https://doi.org/10.1016/j.cvsm.2016.11.015.

Centre, S.A., Randolph, J.F., Warner, K.L. et al. (2022). Clinical features, concurrent disorders, and survival time in cats with suppurative cholangitis-cholangiohepatitis syndrome. *Journal of the American Veterinary Medical Association* 260 (2): 212–227. https://doi.org/10.2460/javma.20.10.0555.

Jaffey, J.A. (2022). Feline cholangitis/cholangiohepatitis complex. *The Journal of Small Animal Practice* 63 (8): 573–589. https://doi.org/10.1111/jsap.13508.

40

Exocrine Pancreas

40.1

Physiological Functions and General Pathophysiology of Organ Insufficiency

Functions

Two main functions of the pancreas can be differentiated, the endocrine and the exocrine function. The endocrine function of the pancreas is explained in Chapter 43.5.1. Here we explain the exocrine function (Figure 40.1.1).

Formation of the Digestive Secretion

The pancreas is a lobulated organ that lies adjacent to the duodenum and secretes an alkaline secretion into the lumen of the small intestine via a branched duct system. At the beginning of each duct is an acinus with enzyme-producing acinar cells. These produce precursors of digestive enzymes and store them in vacuoles on the apical cell membrane.

To protect the pancreas from self-digestion, the enzymes are synthesised in an inactive form, stored in vacuoles and blocked by protease inhibitors of the acinar cells (Table 40.1.1, Figure 40.1.2).

Control of Pancreatic Secretion

The formation of the enzyme precursors is stimulated by parasympathetic activity or hormones (secretin, cholecystokinin), the release of which is associated with food intake. The effect on the acinar cells is given by receptors on their basal cell membrane. The hormone influence has a stimulating effect on enzyme synthesis via a receptor and a second messenger (e.g. cAMP). The storage of the enzymes takes place as inactive precursors, which are stored in vesicles at the apical membrane. Under the influence of Ca^{2+}, these fuse with the cell membrane and the enzymes are released into the ductal system via exocytosis. The secretion of the acinar cells is rich in enzymes and salts. Chloride ions are secreted by the acinar cells via $Na^+/K^+/Cl^-$ cotransport. Sodium ions follow the negative charge gradient established by the chloride ions and enter the duct lumen via tight-junctions between the acinar cells.

There, the secretion becomes more voluminous and alkaline due to a bicarbonate and water secretion of the duct epithelia.

The bicarbonate secretion is influenced by parasympathetic activity, gastrointestinal hormones and luminal factors. Luminal factors include intraductal pressure and Ca^{2+} concentration. Calcium influences bicarbonate secretion via a secretin-dependent receptor on the basal epithelial cell membrane that uses cAMP as a second messenger (Ishiguro et al. 2012).

Pancreatic bicarbonate secretion makes more protons available for the synthesis of gastric acid (Figure 40.1.3).

Textbook of Small Animal Pathophysiology, First Edition. Stephan Neumann.
© 2025 John Wiley & Sons Ltd. Published 2025 by John Wiley & Sons Ltd.

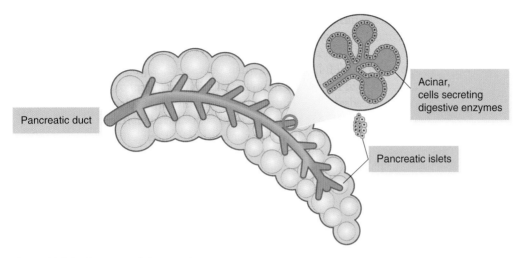

Figure 40.1.1 Structure of the exocrine pancreas.

Table 40.1.1 Pancreatic digestive enzymes.

Protein	Carbohydrate	Lipid	DNA/RNA
Trypsin	Amylase	Lipase	DNAsen
Chymotrypsin		Phospholipase	RNAsen
Elastase			
Carboxypeptidase A and B			

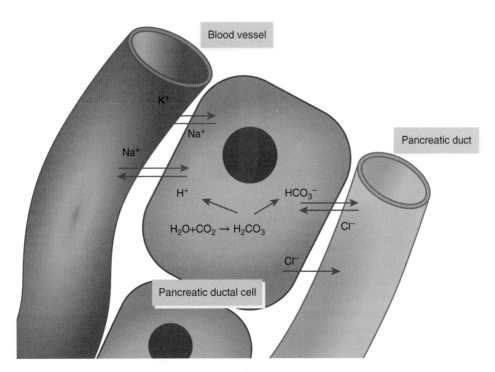

Figure 40.1.2 Mechanism of bicarbonate secretion.

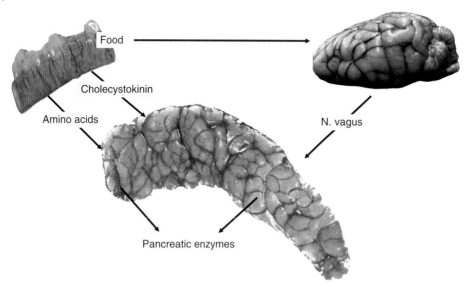

Figure 40.1.3 Control of pancreatic juice secretion.

Digestion of the Nutrients

The secretion of pancreatic juice is intended to support the digestion of nutrients and, at the same time, buffer the acidic chyme coming from the stomach via its high bicarbonate concentration. Digestion is performed by the enzymes of the pancreatic juice, which are activated in the intestinal lumen. Activation occurs by several mechanisms. The activation and function of individual pancreatic enzymes are explained here.

Trypsin is an endopeptidase that cleaves protein molecules at specific sites within the protein chain. Trypsin cleaves peptides after lysine or arginine, at a pH optimum of 7–8. The enzymatic action of trypsin is not selective, which means that not specific proteins, but all proteins are cleaved. This is important for the digestion process, as there are many proteins of different structure in the food.

The intestinal enzyme enteropeptidase of the enterocytes controls the activation of trypsinogen to trypsin. The formed trypsin activates itself (positive feedback) and converts chymotrypsinogen, proelastase, as well as procarboxypeptidase and other inactive enzymes into their active forms (chymotrypsin, elastase and carboxypeptidase).

Chymotrypsin is a second pancreatic protease that cleaves peptides after tyrosine, tryptophan and phenylalanine. Chymotrypsin is activated by trypsin.

Pancreatic lipase breaks down dietary fats into fatty acids, glycerol and mono- and diacylglycerols. These can then be absorbed into the enterocytes in the form of micelles together with the help of bile salts. The activation of pancreatic lipase takes place via trypsin.

The **amylases** occur in different forms and serve the digestion of carbohydrates. They act as endo- and exohydrolases, which means that they can cleave carbohydrates from the inside and from the end of the molecule. Mono- and disaccharides are formed in the process.

Reference

Ishiguro, H., Yamamoto, A., Nakakuki, M. et al. (2012). Physiology and pathophysiology of bicarbonate secretion by pancreatic duct epithelium. *Nagoya Journal of Medical Science* 74 (1–2): 1–18.

Further Reading

Leung, P.S. (2010). Physiology of the pancreas. *Advances in Experimental Medicine and Biology* 690: 13–27. https://doi.org/10.1007/978-90-481-9060-7_2.

40.2

Acute Pancreatitis

Definition

Acute pancreatitis is defined as an acute inflammatory reaction of the pancreatic tissue after a mostly idiopathic trigger.

Aetiology

Although some causalities are described in the literature, many cases of acute pancreatitis in dogs and cats remain idiopathic. An essential key mechanism for pancreatitis appears to be tissue ischaemia. This is caused by numerous morphological and metabolic factors. Breed predisposition are described especially for the dog. The disease occurs in dogs and cats (Table 40.2.1).

Pathogenesis

The essential step in the development of pancreatitis is the premature activation of pancreatic enzymes. Numerous protective measures, such as formation as an inactive precursor, storage in vacuoles and intracellular activity of protease inhibitors, such as trypsin inhibitors or serine inhibitors are supposed to prevent this step. An increased Ca^{2+} concentration in the acinar cells is assumed to be the triggering factor for activation. This in turn may be the result of hypoxia, which impedes the energy-consuming Na^+/Ca^{2+} exchange at the cell membrane (Ward et al. 1995).The increased Ca^{2+} concentration in the acinar cells activates trypsinogen to form trypsin; this was shown experimentally by measuring the activation factor trypsinogen activation peptide (TAP) in acinar cells after calcium addition (Frick et al. 1997). Activated trypsin leads to the cascade-like activation of further enzymes, such as elastase and phospholipase A2, and to further excessive calcium release from intracellular calcium stores.

Hypoxia in turn can be explained by the aetiologies described. Anaesthesia, surgery, shock and trauma can cause local hypoxia in the pancreas by disturbing systemic and local circulation.

Endocrinopathies or lipaemia cause microcirculatory disturbance of the pancreas through increased production of vasoactive factors (e.g. thromboxane), intravascular coagulation and leucocyte adherence. In addition, pancreatic blood flow may slow down and stasis may develop (Guo et al. 2019) (Figure 40.2.1).

Diagnostics

Clinical signs	Clinical pathology	Imaging	Histopathology	Microbiology
Inappetence Abdominal pain Vomiting	**Lipase** measurement as DGGR-lipase or c/fPLI	**Ultrasonography** Imaging of pancreatic enlargement and hypoechogenicity	Not necessary	Not necessary

Textbook of Small Animal Pathophysiology, First Edition. Stephan Neumann.
© 2025 John Wiley & Sons Ltd. Published 2025 by John Wiley & Sons Ltd.

Table 40.2.1 Causes of pancreatitis in dogs and cats.

Genetic	Metabolic	Morphologic
Mini Schnauzer (D)	Lipaemia (C/D)	Surgery (C/D)
Terriers (D)	Endocrinopathy (D)	Anaesthesia (C/D)
Siam cat (C)	Hypercalcaemia (C/D)	Trauma (C/D)
	Inflammatory gastrointestinal disease (C)	Shock (C/D)

D-dog C-cat

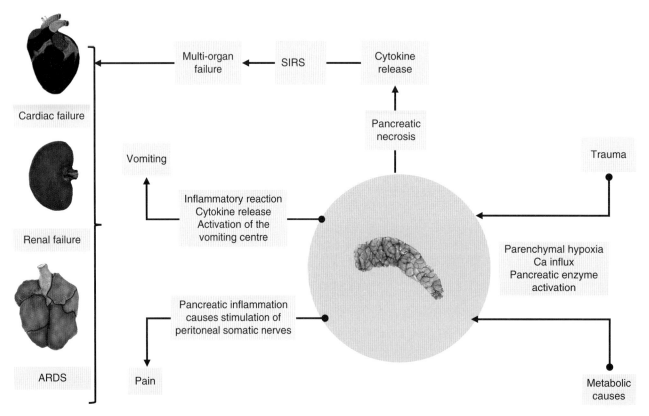

Figure 40.2.1 Pathogenesis and pathophysiologic consequences of acute pancreatitis.

Pathophysiologic Consequences

Major pathophysiologic consequences arise in connection with the massive inflammatory reaction.

Influenced organ systems	Clinical symptoms	Clinical pathological alterations
Cardiovascular system	Anorexia	Leucocytosis
Gastrointestinal system	Abdominal pain	Increased lipase
Hepatobiliary system	Vomitus	Increased ALT, ALP, GLDH
Pancreas	Dehydration	Bilirubinaemia
Systemic		Hypoalbuminaemia
	Shock	
	SIRS	
	ARDS	

Source: Hill and Van Winkle (1993) and Hess et al. (1998).

Enzyme activation within the pancreatic tissue is thought to be the essential step in the initiation of acute pancreatitis. Activated trypsin can activate other enzymes and cause pancreatic autodigestion and local fat necrosis. This initiates an inflammatory response in which macrophages and granulocytes infiltrate locally. These release proinflammatory cytokines (IL-1, IL-6, TNF-α) and recruit further inflammatory cells, which increases the local tissue destruction of the pancreas. In addition, the systemic increase in cytokines can cause a so-called 'cytokine storm', which can eventually lead to a systemic inflammatory response (**SIRS**). The consequence can be systemic multi-organ failure. Increased concentrations of activated pancreatic enzymes, such as phospholipase, can lead to acute respiratory syndrome (**ARDS**) via an inhibitory effect on the surfactant in the alveoli.

Local consequences would be an inflammation-associated increase in vascular permeability, which can eventually lead to haemorrhagic pancreatitis or pancreatic necrosis. Another phenomenon of altered permeability can be a disruption of the intestinal bacterial barrier, with the consequence of bacteria migrating out of the intestine and local infection (Mifkovic et al. 2006).

Anorexia or inappetence are systemic consequences of pancreatitis and are probably due to a direct central effect of the proinflammatory cytokines IL-1, IL-6 and TNF-α. These act directly on hypothalamic neurons. This stimulates the activity of anorectic neurons and inhibits orexigenic neurons (Braun and Marks 2010).

Abdominal pain is a symptom frequently observed in dogs with pancreatitis. Numerous molecular and morphological changes in intrapancreatic and extrapancreatic regions are causally responsible for the pain. Irritation of intrapancreatic nociceptors is one mechanism, although the triggers are not known; substances released from destroyed acinar cells, such as serotonin, bradykinin or calcium are suspected. More recent studies focus on neurotrophic factors, such as nerve growth factor (NGF) or artemin (Demir et al. 2011).

The development of **vomiting** in cases of pancreatitis is explained by the 'cytokine storm' occurring in connection with pancreatitis or local peritonitis. The latter can trigger vomiting via vagus irritation (Fajgenbaum and June 2020).

Dehydration is a consequence of vomiting and anorexia.

Another phenomenon that is observed in connection with advanced pancreatitis is **paralytic ileus**. This is explained by the local inflammatory reaction. Inflammatory cells are attracted by proinflammatory cytokines, which also invade the intestinal wall muscularis. Infiltration inhibits the activity of smooth muscle cells in the tunica, resulting in ileus. As a result of the delayed peristalsis, ingestastasis, bacterial overgrowth and a recurrent inflammatory response occur. Another mechanism for the development of paralytic ileus is hypokalaemia resulting from vomiting. This develops partly through a direct loss of potassium during vomiting, but also as a result of the alkalosis that develops during vomiting. In the case of alkalosis, cells secrete protons in return for potassium ions to compensate for the alkalosis.

The consequence of hypokalaemia is reduced neuromuscular excitability and thus paralysis of the smooth muscle cells (Figure 40.2.2).

Due to the massive inflammatory reaction in pancreatitis, **leucocytosis** and an increased C-reactive protein (CRP) concentration are present in the blood. **Hypoalbuminaemia** could also be a consequence of the acute inflammatory reaction, since albumin, as a negative acute phase protein, is synthesised in the liver at a reduced level at the beginning of inflammation.

The increase in pancreatic enzymes, especially **lipase,** is seen as a result of the premature activation of enzymes in the pancreatic tissue, as well as the destruction of acinar cells. Elevated liver enzymes again are related to the local inflammatory response or to outflow disturbances from the common bile and pancreatic duct in cases of pancreatitis. This stasis explains the increased expression of cholestatic ALP and bilirubin.

The diagnosis of pancreatitis can be confirmed by laboratory diagnostics using two parameters. The DGGR-lipase is the detection of pancreas-specific lipase activity. This can be measured by using the DGGR ester as a substrate, which significantly improves the sensitivity and specificity of the measurement.

When measuring canine- or feline-specific pancreatic lipase, lipase activity is determined using an immunoassay (Table 40.2.2).

Therapy

Symptom	Therapy
Shock	Infusion
Pain	Analgesics (e.g. Morphine)
Vomiting	Antiemetics (e.g. Maropitant, Metoclopramide, Ondansetron)

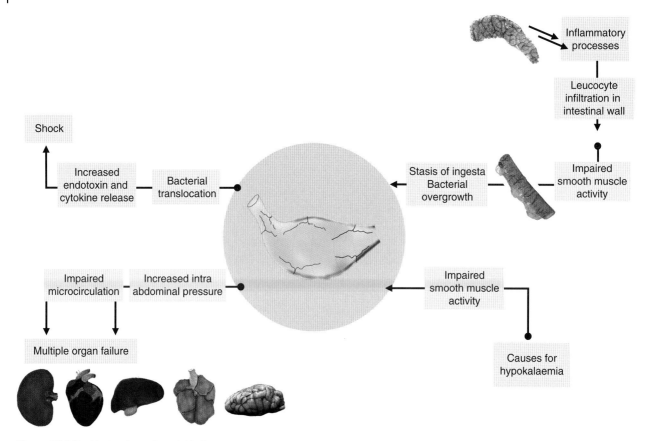

Figure 40.2.2 Mechanism of paralytic ileus.

Table 40.2.2 Differentiation of different tests for the diagnosis of pancreatitis.

	c/fPLI	c/fTLI	DGGR-lipase	Lipase	Amylase
Pancreatitis	+	(+)	+	(+)	–

References

Braun, T.P. and Marks, D.L. (2010). Pathophysiology and treatment of inflammatory anorexia in chronic disease. *Journal of Cachexia, Sarcopenia and Muscle* 1 (2): 135–145. https://doi.org/10.1007/s13539-010-0015-1.

Demir, I.E., Tieftrunk, E., Maak, M. et al. (2011). Pain mechanisms in chronic pancreatitis: of a master and his fire. *Langenbeck's Archives of Surgery* 396 (2): 151–160. https://doi.org/10.1007/s00423-010-0731-1.

Fajgenbaum, D.C. and June, C.H. (2020). Cytokine storm. *The New England Journal of Medicine* 383 (23): 2255–2273. https://doi.org/10.1056/NEJMra2026131.

Frick, T.W., Fernández-del Castillo, C., Bimmler, D., and Warshaw, A.L. (1997). Elevated calcium and activation of trypsinogen in rat pancreatic acini. *Gut* 41 (3): 339–343. https://doi.org/10.1136/gut.41.3.339.

Guo, Y.Y., Li, H.X., Zhang, Y., and He, W.H. (2019). Hypertriglyceridemia-induced acute pancreatitis: progress on disease mechanisms and treatment modalities. *Discovery Medicine* 27 (147): 101–109.

Hess, R.S., Saunders, H.M., Van Winkle, T.J. et al. (1998). Clinical, clinicopathologic, radiographic, and ultrasonographic abnormalities in dogs with fatal acute pancreatitis: 70 cases (1986–1995). *Journal of the American Veterinary Medical Association* 213 (5): 665–670.

Hill, R.C. and Van Winkle, T.J. (1993). Acute necrotizing pancreatitis and acute suppurative pancreatitis in the cat. A retrospective study of 40 cases (1976–1989). *Journal of Veterinary Internal Medicine* 7 (1): 25–33. https://doi.org/10.1111/j.1939-1676.1993.tb03165.x.

Mifkovic, A., Pindak, D., Daniel, I., and Pechan, J. (2006). Septic complications of acute pancreatitis. *Bratislavske lekarske listy* 107 (8): 296–313.

Ward, J.B., Petersen, O.H., Jenkins, S.A., and Sutton, R. (1995). Is an elevated concentration of acinar cytosolic free ionised calcium the trigger for acute pancreatitis? *Lancet (London, England)* 346 (8981): 1016–1019. https://doi.org/10.1016/s0140-6736(95)91695-4.

Further Reading

Watson, P. (2015). Pancreatitis in dogs and cats: definitions and pathophysiology. *The Journal of Small Animal Practice* 56 (1): 3–12. https://doi.org/10.1111/jsap.12293.

Xenoulis, P.G. (2015). Diagnosis of pancreatitis in dogs and cats. *The Journal of Small Animal Practice* 56 (1): 13–26. https://doi.org/10.1111/jsap.12274.

40.3

Chronic Pancreatitis

Definition

Chronic pancreatitis arises from acute pancreatitis and is associated with tissue remodelling, in the sense of parenchyma fibrosis. Accordingly, the changes are partly irreversible and cause organ insufficiency.

Aetiology

Mainly, chronic pancreatitis arises from the acute form. Independent causes are always associated with long-term irritation of the parenchyma. The disease occurs in dogs and cats.

Inflammatory	Obstructive
Acute pancreatitis	Pancreatic duct obstruction

Pathogenesis

If acute pancreatitis persists or recurs, it can develop into chronic pancreatitis. In contrast to the acute form, this is characterised by a morphological remodelling of the parenchyma in the sense of fibrosis.

A clear distinction between acute and chronic pancreatitis is made difficult by the fact that chronic pancreatitis is also accompanied by acute episodes. However, the initial situation is as already described for acute pancreatitis.

There are different hypotheses on the development of chronic pancreatitis.

On the one hand, oxidative stress in the acinar cells due to different triggers is seen as responsible for cell damage in the acinus with enzyme activation. Obstructions in the area of the pancreatic ducts cause a stasis of the pancreatic juice, which leads to a premature activation of pancreatic enzymes in the pancreatic parenchyma.

In chronic pancreatitis, recurrent inflammation leads to an increase in extracellular matrix, especially collagen types I and III. The mechanism is based on growth factor-controlled activation of sessile connective tissue cells, the pancreatic stellate cells. The growth factors are, for example, transforming growth factor β1, TGFβ1 or platelet-derived growth factor (PDGF).

Similar to the stellate cells in the liver, the pancreatic stellate cells are able to metamorphose into myofibroblasts. This process is controlled by a causative inflammatory process and the activation of growth factors in the healing phase. However, this can lead to reparation in the sense of fibrosis instead of restitution.

Textbook of Small Animal Pathophysiology, First Edition. Stephan Neumann.
© 2025 John Wiley & Sons Ltd. Published 2025 by John Wiley & Sons Ltd.

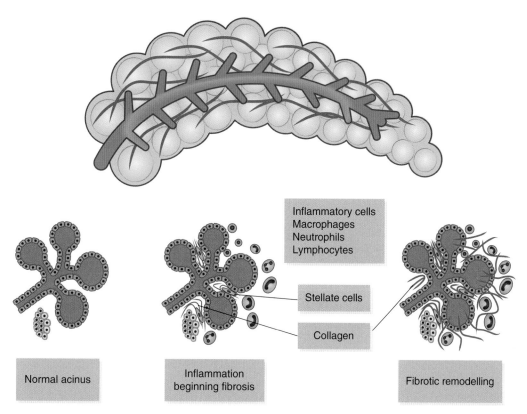

Figure 40.3.1 Pathogenesis of chronic pancreatitis.

In the development of fibrosis, the stellate cells are activated. This is morphologically indicated by a loss of lipid vacuoles and a change in the cytoskeleton with increased expression of α-SMA and synthesis of collagens, such as type I and III (Figure 40.3.1).

Diagnostics

Clinical signs	Clinical pathology	Imaging	Histopathology	Microbiology
Non-specific	DGGR-lipase; c/fPLI	**Ultrasonography** Visualisation of morphological parenchymal remodelling	Not necessary	Not necessary

Pathophysiologic Consequences

The pathophysiologic consequences of chronic pancreatitis are similar to those of the acute form, especially when the chronic form suffers an acute episode. In the non-acute phase of chronic inflammation, rather discreet symptoms are found.

Influenced organ systems	Clinical symptoms	Clinical pathological alterations
Gastrointestinal system	Anorexia	Leucocytosis
Hepatobiliary system	Abdominal pain	Increased lipase
Pancreas	Diabetes mellitus	Increased ALT, AST
	Exocrine pancreatic insufficiency	Hyperbilirubinaemia
	Triaditis	Increased ALP
		Hypoalbuminaemia

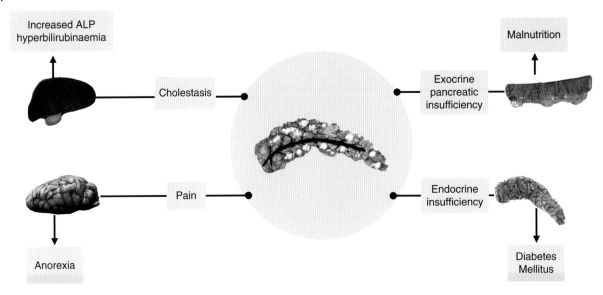

Figure 40.3.2 Pathophysiologic consequences of chronic pancreatitis.

In the acute phase of chronic pancreatitis, **anorexia** and **pain** may occur. The anorexia may be a consequence of the pain or may result from the release of inflammatory cytokines that act on the hunger centre. The pain is a consequence of the irritation of regional nociceptors. A connection between chronic pancreatitis and **diabetes mellitus** has been found, especially in cats. Infiltration of the islet apparatus with inflammatory cells is seen as the cause (Caney 2013; Davison 2015).

The loss of active pancreatic parenchyma due to fibrotic remodelling is associated with developing **pancreatic insufficiency**. Finally, chronic pancreatitis is causally related to cholangiohepatitis and IBD as a so-called **triaditis** in the cat. So both latter diseases have to be considered in cats with chronic pancreatitis.

The increased **lipase activity** results from a release from destroyed acinar cells. An increase in liver enzymes is observed primarily for hepatocellular enzymes, such as **ALT** and **AST**. This may be due to a consequence of the systemic inflammatory response syndrome (SIRS) that may occur. However, this is more a symptom of acute pancreatitis. Obstructions of the pancreatic duct can lead to cholestasis, as the pancreatic duct joins the choledochal duct in the small intestine. This can also lead to **hyperbilirubinaemia**, as well as an increase in **ALP** serum activity. Insufficiencies in pancreatic function can cause maldigestion and **hypoalbuminaemia**.

Leukocytosis reflects the pancreatic inflammatory process. Inflammation is also present in chronic pancreatitis and its extent increases when acute phases are added (Figure 40.3.2).

Therapy

Symptom	Therapy
Diabetes mellitus	Insulin, diet
Pancreatic insufficiency	Pancreatic enzymes
Acute phases	Infusions, painkillers, antiemetics

References

Caney, S.M. (2013). Pancreatitis and diabetes in cats. *The Veterinary Clinics of North America. Small Animal Practice* 43 (2): 303–317. https://doi.org/10.1016/j.cvsm.2012.12.001.

Davison, L.J. (2015). Diabetes mellitus and pancreatitis—cause or effect? *The Journal of Small Animal Practice* 56 (1): 50–59. https://doi.org/10.1111/jsap.12295.

Further Reading

Armstrong, P.J. and Williams, D.A. (2012). Pancreatitis in cats. *Topics in Companion Animal Medicine* 27 (3): 140–147. https://doi.org/10.1053/j.tcam.2012.09.001.

Bazelle, J. and Watson, P. (2014). Pancreatitis in cats: is it acute, is it chronic, is it significant? *Journal of Feline Medicine and Surgery* 16 (5): 395–406. https://doi.org/10.1177/1098612X14523186.

Bostrom, B.M., Xenoulis, P.G., Newman, S.J. et al. (2013). Chronic pancreatitis in dogs: a retrospective study of clinical, clinicopathological, and histopathological findings in 61 cases. *Veterinary journal (London, England: 1997)* 195 (1): 73–79. https://doi.org/10.1016/j.tvjl.2012.06.034.

Forman, M.A., Steiner, J.M., Armstrong, P.J. et al. (2021). ACVIM consensus statement on pancreatitis in cats. *Journal of Veterinary Internal Medicine* 35 (2): 703–723. https://doi.org/10.1111/jvim.16053.

Hashimoto, A., Karim, M.R., Izawa, T. et al. (2017). Immunophenotypical analysis of pancreatic interstitial cells in the developing rat pancreas and myofibroblasts in the fibrotic pancreas in dogs and cats. *The Journal of Veterinary Medical Science* 79 (12): 1920–1926. https://doi.org/10.1292/jvms.17-0423.

Watson, P. (2012). Chronic pancreatitis in dogs. *Topics in Companion Animal Medicine* 27 (3): 133–139. https://doi.org/10.1053/j.tcam.2012.04.006.

Watson, P. (2015). Pancreatitis in dogs and cats: definitions and pathophysiology. *The Journal of Small Animal Practice* 56 (1): 3–12. https://doi.org/10.1111/jsap.12293.

Xenoulis, P.G., Suchodolski, J.S., and Steiner, J.M. (2008). Chronic pancreatitis in dogs and cats. *Compendium (Yardley, PA)* 30 (3): 166–181.

40.4

Exocrine Pancreas Insufficiency

Definition

Exocrine pancreatic insufficiency represents functional exhaustion of the organ after exceeding reserve capacity. Consequences are digestion disorders of the small intestine.

Aetiology

The main causes are congenital atrophy of the pancreatic cells, which is more commonly described in dogs, or consequences of chronic pancreatitis, which is more commonly seen in cats.

Genetic	Inflammatory
Pancreatic acinar atrophy (D)	Chronic pancreatitis (C)

D-dog C-cat

Pathogenesis

Canine exocrine pancreatic insufficiency is more commonly described in the German Shepherd dog. The pathomorphological changes describe an atrophy of the pancreatic tissue with loss of the glandular structure of the parenchyma. Histopathologically, hardly any acini are recognisable in the advanced stage, but these are largely replaced by fatty tissue. Sporadically, lymphocytes and plasma cells could be found in the atrophic tissue (Wiberg et al. 1999).

Based on inflammatory cell infiltration, it has been hypothesised that the aetiopathogenesis of exocrine pancreatic insufficiency in some breeds of dogs, such as the German Shepherd, is due to an autoimmune reaction (Wiberg et al. 2000; Wiberg 2004).

Pathogenetically, a two-phase course is assumed. In the first phase, lympho-plasma cellular pancreatitis leads to destruction of the acini. In the second phase, the pancreatic parenchyma is replaced by fatty tissue.

In a study, inflammatory cell infiltrates were investigated by immunophenotyping in dogs with exocrine pancreatic insufficiency in phase I and II. In the first phase, CD^{4+} and CD^{8+} T-cells, as well as B lymphocytes and plasma cells could be detected. In the chronic phase, when the replacement of the parenchyma by fat cells takes place, the number of plasma cells and B lymphocytes in particular is reduced (Wiberg 2003).

Chronic pancreatitis, which has also been described in dogs as a possible trigger for pancreatic insufficiency, must be differentiated from this. In these cases, the morphological changes in the pancreatic parenchyma are different from exocrine pancreatic insufficiency and are characterised by a fibrotic remodelling of the organ after the acute inflammatory phase (Watson 2003) (Figure 40.4.1).

Textbook of Small Animal Pathophysiology, First Edition. Stephan Neumann.
© 2025 John Wiley & Sons Ltd. Published 2025 by John Wiley & Sons Ltd.

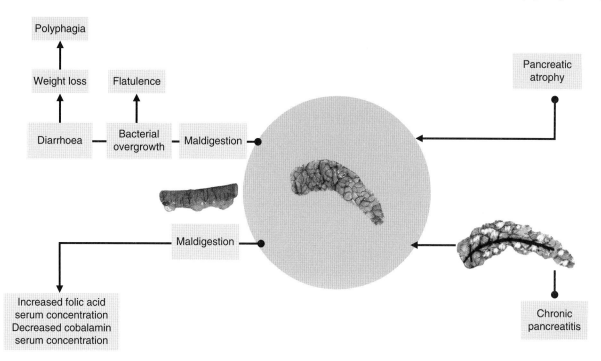

Figure 40.4.1 Mechanism of and pathophysiologic consequences of exocrine pancreatic insufficiency.

Diagnostics

Clinical signs	Clinical pathology	Imaging	Histopathology	Microbiology
Chronic diarrhoea	**TLI test**	Difficult to perform because of pancreas atrophy	Not necessary	Not necessary

Pathophysiologic Consequences

The consequences of pancreatic insufficiency primarily affect the gastrointestinal tract. The consequence of maldigestion, however, has systemic consequences.

Influenced organ systems	Clinical symptoms	Clinical pathological alterations
Systemic	Small bowel diarrhoea	Low cobalamin
	Flatulence	High folate
	Weight loss	
	Polyphagy	
	Coprophagia	

The main symptom is small intestinal diarrhoea due to maldigestion. This is light in colour, soft in consistency and large in volume. The diarrhoea follows the mechanism of **osmotic diarrhoea**. This occurs due to an increased concentration of osmotically active molecules in the intestinal lumen. These build up an osmotic gradient between the intestinal lumen and the extraintestinal area and prevent water reabsorption by the enterocytes. The causes are usually osmotically active molecules that remain in the intestinal lumen due to insufficient breakdown (maldigestion, malabsorption). These can be part of the food or result from insufficient activity of digestion processes. The latter can result from reduced microbial breakdown or reduced activity of digestive enzymes on the enterocyte membrane.

Table 40.4.1 Influence of SIBO and IBD on serum concentrations of folic acid and vitamin B12.

Cobalamin	Increased	Normal	Decreased
Folic acid			
Increased	SIBO	SIBO	SIBO
Normal			SIBO
Decreased	IBD	IBD	IBD

Due to the high concentration of nutrients in the intestinal lumen, small intestinal bacterial overgrowth (SIBO) can occur. Small intestinal bacterial overgrowth is an uncontrolled and high-grade proliferation of bacteria in the small intestine.

The disease is assumed to occur at a bacterial concentration of $>10^5$ CFU (colony forming units)/ml. The predominant bacterial species are coliforms, *Staphylococci*, *Enterococci*, *Clostridium* and *Bacteroides* spp. There is a marked increase in anaerobic germs. Due to the increased gas formation, one symptom of SIBO is **flatulence**. Maldigestion also leads to reduced absorption of nutrients, resulting in weight loss and the deficiency and imbalance of certain nutrients.

The bacterial overgrowth leads, among other things, to an altered metabolism of folic acid and vitamin B12, which is also used diagnostically. **Folic acid** cannot be synthesised by dogs and cats. In contrast, bacteria are capable of synthesising this vitamin. The resource for folic acid in dogs and cats is folic acid ingested through food. This is predominantly absorbed as polyglutamate. In the proximal small intestine, glutamate is enzymatically cleaved from the folic acid and at the membrane of the enterocytes, primarily in the jejunum, folic acid is reduced via dihydrofolic acid to tetrahydrofolic acid and then reabsorbed. The latter form is also found in serum. There, folic acid is transported via transport proteins to the target cells where it is absorbed via an active transport mechanism. Due to the bacterial synthesis of folic acid, its concentration in the serum is increased in SIBO.

The absorption of **vitamin B12** takes place in several steps. First, the vitamin is released from the food in the stomach by the influence of gastric acid. It binds to a protein secreted by the fundus cells (R-protein). In the small intestine, the R-protein is detached by intestinal proteinases. The vitamin B12 now binds to another protein, the so-called 'intrinsic factor', which is essential for vitamin B12 absorption. In dogs, the intrinsic factor comes from enterocytes or from the pancreas, and in cats mainly from the pancreas. In the ileum, the complex of vitamin B12 intrinsic factor reacts with a receptor of the enterocyte membrane. After cellular uptake, vitamin B12 is bound to transcobalamin, transported to the apical cell membrane and released into the blood. Transport to the target cells also takes place bound to transcobalamin. SIBO can influence the vitamin B12 metabolism. Numerous intestinal bacteria also reabsorb vitamin B12. This leads to competition between bacteria and macro-organisms in the case of SIBO (Table 40.4.1).

In animals with exocrine pancreatic insufficiency, **poly-** or even **coprophagia is** observed. Both symptoms are explained by the increased feed requirement of the animals resulting from maldigestion.

Therapy

Symptom	Therapy
Maldigestion	Pancreatic enzymes
Weight loss	Diet
Cobalamin deficiency	Cobalamin

References

Watson, P.J. (2003). Exocrine pancreatic insufficiency as an end stage of pancreatitis in four dogs. *The Journal of Small Animal Practice* 44 (7): 306–312. https://doi.org/10.1111/j.1748-5827.2003.tb00159.x.

Wiberg, M. E. (2003). Pancreatic acinar atrophy in German shepherd dogs and rough-coated collies. *PhD thesis*.

Wiberg, M.E. (2004). Pancreatic acinar atrophy in German Shepherd dogs and Rough-coated Collies. Etiopathogenesis, diagnosis and treatment. A review. *The Veterinary Quarterly* 26 (2): 61–75. https://doi.org/10.1080/01652176.2004.9695169.

Wiberg, M.E., Saari, S.A., and Westermarck, E. (1999). Exocrine pancreatic atrophy in German Shepherd dogs and Rough-coated Collies: an end result of lymphocytic pancreatitis. *Veterinary Pathology* 36 (6): 530–541. https://doi.org/10.1354/vp.36-6-530.

Wiberg, M.E., Saari, S.A., Westermarck, E., and Meri, S. (2000). Cellular and humoral immune responses in atrophic lymphocytic pancreatitis in German Shepherd dogs and Rough-coated Collies. *Veterinary Immunology and Immunopathology* 76 (1–2): 103–115. https://doi.org/10.1016/s0165-2427(00)00202-6.

Further Reading

Kennedy, O.C. and Williams, D.A. (2012). Exocrine pancreatic insufficiency in dogs and cats: online support for veterinarians and owners. *Topics in Companion Animal Medicine* 27 (3): 117–122. https://doi.org/10.1053/j.tcam.2012.05.001.

Xenoulis, P.G., Zoran, D.L., Fosgate, G.T. et al. (2016). Feline exocrine pancreatic insufficiency: a retrospective study of 150 cases. *Journal of Veterinary Internal Medicine* 30 (6): 1790–1797. https://doi.org/10.1111/jvim.14560.

41

Urinary System

41.1

Physiological Functions of the Kidneys and General Pathophysiology of Organ Insufficiency

Functions

The kidneys are important excretory organs. As a result, they significantly regulate the water balance, the electrolyte balance and the acid-base balance. In this way, the kidneys influence different regulatory mechanisms in the body (Table 41.1.1).

Kidney function depends largely on renal circulation. Accordingly, the kidneys are best supplied with blood; in dogs at rest about 20% of the arterial cardiac output is supplied to the kidneys, which corresponds to about 400 ml/min in a 20 kg dog. The arterial blood reaches the kidneys via a short renal artery. Within the kidneys, the arteries branch into arterioles, which end as afferent arterioles in the glomerulum. There, the arterioles branch into capillaries, which combine to form efferent arterioles to build up a peritubular capillary network. From there, the capillaries combine to form venules, which in turn flow into the vena renalis, which is drained into the vena cava.

The glomerulum is surrounded by a capsule, the Bowman's capsule, which merges into a tubule system with proximal part, Henle's loop and distal part. Finally, the distal tubule flows into the collecting tubes, which drain into the renal pelvis. The entire anatomical unit is called the 'nephron', and it represents the functional structure of the kidneys (Figure 41.1.1).

In the glomerulum, an essential function of the kidneys, excretion, takes place. For this purpose, blood plasma is filtered into the glomerula. The following factors influence the glomerular filtration:

Blood pressure in the capillaries
Blood pressure in the Bowman's capsule
Semipermeability of glomerular membranes
Osmotic pressure in the capillaries

Blood pressure in the capillaries is the essential filtration pressure for the formation of the filtrate. This is about 60 mmHg. Within the Bowman's capsule there is a pressure of about 15 mmHg, which is opposed to the filtration pressure. The semipermeable membrane of the glomerulum also influences filtration under physiological conditions. The passage of large molecules (>4 nm; >50 kDa) and negatively charged molecules is restricted. As a result, there is a negative excess of charge in the capillaries (Gibbs-Donnan potential), which reduces the filtration of cations and increases the filtration of anions. At the same time, an osmotic pressure (30 mmHg) occurs, which is opposed by the filtration pressure. In sum, the following applies:

$$\text{Total pressure} = \text{filtration pressure} - \text{pressure}\left(\text{Bowman's capsule}\right) - \text{osmotic pressure}$$

The glomerular filtrate corresponds to about 80 l/day for a dog of about 20 kg and about 20 l/day for a cat. However, urine is excreted in an amount of about 500–1000 ml/day in a 20 kg dog and of about 100–200 ml/day in the cat. Accordingly, 98–99% of the primary urine is reabsorbed. This process takes place in the tubular system. Within the tubular system, reabsorption of components of the glomerular filtrate is located. In addition, individual molecules in this section of the nephron can be secreted.

Textbook of Small Animal Pathophysiology, First Edition. Stephan Neumann.
© 2025 John Wiley & Sons Ltd. Published 2025 by John Wiley & Sons Ltd.

Table 41.1.1 Kidney functions.

Excretion	Electrolyte metabolism	Acid-base-balance	Bone metabolism	Blood pressure	Erythropoiesis Thrombopoiesis	Gluconeogenesis
Urea	Sodium	Proton	Calcium	Blood volume	Erythropoietin	Glutamate
Creatinine	Potassium	Bicarbonate	Phosphates		Thrombopoietin	
Uric acid	Calcium		Calcitriol			
Allantoin						
Ammonia hippuric acid						

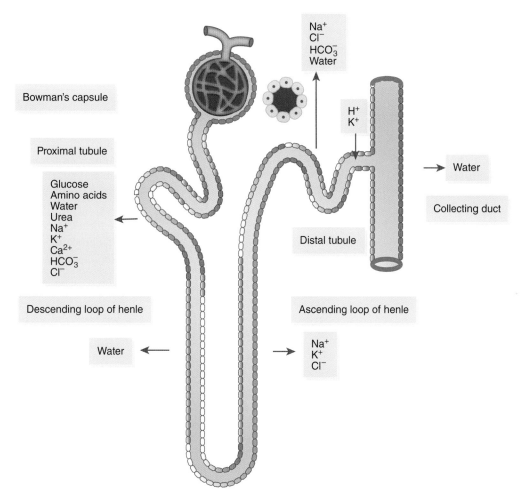

Figure 41.1.1 Nephron – the shortest functional unit of the kidneys.

Especially in the proximal tubule, numerous molecules of the glomerular filtrate are partially or completely reabsorbed. The reabsorption of sodium plays an important role here. This is reabsorbed in the proximal tubule to about 60% by an active transport process. There is a symport together with glucose, amino acids and organic acids. Glucose and amino acids are reabsorbed as so-called 'threshold substances' at physiological plasma concentration to almost 100% in the proximal tubule. Increased plasma concentrations overwhelm the transport capacities in the proximal tubule, resulting in excretion in the urine. Through the reabsorption processes in the proximal tubule, an osmotic gradient develops, which is followed by water. This in turn can take dissolved ions with it (solvent drag). About 50% of urea is reabsorbed in the proximal tubules coupled to transport proteins; a reabsorption of creatinine does not take place.

Table 41.1.2 Secretion and reabsorption in the tubular system.

Location	Secretion	Reabsorption
Proximal tubule	Creatinine, SO_4^-, H^+	Urea, H_2O, glucose, Na^+, K^+, Ca^+, Mg^+, PO_4^-, HCO_3^-
Descending limb		H_2O, urea
Ascending limb		Na^+
Distal tubule	K^+, H^+, NH_3^+	K^+, Na^+, H_2O, urea
Collecting duct		H_2O

In the further course of the tubule system, the Henle's loop, the concentration of the filtrate is located. This essentially leads to reabsorption of water along an osmotic gradient between the tubular lumen and the interstitial space. The osmotic gradient is built up by the accumulation of urea and NaCl in the interstitial. While in the renal cortex a tissue osmolality as in the blood plasma (about 290 mosmol/kg) prevails, this rises in the renal medulla to about 1200 mosmol/kg.

In the distal tubule and in the collecting tube, NaCl, urea, calcium and water are reabsorbed and potassium and protons are secreted. This leads to the final influence on the urine composition (Table 41.1.2).

Acid-Base Regulation

Numerous metabolic processes in the body lead to the formation of acids. Buffering these and compensating their negative influence is the task of the acid-base balance. The kidneys affect this system by resorption of phosphate and bicarbonate and secretion of protons.

In the proximal tubule, protons are exchanged for sodium ions via a Na^+/H^+ antiport. Thus, protons enter the tubular lumen, where they react under the catalysis of a membrane-bound carboanhydrase with bicarbonate to form CO_2, which diffuses into the tubule cells. There, the synthesis of bicarbonate also takes place under the catalysis of the carboanhydrase, which enters the blood plasma via an Na^+-symport at the basal tubular cell membrane. In the distal tubule, protons are secreted from carbonic acid and form ammonium ions with ammonia.

Bone Metabolism

A link between kidney function and bone metabolism is given by the excretion of calcium and phosphate via the kidneys. In the case of calcium deficiency in the blood, there is the secretion of parathyroid hormone from the main cells of the parathyroid gland. This promotes renal calcium reabsorption in the distal tubule and phosphate secretion. In addition, the kidney is an important synthesis site of calcitriol, in addition to epithelial cells and macrophages. This in turn promotes calcium and phosphate reabsorption in the intestine and kidneys (Figure 41.1.2).

Blood Pressure

The kidneys control blood pressure through the renin-angiotensin-aldosterone system. The trigger is a drop in blood pressure, which initially increases peripheral vascular resistance by activating the sympathicus via alpha receptors. The result is a reduced renal circulation. This leads to the secretion of renin from epithelial cells of the juxtaglomerular apparatus. Renin is a protease that converts angiotensinogen formed in the liver or adipose tissue into angiotensin I by cleaving a decapeptide. This in turn is converted by proteolytic angiotensin-converting-enzyme (ACE inhibitors) into angiotensin II by cleavage of an octapeptide. Angiotensin II acts via angiotensin receptors and is able to increase blood pressure by contraction of smooth vascular muscle cells. At the same time, it stimulates sodium reabsorption in the proximal tubule and aldosterone synthesis in the adrenal cortex. Aldosterone, in turn, promotes sodium reabsorption in the distal tubule and in the collecting tubes. In both cases, water follows the built-up osmotic guard. Angiotensin II also increases the secretion of ADH in the posterior pituitary gland. This in turn causes water reabsorption in the collecting tubule via so-called 'aquaporins'.

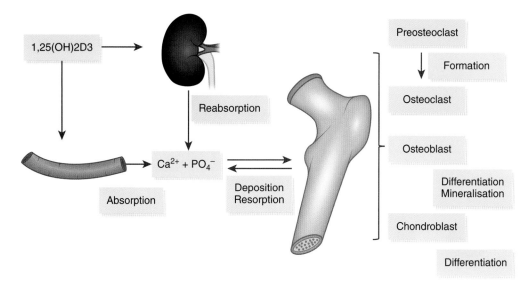

Figure 41.1.2 Kidney and bone metabolism.

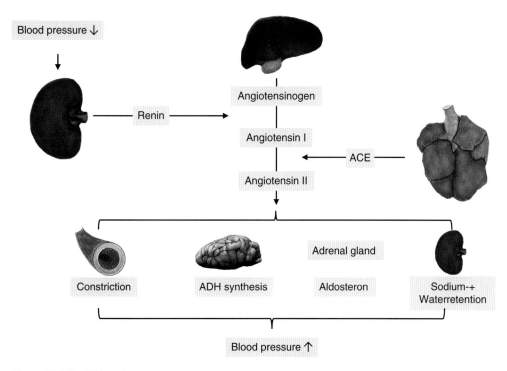

Figure 41.1.3 RAA-system.

Finally, angiotensin II causes a feeling of thirst. All these mechanisms increase the volume of blood and thus blood pressure (Figure 41.1.3).

Erythropoiesis

Hypoxia induces erythropoiesis; the peptide hormone erythropoietin is significantly involved in the stimulation of erythropoiesis. A reduced supply of oxygen to specialised fibroblasts in the proximal tubules induces the synthesis of the transcription factor hypoxia-inducible factor (HIF). This causes the increased transcription of the erythropoietin gene.

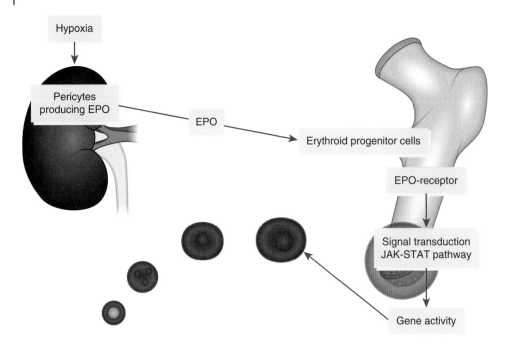

Figure 41.1.4 Erythropoietin pathway.

Oxygen reduction may be due to decreased renal perfusion, reduction of erythrocytes or reduced oxygen uptake in the lungs. Erythropoietin itself acts via an erythropoietin receptor on nucleated erythrocyte progenitor cells. By binding erythropoietin to the receptor, the apoptosis of erythrocyte progenitor cells is suppressed by intracellular tyrosine kinases. The result is a proliferation and differentiation of these cells into erythrocytes. The process leads to reticulocytosis with a time delay of three to four days (Figure 41.1.4).

A subordinate but existing renal function is given by the formation of thrombopoietin, which induces the differentiation of megakaryocytes and thus affects blood clotting.

Gluconeogenesis

Finally, the kidneys also have a metabolic function via gluconeogenesis. In the tubular cells, the amino acid glutamine can be deaminated. The resulting glutamate is built up into glucose via oxoglutarate. The resulting amino groups can contribute to acid elimination by synthesis of ammonium ions and thus support the function of the kidneys in the acid-base balance. Further, glucose synthesis from lactate is possible. In the case of metabolic acidosis, gluconeogenesis in the kidney can be increased.

Further Reading

Rastogie, S.C. (2007). *Essentials of Animal Physiology*. New Age International Publishers.

Schmidt, R.F., Lang, F., and Heckmann, M. (2010). *Human Physiology*. Springer Verlag.

Sjaastad, O.V., Sand, O., and Hove, K. (2016). Physiology of Domestic Animals. Scandinavian Veterinary Press.

Wei, K., Yin, Z., and Xie, Y. (2016). Roles of the kidney in the formation, remodeling and repair of bone. *Journal of Nephrology* 29 (3): 349–357. https://doi.org/10.1007/s40620-016-0284-7.

41.2

Glomerulonephritis/Nephrotic Syndrome

Definition

Glomerulonephritis is usually the consequence of an inflammatory response to the deposition of antigen-antibody complexes in the glomerulum. It is the most common form of glomerulopathy and leads to chronic renal insufficiency by reducing glomerular filtration. *Nephrotic syndrome* is a special form of glomerulopathy with a defined combination of the symptoms hypoalbuminaemia, proteinuria, oedema and hypercholesterolaemia. Not every glomerulonephritis develops the complete symptomatology of a nephrotic syndrome.

Aetiology

The causes of glomerulonephritis are usually infectious or non-infectious inflammatory processes. In any case, the formation of soluble antigen-antibody complexes is a prerequisite for the inflammatory reaction in the glomerulum. Few neoplastic and some congenital diseases are also causative of glomerulonephritis. Apart from the known causalities, many glomerulonephritides are idiopathic. Both species, dogs and cats, can be affected, but it is more often seen in dogs.

Infection	Non-infectious inflammation	Neoplasia	Congenital
Babesiosis (D)	Systemic lupus erythematosus (SLE) (D)	Lymphoma (D/C)	Spaniels
Dirofilariasis (D)	Pancreatitis (D)	Mast cell tumour (D/C)	Wheaten Terriers
Ehrlichiosis (D)			Newfoundland dogs
Hepatozoonosis (D)			
Leishmaniasis (D)			
Lyme disease (D)			
Brucellosis (D)			
FeLv (C)			
FIV (C)			
FIP (C)			

D – Dog, C – Cat

Pathogenesis

The essential pathogenetic step in the development of glomerulonephritis is the deposition of soluble immune complexes in the glomerular area. Rarely, the disease develops through synthesis of antibodies against structures of the glomerulum. Immune complexes are differentiated according to molecular weight and charge. Very large immune complexes lead less

Textbook of Small Animal Pathophysiology, First Edition. Stephan Neumann.
© 2025 John Wiley & Sons Ltd. Published 2025 by John Wiley & Sons Ltd.

Table 41.2.1   Cells and mediators in the pathogenesis of glomerulonephritis.

Effector	Mediator	Target cell
Podocyte	Cytokines (IL-1, IL-6, TNF, TGF, PDGF) Prostaglandins, Leukotrienes, Proteases	Glomerular epithelial cells and endothelial cells
Macrophage		
Neutrophilic granulocyte		
Platelet		

Source: Adapted from Breshears and Confer (2017).

frequently to glomerulonephritis because they are already eliminated in the blood vessels by phagocytosis. Smaller and medium complexes reach the glomerular vessels. Mediated by the release of vasoactive mediators from sessile mast cells and basophilic granulocytes, the immune complexes pass from the vessel into the glomerular area. The mediator release is determined by the interaction of the immune complexes with cellular surface receptors.

The next step in pathogenesis is the initiation of an inflammatory process. This is initiated by complement activation following the reaction of complement with the immune complex (Table 41.2.1).

Subsequently, an inflammatory response mediated by macrophages and neutrophilic granulocytes develops. Aggregation of platelets and activation of the intrinsic coagulation cascade leads to thrombus formation and glomerular ischaemia, which also influences disease progression.

Morphologically, depending on the localisation of the immune complexes, membranous glomerulonephritis with subepithelial deposition of immune complexes, between the basement membrane and the podocytes mesangioproliferative glomerulonephritis with immune complexes in the mesangium and membranoproliferative glomerulonephritis with immune complex deposits in the mesangium and along the glomerular capillary walls can be distinguished.

The morphological changes in glomerulonephritis can be reversible. Progressive inflammatory processes eventually lead to fibrotic remodelling of the glomerulus (Figure 41.2.1).

Glomerulonephritis of various causes, such as lupus erythematosus, amyloidosis or various infections can develop into a nephrotic syndrome. This leads to a pronounced destruction of components of the glomerular filtration barrier. This consists of the endothelial cells of the glomerular capillaries, a basement membrane consisting of collagens and proteoglycans, such as heparan sulphates, and a layer of podocytes. All components of the glomerular filtration barrier prevent the filtration of molecules of certain size and negative charge.

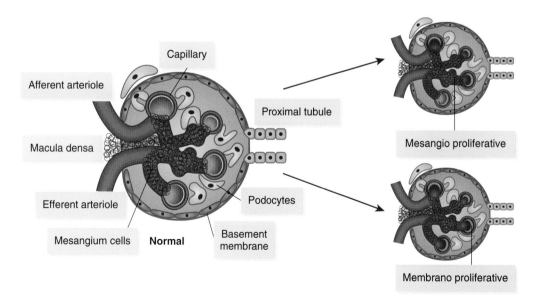

Figure 41.2.1   Different forms of glomerulonephritis.

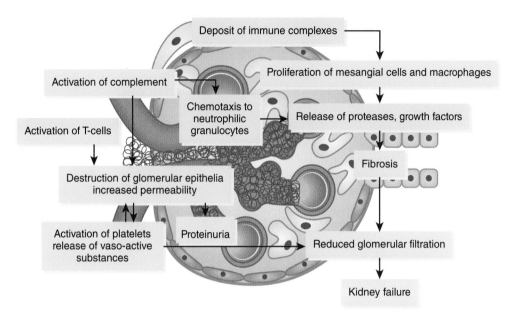

Figure 41.2.2 Pathogenesis of glomerulonephritis with nephrotic syndrome.

The consequences of destruction are loss of negative charge carriers (e.g. heparan sulphates), which leads to proteinuria, since proteins as negatively charged molecules are also protected from glomerular loss by the charge-associated barrier. Furthermore, filtration areas are lost due to the destruction, which are compensated by an increased filtration pressure in functional glomeruli. Glomerular hypertension leads to proteinuria even in still intact glomerulus. Increased tubular protein concentration, in turn, induces tubular cytokine expression and complement activation. This results in further loss of active nephrons (Abbate et al. 2006).

In the further course, there is a loss of primarily non-urinary molecules. These include proteins, such as albumin, immunoglobulins, antithrombin III, etc. This loss is the reason for the pathophysiologic consequences of the nephrotic syndrome (Figure 41.2.2).

Diagnostics

Clinical signs	Clinical pathology	Imaging	Histopathology	Microbiology
Non-specific; PU/PD	Proteinuria; Increased urine protein-creatinine ratio	Non-specific	If necessary to confirm the diagnosis	Not necessary

Pathophysiologic Consequences

The pathophysiologic consequences of glomerulonephritis can be explained primarily by the loss of functional molecules across the glomerular filtration barrier. In addition to the urinary system, they also affect the cardiovascular system and metabolism.

Influenced organ systems	Clinical symptoms	Clinical pathological alterations
Urinary tract	Weight loss	Hypoalbuminaemia
Cardiovascular system	Lethargy	Proteinuria
Metabolism	Oedema	Hypercholesterolaemia
	Dyspnoea	Azotaemia

Proteinuria and **hypoalbuminaemia** are the main pathophysiologic consequences of glomerulonephritis.

Weight loss in patients with glomerulonephritis and nephrotic syndrome may develop from the underlying disease. Inflammatory reactions can lead to a reduction in body mass. On the one hand, proinflammatory cytokines such as TNF-α or IL-1 induce a catabolic metabolic state. One mechanism is the activation of the hypothalamus-hypophysis axis with the consequence of increased corticoid synthesis, which causes a catabolic metabolic state. Furthermore, inflammatory cells have a direct influence on the metabolic state (Baazim et al. 2022). In addition, proteinuria leads to hypoalbuminaemia, which in turn induces albumin synthesis in the liver. At the same time, the liver is the site of synthesis for acute phase proteins that are active in glomerulonephritis. Both lead to an increase in protein synthesis in the liver. The resource for amino acids is the muscles. This leads to muscle wasting and weight loss due to increased liver synthesis to compensate for the hypoalbuminaemia (Argilés et al. 2015).

Lethargy is characterised by decreased activity, increased somnolence and increased tolerance to irritation. It is a symptom that is related to the extent of the disease and can have different causalities. Causes of lethargy include reduced oxygen supply, for example in anaemia or dyspnoea, increased intracranial pressure in disorders of fluid balance, or a lack of energy-providing metabolites. All causalities can come into play in glomerulonephritis.

Another consequence of glomerulonephritis with nephrotic syndrome is **oedema** formation. The pathomechanism begins with a reduction in oncotic pressure due to albumin loss via the kidneys. This leads to a reduction in blood volume. According to the 'underfill' theory, this in turn leads to activation of the RAAS and increased ADH secretion, resulting in increased sodium and water reabsorption in the proximal tubule, as well as increased water reabsorption in the distal tubule and collecting tube. According to the 'overfill' theory, glomerulonephritis results in an independent activation of sodium reabsorption due to a reduced effect of ANP in the proximal tubule. Both theories lead to hyperhydration. As the oncotic pressure in the vascular system is reduced, oedema develops. Oedema formation is possible at albumin concentrations below 2.0 mg/dl in dogs and cats (Bockenhauer 2013).

The glomerular loss of proteins also affects antithrombin III, a glycoprotein with a molecular weight of 58 kDa that is produced in the liver. It belongs to the serine protease inhibitors, which is involved in the inhibition of clotting by inactivating the clotting factors, e.g. thrombin, factor IXa, Xa, XIa and XIIa. Glomerular loss of antithrombin III interferes with fibrinolysis and promotes platelet aggregation. Both lead to hypercoagulability and thrombus formation. If thrombi form in the pulmonary arteries, a pulmonary embolism is present and can cause **dyspnoea**.

Other glomerular protein losses with possible pathophysiologic consequences include loss of immunoglobulins with a possible increased risk of infection. Glomerular loss of thyroxine-binding globulin can lead to a reduction in protein-bound thyroid hormones. Although these are hormonally inactive, they generate the free biologically active forms. This could help explain the euthyroid state with reduced T4 at normal TSH observed in chronic diseases.

Renal loss of transferrin and iron can cause microcytic hypochromic iron deficiency anaemia.

Finally, vitamin D-binding protein is also lost in glomerulonephritis. As a result, vitamin D deficiency develops and affects calcium metabolism.

The renal protein loss and thus the reduction of oncotic pressure induces hepatic protein synthesis, whereby lipoproteins are formed in addition to albumins. For example, the reduction of oncotic pressure leads directly to the expression of apolipoprotein B. This is a structural protein of VLDL and LDL. Since lipoproteins are hardly filtered even in the damaged glomerulum, both processes lead to their increase in the blood. Cholesterol is a component of these lipoproteins, which is why **hypercholesterolaemia** develops.

Renal loss of other molecules implies additional symptoms of glomerulonephritis (Table 41.2.2).

The morphological remodelling processes with disturbances of the glomerular filtration process may also affect renal function in terms of excretion of urinary molecules and thus cause **azotaemia** (Figure 41.2.3).

Table 41.2.2 Summary of possible glomerular protein losses.

Molecule	Clinical consequence
IgG	Susceptibility to infections
Thyroxine-binding globulin	Hypothyroidism
Transferrin	Anaemia
Iron	Anaemia
Vitamin D	Osteomalacia

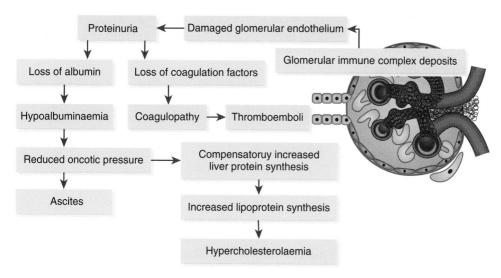

Figure 41.2.3 Pathophysiologic consequences of glomerulonephritis with nephrotic syndrome.

Therapy

Symptom	Therapy
Proteinuria	ACE inhibitors, angiotensin receptor blockers
Hypoalbuminaemia, oedema	Diet
Thromboembolism	Inhibition of thrombocyte aggregation (e.g. acetylsalicylic acid, clopidogrel)

References

Abbate, M., Zoja, C., and Remuzzi, G. (2006). How does proteinuria cause progressive renal damage? *Journal of the American Society of Nephrology: JASN* 17 (11): 2974–2984. https://doi.org/10.1681/ASN.2006040377.

Argilés, J.M., Stemmler, B., López-Soriano, F.J., and Busquets, S. (2015). Nonmuscle tissues contribution to cancer cachexia. *Mediators of Inflammation* 2015: 182872. https://doi.org/10.1155/2015/182872.

Baazim, H., Antonio-Herrera, L., and Bergthaler, A. (2022). The interplay of immunology and cachexia in infection and cancer. *Nature Reviews. Immunology* 22 (5): 309–321. https://doi.org/10.1038/s41577-021-00624-w.

Bockenhauer, D. (2013). Over- or underfill: not all nephrotic states are created equal. *Pediatric Nephrology (Berlin, Germany)* 28 (8): 1153–1156. https://doi.org/10.1007/s00467-013-2435-6.

Breshears, M.A. and Confer, A.W. (2017). The urinary system. In: *Pathologic Basis of Veterinary Disease*, 6e (ed. J.F. Zachary), 645. Elsevier.

Further Reading

Littman, M.P., Gerber, B., Goldstein, R.E. et al. (2018). ACVIM consensus update on Lyme borreliosis in dogs and cats. *Journal of Veterinary Internal Medicine* 32 (3): 887–903.

Slauson, D.O. and Lewis, R.M. (1979). Comparative pathology of glomerulonephritis in animals. *Veterinary Pathology* 16 (2): 135–164.

Vaden, S.L. (2011). Glomerular disease. *Topics in Companion Animal Medicine* 26 (3): 128–134.

Vaden, S.L. and Elliott, J. (2016). Management of proteinuria in dogs and cats with chronic kidney disease. *The Veterinary Clinics of North America. Small Animal Practice* 46 (6): 1115–1130.

41.3

Tubular Disease/Fanconi Syndrome

Definition

Fanconi syndrome describes a resorption disorder of the proximal tubule. As a result, substances requiring absorption appear in the urine.

Aetiology

In dogs, mainly Basenjis are affected by this disease, which suggests a congenital defect. Intoxication caused by the ingestion of duck, chicken or turkey meat produced in China led to an increase in the number of cases described in the 2010s. Finally, drug-induced tubulopathies are possible after the administration of gentamycin or chlorambucil. The disease occurs very rarely in dogs and cats.

Congenital	Intoxication
Basenji	Chicken jerkys (D)
	Gentamycin (D)
	Chlorambucil (C)

D – Dog, C – Cat

Pathogenesis

Isolated tubulopathies are rare in dogs and cats. The molecular cause of Fanconi syndrome is a resorption disorder in the tubule of unknown genesis. This leads to an excretion of substances requiring resorption, such as some amino acids (COLA: cystine, ornithine, lysine, arginine), glucose, bicarbonate, phosphate and sodium. The absorption of these substances is associated with a transmembrane Na^+ gradient between tubule lumen and intracellular space, which in turn is maintained by an Na^+/K^+-ATPase of the basolateral membrane. Disturbances of the Na^+/K^+-ATPase could therefore be responsible for the resorption disturbances and the increased excretion (Figure 41.3.1).

Another possible mechanism could be due to impaired megalin endocytosis. Megalin is a transmembrane protein that, together with cubilin, enables membranous endocytosis in epithelia, such as the proximal tubule. In this way, molecules such as peptides are reabsorbed into the tubule. For this purpose, the molecules attach themselves to the receptor. The resulting complex is taken up intracellularly via membrane invagination. The receptor can be regenerated from the complex by the influx of protons into the vesicle. The absorbed molecule undergoes lysosomal catabolism. Disturbances of this process are possibly causative of proximal tubular resorption disorders (Nielsen et al. 2016).

Textbook of Small Animal Pathophysiology, First Edition. Stephan Neumann.

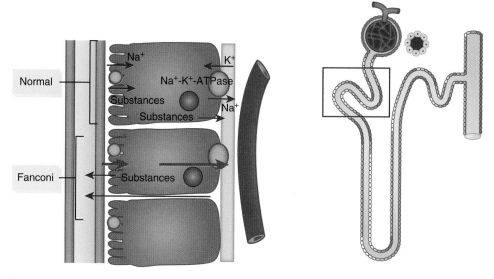

Figure 41.3.1   Resorption disorders in Fanconi syndrome.

Diagnostics

Clinical signs	Clinical pathology	Imaging	Histopathology	Microbiology
Non-specific	Aminoaciduria (COLA) Glucose uria with normal serum glucose	Non-specific	Not necessary	Not necessary

Pathophysiologic Consequences

The disease primarily affects the urinary system and metabolism.

Influenced organ systems	Clinical symptoms	Clinical pathological alterations
Urinary tract	Lethargy	Metabolic acidosis
Metabolism	Weight loss PU/PD	Urinary loss of cystine, ornithine, lysine, arginine, glucose, bicarbonate, phosphate and sodium

The loss of amino acids and glucose as a source of energy induces the clinical symptoms of **lethargy** and **weight loss**. Similarly, the symptoms of **PU/PD** are explained by glucosuria, which leads to osmotic diuresis due to the water-binding capacity of glucose. The polyuria leads to a loss of volume, which lowers the blood pressure and implies, among other things, the formation of ADH. This in turn increases the blood volume by increasing water reabsorption via aquaporins and by inducing the feeling of thirst, which leads to polydipsia.

The respective losses of substances that are proximally tubularly reabsorbed explain their excretion via the urine. In particular, the loss of buffer substances, such as bicarbonate or phosphate is responsible for the **metabolic acidosis** in Fanconi syndrome. This also leads to reduced sodium and potassium reabsorption. This in turn causes hyponatraemia and hypokalaemia and is also responsible for the systemic symptomatology of lethargy (Figure 41.3.2).

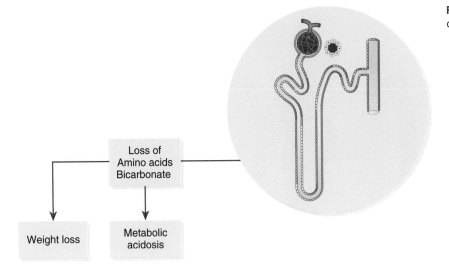

Figure 41.3.2 Pathophysiologic consequences of Fanconi syndrome.

Therapy

Symptom	Therapy
Weight loss	Diet
Metabolic acidosis	Infusion with bicarbonate

Reference

Nielsen, R., Christensen, E.I., and Birn, H. (2016). Megalin and cubilin in proximal tubule protein reabsorption: from experimental models to human disease. *Kidney International* 89 (1): 58–67. https://doi.org/10.1016/j.kint.2015.11.007.

Further Reading

Carmichael, N., Lee, J., and Giger, U. (2014). Fanconi syndrome in dogs in the UK. *The Veterinary Record* 174 (14): 357–358.

Igase, M., Baba, K., Shimokawa Miyama, T. et al. (2015). Acquired Fanconi syndrome in a dog exposed to jerky treatments in Japan. *The Journal of Veterinary Medical Science* 77 (11): 1507–1510.

Reinert, N.C. and Feldman, D.G. (2016). Acquired Fanconi syndrome in four cats treated with chlorambucil. *Journal of Feline Medicine and Surgery* 18 (12): 1034–1040.

41.4

Acute Renal Failure

Definition

Acute kidney failure is defined as an abrupt reduction in the function of the kidneys with an accumulation of substances excreted in the urine in the body.

Aetiology

The causes of acute renal failure are mainly due to reduced perfusion of the kidneys or toxic-inflammatory damage to the kidney tissue. Acute renal failure occurs in dogs and cats.

Renal ischaemia	Nephrotoxins	Inflammation
Adrenal insufficiency (D)	Aminoglycosides (D,C)	Glomerulonephritis (D)
Anaesthesia (D,C)	Ethylene glycols (D,C)	Interstitial nephritis (C)
Congestive heart failure (D,C)		Pancreatitis (D,C)
Shock (D,C)		Sepsis (D,C)

D – Dog, C – Cat

The consequence is impaired kidney function with an accumulation of substances excreted in the urine. In addition to urea and creatinine, both of which are used in laboratory diagnostics as parameters of kidney function, these include over 100 so-called 'substances excreted in the urine'. Many of these are the so-called 'biogenic amines' which, when they accumulate in the body, lead to symptoms of intoxication, i.e. uraemia. The uraemic toxins are divided into small water-soluble, non-protein-bound substances (e.g. urea, creatinine, polyamines, oxalates), protein-bound substances (e.g. cresol, homocysteine, indoles) and higher molecular substances (e.g. parathormone, leptin, cytokines).

Pathogenesis

The triggering factors can cause acute renal failure via three morphologically differentiated localisations. In **pre-renal acute renal failure**, the cause lies in the area of renal perfusion. The reduction of renal perfusion, for example in shock, reduces renal perfusion. The consequence is a reduction in blood pressure in the afferent arterioles. This leads to constriction of the vasa afferentia. As a result, the filtration pressure and thus the glomerular filtration rate is reduced. At the same time, the glomeruli swell, reducing permeability at the glomerular filtration barrier, which further lowers GFR. In the course of the disease, the reduction in post-glomerular blood flow leads to ischaemia of the proximal and distal tubule.

Textbook of Small Animal Pathophysiology, First Edition. Stephan Neumann.
© 2025 John Wiley & Sons Ltd. Published 2025 by John Wiley & Sons Ltd.

This reduces active reabsorption processes. Necrotic tubular epithelia detach from the tubule and can lead to obstruction of the tubule with a further reduction in urine production.

The organism tries to increase renal perfusion again through three different mechanisms. Firstly, a reflex relaxation of the smooth vascular musculature of the afferent arterioles leads to vascular dilatation, as a result of which glomerular perfusion increases. Another mechanism is based on the increased secretion of ADH. This is produced in the supraoptic nucleus and paraventricularly in the hypothalamus and reaches the posterior pituitary via nerve axons. An increase in plasma osmolarity measured at osmoreceptors in the hypothalamus or a reduction in volume measured at baroreceptors in the right atrium leads to ADH secretion. ADH initiates the synthesis of aquaporins, water tubules, in the distal tubule and collecting duct via a membrane receptor and cAMP as a second messenger. In this way, water reabsorption in the tubule system is increased, and the blood volume increases with the consequence of an increase in blood pressure. Finally, the third mechanism activates the RAAS. The following activators have been described, a decreased glomerular filtration and decreased blood pressure in the afferent arterioles measured at baroreceptors. Renin activates angiotensinogen to angiotensin I, which is activated by angiotensin-converting enzymes to angiotensin II, which leads to smooth muscle constriction in the efferent arterioles, resulting in an increase in glomerular blood pressure and glomerular filtration. Angiotensin II promotes the secretion of ADH and simultaneously that of aldosterone. The latter is formed in the zona glomerulosa of the adrenal cortex. Aldosterone initiates the synthesis of sodium tubules on the luminal and sodium transport proteins on the basal side of the tubule cells in the distal tubule. The result is increased sodium reabsorption, which increases water uptake via a symport and thus blood volume and blood pressure. If the described compensatory mechanisms are overtaxed, acute kidney failure develops.

In renal **acute renal failure**, the causal pathological change is found in the renal parenchyma. This can affect the glomeruli as glomerulonephritis, the interstitium as interstitial nephritis or the tubules as tubulopathy. The causes of glomerulonephritis are in many cases immune-mediated. Soluble antigen-antibody complexes are deposited in the glomerulum. This induces a complement-mediated inflammatory response. This results in complement activation and infiltration of neutrophilic granulocytes and macrophages. Secreted lysosomal enzymes and free radicals damage the endothelial cells of the vessel wall and the basement membrane, resulting in a reduced filtration surface. At the same time, platelet aggregation and thrombus formation develops. Secretion of vasoactive substances by platelets further reduces blood flow to the glomeruli. Contraction of the mesangial cells by the action of the inflammatory mediators further impedes glomerular perfusion and filtration. The anionic charge of the capillary wall decreases, the filtration pores become larger, allowing proteinuria despite hypofiltration. The result is a membranous, mesangioproliferative or membranoproliferative remodelling in the glomerulum (Figure 41.4.1).

Interstitial nephritis usually develops from an infectious event in the tubulo-interstitial area. An example of tubulo-interstitial nephritis is leptospirosis (see Chapter 48.3.4).

The inflammatory process damages the tubular epithelia via cytokines and other mediators. This leads to an alteration of the cytoskeleton. In consequence, there is a loss of the microvilli, a destruction of the tight-junctions to the neighbouring tubule epithelial cells and dissolution of the connection between the tubule epithelial cells and the extracellular matrix. Everything leads to necrotic or apoptotic cell death (Sancho-Martínez et al. 2015) (Figure 41.4.2).

Post-renal acute renal failure represents the third localisation that can lead to renal failure. Urinary outflow disorders are causally present. They can be localised as tumour diseases in the area of the urinary tract, e.g. at the transitional epithelial carcinoma at the bladder neck. More frequently, obstructions of the urethra caused by calculi are causal. Neurogenic bladder emptying disorders can also lead to post-renal acute kidney failure. In all cases, glomerular filtration is reduced. This in turn activates the compensatory mechanisms described in pre-renal acute renal failure. In addition, urinary reflux into the renal tubules increases the pressure and thus promotes necrosis of the tubular epithelial cells, which is described as a causality in renal acute kidney failure. Consequences of obstruction include nephron loss, altered renal expression of growth factors and cytokines and apoptosis of glomerular, tubular and vascular cells (Chevalier et al. 2010).

Acute renal failure is a morphologically functionally dynamic process.

The main initiating mechanisms are ischaemia caused by reduced perfusion and consequent hypoxia of the tubular cell structures, as well as reduced glomerular filtration rate due to reduced filtration.

This leads to the:

Destruction of capillary endothelial cells, which causes medullary congestion
Constriction of the vas afferens and dilatation of the vas efferens (= shunt)

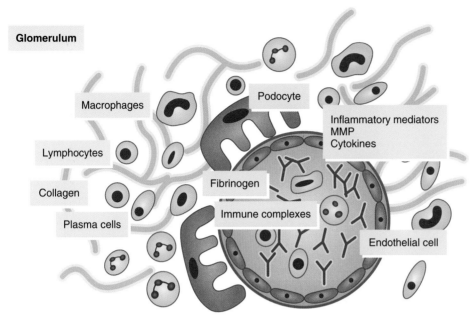

Figure 41.4.1 Mechanism of glomerular damage.

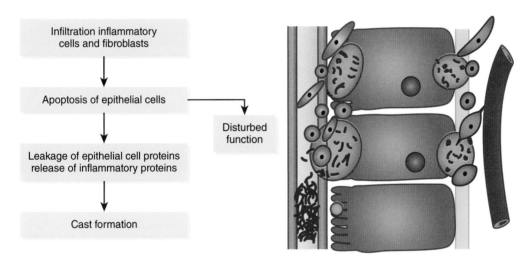

Figure 41.4.2 Mechanism of tubule damage.

Reperfusion damage to epithelial cells with accumulation of free radicals, lysosomal enzymes and mediators, such as prostaglandins, leukotrienes and endothelin.

This causes the tubular epithelial cells to lose their polarity and undergo apoptosis or necrosis. The detached cells form cylinders in the lumen, causing occlusions and proximal fluid back-flow (back-leak). In severe cases, damage to the basement membrane occurs in addition to epithelial damage and is irreversible (Figure 41.4.3).

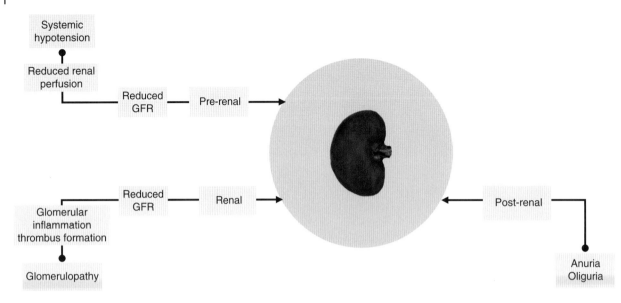

Figure 41.4.3 Pathogenesis of acute renal failure.

Diagnostics

Clinical signs	Clinical pathology	Imaging	Histopathology	Microbiology
Disturbed general condition Oliguria	Elevated kidney parameters Urea, creatinine, phosphorus, Symmetric dimethylarginine (SDMA)	**Ultrasonography** Enlargement of the kidneys, structural changes of the parenchyma	Not necessary	Not necessary

Pathophysiologic Consequences

The consequences of acute kidney failure are local and systemic. Besides the urinary system, the cardiovascular system, the respiratory system and the gastrointestinal tract are affected.

Influenced organ systems	Clinical symptoms	Clinical pathological alterations
Cardiovascular system	Lethargy	Variable PCV
Respiratory system	Anorexia	Leucocytosis
Gastrointestinal system	Vomiting	Increased
Urinary tract	Diarrhoea	Urea
	Bradycardia	Creatinine
	Tachypnoea	Phosphorus
	Oliguria	Potassium
		Metabolic acidosis
		Proteinuria
		Glucosuria
		Casts

Acute renal failure is clinically divided into two phases. The primary oliguric phase is characterised by reduced glomerular filtration and is accompanied by anuria or oliguria. The secondary polyuric phase reflects the recovery of the nephron, in which glomerular filtration slowly becomes physiological again. In some causalities, such as heavy metals, the primary phase may already be polyuric.

Major factors determining the clinical consequences of acute renal failure are hyperhydration due to reduced glomerular filtration, metabolic acidosis, retention of uraemic toxins and disturbances of electrolyte balance, especially hyperkalaemia.

The disturbance of fluid balance in acute renal failure results from reduced glomerular filtration and compensatory activation of the RAAS. As a result, water retention in the third space may occur and oedema may develop. Water retention in the lung parenchyma can cause **tachypnoea** due to impaired ventilation. In this case, alveolar oxygen uptake is reduced. The developing hypoxia leads to stimulation of peripheral chemoreceptors in the carotid artery. The reaction is an increase in respiratory rate. This is exacerbated by respiratory compensation for **metabolic acidosis**. If the pH value in the blood drops, central chemoreceptors in the brain stem initiate hyperventilation through tachypnoea, which has the function of reducing the pCO_2 in the blood.

Hyperhydration in the intestinal mucosa leads to a dysfunction of the intestinal wall and possibly a disturbance of the intestinal wall barrier with translocation of intestinal bacteria. Bacterial toxins also enter the body's systems, which, due to the reduced glomerular filtration in acute renal failure, also act as uraemic toxins. Indoxyl sulphate or p-cresyl sulphate are two examples of uraemic toxins from the intestinal microbiome. Intestinal dysfunction, in turn, is responsible for the clinical symptom **diarrhoea**. The cause of **vomiting** in acute renal failure may be hypergastrinaemia due to impaired excretion. Gastrin acts on the parietal cells in the gastric mucosa and influences the activity of the proton pump. The result is an increase in gastric acid. This can lead to gastritis and vomiting. The central effect of uraemic toxins on the vomiting centre also has an influence (Rosner et al. 2021). The formation of uraemic toxins has a significant influence on the symptoms of renal failure. These are divided into different groups (Table 41.4.1).

Table 41.4.1 Uraemic toxins.

Small, water soluble	Protein bound	Medium-sized molecules
Asymmetric dimethylarginine	3-Deoxyglucosone	Adrenomedullin
Benzylalcohol	Fructoselysine	Atrial natriuretic peptide
ß-Guanidinopropionic acid	Glyoxal	ß-microglobulin
ß-Lipotropin	Hippuric acid	ß-endorphin
Creatinine	Homocysteines	Cholecystokinin
Cytidine	Hydroquinone	Clara cell protein
Guanidine	Indole-3-acetic acid	Complement factor D
Guanidinoacetic acid	Indoxyl sulphate	Cystatin
Guanidinosuccinic acid	Kinurenine	Degranulation inhibiting protein I
Hypoxanthine	Kynurenic acid	Endothelin
Malondialdehyde	Methylglyoxal	Hyaluronic acid
Methylguanidine	N-carboxymethyllysine	IL-1
Myoinositol	P-cresol	IL-6
Orotic acid	Pentosidine	κ-Ig light chain
Orotidine	Phenol	λ-Ig light chain
Oxalate	Hippuric acid	Leptin
Pseudouridine	Quinolinic acid	Methionine- enkephalin
Symmetric dimethylarginine	Spermidine	Neuropeptide Y
Uric acid	Spermine	Parathyroid hormone
Xanthine		Retinol binding protein
		TNF-alpha

Source: Adapted from Vanholder et al. (2003).

Effects of the toxins are possible on different organ systems. Central effects of the toxins on the CNS are also held responsible for the generalised symptoms of **lethargy** and **anorexia** (Kellum et al. 2021).

The main disturbance of the electrolyte balance in acute kidney failure is the reduced excretion of potassium. The consequences of hyperkalaemia are, for example, disturbances of cardiac function up to **bradycardia**.

The biochemical parameter in acute renal failure is a variable **haematocrit**. In particular, the increase in haematocrit may be the cause rather than the consequence of renal failure. Increases in red blood cell count are associated with numerous consequences due to altered blood flow properties. The increased viscosity slows blood flow and can activate the intrinsic blood coagulation cascade, which can lead to microthrombi resulting in vascular occlusion and tissue ischaemia. Clinical symptoms develop depending on the organ in which the tissue ischaemia occurs. For example, neurological symptoms, such as **lethargy** and **weakness** have been described (Cuthbert and Stein 2019). The pathological mechanisms in acute renal failure inherently induce an inflammatory response with **leukocytosis**. Resident dendritic cells also initiate a strong chemotactic gradient for neutrophil recruitment, through secretion of TNF-α, IL-6, MCP-1, IL-8. Through secretion of proinflammatory cytokines, neutrophilic granulocytes recruit other inflammatory cells, such as natural killer cells, monocytes and macrophages (Han and Lee 2019).

The main biochemical consequence of acute kidney failure is the accumulation of substances physiologically excreted via the urine. Laboratory diagnostics classically measure **urea**, **creatinine** and **phosphorus**. The mechanism underlying **hyperkalaemia** is explained by the reduced filtration capacity of the kidney. The increased extracellular potassium concentration leads to a disturbance of the membrane potential. The membrane potential at the cell membrane results from a potassium transport directed to the extracellular area. With an increased extracellular potassium concentration, this mechanism is disturbed, resulting in a permanent membrane depolarisation. This prevents the excitability of the cells; usually the heart and skeletal muscle cells are affected. Such disturbances are to be expected at serum concentrations of potassium >6–8 mmol/l. Clinical consequences on the heart are disturbances recognisable in the ECG, such as prolonged PR intervals, a widened QRS complex or a peaked T-wave. In the most severe cases, hyperexcitability initially occurs because the membrane potential approaches the threshold potential due to increasing depolarisation and action potentials are triggered in the meantime, which manifests itself in ventricular fibrillations. In the further course, asystole occurs.

The consequences of depolarised skeletal muscles are muscle cramps, muscle weakness and paralysis. Central nervous structures are protected from the consequences of hyperkalaemia by the blood-brain barrier. In addition, potassium-associated depolarisation can stimulate the secretion of various hormones, such as insulin, aldosterone or corticoids (Hunter and Bailey 2019).

Metabolic acidosis occurs as a consequence of acute renal failure, as the regulation of proton excretion via the nephron is suppressed. The consequences of metabolic acidosis are an increased influx of protons into the cells. This inhibits the ATP-dependent Na^+-K^+ pump. The consequence is an increased intracellular retention of sodium ions, a water shift leads to cell swelling and thus to a disturbance of cell function. Furthermore, inhibition of the ATP-dependent Na^+-K^+ pump supports the extracellular retention of potassium ions, which promotes hyperkalaemia. Finally, protons displace intracellular potassium from protein binding, thereby increasing cellular potassium efflux. The cellular disruption and promoted hyperkalaemia induced by acidosis affects different organs. A reduction in contractile force develops in the heart. Bone demineralisation occurs as a result of acidosis, as the alkaline bone salts are dissolved under the influence of acid (Kim 2021).

Renal consequences of acute renal failure may include proteinuria, glucosuria and be the formation of casts. Casts occur as cell-rich or cell-free aggregates and form in the tubules. On the one hand, proteins are involved in the formation, which arise in acute renal failure due to tubulopathy and are a consequence of inflammation or tubular epithelial cell necrosis. The protein backbone shows osmotic properties and can hinder the secretion and reabsorption processes in the tubule. In addition, casts that are formed sometimes also induce an inflammatory process. In severe cases, the nephron becomes blocked (Basnayake et al. 2011). This leads to atrophy of the nephron with functional insufficiency (Figure 41.4.4).

Therapy

Symptom	Drug
Induction of diuresis	Infusion
	Diuretics
	Dopamine
Equalisation of acidosis	Infusion with buffer (bicarbonate)
Equalisation of hyperkalaemia	Bicarbonate infusion
	Loop diuretics

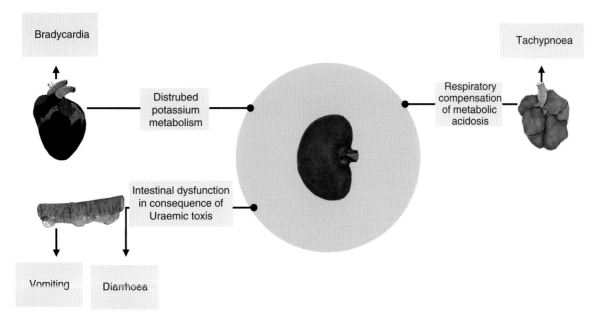

Figure 41.4.4 Pathophysiologic consequences of acute renal failure.

References

Basnayake, K., Stringer, S.J., Hutchison, C.A., and Cockwell, P. (2011). The biology of immunoglobulin free light chains and kidney injury. *Kidney International* 79 (12): 1289–1301. https://doi.org/10.1038/ki.2011.94.

Chevalier, R.L., Thornhill, B.A., Forbes, M.S. et al. (2010). Mechanisms of renal injury and progression of renal disease in congenital obstructive nephropathy. *Pediatric Nephrology* 25: 687–697. https://doi.org/10.1007/s00467-009-1316-5.

Cuthbert, D. and Stein, B.L. (2019). Polycythemia vera-associated complications: pathogenesis, clinical manifestations, and effects on outcomes. *Journal of Blood Medicine* 10: 359–371. https://doi.org/10.2147/JBM.S189922.

Han, S.J. and Lee, H.T. (2019). Mechanisms and therapeutic targets of ischemic acute kidney injury. *Kidney Research and Clinical Practice* 38 (4): 427–440. 10.23876/j.krcp.19.062.

Hunter, R.W. and Bailey, M.A. (2019). Hyperkalemia: pathophysiology, risk factors and consequences. *Nephrology, Dialysis, Transplantation: Official Publication of the European Dialysis and Transplant Association – European Renal Association* 34 (Suppl 3): iii2–iii11. https://doi.org/10.1093/ndt/gfz206.

Kellum, J.A., Romagnani, P., Ashuntantang, G. et al. (2021). Acute kidney injury. *Nature Reviews. Disease Primers* 7 (1): 52. https://doi.org/10.1038/s41572-021-00284-z.

Kim, H.J. (2021). Metabolic acidosis in chronic kidney disease: pathogenesis, clinical consequences, and treatment. *Electrolyte & Blood Pressure: E & BP* 19 (2): 29–37. https://doi.org/10.5049/EBP.2021.19.2.29.

Rosner, M.H., Reis, T., Husain-Syed, F. et al. (2021). Classification of uremic toxins and their role in kidney failure. *Clinical Journal of the American Society of Nephrology: CJASN* 16 (12): 1918–1928. 10.2215/CJN.02660221.

Sancho-Martínez, S.M., López-Novoa, J.M., and López-Hernández, F.J. (2015). Pathophysiological role of different tubular epithelial cell death modes in acute kidney injury. *Clinical Kidney Journal* 8 (5): 548–559. https://doi.org/10.1093/ckj/sfv069.

Vanholder, R., Glorieux, G., De Smet, R. et al. (2003). New insights in uremic toxins. *Kidney International. Supplement* 84: S6–S10. https://doi.org/10.1046/j.1523-1755.63.s84.43.x.

Further Reading

Basile, D.P., Anderson, M.D., and Sutton, T.A. (2012). Pathophysiology of acute kidney injury. *Comprehensive Physiology* 2 (2): 1303–1353. https://doi.org/10.1002/cphy.c110041.

Chen, H., Dunaevich, A., Apfelbaum, N. et al. (2020). Acute on chronic kidney disease in cats: etiology, clinical and clinicopathologic findings, prognostic markers, and outcome. *Journal of Veterinary Internal Medicine* 34 (4): 1496–1506.

Dunaevich, A., Chen, H., Musseri, D. et al. (2020). Acute on chronic kidney disease in dogs: etiology, clinical and clinicopathologic findings, prognostic markers, and survival. *Journal of Veterinary Internal Medicine* 34 (6): 2507–2515.

Keir, I. and Kellum, J.A. (2015). Acute kidney injury in severe sepsis: pathophysiology, diagnosis, and treatment recommendations. *Journal of Veterinary Emergency and Critical Care (San Antonio, Tex.: 2001)* 25 (2): 200–209.

Monaghan, K., Nolan, B., and Labato, M. (2012). Feline acute kidney injury: 1. Pathophysiology, etiology and etiology-specific management considerations. *Journal of Feline Medicine and Surgery* 14 (11): 775–784.

Ross, L. (2011). Acute kidney injury in dogs and cats. *The Veterinary Clinics of North America. Small Animal Practice* 41 (1): 1–14.

Ross, L. (2022). Acute kidney injury in dogs and cats. *The Veterinary Clinics of North America. Small Animal Practice* 52 (3): 659–672. https://doi.org/10.1016/j.cvsm.2022.01.005.

41.5

Chronic Kidney Disease

Definition

Chronic kidney disease (CKD) is, by definition, a chronic, non-reversible, degenerative kidney disease with a progressive course for at least three months. The causes of the disease are usually no longer apparent at the time of diagnosis.

Aetiology

Chronic kidney disease can develop from numerous underlying renal diseases of different aetiologies. Glomerulonephritis with or without nephrotic syndrome can lead to CKD. Many cases of CKD, however, are idiopathic, which is also due, in particular, to their progression over several months. Known causes are infections, neoplasia and congenital diseases. The clinical picture occurs in dogs and cats, but is very common in old cats.

Infection	Neoplasia	Congenital
Canine adenovirus (D)	Lymphoma (D/C)	Amyloidosis (D/C)
Ehrliochiosis (D)		Polycystic kidney disease (D/C)
Leptospirosis (D)		
FIV (C)		
Paramyxovirus (C)		

D – Dog, C – Cat

Pathogenesis

The pathogenesis of CKD is similar to that of other degenerative processes in the organism, such as liver cirrhosis. Here, too, the trigger is a chronic activation of the immune system, primarily of the non-specific macrophage system with the formation of extracellular matrix. For this purpose, macrophages first migrate into the parenchyma as a result of an insult. This process is initiated by mediators of inflammation, e.g. cytokines. Among others, the interleukins IL-1 and IL-6, as well as TNF-α, lead to an inflammatory reaction. Macrophages and migrated fibroblasts are activated. The result is the release of growth factors, such as transforming growth factor (TGF). Under the effect of the growth factors, the fibroblasts form extracellular matrix, mostly in the form of collagens. This is the beginning of the remodelling of the parenchymal architecture, with subsequent problems for the synthesis capacity and vascularisation of the parenchyma. Eventually, there is a loss of organ function. The remodelling is progressive and, at least in the beginning, reversible. In the advanced stage, reversibility is lost.

Chronic renal failure is a common disease of ageing cats. In most cases, the underlying aetiology is unknown and the pathological changes manifest as tubulo-interstitial fibrosis. In dogs, glomerular sclerosis is more likely to be found.

The progression of CKD depends on different factors.

Textbook of Small Animal Pathophysiology, First Edition. Stephan Neumann.
© 2025 John Wiley & Sons Ltd. Published 2025 by John Wiley & Sons Ltd.

Loss of functional glomeruli, systemic hypertension due to activation of the RAAS and local inflammatory mediators such as prostaglandins increase the hydrostatic pressure of the remaining glomeruli and lead to hyperfiltration.

The increased amount of ultrafiltrate generates mechanical forces that deform the molecular cell association of the podocytes and stretch the basement membrane. As a result, the podocytes react with compensatory hypertrophy. If the stretching of the basement membrane exceeds the compensatory possibilities of the podocytes, synechiae develop between the capillary walls and Bowman's capsule. Intraglomerular coagulation with fibrin formation develops due to platelet activation (Chagnac et al. 2019).

In the presence of associated renal hyperparathyroidism, renal Ca deposition leads to sclerosis of the fibrin.

Hyperlipidaemia, which can also be a concomitant factor in nephrotic syndrome, induces proliferation of mesangial cells and leads to a decrease in negative charge at the basement membrane, thereby increasing permeability. Mesangial cells are specialised, contractile cells on the glomerulum. Together with the surrounding extracellular matrix, they form the mesangium. The mesangium is a supporting scaffold of the glomerulus and is involved in the regulation of intracapillary pressure by secreting vasoactive mediators, such as prostaglandins. In addition, the cells also show a non-specific defence function through the secretion of cytokines and the ability to phagocytose.

A major progressive factor in CKD is proteinuria. This increases intraglomerular pressure and activates the mesangial cells leading to the synthesis of mesangial matrix. The process leads to glomerulosclerosis. Increased protein filtration is followed by increased protein resorption in the proximal tubules.

The proteins damage the tubules by promoting the release of lysosomal enzymes and the production of inflammatory and vasoactive proteins. These include proteins, such as osteopontin and endothelin, which initiate parenchymal fibrosis (Figures 41.5.1 and 41.5.2).

Diagnostics

Clinical signs	Clinical pathology	Imaging	Histopathology	Microbiology
Non-specific	Elevated kidney parameters	Ultrasonography	Not necessary	Not necessary
PU/PD	Urea, creatinine, phosphorus, SDMA	Reduced size		
Cachexia		Changes of parenchymal structure, fibrosis		

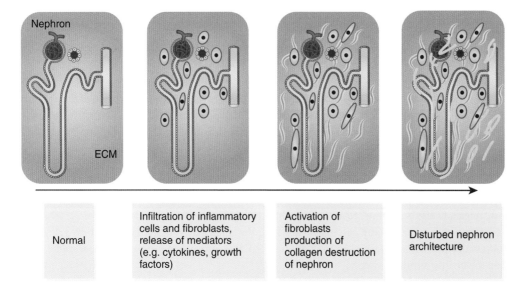

Figure 41.5.1 Pathogenesis of chronic renal failure, morphology.

Figure 41.5.2 Pathogenesis of chronic renal failure, function.

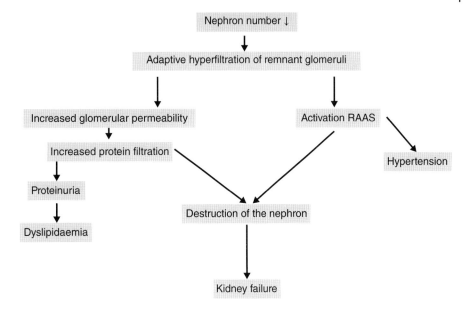

Pathophysiologic Consequences

The consequences of chronic kidney failure affect not only the organs of the urinary system, but also the cardiovascular system, haematopoiesis and the skeleton, in particular.

Influenced organ systems	Clinical symptoms	Clinical pathological alterations
Urinary tract	Inappetence	Azotaemia
Haematological system	Cachexia	Anaemia
Bones, joints	Dehydration	Hypokalaemia
Cardiovascular system	Polydipsia/polyuria	Hyperphosphataemia
	Hypertension	Proteinuria
		Acidosis

Source: Elliott and Barber (1998); Elliott et al. (2003); Chalhoub et al. (2011).

Cachexia and **inappetence** are related to each other. The emaciation can not only be explained by the reduced food intake, but also by the protein catabolism, especially in advanced cases. The latter, in turn, results essentially from metabolic acidosis, which about 50% of cats with advanced CKD show. Inappetence, in turn, develops from nausea due to uraemic toxins. These also include anorectic factor, which helps trigger the inappetence. Finally, about 80% of cats with advanced CKD also have gastropathy. This is primarily reflected in mineralisation and fibrosis of the stomach wall (McLeland et al. 2014). Causally, hypergastrinaemia is seen due to reduced renal gastrine secretion. This promotes the formation of HCl in the stomach. In addition, the increased urea concentration in CKD induces the increased formation of ammonia, promoted by urease-forming bacteria, which can lead to irritation of the gastrointestinal mucosa. Finally, animals with CKD have pyloric incompetence associated with bile reflux into the stomach.

The occurrence of metabolic **acidosis** depends on the degree of CKD (10% in moderate forms, 50% in severe forms). The cause is the impaired excretion of protons. The excretion of protons via the kidneys is an important element for the regulation of the acid–base balance and can be regulated via phosphate and ammonium excretion, as well as bicarbonate reabsorption. Phosphate dissociates in the blood to 80% in HPO_4^{2-}. In the tubule, this secondary phosphate meets a proton and $H_2PO_4^-$ is formed. The primary phosphate now formed can no longer be absorbed and a proton is excreted with the help of phosphate excretion. The impaired phosphate excretion in CKD prevents this mechanism. In contrast, filtered bicarbonate is reabsorbed in the proximal tubule. From the filtered HCO_3^- and secreted H^+ from the tubular cell (Na-H exchanger), H_2CO_3 is formed with the assistance of luminal carbonic anhydrase, which breaks down into CO_2 and H_2O. The CO_2 crosses the tubular cell membrane and combines with OH^- (remnant of H^+ secretion) within the tubular cell to form HCO_3^-. Through an Na^+/HCO_3^- cotransporter at the basolateral membrane, the bicarbonate is returned to the circulation. In the case of CKD, the intake of bicarbonate decreases. Finally, ammonium excretion binds protons, which is also reduced in the case of CKD.

The consequences of metabolic acidosis are different metabolic alterations (Table 41.5.1).

Polydipsia and dehydration are closely related to **polyuria**. This is caused in CKD due to increased natriuresis; sodium binds water and this is lost with natriuresis. In addition, animals with CKD show reduced sensitivity of the ADH receptors in the distal tubule and the collecting tube, resulting in increased diuresis. Finally, in CKD, the medulla osmolality in the renal parenchyma is reduced. This reduces the osmotic gradient for water reabsorption in Henle's loop.

The loss of water reduces the blood pressure, ADH is produced more frequently and the feeling of thirst is increased, resulting in **polydipsia**. However, in most cases this is not completely compensatory, so that the animals still develop **dehydration**.

The **anaemia** in CKD is a non-regenerative form, which reflexes an anaemia of chronic disease. Here, chronic inflammatory reactions lead to the activation of T lymphocytes and monocytes. These, in turn, secrete IL-1, IL-6, TNF-α and IFN-γ, which cause the inhibition of duodenal iron reabsorption, the increased iron uptake in macrophages and decreased iron release to erythrocytic progenitor cells. Reduced serum iron concentrations are found in dogs and cats with CKD (Neumann 2003).

Furthermore, animals with CKD have an erythropoietin deficiency which negatively affects erythropoiesis. In addition, animals with CKD show increased gastrointestinal bleeding due to platelet dysfunction caused by uraemic toxins, which can also contribute to anaemia.

While severe renal insufficiencies tend to show hyperkalaemia, **hypokalaemia** is present in moderate forms. This develops from reduced tubular reabsorption. The consequences are disturbances of the membrane potential with cardiac arrhythmias and muscle weakness. **Azotaemia** and **hyperphosphataemia** are criteria for the diagnosis of CKD, and are therefore present in all cases. Hyperphosphataemia affects bone metabolism. Consequences of CKD are phosphate accumulation, this induces parathyroid hormone release. It promotes phosphate excretion by inhibiting its reabsorption from the proximal tubule. At the same time, PTH promotes the release of calcium from bone resulting in demineralisation and the clinical syndrome of secondary renal hyperparathyroidism.

Chronic kidney disease also leads to reduced synthesis of calcitriol. As a result, intestinal absorption of calcium decreases. Finally, phosphate and calcium accumulate in various soft tissues and lead to their calcification.

Proteinuria is a consequence of impaired glomerular function and is described in its pathophysiologic consequences in Chapter 41.2. Proteinuria plays an essential role in the pathogenesis of CKD, as it induces the remodelling processes in the glomerulum. The described sodium retention and activation of the RAAS in CKD causes **hypertension**. This in turn can lead to haemorrhages and thus symptoms in the CNS or the eyes (Figure 41.5.3).

Table 41.5.1 Metabolic acidosis consequences.

Organ	Consequence
Liver	Reduced albumin synthesis
	Reduced IGF I synthesis
Bone	Increased PTH
	Reduced calcitriol
	Disturbed bone mineralisation
Metabolism	Increased cortisol production
	Increased insulin resistance

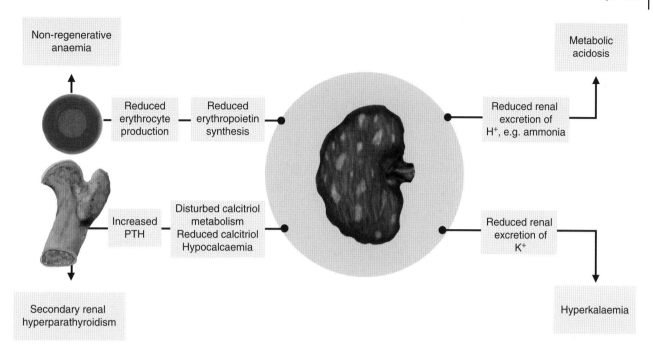

Figure 41.5.3 Pathophysiologic consequences of chronic renal failure.

Therapy

Symptom	Therapy
Nausea	Antiemetic drugs (e.g. Metoclopramide, Maropitant, Ondansetron)
Inappetence	Appetite inducer (e.g. Mirtazepine)
Gastritis	Blockers of gastric acid (e.g. Ranitidine, Omeprazole)
Acidosis	Infusion, bicarbonate, diet
Dehydration	Infusion
Anaemia	Erythropoietin, iron
Hypokalaemia	Infusion
Hyperphosphataemia	Phosphates binder (e.g. aluminium hydroxide, lanthanum carbonate, calcium carbonate)
Proteinuria	ACE inhibitors, angiotensin receptor inhibitor
Hypertension	ACE inhibitors, Amlodipine

References

Chagnac, A., Zingerman, B., Rozen-Zvi, B., and Herman-Edelstein, M. (2019). Consequences of glomerular hyperfiltration: the role of physical forces in the pathogenesis of chronic kidney disease in diabetes and obesity. *Nephron* 143 (1): 38–42. https://doi.org/10.1159/000499486.

Chalhoub, S., Langston, C., and Eatroff, A. (2011). Anemia of renal disease: what it is, what to do and what's new. *Journal of Feline Medicine and Surgery* 13 (9): 629–640. https://doi.org/10.1016/j.jfms.2011.07.016.

Elliott, J. and Barber, P.J. (1998). Feline chronic renal failure: clinical findings in 80 cases diagnosed between 1992 and 1995. *The Journal of Small Animal Practice* 39 (2): 78–85. http://dx.doi.org/10.1111/j.1748-5827.1998.tb03598.x.

Elliott, J., Syme, H.M., Reubens, E., and Markwell, P.J. (2003). Assessment of acid-base status of cats with naturally occurring chronic renal failure. *The Journal of Small Animal Practice* 44 (2): 65–70. http://dx.doi.org/10.1111/j.1748-5827.2003.tb00122.x.

McLeland, S.M., Lunn, K.F., Duncan, C.G. et al. (2014). Relationship among serum creatinine, serum gastrin, calcium-phosphorus product, and uremic gastropathy in cats with chronic kidney disease. *Journal of Veterinary Internal Medicine* 28 (3): 827–837. https://doi.org/10.1111/jvim.12342.

Neumann, S. (2003). Serum iron level as an indicator for inflammation in dogs and cats. *Comparative Clinical Pathology* 12: 90–94. https://doi.org/10.1007/s00580-003-0481-3.

Further Reading

Bartges, J.W. (2012). Chronic kidney disease in dogs and cats. *The Veterinary Clinics of North America. Small Animal Practice* 42 (4): 669–692.

Foster, J.D. (2016). Update on mineral and bone disorders in chronic kidney disease. *The Veterinary Clinics of North America. Small Animal Practice* 46 (6): 1131–1149.

Grauer, G.F. (2005). Early detection of renal damage and disease in dogs and cats. *The Veterinary Clinics of North America. Small Animal Practice* 35 (3): 581–596.

Polzin, D.J. (2011). Chronic kidney disease in small animals. *The Veterinary Clinics of North America. Small Animal Practice* 41 (1): 15–30.

41.6

Urinary Tract Infection

Definition

A *urinary tract infection* (UTI) is a condition in which bacteria invade and grow in the whole urinary tract (the kidneys, ureters, bladder and urethra). Most UTIs are located in the bladder.

Aetiology

Beside some primary pathogenic bacteria, often infections of the urinary tract will be predisposed by other diseases. Dogs and cats are equally affected by this clinical picture.

Primary disease	Pathogens
Diabetes mellitus (D/C)	*Escherichia coli*
Hyperadrenocorticism (D)	*Staphylococcus* spp.
Hyperthyroidism (C)	*Proteus*
Kidney disease (D/C)	*Klebsiella*
Urinary tract neoplasia (D/C)	*Enterococcus* spp.
Urolithiasis (D/C)	*Streptococcus* spp.
Prostatic disease (D)	
Spinal cord disease (D/C)	

D – Dog, C – Cat

Pathogenesis

Bacterial infections of the urinary tract can be asymptomatic or cause a clinically manifest UTI. Most bacteria that lead to a UTI originate from the colon or the skin. Accordingly, ascending infections via the urethra are more often the cause of a UTI than haematogenously spread pathogens, which also explains why females with an anatomically shorter and wider urethra are predisposed to such infections. Different defence mechanisms are designed to prevent infection in the urinary bladder. These include continuous urination, which washes away the bacteria with the flow of urine. Consequently, diseases with a restricted urine output, such as paralysis, lead to UTI. Other defence mechanisms include antibacterially active molecules in the urine, such as IgA, defensins or even mucins, which prevent bacterial adhesion to the bladder wall. Finally, a lowered pH value can have an antibacterial effect.

Impaired defence mechanisms, for example, due to primary underlying diseases or pathogenicity characteristics of the bacteria, can lead to UTI.

The bacteria can be found unbound in the bladder or attached to the bladder wall in a biofilm. The latter causality is more often associated with the placement of indwelling catheters. The biofilm is a protective layer that surrounds bacterial

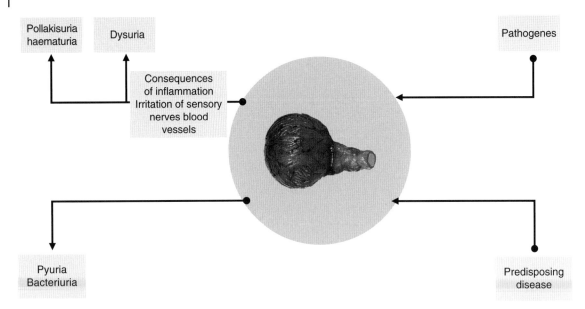

Figure 41.6.1 Pathomechanism and clinical consequences of bacterial cystitis.

colonies at sites of infection. The composition is based on the type of bacteria and the type of tissue infected. Polysaccharides are often involved in the protective film. The consequence is a protection of the bacteria against defence measures of the organism or therapy, such as antibiotic administration.

Bacterial infection of the bladder epithelium down to the lamina propria results in the secretion of proinflammatory cytokines (IL-1, IL-6, IL-8, TNF-α) from the bladder epithelial cells. This results in the recruitment of inflammatory cells, such as neutrophilic granulocytes or macrophages. This can result in haemorrhagic or necrotic-ulcerative cystitis. Cystitis can be acute or chronic. The latter process is often associated with fibrosis of the bladder wall, which leads to a palpable thickening. Such remodelling processes hinder the defence mechanisms described above and predispose to further infections. The mechanism of bladder wall remodelling in chronic cystitis is similar to that of chronic inflammation in other organs. The inflammatory process leads to an activation of myofibroblasts and their synthesis of connective tissue consisting mainly of collagens. This, in turn, results in morphological alteration due to collagen retraction and bladder wall thickening (Figure 41.6.1).

Diagnostics

Clinical signs	Clinical pathology	Imaging	Histopathology	Microbiology
Dysuria, pollakisuria, haematuria	Urinalysis, sediment	**Ultrasonography** Thickened bladder wall	Not necessary	Necessary for germ detection and antibiogram

Pathophysiologic Consequences

The consequences of bacterial cystitis are mainly concentrated on the urinary apparatus or the bladder. In some cases, however, symptoms of predisposing underlying diseases can also come to the fore.

Influenced organ systems	Clinical symptoms	Clinical pathological alterations
Urinary tract	Dysuria	Leucocytosis
	Pollakisuria	Pyuria
	Haematuria	Bacteriuria

The clinical symptoms of UTI can be explained primarily by the inflammatory reaction in the bladder. **Dysuria** describes difficult and painful micturition and **pollakisuria** describes frequent passing of small amounts of urine. Both are due to the infiltration of inflammatory cells, release of mediators and irritation of nociceptors in the bladder wall. Vascular alteration during inflammation causes **haematuria** to develop. Laboratory diagnostic findings of UTI usually show up in the urine sediment and consist of the detection of inflammatory cells (**pyuria**) or bacteria (**bacteriuria**). A systemic inflammatory reaction with **leucocytosis** does not occur in all cases.

Therapy

Symptom	Therapy
Dysuria	Analgesics
Bacteriuria	Antibiotics

Further Reading

Byron, J.K. (2019). Urinary tract infection. *The Veterinary Clinics of North America. Small Animal Practice* 49 (2): 211–221.

Dorsch, R., Teichmann-Knorrn, S., and Sjetne Lund, H. (2019). Urinary tract infection and subclinical bacteriuria in cats: a clinical update. *Journal of Feline Medicine and Surgery* 21 (11): 1023–1038.

Johnstone, T. (2020). A clinical approach to multidrug-resistant urinary tract infection and subclinical bacteriuria in dogs and cats. *New Zealand Veterinary Journal* 68 (2): 69–83.

Olin, S.J. and Bartges, J.W. (2015). Urinary tract infections: treatment/comparative therapeutics. *The Veterinary Clinics of North America. Small Animal Practice* 45 (4): 721–746.

Weese, J.S., Blondeau, J., Boothe, D. et al. (2019). International Society for Companion Animal Infectious Diseases (ISCAID) guidelines for the diagnosis and management of bacterial urinary tract infections in dogs and cats. *Veterinary Journal (London, England: 1997)* 247: 8–25.

41.7

Urolithiasis

Definition

Urolithiasis is defined as the formation of concrements in the urinary organs.

Aetiology

Causally, concrements with different chemical composition and pathogenesis are formed during crystal and stone formation. The following table lists the most common concrements in dogs and cats. Since the urine pH has an influence on concrements formation, the concrements are differentiated according to the predominant urine pH. The clinical picture occurs equally in dogs and cats.

pH	Genetic	Infectious	Metabolic
<pH 7	Cystine		Oxalate
	Urate		
>pH 7		Struvite	

Pathogenesis

Different theories on the development of concrements in the urinary tract are discussed. In principle, two geneses are distinguished. According to the matrix hypothesis, every concrement is based on an organic matrix which, as a crystallisation nucleus, induces the binding of inorganic molecules and thus promotes concrement growth. High-molecular proteins or glucosaminoglycans are primarily discussed as matrix molecules. The ions bind to these molecules via covalent bonds and thus first form crystals and later stones.

The crystallisation hypothesis assumes an absolute or relative supersaturation of the urine with ions. If the ion concentration exceeds the saturation product, crystallisation follows and later stone formation. In the case of relative supersaturation, the ion concentration to be achieved is lowered by the presence of crystallisation nuclei. Organic substances also act as crystallisation nuclei in this hypothesis.

Another hypothesis focuses on the importance of the renal tubules in the development of calculi. Especially for calcium oxalate stones in humans, the development of the so-called 'Randall plaques' has been described as a causality. This is also discussed for the development of calcium oxalates in dogs and cats (O'Kell et al. 2017). Randall plaques are Ca deposits on the basement membrane in the thin limp of Henle's loop. In combination with organic substances, such as glucosaminoglycans, these plaques develop. Once formed, the plaque develops by crystallisation in the collagen matrix of the basement membrane of Henle's loop and further in the subepithelial tissue (Green and Ratan 2013).

Textbook of Small Animal Pathophysiology, First Edition. Stephan Neumann.
© 2025 John Wiley & Sons Ltd. Published 2025 by John Wiley & Sons Ltd.

Both crystal formation and stone formation are supported by promoters and prevented by inhibitors. An essential promoter for the formation of crystals and stones is the pH value of the urine. This affects the solubility of crystals. Depending on the type of crystal, acidic or alkaline pH can be seen as a promoter. In the case of the frequently observed struvite crystals, an alkaline pH value promotes crystal formation, while in the case of oxalate crystals, a more acidic pH value supports crystal formation. Inhibitors of crystal formation can be food components that are excreted in the urine. These include phytates, which inhibit the formation of calcium salts in the animal model (Grases et al. 2007).

Inhibitors that influence crystallisation within the nephrons are to be distinguished from this. These include some glucoproteins. An inhibitory effect on the formation of oxalates was described for osteopontin, Tamm-Horsfall protein and urinary prothrombin fragment 1. The effect is probably due to a high number of sulphated amino acids in the inhibitors, which prevent calcium salt binding (Kumar et al. 2003; Ratkalkar and Kleinman 2011) (Figure 41.7.1).

The development of the most common urinary calculi will now be presented in detail:

Struvite crystals (magnesium ammonium phosphate) are sometimes associated with urinary tract infections, especially in dogs. Urea excreted in the urine is broken down into ammonia and ammonium ions by bacteria that produce urease, such as *Staphylococcus* or *Proteus*. The ammonium ions in turn increase the pH value in the urine, and dihydrogen phosphate is reduced to phosphate. Thus, two molecular components of the struvite crystals are formed, which combine with magnesium ions. The mechanism of non-infection-related struvite crystals is probably due to an increase in urine pH caused by the so-called 'alkalogenic cations', such as magnesium.

Calcium oxalate crystals are the result of supersaturation of the urine with both components and occur as whewellite (calcium oxalate monohydrate) and weddellite (calcium oxalate dihydrate). A vitamin B6 deficiency and a deficiency of the so-called 'crystallisation inhibitors' are described as predisposing factors (Grimm et al. 1988; Worcester 1994).

Cystine is composed of two cysteine molecules. The former is filtered glomerularly together with other amino acids (lysine, arginine, ornithine) and reabsorbed in the proximal tubule. A disturbance of reabsorption can be caused by a genetic deficiency of the transporter, which is presumably inherited in an autosomal recessive manner. The result is an supersaturation of the urine with the amino acid, which causes stone formation.

Urate crystals form when the breakdown of purines is not continued to allantoin in the course of purine metabolism. The result is an increased uric acid concentration. In Dalmatians and possibly in other dog breeds, a genetic defect underlies the reduced uric acid degradation. Another important mechanism is liver dysfunction (cirrhosis) or porto-systemic shunt bypasses of the liver. In such cases, the uric acid concentration in the body also increases.

The consequence of both causalities is hyperuricosaemia, which leads to increased glomerular uric acid filtration. Uric acid is partially reabsorbed in the proximal tubule and secreted in the distal tubule. However, the consequence of the increased blood concentration and greatly increased glomerular filtration is a supersaturation of the urine with uric acid. This induces crystal formation.

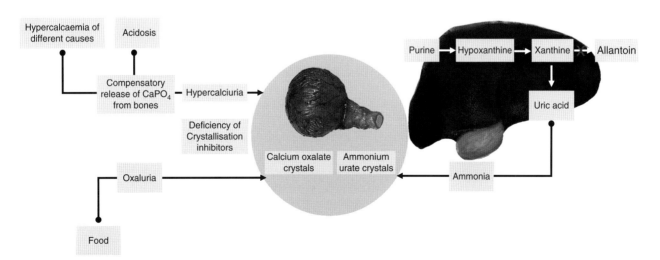

Figure 41.7.1 Mechanism of stone formation using the example of calcium oxalate stones and urate stones.

Diagnostics

Clinical signs	Clinical pathology	Imaging	Histopathology	Microbiology
Dysuria	Crystalluria	**Ultrasonography**	Not necessary	Germ detection and antibiogram
Haematuria	Bacteriuria	Crystal detection, bladder wall thickness		

Pathophysiologic Consequences

The consequences of crystal or stone formation are mainly concentrated in the urinary system. In case of complete obstruction, systemic symptoms may also develop via post-renal failure.

Influenced organ systems	Clinical symptoms	Clinical pathological alterations
Urinary tract	Dysuria	Azotaemia
Systemic	Pollakisuria	Phosphataemia
	Oliguria	Uraemia
	Haematuria	Hypercalcaemia
	Shock	Acidosis
		Proteinuria
		Haematuria

The main pathophysiologic consequences of urinary calculi are inflammation of the urinary bladder or obstruction of the urinary tract organs. The former may be the cause or the consequence. Inflammation in the bladder could form a matrix that acts as a crystallisation centre. This is rarely the single cause. However, if infections are present, especially with urease-forming bacteria, the formation of struvite stones is particularly possible. In addition to initiation, cystitis is often the result of concrement formation. Acute inflammation is characterised by vasodilation and increased vascular permeability, leukocyte migration and activation of the inflammatory cascade, with release of mediators, such as cytokines, histamines, kinins, complement factors, coagulation factors, nitric oxide and proteases. In acute cystitis, these mediators cause inflammatory swelling and ulceration of the bladder mucosa, which bleeds easily and leads to **haematuria** and **proteinuria.** In addition, these mediators cause bladder mucosal irritation, causing **dysuria** and **pollakisuria** (Grover et al. 2011).

If the concrements lead to stone formation, there is a risk of obstruction of the urinary tract in addition to the inflammatory reaction in the bladder. In the case of a partial obstruction, the animals continue to pass small amounts of urine. This can result in **oliguria**, **dysuria** and **pollakisuria**. In the case of complete loss, excretion of urinary substances is lost and renal failure develops within about 24 hours. This is increasingly associated with **shock** symptoms of **azotaemia** due to a reduction in the excretion of urea and creatinine, **uraemia** due to reduced excretion of uraemic toxins and finally **hyperkalaemia** and **acidosis.**

In most cases, obstruction develops in the urethra, for which there are some predilection sites due to anatomical stenosis, such as the beginning of the urethra, the localisation of the bulbourethral gland as well as the tip of the penis in males and the area of the penile bone in male dogs. The increase in bladder pressure after urethral obstruction leads to a reduced blood supply to the bladder wall with hypoxia of the bladder wall epithelia, this implies a reduced ATP formation, thus the function of the Na^+-K^+ pump is reduced, the consequence is a reduced excretion of Na^+ ions, these hold water in the cell, hydropic swelling with loss of function of the epithelial cells occurs. In advanced severe cases, urinary bladder wall rupture may occur.

The overstretching of the contractile elements of the bladder wall can in turn lead to atony of the bladder wall muscles with micturition disorders. The severe increased CK- serum activity in cases of acute urethral obstruction may be due to overstretching of the bladder wall muscles.

In the proximal urinary tract, the increase in pressure after urethral obstruction creates an increased pressure in Bowman's capsule, which opposes the filtration pressure in the glomerulus, resulting in a decrease in glomerular filtration. This process is supported by the fact that after an initial phase of dilatation of afferent arterioles due to the release of vasodilator prostaglandins, these are subsequently under the influence of vasoconstrictive thromboxanes and angiotensins, which leads to vasoconstriction with a reduction in glomerular filtration. In the tubular system, increased pressure after urethral obstruction leads to disturbances in urine concentration due to reduced reabsorption of water and salts. Furthermore, the excretion of bicarbonate and potassium is disturbed. The disturbance of water reabsorption in the loop of Henle, as well as the distal tubule and the collecting tube, seems to be based on two functional disturbances. Firstly, kidneys in the obstructive phase show a medullary washout with reduction of the osmotic gradient between the tubule and the renal interstitium, and the reabsorption pressure for water decreases accordingly. A second mechanism seems to reduce water reabsorption through a reduced response of the distal tubule and collecting duct to ADH.

The renal function of the acid-base balance is disturbed in obstructive urethral diseases because the excretion of protons is reduced. In addition, the increasing shock in these patients leads to hypovolaemia with cellular hypoxia. The consequence is a switch to anaerobic glycolysis as a form of energy production, resulting in increased lactate formation, which promotes the genesis of **metabolic acidosis.** The frequently observed hyperkalaemia is partly a consequence of the reduced renal excretion of potassium in the case of obstruction. Another mechanism is metabolic acidosis, which leads to hyperkalaemia. Here, the high extracellular concentrations of protons promote an exchange with intracellularly concentrated potassium. As a result, the extracellular potassium concentration increases. Consequences of hyperkalaemia include cardiac arrhythmias (see Chapter 36.6) (Bartges et al. 1996) (Figure 41.7.2).

Therapy

Symptom	Therapy
Obstruction	Removal
Acidosis, hypercalcaemia, uraemia	Infusion, buffered NaCl solution
Prevention	Diet

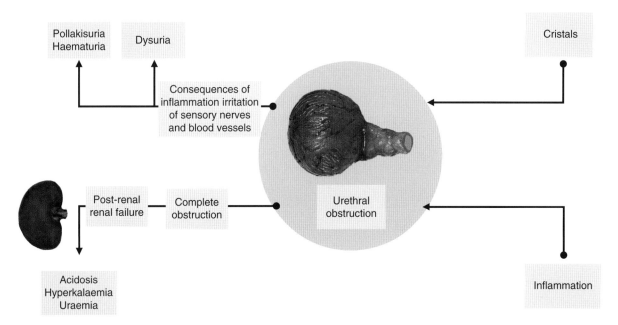

Figure 41.7.2 Pathophysiologic consequences of urethral obstruction.

References

Bartges, J.W., Finco, D.R., Polzin, D.J. et al. (1996). Pathophysiology of urethral obstruction. *The Veterinary Clinics of North America. Small Animal Practice* 26 (2): 255–264.

Grases, F., Isern, B., Sanchis, P. et al. (2007). Phytate acts as an inhibitor in formation of renal calculi. *Frontiers in Bioscience: a Journal and Virtual Library* 12: 2580–2587. https://doi.org/10.2741/2256.

Green, W. and Ratan, H. (2013). Molecular mechanisms of urolithiasis. *Urology* 81 (4): 701–704. https://doi.org/10.1016/j.urology.2012.12.039.

Grimm, U., Steinhauser, I., Wulff, K. et al. (1988). Tryptophan metabolism studies in calcium oxalate urolithiasis [Studies on tryptophan metabolism in calcium oxalate urolithiasis]. *Zeitschrift fur Urologie und Nephrologie* 81 (5): 299–303.

Grover, S., Srivastava, A., Lee, R. et al. (2011). Role of inflammation in bladder function and interstitial cystitis. *Therapeutic Advances in Urology* 3 (1): 19–33. https://doi.org/10.1177/1756287211398255.

Kumar, V., Farell, G., and Lieske, J.C. (2003). Whole urinary proteins coat calcium oxalate monohydrate crystals to greatly decrease their adhesion to renal cells. *The Journal of Urology* 170 (1): 221–225. https://doi.org/10.1097/01.ju.0000059540.36463.9f.

O'Kell, A.L., Grant, D.C., and Khan, S.R. (2017). Pathogenesis of calcium oxalate urinary stone disease: species comparison of humans, dogs, and cats. *Urolithiasis* 45 (4): 329–336. https://doi.org/10.1007/s00240-017-0978-x.

Ratkalkar, V.N. and Kleinman, J.G. (2011). Mechanisms of stone formation. *Clinical Reviews in Bone and Mineral Metabolism* 9 (3–4): 187–197. https://doi.org/10.1007/s12018-011-9104-8.

Worcester, E.M. (1994). Urinary calcium oxalate crystal growth inhibitors. *Journal of the American Society of Nephrology: JASN* 5 (5 Suppl 1): S46–S53. https://doi.org/10.1681/ASN.V55s46.

Further Reading

Bartges, J.W. and Callens, A.J. (2015). Urolithiasis. *The Veterinary Clinics of North America. Small Animal Practice* 45 (4): 747–768.

Lahme, S. (2003). *Untersuchungen zur Bedeutung des Nierentubulus für die Harnsteingenese*. Habilschrift Universität Tübingen.

Langston, C., Gisselman, K., Palma, D., and McCue, J. (2008). Diagnosis of urolithiasis. *Compendium (Yardley, PA)* 30 (8): 447–455.

Lulich, J.P., Berent, A.C., Adams, L.G. et al. (2016). ACVIM small animal consensus recommendations on the treatment and prevention of uroliths in dogs and cats. *Journal of Veterinary Internal Medicine* 30 (5): 1564–1574.

McCue, J., Langston, C., Palma, D., and Gisselman, K. (2009). Urate urolithiasis. *Compendium (Yardley, PA)* 31 (10): 468–475.

42

Electrolyte System and Acid-Base Balance

42.1

Acid-Base Balance

Physiology

The physiological processes in the organism are closely linked to the formation of metabolites that are active as proton donors (acids) or acceptors (bases). As a result, the pH value intra- and extracellularly is subject to constant influence.

Under physiological conditions, the pH value in the organism is stabilised in a very narrow, slightly alkaline range of approximately 7.35. This is necessary because, for example, the activity of enzyme systems depends on the pH value; the same applies to the distribution of ions between the intracellular and extracellular space, which in turn influences the formation and transmission of impulses. Against this background, it is understandable that the organism stabilises the pH value within narrow limits.

In principle, three systems are available for this purpose:

The Buffering of Protons

A buffer is a molecule or mixture of substances that is capable of absorbing or releasing protons in an appropriate environment. Accordingly, buffers consist of weak acids or bases. The consequence of buffering is the binding or release of protons and thus stabilisation of the pH value in a narrower range than an unbuffered mixture can.

In the blood, protons can be bound and thus eliminated by the hydrogen carbonate buffer, haemoglobin, proteins and phosphates. Bicarbonate can absorb protons and thus becomes carbonic acid, which in turn dissolves into carbon dioxide and water. The former can be exhaled through the lungs and thus regenerate the buffer.

The buffering reaction in the bicarbonate buffer:

$$HCO_3^- + H^+ > H_2CO_3 > CO_2 + H_2O$$

Haemoglobin and proteins both act as weak acids that bind protons when the pH value drops and thus buffer them. The phosphate buffer is composed of dihydrogen phosphate and hydrogen phosphate. The buffering principle is based on the absorption of protons in the event of an increase in acidity. The phosphate buffer is more important as a buffer system in urine than in blood.

The buffering reaction in the phosphate buffer:

$$HPO_4^{2-} + H^+ > H_2PO_4^-$$

The Elimination of CO_2 via the Lungs (Respiratory Regulation)

Carbon dioxide diffuses out of tissue cells to surrounding capillary blood. A small proportion dissolves in blood plasma and is transported to the lungs unchanged.

Textbook of Small Animal Pathophysiology, First Edition. Stephan Neumann.

$$CO_2 + H_2O \rightleftharpoons H_2CO_3 \rightleftharpoons H^+ + HCO_3^- \rightleftharpoons HCO_3^-$$ **Figure 42.1.1**   Function of bicarbonate buffering.

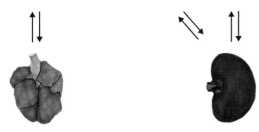

But most diffuses into red cells where it combines with water to form carbonic acid. The acid dissociates with production of hydrogen ions and bicarbonate. Hydrogen ions combine with deoxygenated haemoglobin (haemoglobin is acting as a buffer here), preventing a dangerous fall in cellular pH, and bicarbonate diffuses along a concentration gradient from red cell to plasma.

Thus, most of the carbon dioxide produced in the tissues is transported to the lungs as bicarbonate in blood plasma.

At the alveoli in the lungs, the process is reversed. Hydrogen ions are displaced from haemoglobin as it takes up oxygen from inspired air. The hydrogen ions are now buffered by bicarbonate which diffuses from plasma back into red cell, and carbonic acid is formed. As the concentration of this rises, it is converted to water and carbon dioxide.

Finally, carbon dioxide diffuses down a concentration gradient from red cell to alveoli for excretion in expired air (Figure 42.1.1).

Elimination of Protons via the Kidney and Reabsorption of Bicarbonate (Renal Regulation)

The influence of the kidneys with regard to the acid-base balance consists, on the one hand, in the elimination of protons. At the same time, the kidneys control the acid-base balance through the elimination and synthesis of bicarbonate.

An essential mechanism is the synthesis of carbonic acid from $CO_2 + H^+ + H_2O$ in the tubule cells under the catalysis of the enzyme carbonic anhydrase. This in turn releases protons as a weak acid and can be absorbed by the blood as bicarbonate, where it stabilises the pH value.

The physiological adaptations of the lungs and kidneys to changes in the acid-base balance consist of a respiratory change in ventilation. In the case of an existing metabolic acidosis, central chemoreceptors are stimulated by the protons, resulting in hyperventilation with a reduction in pCO_2. To maintain the balance of the carbonic acid buffer, protons are bound by bicarbonate to regenerate CO_2.

$$HCO_3^- + H^+ > H_2CO_3 > CO_2 + H_2O$$

The opposite, hypoventilation, occurs when the pH in the blood rises, metabolic alkalosis develops.

Renal compensation takes place through the excretion of protons as ammonium ions (NH_4^+) or as phosphate (H_3PO_4). Furthermore, the kidneys can have a stabilising effect on the pH value through the synthesis of bicarbonate.

Disorders in the Acid-Base Balance

Disturbances in the physiological balance of acids and bases result from an increased synthesis of active molecules (acids or bases) and as a consequence of the disturbed regulatory systems. Depending on the localisation of the disturbance, we speak of respiratory or metabolic acidosis or alkalosis.

The most common form of a pathological imbalance of the acid-base balance is **metabolic acidosis**. This is based on an increased synthesis of acids. Lactic acidosis, as a consequence of increased lactate formation during a change from aerobic to anaerobic glycolysis, and ketoacidosis, as a consequence of excessive ketone body formation in diabetes mellitus, are considered clinically most common. In addition to increased acid formation, reduced acid excretion is also a possible cause of metabolic acidosis. This is often due to a disturbance in renal excretion. Another complex of causes for the formation of metabolic acidosis is the loss of bicarbonate. This is usually lost during diarrhoea. Less frequent are renal losses, for example, in tubulopathy.

In the case of metabolic acidosis, the following compensatory mechanisms become active:

1) buffering of the protons in the blood
2) respiratory compensation by increasing ventilation.
3) renal compensation through increased proton excretion and increased bicarbonate synthesis.

In case of insufficient compensation, numerous symptoms develop based on acidosis.
The pathophysiologic consequences of metabolic acidosis are manifold and depend on the degree of acidosis and its duration.

Pathophysiologic Consequences

Influenced organ systems	Consequences
Cardiovascular system	Catecholamine resistance
Central nervous system	Reduced heart contraction
Systemic	Arterial vasodilation
	Venoconstriction
	Reduced oxygen binding to haemoglobin
	Immunosuppression
	Insulin resistance
	Electrolyte shift
	Apoptosis

The cardiovascular consequences lead to decreased **cardiogenic output** and vasodilation. Both induce hypotension. One of the causes is a reduced response to **catecholamines**. This can occur because acidosis can impair the binding of catecholamines to their receptors on target cells, or because it can interfere with the downstream signalling pathways that these hormones activate. In addition, acidosis can also lead to a decrease in the release of catecholamines from the adrenal glands, which can further reduce their effectiveness.

Furthermore, the formation of impulses at the cardiac muscle cells can be influenced by associated hyperkalaemia. Central nervous symptoms can also be explained by shifts in electrolytes. Reduced oxygen binding by **haemoglobin** contributes to cerebral hypoxia. In the presence of acidosis, the concentration of hydrogen ions in the blood increases, which leads to the formation of protonated haemoglobin. This form of haemoglobin has a reduced affinity for oxygen, meaning that it is less likely to bind to oxygen molecules. This is because the positive charge of the protonated haemoglobin interferes with the binding of oxygen to the iron atoms in the haeme groups of haemoglobin.

Additionally, acidosis can also cause a shift in the oxygen dissociation curve of haemoglobin. This means that at any given partial pressure of oxygen, haemoglobin releases less oxygen to the tissues. This effect is known as the 'Bohr effect' and is due to the fact that the increased concentration of hydrogen ions in the blood causes a decrease in pH, which reduces the affinity of haemoglobin for oxygen.

Due to a suppressive effect of acidosis on the formation of **macrophages** and the function of **lymphocytes**, acidosis can lead to an increased susceptibility to infections. Acidosis impairs the ability of these cells to phagocytose and kill pathogens. Acidosis can affect the production and release of cytokines, leading to alterations in the balance between pro- and anti-inflammatory responses. Acidosis can impair the activation and proliferation of T-cells, which are critical for an effective immune response against pathogens. Acidosis can also impair the function of B cells, which produce antibodies, leading to a decreased ability to clear infections.

Chronic acidosis affects muscle metabolism by impairing protein synthesis or stagnating energy supply, due to the reduced **insulin** action in acidosis. The interference with protein synthesis may contribute to amyloidosis via increased synthesis of microglobulins. Finally, metabolic acidosis causes increased cell apoptosis by disrupting cellular metabolism.

Respiratory acidosis is the result of a disturbed respiratory gas exchange in which carbon dioxide is insufficiently exhaled. This leads to the development of carbonic acid, which dissociates into bicarbonate and protons. Diseases that lead to insufficient CO_2 exhalation are stenoses in the upper airway, aspiration or pneumonia of other origin, as well as central nervous diseases affecting the respiratory centre or diseases of the respiratory muscles. In chronic respiratory acidosis, the excretion of protons via the kidneys can be increased as a compensatory measure.

The clinical consequences of respiratory acidosis are often also due to the associated hypoxia. Cardiologically, hypercapnia leads to increased activity of the sympathetic nervous system, which has a positive chronotropic effect, but the simultaneous negative ionotropic effect does not lead to a significant change in blood pressure. Furthermore, presumably due to increased ADH release, sodium and water retention takes place in hypercapnia. Finally, hypercapnia combined with hypoxia leads to cerebral vasodilation and increased intracranial pressure, which causes neurological symptoms, such as disorientation or loss of consciousness.

In contrast to acidotic changes, acaloses can also develop as metabolically and respiratory caused. **Metabolic alkalosis** is characterised by an increased bicarbonate serum concentration. A major cause is hypokalaemia of different genesis. In the case of low serum potassium, intracellular potassium ions are increasingly transported into the extracellular space. This leads to an increased influx of protons in the sense of electroneutrality. Extracellularly, a proton deficiency develops an alkalosis. Tubularly, the activity of the proton pump is increased and promotes the excretion of protons. Another cause is due to a loss of chloride, for example during vomiting. Chloride loss leads to reduced bicarbonate excretion. In contrast to these so-called 'loss alkaloses', metabolic alkalosis can also be the consequence of increased bicarbonate reabsorption in the tubule. This form of the so-called 'addition alkalosis' occurs in hyperaldosteronism.

Symptoms develop cardiogenically as arrhythmias, which are, however, more likely in the hypokalaemia. A reduction of ionised calcium due to a stronger albumin binding in the case of alkalosis also leads to cardiological and also neuromuscular symptoms, such as tetanic spasms.

Respiratory alkalosis is the result of hyperventilation with increased exhalation of carbon dioxide. Thus, the disease is related to an increase in activity in the respiratory centre, for example during stress or hypermetabolism (e.g. hyperthyroidism). The cellular proton release can be increased in a compensatory manner. The symptoms correspond to those of metabolic alkalosis (Figures 42.1.2 and 42.1.3).

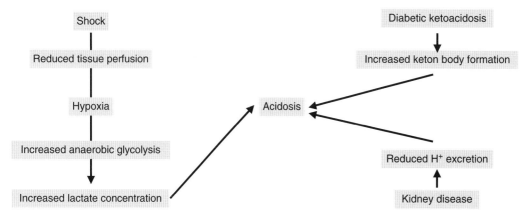

Figure 42.1.2 Pathogenesis of metabolic acidosis.

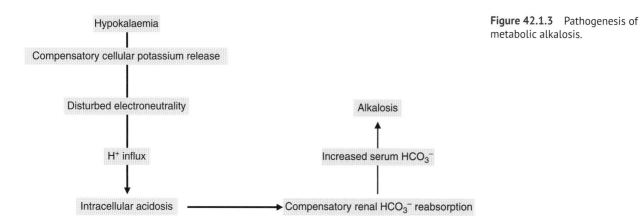

Figure 42.1.3 Pathogenesis of metabolic alkalosis.

Due to causalities and compensations, the primary changes in the acid-base balance are to be determined by measuring plasma bicarbonate and plasma pH. In the case of metabolic acidosis, pH is low <7.3 and bicarbonate is also decreased <15 mmol/l. In the case of respiratory acidosis, the pH is comparable to that of metabolic acidosis. However, the bicarbonate is elevated >25 mmol/l. In contrast, metabolic alkalosis is associated with a pH increase >7.4 and a bicarbonate concentration >25 mmol/l. Respiratory alkalosis has a comparable pH value, but bicarbonate is <20 mmol/l.

Therapy

Metabolic Acidosis	Sodium bicarbonate infusion (Calculation of the Bicarbonate deficit (mEq) = Base excess (BE) × body weight (kg) × 0.3
Metabolic Alkalosis	Is typically associated with hypokalemia. Infusion therapy with potassium if necessary
	Respiratory Acidosis (Hypoventilation) Intubation and support with positive pressure ventilation.
Respiratory Alkalosis (Hyperventilation)	Oxygen supplementation (hypoxia). Sedation.

Further Reading

Hopper, K. (2023). Acid-base. *The Veterinary Clinics of North America. Small Animal Practice* 53 (1): 191–206. https://doi.org/10.1016/j.cvsm.2022.07.014.

Kraut, J.A. and Madias, N.E. (2010). Metabolic acidosis: pathophysiology, diagnosis and management. *Nature Reviews. Nephrology* 6 (5): 274–285. https://doi.org/10.1038/nrneph.2010.33.

Rubash, J.M. (2001). Metabolic acid-base disorders. *The Veterinary Clinics of North America. Small Animal Practice* 31 (6): 1323.-viii. https://doi.org/10.1016/s0195-5616(01)50105-9.

42.2

Hypo-/Hypernatraemia

Physiology

Sodium is absorbed into the body through food. In the process, the effect of the RAAS can promote the absorption of NaCl through the so-called 'salt starvation'. When sodium reaches the small intestine, it is almost completely absorbed. Only about 5% of the sodium absorbed through food is lost through the faeces.

The establishment of an intracellular concentration gradient is essential for resorption through the apical enterocyte membrane. This is achieved by the Na^+-K^+-ATPase in the basal membrane constantly shifting sodium from the enterocytes into the interstitium. Different forms of sodium resorption take place in the various intestinal segments.

In the jejunum, sodium is reabsorbed in a cotransport with glucose and other nutrients. In the ileum, sodium reabsorption occurs in cotransport and exchange with chloride, proton and bicarbonate ions. Another resorption mechanism for sodium is possible through paracellular diffusion.

Sodium is distributed in the body in different compartments. In the extracellular space, 55% of the sodium remains. About 40% of the sodium is stored in the bone tissue and the remaining 10% is intracellular.

The excretion of sodium mainly takes place via the kidneys. Sodium is freely filtered in the glomerulus. In the proximal tubule, 65% of the freely filtered sodium is reabsorbed. Reabsorption is driven by a concentration gradient generated by the action of basolateral Na^+/K^+-ATPase. Apical resorption with the concentration gradient occurs in a sodium-proton exchange.

Further reabsorption takes place in the ascending limb of Henle's loop, which is permeable to ions but not to water. Finally, the remaining sodium is reabsorbed in the distal tubule and the collecting tube. These processes are controlled by aldosterone.

Sodium balance is controlled by a variety of hormones (Table 42.2.1).

The functions of sodium are essentially concentrated on the formation of the membrane potential and the control of the water balance. In this way, sodium indirectly influences blood pressure.

Hypernatraemia

The causes of hypernatraemia are often based on increased water loss and thus on a shift in the sodium-H_2O ratio. This can be caused by a reduced water intake or an increased loss. The latter is particularly the case when water continues to be released via the kidneys, lungs or sweat glands despite reduced intake. This results in dehydration with increased sodium serum concentration. In diabetes insipidus, there is a so-called 'pure water loss', i.e. an increased renal water release, which can lead to hypernatraemia. The same happens when osmotic diuresis or diarrhoea lead to water loss. In cases of increased

Textbook of Small Animal Pathophysiology, First Edition. Stephan Neumann.
© 2025 John Wiley & Sons Ltd. Published 2025 by John Wiley & Sons Ltd.

Table 42.2.1 Hormones with sodium control.

Hormone	Trigger	Effect
Aldosterone	RAAS	Increase of sodium channel expression and Na^+-K^+-ATPase activity in the distal tubule
ANP	Atrial dilatation	Reduction of sodium resorption in the distal tubule
Catecholamines	Reduction of the blood volume	Increase in sodium reabsorption in the proximal tubule

aldosterone concentration, sodium reabsorption in the distal tubule and the collecting tube is increased, which can also increase the serum concentration of sodium.

Causes of Hypernatraemia

Water loss	Hormonal disorder
Pure water loss	Hyperaldosteronism
Diabetes insipidus	
Central	
Nephrogenic	
High environmental temperature	
Fever	
Hypotonic water loss	
Gastrointestinal	
Vomiting	
Diarrhoea	
Third-space loss peritonitis	
Renal	
Osmotic diuresis	
Diabetes mellitus	
Chronic renal failure	

Pathophysiologic Consequences

Weakness	Drinking behaviour
Weakness	Thirst
Seizures	Oliguria
Coma	

The consequences of hypernatraemia are based on influencing the membranous ion distribution and on disturbances of the water distribution. The latter can influence cell structure and function via a water shift from the interior of the cell. Compensatory mechanisms of hypernatraemia, which also become clinically visible, are increased thirst or olguria. Both lead to dilution of the high sodium concentration (Figure 42.2.1).

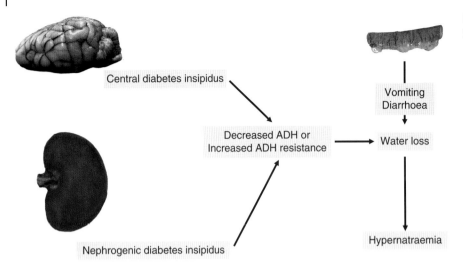

Figure 42.2.1 Pathomechanisms of hypernatraemia.

Hyponatraemia

Hyponatraemia is often the result of increased sodium loss. This can occur with or without altered osmolality. Accordingly, different mechanisms come into play.

Normal osmolality	Increased osmolality	Decreased osmolality
Hyperlipemia	Hyperglycaemia	Nephrotic syndrome
Hyperproteinaemia		Psychogenic polydipsia
		Gastrointestinal loss
		Vomiting
		Diarrhoea
		Third-space loss peritonitis
		Pleural effusion
		Hypoadrenocorticism

The consequences of hyponatraemia develop through disturbance of osmolality in the extracellular space. Hyponatraemia creates an osmotic imbalance in the brain, as the concentration of solutes in the blood is lower than that in the brain. This can lead to an influx of water into the brain cells, causing them to swell and leading to cerebral oedema. The swelling of the brain cells can lead to an increase in intracranial pressure, which can cause symptoms, such as seizures, disorientation, coma and vomiting.

Disruption of neurotransmitter function: Sodium ions play a critical role in the function of neurotransmitters, which are molecules that transmit signals between brain cells. In hyponatraemia, the low concentration of sodium ions can impair the function of neurotransmitters, such as glutamate and GABA, leading to altered neuronal activity and cerebral dysfunction. Sodium ions are also involved in various metabolic processes in the brain, including the production of ATP as a cofactor. In hyponatraemia, the low concentration of sodium ions can impair cellular metabolism, leading to a decrease in ATP production and cellular dysfunction. Hyponatraemia can also impair the function of the blood-brain barrier, which is a protective barrier that separates the brain from the blood. This can lead to the leakage of substances into the brain that can cause inflammation and cerebral dysfunction.

Therapy

Hypernatraemia	Intravenous fluids to replace lost water or dilute sodium.
Hyponatraemia	Intravenous fluids to replace body sodium. Use only 0.9% saline

Further Reading

Ames, M.K., Atkins, C.E., and Pitt, B. (2019). The renin-angiotensin-aldosterone system and its suppression. *Journal of Veterinary Internal Medicine* 33 (2): 363–382. https://doi.org/10.1111/jvim.15454.

Borrelli, S., Provenzano, M., Gagliardi, I. et al. (2020). Sodium intake and chronic kidney disease. *International Journal of Molecular Sciences* 21 (13): 4744. https://doi.org/10.3390/ijms21134744.

Burton, A.G. and Hopper, K. (2019). Hyponatremia in dogs and cats. *Journal of Veterinary Emergency and Critical Care (San Antonio, Tex.: 2001)* 29 (5): 461–471. https://doi.org/10.1111/vec.12881.

Robert, A., Cheddani, L., Ebel, A. et al. (2020). Métabolisme du sodium: une mise au point en 2019 [Sodium metabolism: an update in 2019]. *Nephrologie & Therapeutique* 16 (2): 77–82. https://doi.org/10.1016/j.nephro.2019.06.004.

42.3

Hypo-/Hyperkalaemia

Physiology

Potassium intake takes place through food. Since potassium is the intracellular conducting cation, it is supplied to the body in particular via the absorption of organic tissue. Potassium is absorbed from food in the stomach and proximal small intestine via passive transport. Approximately 90% of the ingested potassium is absorbed and 10% leaves the organism unused in the faeces. After resorption, potassium is distributed. From the extracellular potassium pool, potassium is excreted via the kidneys or absorbed cellularly.

The cellular uptake is realised via Na^+-K^+-ATPase. An energy-consuming mechanism is necessary here, since the Na^+ and K^+ transport takes place against the concentration gradient. The Na^+-K^+-ATPase is composed of two polypeptides (α- and β-subunit). The α-element is the functional unit and the β-element serves to bind the protein in the cell membrane. The Na^+-K^+-ATPase exists in several isoforms with different cellular distribution. The transport mechanism is based on phosphorylation of an aspartate residue of the α-subunit. This leads to a conformational change of the protein and three Na^+ ions are trapped and transported into the extracellular area. There, the three Na^+ ions are exchanged for two K^+ ions. The latter are transported into the cell. One ATP molecule is cleaved per exchange.

The total distribution of potassium within the organism is 98% intracellular, 2% extracellular, of which 0.4% is present in the serum.

The functions of potassium lie primarily in the maintenance of the cellular membrane potential. This is the tension that exists between the inside and outside of a semipermeable membrane, in this case the cell membrane. It results from a different distribution of ions between the intracellular and extracellular space.

Due to the high intracellular potassium concentration, which is maintained by the Na^+-K^+-ATPase, a chemical gradient for potassium exists at the cell membrane. Following this gradient, K^+ ions diffuse outwards. As a result, cations are lost from the cell and the electrical balance is disturbed. An electrical gradient develops in the opposite direction to the chemical gradient. In the state of equilibrium of both gradients, the potassium movement comes to a standstill. The membrane potential present at this time, which corresponds to approximately $-70\,mV$, is called the 'rest potential'.

The maintenance of the potassium pool depends not only on the intake but also on the excretion of potassium. This occurs predominantly via the kidneys. Potassium is freely filtered glomerularly and predominantly reabsorbed in the proximal tubule. In the initial part of the proximal tubule, potassium follows the paracellular water reabsorption, the so-called 'solvent drag'. In the further course, the luminal charge changes due to reabsorption processes. The predominant positive charge in the distal part of the proximal tubule allows further paracellular potassium reabsorption along an electrical gradient.

In the distal tubule, further potassium regulation takes place under the control of aldosterone.

Aldosterone belongs to the mineralocorticoids and is synthesised in the adrenal cortex, the zona glomerulosa. The release of aldosterone is initiated by a reduction in blood volume and/or blood pressure via renin and angiotensin. Hyperkalaemia also increases the secretion of aldosterone, while hypernatraemia inhibits the secretion. Aldosterone regulates luminal potassium levels by inhibiting potassium reabsorption or causing luminal secretion.

For this purpose, aldosterone binds to mineralocorticoid receptors of the tubule cells and causes an increased formation of sodium tubules at the luminal membrane and of Na^+-K^+-ATPase at the basal tubule membrane. The result is increased sodium reabsorption and potassium secretion.

Further control of the potassium balance takes place via insulin, catecholamines and the acid-base balance (Table 42.3.1).

Textbook of Small Animal Pathophysiology, First Edition. Stephan Neumann.
© 2025 John Wiley & Sons Ltd. Published 2025 by John Wiley & Sons Ltd.

Table 42.3.1 Metabolic control of the potassium balance.

Insulin	Catecholamines	Acid-base balance
Increases cellular potassium uptake through simultaneous glucose uptake	Increases cellular potassium uptake in the long term by activating Na^+-K^+-ATPase	In acidosis, hydrogen ions increasingly penetrate the cell membrane and lower the intracellular pH. This inhibits the Na^+-K^+-ATPase
		Acidosis, therefore, lowers the uptake of potassium into the cell and leads to a redistribution of potassium from the intra- to the extracellular space

Hyperkalaemia

The **causes** of hyperkalaemia can be divided into increased absorption, translocation between the intracellular and extracellular areas and reduced excretion. A special form, pseudohyperkalaemia, occurs when erythrocytes are increasingly destroyed by haemolysis or when there is a massive increase in the number of thrombocytes (Table 42.3.2).

Increased potassium intake is an unlikely cause of hyperkalaemia, because in the case of hyperkalaemia the aldosterone-controlled increased potassium excretion would be activated immediately.

Translocation due to **acidosis** is based on the increased extracellular proton concentration. This leads to increased cellular proton uptake and thus to a drop in cellular pH. This inhibits the activity of Na^+-K^+-ATPase, which hinders cellular potassium uptake. Furthermore, protons replace the protein-bound potassium in the intracellular area, resulting in an increased release of potassium, which leaves the cell via potassium channels and leads to an increase in the extracellular potassium concentration.

The **insulin-dependent** translocation of potassium is due to the hyperosmolality that develops as a result of reduced cellular glucose uptake in insulin deficiency. In the serum, the glucose concentration increases, thus an osmotic gradient develops between the cell interior and the extracellular space, which leads to a water shift from intracellular to extracellular. This solvent drag is followed by potassium into the extracellular area.

Solvent drag refers to passive, paracellular absorption. The active transport of electrolytes and/or organic molecules creates an osmotic suction. This causes a passive para- and transcellular water movement into the interstitium. Ions dissolved in the water are transported along with it.

Hyperkalaemia due to massive **cell lysis** occurs predominantly in tumour cell lysis. This develops in fast-growing tumours whose vascular supply becomes insufficient. The resulting tumour cell necrosis leads to the increased release of cellular ions, such as potassium.

Excretion disorders that lead to hyperkalaemia are mainly associated with **urinary retention disorders**. If urine remains in the organism, dissolved potassium also remains in it. Accordingly, the decreasing glomerular filtration associated with renal failure leads to retention of potassium through its reduced glomerular filtration. The same applies to urethral obstruction, which reduces glomerular filtration post-renally. Finally, in the case of bladder rupture, potassium-rich urine can enter the abdominal cavity and be reabsorbed there, which corresponds to increased reabsorption.

In **hypoadrenocorticism**, hypovolaemia with associated reduced glomerular filtration is one mechanism.

Table 42.3.2 Causes of hyperkalaemia.

Uptake	Translocation	Reduced excretion
Unlikely	Acidosis	Urethral obstruction
	Insulin deficiency	Bladder rupture
	Tumour lysis	Kidney failure
		Hypoadrenocorticism

Pathophysiologic Consequences

The **consequences** of hyperkalaemia develop primarily in the heart and skeletal muscles due to depolarisation. Another consequence occurs in the kidneys.

Heart	Skeletal muscle	Kidneys
Bradycardia	Muscle weakness	Metabolic acidosis
AV block	Paralysis	
Asystole		

If the extracellular potassium concentration increases, this causes a reduction of the chemical potassium gradient intra- to extracellularly. As a result, the resting membrane potential decreases. Initially, this leads to easier formation of an action potential. However, chronic membrane depolarisation causes a reduction in the sensitivity of the Na^+ channels and thus a reduced generation of an action potential and overall excitability of the cell membrane.

The electrical conduction between the cardiomyocytes is reduced. This leads to conduction disturbances in the form of atrioventricular block (AV block). As a result, cardiac output decreases, causing organ diminished perfusion. This produces clinical symptoms, such as fatigue, dyspnoea or even syncope. In the heart itself, the reduced conduction leads to a prolonged PR interval. From a serum potassium concentration of $>5.5\,mmol/l$, myocardial repolarisation accelerates, resulting in a markedly increased T-wave in the ECG, which in turn is characteristic of hyperkalaemia.

In the **skeletal muscles**, stimulus formation and transmission are also negatively affected by hyperkalaemia, causing symptoms, such as weakness and paralysis to develop.

Renally, hyperkalaemia causes increased uptake by the tubule cells. This drives protons into the tubule lumen. In the tubule lumen, decreased pH causes reduced glutamate deamination. This decreases the luminal NH_3 concentration. In the collecting tube, NH_3 takes up protons and promotes their renal excretion. If this mechanism is reduced, the protons remain in the organism and lead to metabolic acidosis (Figure 42.3.1).

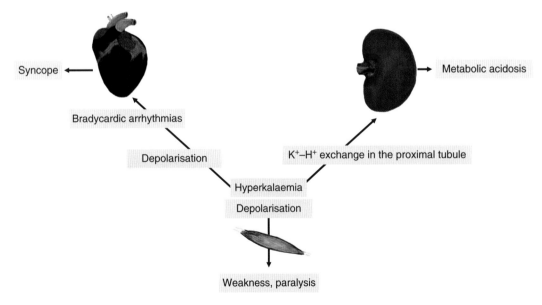

Figure 42.3.1 Pathophysiologic consequences of hyperkalaemia.

Hypokalaemia

The causes of hypokalaemia are due to reduced uptake, translocation from the extra- to the intracellular space or increased excretion.

Uptake	Translocation	Increased excretion
Unlikely	Alkalosis	Gastrointestinal loss
		Vomiting
		Diarrhoea
		Renal loss
		Polyuric renal failure
		Mineralocorticoid excess
		Hyperadrenocorticism

Due to the high concentration of potassium in dog and cat food, an undersupply is unlikely.

The translocation in **alkalosis** corresponds to the opposite processes in acidosis. Alkalosis preserves the function of the Na^+-K^+-ATPase at the cell membrane, and at the same time there is no replacement of potassium ions by protons in intracellular proteins, whereby potassium output would increase the extracellular potassium concentration.

The increased loss of potassium, especially during **vomiting**, is due to a shift in bicarbonate as a result of vomiting. Vomiting causes increased loss of protons from the stomach acid. This leads to an increased concentration of plasma bicarbonate (HCO_3^-). As a result, the tubular bicarbonate concentration increases. An electrical gradient is created to the tubular lumen due to the increased negative charges there. This shifts potassium ions into the tubular lumen and promotes their excretion.

The renal loss is due to increased urine output and potassium ions dissolved in it. During **mineralocorticoid excess**, increased potassium is excreted renally due to the increased aldosterone effect.

Pathophysiologic Consequences

The **consequences** of hypokalaemia also cause disturbances at the cell membrane, like hyperkalaemia already does.

Heart	Skeletal muscle	Kidneys
Arrhythmia	Muscle weakness	Metabolic alkalosis
	Paralysis	

The consequences on the heart and skeletal muscles are caused by hyperpolarisation due to hypokalaemia. Clinically, muscle weakness and paralysis develop, as well as cardiac arrhythmias. Intestinal ileus may develop due to hypokalaemia (Figure 42.3.2).

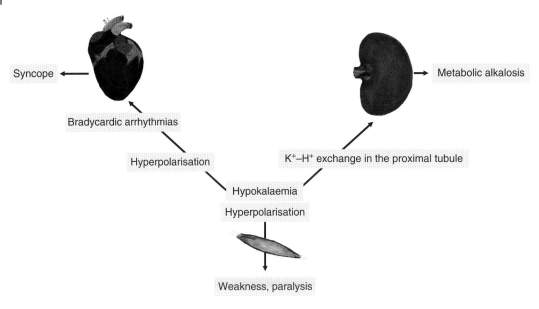

Figure 42.3.2 Pathophysiologic consequences of hypokalaemia.

Therapy

Hyperkalaemia	1) Mild hyperkalaemia (5.5–7.0 mEq/L) Infusion with crystalloid fluids.
	2) If the patient is not in renal failure and is not dehydrated, furosemide
	3) Administer glucose 20%, 1–2 mL/kg IV over 30–60 minutes.
Hypokalaemia	Acute or severe. Potassium chloride in intravenous fluids (generally not exceed 0.5 mEq/kg/h IV) in a crisis increase to 1.5 mEq/kg/h under direct ECG monitoring.

Further Reading

Hunter, R.W. and Bailey, M.A. (2019). Hyperkalemia: pathophysiology, risk factors and consequences. *Nephrology, Dialysis, Transplantation: Official Publication of the European Dialysis and Transplant Association – European Renal Association* 34 (Suppl 3): iii2–iii11. https://doi.org/10.1093/ndt/gfz206.

Palmer, B.F. and Clegg, D.J. (2019). Physiology and pathophysiology of potassium homeostasis: core curriculum 2019. *American Journal of Kidney Diseases: The Official Journal of the National Kidney Foundation* 74 (5): 682–695. https://doi.org/10.1053/j.ajkd.2019.03.427.

43

Endocrine System

43.1

General Physiology

Higher organisms have coordinating systems to maintain the homeostasis and to react to external and internal factors. The nervous system has a superordinate function in this. The hormone system is controlled by the nervous system and supports homeostasis. The endocrine system is composed of a number of glands whose secretions reach the site of action via the blood. The term 'internal secretion' describes this activity.

The essential link between the nervous system and the hormonal system is located in the hypothalamus. This is a structure in the diencephalon which, as a switching point, receives afferents from different areas of the brain, for example, the thalamus and the hippocampus, but also information from the periphery, for example, with regard to blood pressure and body temperature.

In the hypothalamus, the information received can lead to the secretion of various hormones. A distinction is made between effector hormones, such as oxytocin or antidiuretic hormone, which directly influence control processes in the periphery, and the so-called 'regulatory hormones', whose effect is mediated via the pituitary gland. Through secretion of the so-called 'releasing hormones', the hypothalamus can induce the release of regulatory hormones for peripheral organs in the pituitary gland, for example, TSH or ACTH (Table 43.1.1).

The pituitary gland is subordinate to the hypothalamus. It lies extradurally in a connective tissue capsule in the hypophysial fossa as part of the sella turcica on the inner side of the sphenoidal bone. The pituitary gland can be anatomically divided into sections. The infundibulum connects the hypothalamus with the pituitary gland. Cranially lies the anterior pituitary lobe, the adenohypophysis. It has five endocrine gland types and is responsible for the syntheses and secretion of the glandotropic hormones thyrotropin (TSH), luteinising hormone (LH) and adrenocorticotropic hormone (ACTH) as well as the non-glandotropic hormones growth hormone (GH, somatotropin) and prolactin (PRL). Glandotropic hormones are hormones that regulate the hormone production of other endocrine organs; in contrast, the two non-glandotropic hormones act directly on the target organs.

The posterior pituitary, the neurohypophysis, is the storage organ for the hormones oxytocin and ADH, which were originally synthesised in the hypothalamus.

The peripheral endocrine organs are controlled from the pituitary gland. These include the thyroid gland, the adrenal gland and the hormone-producing sex organs (Figure 43.1.1).

The functions of the peripheral endocrine organs are described in the respective chapters.

Endocrine organs act via hormones, which are molecules that influence cell metabolism and the expression of proteins. The hormones can be divided into peptide hormones, amino acid hormones and steroid hormones. Depending on their chemical structure, the hormones activate the protein expression of the target cell via two receptors.

Receptors in the cell membrane interact with hormones, such as adrenaline, noradrenaline and most peptide hormones (e.g. glucagon, ACTH, TRH, TSH).

Receptors for steroid hormones or thyroxines and calcitriol are located in the cytosol or in the cell nucleus. A functional difference between the two receptor effects is the reaction time and duration of action. Membrane receptors usually exert an immediate effect that becomes measurable in the cells within seconds or minutes and then rapidly decreases. The intracellular hormone receptors, on the other hand, usually only take effect after several minutes or hours, but their effect usually lasts longer.

Textbook of Small Animal Pathophysiology, First Edition. Stephan Neumann.

Table 43.1.1 Hormones of hypothalamus.

Name	Abbreviation	Target organ	Function
Thyrotropin-releasing hormone	TRH	Pituitary gland	Release of TSH
Corticotropin releasing hormone	CRH	Pituitary gland	Release of ACTH
Gonadotropin releasing hormone	GnRH	Pituitary gland	Release of LH and FSH
Somatotropin		Pituitary gland	Release from GH
Somatostatin		Pituitary gland	Inhibition of the release of GH
Prolactin releasing peptide	PRP	Pituitary gland	Release of prolactin
Dopamine		Pituitary gland	Inhibition of the release of prolactin
Oxytocin		Uterus/mammary gland	Contraction of the smooth muscle fibres
Antidiuretic hormone	ADH	Kidney	Water reabsorption

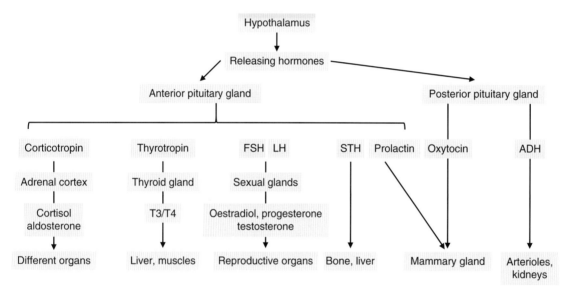

Figure 43.1.1 Hierarchy of hormones.

The membrane receptors transmit the hormonal signal into the interior of the cell. In the process, amplification of the signal also takes place. According to current knowledge, this signal transmission takes place via three different pathways: (1) via G-protein-coupled receptors, (2) via enzyme-coupled receptors or (3) via ligand-dependent ion channels.

1) G-protein-coupled membrane receptors. These receptors lie transmembranously and are intracellularly connected to the so-called 'G-proteins'. They bind either GDP (inactive state) or GTP (active state). The binding of the hormone to the receptor leads to the exchange of GDP by GTP in the G-protein. The G-protein activated in this way binds and activates an enzyme that is required to produce a second messenger, such as cyclic AMP (cAMP) or cyclic GMP (cGMP). These activate protein kinases, which can eventually activate further cellular proteins through phosphorylation. In this way, the hormone effect is implemented cellularly. Examples of G-protein-coupled membrane receptors are: Adrenalin receptors, ACTH, TSH and TRH receptors (Table 43.1.2).
2) Enzyme-coupled membrane receptors.
   A second family of membrane receptors has a direct enzyme function that is activated by hormone binding. For example, the insulin receptor has tyrosine kinase activity, whereby the receptor autophosphorylates tyrosine residues after insulin binding. These bind to cellular enzymes which are thus activated and induce intracellular metabolic processes.
3) Ligand-dependent ion channels.

Table 43.1.2 Examples of cAMP-induced cell metabolic processes.

Target molecule	Effect
Calcium channel protein	Calcium channel opening
Myosin kinase	Muscle relaxation
Transcription factors	Gene expression
Enzymes of glycogenolysis	Glycogen degradation
Enzymes of lipolysis	Lipolysis

These receptors carry out a conformational change after hormone binding and thus allow an ion flow. This activates the cell, for example, by forming an action potential. The acetylcholine receptor, for example, is a subunit of an ion channel. Binding of acetylcholine leads to the temporary opening of the channel, whereupon the influx of positively charged sodium ions is enabled. This in turn leads to a depolarisation of the membrane with possible consequences: such as, triggering an action potential or secretion of hormones, cytokines or growth factors.

The intracellular receptors are to be differentiated from the membrane receptors. Intracellular receptors are localised in the cytosol or nucleus. Hormones that act intracellularly are steroid hormones, thyroid hormones or 1,25-dihydroxycholecalciferol, whereby the steroid hormone receptors are cytosolic and the thyroid hormone or 1,25-dihydroxycholecalciferol receptors are localised in the nucleus. The cytosolic hormone receptors are transported to the nucleus after activation by a hormone. The nuclear receptors are already localised at the cell nucleus. The intracellular hormones control the expression of genes. They are active over a period of hours or days and influence the growth and differentiation of cells, as well as their enzyme activities.

The hormonal effect is typically regulated through a feedback loop or control circuit.

In simple pathway, the end product controls hormone release. In complex control loops, the control takes place via the hypothalamus and pituitary gland. As a rule, hormone release is controlled by a negative feedback mechanism in which the secreted hormone or the target product of hormone release prevents its synthesis. An example of negative feedback is found in the thyroid gland. Here, a high concentration of thyroid hormones leads to an inhibited secretion of thyrotropin-releasing hormone (TRH) in the hypothalamus, which indirectly results in a decrease in thyroid hormones. However, there are also positive feedback mechanisms in which secreted hormones induce the synthesis of other hormones. An example of this mechanism is oestrogen, which, when secreted more often, leads to increased LH secretion from the pituitary gland. The positive feedback causes a rapid increase in hormone concentration.

Further Reading

Reddy, S.S. (2006). Endocrinology update 2006. *Cleveland Clinic Journal of Medicine* 73 (11): 1019–1024. https://doi.org/10.3949/ccjm.73.11.1019.

van den Beld, A.W., Kaufman, J.M., Zillikens, M.C. et al. (2018). The physiology of endocrine systems with ageing. *The Lancet. Diabetes & Endocrinology* 6 (8): 647–658. https://doi.org/10.1016/S2213-8587(18)30026-3.

43.2

Pituitary Gland

43.2.1

Acromegaly

Definition

Acromegaly is a condition in which the body produces too much growth hormone. It is characterised by an extraordinarily strong growth of body size or certain parts of the body.

Aetiology

A common cause in cats and dogs is a growth-hormone-producing tumour of the pituitary gland. Another causality in dogs is externally applied or internally synthesised progesterone. The latter, however, assumes growth hormone production in the mammary gland and not in the pituitary gland.

Tumour	Endocrine
Pituitary gland tumour (D/C)	Progestagens (D)

D – Dog, C – Cat

Pathogenesis

The consequence of a hormone-producing tumour, or hormone production in the mammary gland, is an increased concentration of growth hormone in the blood. Under physiological conditions, growth hormone is released in a pulsatile manner; tumour tissue produces growth hormone permanently. The clinical and laboratory diagnostic consequences based on direct effects of growth hormone or on effects of IGF-1, whose synthesis in the liver is controlled by growth hormone.

In dogs with progesterone induced acromegaly, the feedback mechanism regulating the GH synthesis is disrupted. Progesterone stimulates the production of GH either directly or indirectly. This results in an increase in the synthesis and secretion of GH by the somatotropic cells of the pituitary gland (Table 43.2.1.1).

Diagnostics

Clinical signs	Clinical pathology	Imaging	Histopathology	Microbiology
Organ enlargement	IGF-1 serum concentration	**CT/MRI** Structural alteration of the pituitary gland	Not necessary	Not necessary

Textbook of Small Animal Pathophysiology, First Edition. Stephan Neumann.
© 2025 John Wiley & Sons Ltd. Published 2025 by John Wiley & Sons Ltd.

Table 43.2.1.1   Effects of growth hormone and IGF-1.

Growth hormone	IGF-1
Promote the longitudinal growth of the bones	Anabolic effects of insulin
Promote the growth of muscles and soft tissues	Protein synthesis
Promote the breakdown of fat for energy	Growth of growth plates and cartilage
Increase of the blood sugar level and at the same time increase of the insulin secretion	
Stimulation of calcitriol formation	
Support of the immune defence (via stimulation of T lymphocytes and macrophages)	

Pathophysiologic Consequences

The pathophysiologic consequences of growth hormone excess essentially proceed from the promotion of growth and thus from anatomical changes.

Influenced organ systems	Clinical symptoms	Clinical pathological alterations
Cardiovascular system	Organ enlargement	Hyperglycaemia
Respiratory system	Head	Increased liver enzymes
Hepatobiliary system	Tongue	
Urinary tract	Muscles	
Endocrine system		
Neuromuscular system	PU/PD	
Central nervous system	Dyspnoea	
Bones, joints		
Muscles		

The **organ enlargements** due to growth hormone excess particularly affect the **bones of the head**. Prognathia inferior visibly changes the appearance of the head; this change is more common in the cat. Changes in the **tongue** and larynx lead to voice changes and **dyspnoea**, both observed in dogs and cats.

The essential mechanism of GH action is via the formation of IGF-1 in the liver. Growth hormone binds to a specific growth hormone receptor in the hepatocyte membrane. Via signal transduction through the Jak2/Stat pathway, gene expression of IGF-1 is induced in the cell nucleus and IGF-1 is synthesised. This is released into the blood and transported to the target cells via various binding proteins. There it binds to membrane-bound insulin 1 receptor. This works according to the principle of an enzyme-coupled membrane receptor (see Chapter 43.1).

The consequences of growth hormone excess, or an increased IGF-1 concentration, are first of all increased longitudinal growth of the bones. IGF-1 influences the cell cycle on the one hand and apoptosis on the other. Overall, IGF-1 has a mitogenic effect and is of decisive importance for the proliferation and differentiation of cells. The mitogenic effect of IGF-1 is based on an increase in the expression of cyclin D1, which supports a change in the cell cycle from G1 phase to S phase. The anti-apoptotic effect of IGF-1 is based, among other things, on the stimulation of the expression of Bcl proteins (B-cell lymphoma). These are apoptosis regulators that act by controlling mitochondrial membrane permeability (Le Roith et al. 2001).

IGF-1 is of great importance in the regulation of skeletal muscle. Due to its anabolic effects, there is increased muscle protein synthesis and, in addition, IGF-1 stimulates the proliferation and differentiation of the satellite cells of the skeletal muscles. The anti-apoptotic effect of IGF-1 leads to a reduction in proteolysis and inhibition of the ubiquitin proteasome system in the muscle cell and thus to reduced muscle breakdown (Hong and Forsberg 1994; Chrysis and Underwood 1999).

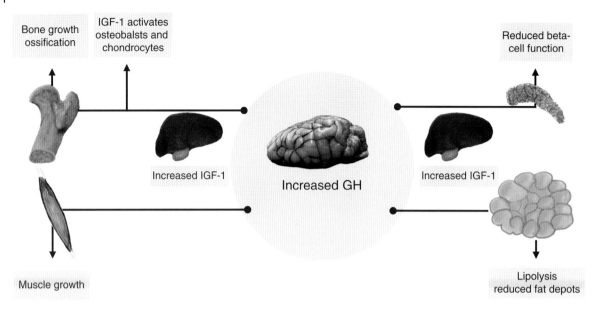

Figure 43.2.1.1 Pathophysiologic consequences of acromegaly.

Furthermore, IGF-1 is important for the growth and differentiation of adipose tissue. It stimulates both the differentiation of adipocyte precursors into mature adipocytes and the growth of mature adipocytes (Blüher et al. 2005). IGF-1 acts on protein metabolism by increasing protein synthesis and inhibiting proteolysis. IGF-1 also has an anabolic effect by increasing the uptake of glucose into the cells.

Outside the musculoskeletal system, enlargements of the **liver** and **kidneys,** in particular, can be observed. Other consequences, such as **PU/PD**, **hyperglycaemia** as well as **weight loss** are due to induced diabetes mellitus. This phenomenon is observed more frequently in the cat than in the dog. The growth hormone excess causes a depression of β-cell function in the endocrine pancreas. In addition, cellular glucose uptake is reduced, but at the same time glycogenolysis and gluconeogenesis are increased (Vila et al. 2019) (Figure 43.2.1.1).

Therapy

Symptom	Therapy
Tumour	Surgery
Diabetes mellitus	Insulin

References

Blüher, S., Kratzsch, J., and Kiess, W. (2005). Insulin-like growth factor I, growth hormone and insulin in white adipose tissue. *Best Practice & Research. Clinical Endocrinology & Metabolism* 19 (4): 577–587. https://doi.org/10.1016/j.beem.2005.07.011.

Chrysis, D. and Underwood, L.E. (1999). Regulation of components of the ubiquitin system by insulin-like growth factor I and growth hormone in skeletal muscle of rats made catabolic with dexamethasone. *Endocrinology* 140 (12): 5635–5641. https://doi.org/10.1210/endo.140.12.7217.

Hong, D. and Forsberg, N.E. (1994). Effects of serum and insulin-like growth factor I on protein degradation and protease gene expression in rat L8 myotubes. *Journal of Animal Science* 72 (9): 2279–2288. https://doi.org/10.2527/1994.7292279x.

Le Roith, D., Bondy, C., Yakar, S. et al. (2001). The somatomedin hypothesis: 2001. *Endocrine Reviews* 22 (1): 53–74. https://doi.org/10.1210/edrv.22.1.0419.

Vila, G., Jørgensen, J.O.L., Luger, A., and Stalla, G.K. (2019). Insulin resistance in patients with acromegaly. *Frontiers in Endocrinology* 10: 509. https://doi.org/10.3389/fendo.2019.00509.

Further Reading

Gouvêa, F.N., Pennacchi, C.S., Assaf, N.D. et al. (2021). Acromegaly in dogs and cats. *Annales d'Endocrinologie* 82 (2): 107–111. https://doi.org/10.1016/j.ando.2021.03.002.

Lidbury, J.A., Cook, A.K., and Steiner, J.M.((2016). Hepatic encephalopathy in dogs and cats. *Journal of Veterinary Emergency and Critical Care (San Antonio, Tex.: 2001)* 26 (4): 471–487.

Rijnberk, A., Kooistra, H.S., and Mol, J.A. (2003). Endocrine diseases in dogs and cats: similarities and differences with endocrine diseases in humans. *Growth Hormone & IGF Research: Official Journal of the Growth Hormone Research Society and the International IGF Research Society* 13 (Suppl A): S158–S164. https://doi.org/10.1016/s1096-6374(03)00076-5.

43.2.2

Pituitary Dwarfism

Definition

Pituitary dwarfism is a growth arrest caused by insufficient secretion of growth hormone. It is the most common form of dwarfism in dogs and cats.

Aetiology

The congenital form of dwarfism is more common in dogs and is a genetic defect that has been described in particular in the German Shepherd dog. Other breeds with pituitary dwarfism are different wolfhound breeds. A mutation in the LHX3 gene is described as the cause. The gene encodes a transcription factor responsible for the development of the anterior and middle pituitary gland and differentiation of the GH-, PRL-, TSH-, LH-, FSH-producing cells (Voorbij et al. 2011).

Independent of this are acquired forms of dwarfism, which develop due to diseases of the pituitary gland, as a result of which a reduction in growth hormone secretion takes place.

Congenital	Acquired
Mutation LHX3 gene	Pituitary gland (D/C)
	Tumour
	Trauma
	Inflammation

Pathogenesis and Pathophysiology

The consequence of all forms of pituitary dwarfism is a short stature in the skeleton, although the proportions remain the same.

This influences the growth of bone length. In long bones, growth originates from epiphyseal joints, which lie between the diaphysis and epiphysis. Chondrocytes are localised within the growth plate as the main cell type. These exist in different variations. As undifferentiated cells, they form the reservoir for growth activity. An increase in the mitotic rate leads to proliferation of the chondrocytes and to columnar growth, which pushes the bone segments apart in the sense of longitudinal growth. Following proliferation, the chondrocytes undergo hypertrophy and then enter an apoptotic phase. The resulting free spaces in the parenchyma are occupied by osteoblasts, which contribute to ossification and thus to the termination of length growth.

Disturbances in length growth and thus the trigger for dwarfism are disturbances during the proliferation of the chondrocytes. These can be influenced by genetic factors. For example, proliferation and differentiation of chondrocytes within

Textbook of Small Animal Pathophysiology, First Edition. Stephan Neumann.
© 2025 John Wiley & Sons Ltd. Published 2025 by John Wiley & Sons Ltd.

the growth plates are controlled by fibroblast growth factor (FGF). After receptor binding, the formation of the transcription factor SOX9 is initiated intracellularly as a second messenger, which controls protein expressions necessary for the cell differentiation of the chondroblasts. Mutations in the FGF receptor gene can thus have a negative influence on the growth of the epiphyseal groove (Ornitz and Legeai-Mallet 2017; Högler and Ward 2020).

In addition, hormonal dysregulation of the pituitary gland leads to dwarfism in dogs and cats. Bone growth is influenced embryonically and postpartum by different hormones, including insulin, thyroid hormones, sex hormones, growth hormone and IGF-1. With the exception of insulin, all other hormones are controlled by the hypothalamic-pituitary axis. Thyroid hormones influence proliferation and differentiation of chondrocytes by positively influencing the hypertrophy of proliferated chondrocytes. At the same time, they promote the differentiation of osteoblasts into osteocytes. In this process, the thyroid hormones act by influencing the growth factors IGF-1 and BMP (Zhu et al. 2022).

Sex hormones have a far-reaching influence on bone growth. Estrogens and testosterone have an effect on bone. The enzyme aromatase can convert testosterone into oestrogen. In this way, both hormones also have an effect on bone metabolism in both sexes. Whereas oestrogens tend to influence the compacta, testosterone affects the trabecular structure. Cellularly, both sex hormones act on osteoblast apoptosis and suppress it. At the same time, osteoclast apoptosis is increased via transcription factor κB (Narla and Ott 2018) (Table 43.2.2.1).

In relation to bone metabolism, the functions of GH and IGF-1 have already been presented in Chapter 43.2.1. In summary, the effects of IGF-1 on bone can be described as promoting the proliferation of chondrocytes and osteoblasts, thus influencing length growth and bone differentiation. Furthermore, the synthesis of matrix molecules (collagens and proteoglycans) as well as the calcium and phosphorus metabolism are influenced by an increased synthesis of vitamin D3.

However, the **pathophysiologic consequences** of dwarfism do not only affect the skeletal system with the growth of bone length but also the skin and reproduction.

Influenced organ systems	Clinical symptoms
Bones, joints	Dwarfism
Muscles	Muscular atrophy
Skin	Soft, woolly coat hyperpigmentation of the skin
Reproduction	Pyoderma
	Anestrus
	Testicular atrophy
	Lethargy

The consequences are based on the deficiency of different pituitary hormones. Skin changes are also caused by the influence of the thyroid hormone balance as well as the sex hormones, while the sex-specific changes are due to the pituitary influence of the sex hormones.

Table 43.2.2.1 Metabolic influence of GH and IGF-1.

Consequence	GH	IGF-1
GH secretion	−	−
IGF-1 secretion	+	−
Insulin secretion	+	−
Gluconeogenesis	+	−
Lipolysis	+	?
Protein synthesis	+	+

Source: Adapted from Rosenbloom (2007).

Diagnostics

Clinical signs	Clinical pathology	Imaging	Histopathology	Microbiology
Dwarfism	**IGF-1** serum concentration	CT/MRI Imaging of the pituitary gland	Not necessary	Not necessary

Therapy

Symptom	Therapy
Dwarfism	Growth hormone

References

Högler, W. and Ward, L.M. (2020). New developments in the management of achondroplasia. New developments in the management of achondroplasia. *Wiener Medizinische Wochenschrift (1946)* 170 (5–6): 104–111. https://doi.org/10.1007/s10354-020-00741-6.

Narla, R.R. and Ott, S.M. (2018). Bones and the sex hormones. *Kidney International* 94 (2): 239–242. https://doi.org/10.1016/j.kint.2018.03.021.

Ornitz, D.M. and Legeai-Mallet, L. (2017). Achondroplasia: development, pathogenesis, and therapy. *Developmental Dynamics: An Official Publication of the American Association of the Anatomists* 246 (4): 291–309. https://doi.org/10.1002/dvdy.24479.

Rosenbloom, A.L. (2007). The physiology of growth. *Annales Nestle* 65: 99–110. http://dx.doi.org/10.1159/000163024.

Voorbij, A.M., van Steenbeek, F.G., Vos-Loohuis, M. et al. (2011). A contracted DNA repeat in LHX3 intron 5 is associated with aberrant splicing and pituitary dwarfism in German shepherd dogs. *PLoS One* 6 (11): e27940. https://doi.org/10.1371/journal.pone.0027940.

Zhu, S., Pang, Y., Xu, J. et al. (2022). Endocrine regulation on bone by thyroid. *Frontiers in Endocrinology* 13: 873820. https://doi.org/10.3389/fendo.2022.873820.

Further Reading

Greco, D.S. (2001). Diagnosis and treatment of juvenile endocrine disorders in puppies and kittens. *The Veterinary Clinics of North America. Small Animal Practice* 31 (2): 401–viii. https://doi.org/10.1016/s0195-5616(01)50212-0.

König, M.L., Henke, D., Adamik, K., and Pérez Vera, C. (2018). Juvenile hyposomatotropism in a Somali cat presenting with seizures due to intermittent hypoglycaemia. *JFMS Open Reports* 4 (1): 2055116918761441. https://doi.org/10.1177/2055116918761441.

43.2.3

Diabetes Insipidus

Definition

Diabetes insipidus is a disorder of the water balance caused by limited water reabsorption in the nephrons.

Aetiology

In principle, a distinction is made in diabetes insipidus between a central and a renal form. Both forms affect the secretion or action of antidiuretic hormone (ADH). The disease occurs in dogs and cats, but is much more common in dogs.

Central	Nephrogenic
Primary	Primary congenital (D)
Congenital (D)	Secondary endocrine (D)
Secondary	Hyperadrenocorticism
Trauma (D/C)	Hypercalcaemia
Neoplasia (D)	Secondary renal (D/C)
	Pyelonephritis
	Chronic kidney disease

D – Dog, C – Cat

Pathogenesis

The synthesis and action of ADH are central part of diabetes insipidus.

ADH is a peptide hormone composed of nine amino acids. It is formed in the nucleus supraopticus and in the nucleus paraventricularis of the hypothalamus as a prohormone and is then transported via axons to the neurohypophysis and stored there.

The essential function of ADH is water reabsorption in the nephron. Accordingly, the release of ADH is initiated when blood volume or blood pressure decrease or when the osmolarity of the blood plasma increases.

The latter is detected by hypothalamic osmoreceptors.

These receptors can absorb water from the interstitium via channels (aquaporins). The amount depends on the osmolarity. If the interstitial fluid is hypoosmolar, there is increased water influx into the receptor cells and the cells swell. This produces hyperpolarisation, which inhibits the release of ADH. In the case of increased osmolarity (hyperosmolar), water flows out of the receptor cells, which shrink, causing depolarisation and initiating release from the pituitary cells.

Textbook of Small Animal Pathophysiology, First Edition. Stephan Neumann.
© 2025 John Wiley & Sons Ltd. Published 2025 by John Wiley & Sons Ltd.

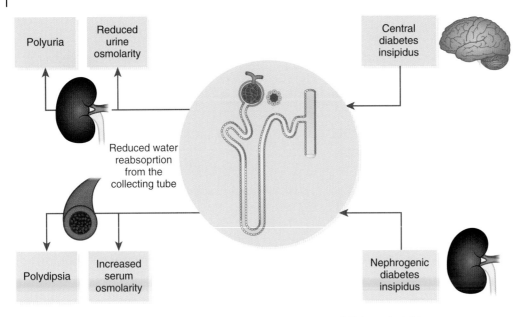

Figure 43.2.3.1   Pathogenesis and pathophysiologic consequences of diabetes insipidus.

Blood volume and blood pressure are detected by baroreceptors, which are particularly localised as arterial baroreceptors in the area of the aorta and carotid artery or as venous baroreceptors in the area of the right atrium. The receptors are located in the media of the vessel wall and can detect wall tension. The ADH secretion is stimulated by vegetative afferents.

Increased osmolarity, reduced blood pressure or reduced blood volume lead to a secretion of ADH in the pituitary gland.

In high concentrations, secreted ADH can cause increased calcium influx via the so-called 'V1 receptors' in the vascular wall, which leads to a contraction of the smooth muscles and thus increases blood pressure. However, this is not the main effect of ADH, which unfolds at the kidney. There, ADH acts via the so-called 'V2 receptors' in the area of the distal tubule and the collecting tube. After ADH binds to the receptor, a G-protein-mediated formation of cAMP occurs as a second messenger. cAMP activates a protein kinase, which activates aquaporin 2 by phosphorylation. This reaches the apical cell membrane via intracellular vesicles and fuses with it. Water can be reabsorbed through the aquaporins.

The different causalities of diabetes insipidus affect the secretion and receptor action of ADH. In the primary congenital form of central diabetes insipidus, there is a congenital defect, which results in reduced ADH synthesis in the hypothalamic cells. In secondary central diabetes insipidus, the hypothalamus or the pituitary gland are restricted in their ADH synthesis or release by different causalities, which ultimately also leads to an overall reduced secretion of ADH.

In primary nephrogenic diabetes insipidus, there is a congenital defect in which the density of the V2 receptor is reduced.

Secondary nephrogenic diabetes insipidus must be differentiated from this. This occurs, for example, in hypercalcaemia. Calcium inhibits the binding of ADH to the V2 receptor, which results in a reduced expression of aquaporins. Bacterial toxins, especially from *Escherichia coli,* can occupy the V2 receptor and thus suppress the binding of ADH. Finally, renal remodelling processes, for example in chronic renal failure, are associated with destruction of the nephrons, which can lead to reduced receptor density (Figure 43.2.3.1).

Diagnostics

Clinical signs	Clinical pathology	Imaging	Histopathology	Microbiology
PU/PD	Urine concentration ability	**CT/MRI** Structural alteration of the pituitary gland	Not necessary	Not necessary

Pathophysiologic Consequences

The consequences of diabetes insipidus are mainly concentrated on the water balance.

Influenced organ systems	Clinical symptoms	Clinical pathological alterations
Urinary tract	PU/PD	Hyposthenuria
Endocrine system	Dehydration	Increased HKT
	Incontinence	Increased serum protein

The clinical symptoms develop primarily due to impaired water reabsorption. This leads to **hyposthenuric** urine. The specific urine weight is <1.006 g/ml in the diabetes insipidus forms. This leads to an increase in plasma osmolarity, which leads to an increased intake of water via the activity of the thirst centre. Accordingly, the clinical symptoms are **polyuria** accompanied by compensatory **polydipsia**. If the polydipsia is insufficient to compensate for the renal water loss, the animals **dehydrate**. This can lead to increased **packed cell volume (PCV)** or increased **serum protein concentrations**. The reduced water reabsorption in diabetes insipidus leads to increased urine volume. This may clinically cause incontinence if the pressure in the urinary bladder exceeds that of the bladder sphincter.

Therapy

Symptom	Therapy
Central DI	Vasopressin (ADH)
Nephrogenic DI	Hydrochlorothiazide

Further Reading

Bovee, K.C. (1977). Diabetes insipidus. *The Veterinary Clinics of North America* 7 (3): 603–611. https://doi.org/10.1016/s0091-0279(77)50060-3.

Greco, D.S. (2012). Pituitary deficiencies. *Topics in Companion Animal Medicine* 27 (1): 2–7. https://doi.org/10.1053/j.tcam.2012.04.002.

Morello, J.P. and Bichet, D.G. (2001). Nephrogenic diabetes insipidus. *Annual Review of Physiology* 63: 607–630. https://doi.org/10.1146/annurev.physiol.63.1.607.

Refardt, J., Winzeler, B., and Christ-Crain, M. (2020). Diabetes insipidus: an update. *Endocrinology and Metabolism Clinics of North America* 49 (3): 517–531. https://doi.org/10.1016/j.ecl.2020.05.012.

43.3

Thyroid Gland

43.3.1

Physiology of the Thyroid Gland

Functions

The thyroid gland is a paired organ consisting of two lobes connected by an isthmus. The thyroid gland is divided into several lobules by septa, which consist of round follicles about 200 μm in size. In the follicular lumen lies the colloid, which consists mainly of thyroglobulin. Surrounding the colloid is a single-layered epithelium consisting of thyrocytes. The follicles are surrounded by a network of capillaries and lymphatic vessels. The thyroid is innervated parasympathetically via branches of the vagus nerve and sympathetically via the cervical medial ganglion.

The thyroid gland is the site of synthesis and storage of the thyroid hormones thyroxine (T4) and triiodothyronine (T3). Both hormones are essentially involved in the energy metabolism of the organism. The thyroid gland synthesises hormones and stores them. Synthesis is located in the thyrocytes and is divided into three phases. The first phase, the exocrine phase, consists of the uptake of iodine from the blood, which is stimulated by thyroid-stimulating hormone (TSH). In the second phase, thyroglobulin is synthesised and in the third phase, iodine is bound.

Iodine, which is ingested with food, absorbed in the intestine and transported to the thyroid gland via the blood, reaches the thyrocytes via an ATP-dependent Na^+ cotransport. At the same time, the synthesis of thyroglobulin takes place under the influence of TSH. For this purpose, TSH binds to a membrane receptor and, mediated by cAMP as a second messenger, the expression of thyroglobulin starts. Thyroglobulin is a glycoprotein with numerous tyrosine residues. This is transported by exocytosis into the follicular space where it binds iodine under the catalysis of thyroid peroxidase. 3-monoiodotyrosine (MIT) and 3,5-diiodotyrosine (DIT) are formed as precursor molecules from the connection with iodine. Through a coupling reaction and with the cleavage of alanine, the thyroid hormone tetraiodothyronine (thyroxine, T4) is formed from two DIT molecules. Also by coupling, the thyroid hormone triiodothyronine (T3) can be formed from one MIT and one DIT molecule. Both molecules initially remain linked to thyroglobulin. After stimulation, the hormones T4 and T3 are taken up by endocytosis from the follicular lumen into the thyrocytes, where they are separated from thyroglobulin by lysosomes, allowing release into the bloodstream. Less than 1% of thyroid hormones are present in the blood unbound. The majority of T3 and T4 is bound to plasma proteins, such as albumin, thyroxine-binding prealbumin and thyroxine-binding globulin. Binding to plasma proteins prolongs the half-life of thyroid hormones and prevents them from being excreted too fast. Protein-bound thyroid hormones are biologically inactive. The thyroid gland secretes mainly T4 and the main part of T3 is produced by extrathyroidal deiodination catalysed by thyroxine deiodinase from T4 to T3 (in the target cell).

The biologically active form of thyroid hormones is T3. The conversion of T4 to T3 occurs in the liver, kidneys or in peripheral cells at the site of action.

The transport of T4 or T3 into the cells is realised via diffusion or bound to carriers. Inside the cell, the thyroid hormones, T3 with higher activity, act via nuclear receptors and induce the gene expression of proteins (Figure 43.3.1.1).

The physiological effect of thyroid hormones is multiple (Table 43.3.1.1).

Overall, the different effects of thyroid hormones can be summarised as metabolic.

Already during embryonic and foetal development, first maternal and later foetal thyroid hormones have an effect on the development with differentiation and growth of the various organs. In particular, cerebral development with the growth of nerve cells and the formation of synapses can be traced back to the function of thyroid hormones.

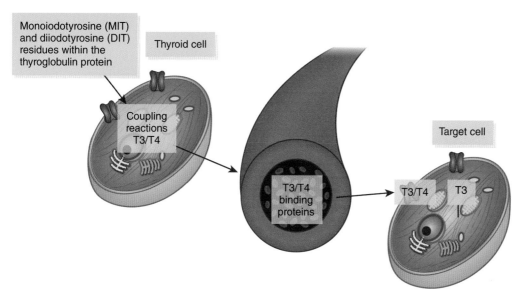

Figure 43.3.1.1 Synthesis and transport of thyroid hormones.

Table 43.3.1.1 Effects of thyroid hormones.

Organ/metabolism	Function
Development	Foetal growth and development
Protein metabolism	Protein synthesis
Carbohydrate metabolism	Glycogenolysis, gluconeogenesis
Fat metabolism	Lipolysis
Energy metabolism	Increased supply of energy, increase in body temperature
Cardiovascular system	Positive chronotropic, positive ionotropic
Respiratory system	Increasing the oxygen supply
Gastrointestinal tract	Increase absorption
Kidneys	Increase glomerular filtration
Musculature	Anabolic
Bones	Anabolic
Skin	Maintenance of the skin metabolism
Sensory organs/nervous system	Development, especially embryonic
Sexual organs	Fertility

Postpartum, thyroid hormones show a positive metabolic function by controlling the provision of energy for metabolic processes. This includes an increased provision of glucose, through an increase in glycogenolysis and gluconeogenesis. Both occurs primarily in the liver. By increasing lipolysis and β-oxidation, more free fatty acids are made available for energy metabolism. In order to optimally use the 'energy carrier' glucose for the formation of ATP, a sufficient supply of oxygen is required. This is achieved by the thyroid hormones via a positive ionotropic and positive chronotropic effect on the heart. The mechanism is based on an increase in the sensitivity of the β-adrenergic receptors to catecholamines, as well as an increase in the supply of calcium in the heart muscle cells.

An influence of thyroid hormones on kidney function is given by the increase in glomerular filtration. This is a consequence of the blood pressure influenced by the thyroid hormones, as well as the post-glomerular vascular resistance. (van Hoek and Daminet 2009; Schairer et al. 2020) A further influence is given via tubular function. Here, thyroid

Table 43.3.1.2 Alterations of the metabolism in hypo- and hyperthyroidism.

Metabolism	Hypothyroidism	Hyperthyroidism
Protein metabolism		
Synthesis	−	+
Proteolysis	−	+
Carbohydrate metabolism		
Glycogenolysis	−	+
Gluconeogenesis	−	+
Fat metabolism		
Lipogenesis	−	+
Lipolysis	−	+

hormones influence the sodium and hydrogen exchange via the activity of the Na^+/K^+-ATPase and, via this, the acid-base balance and the blood volume. A further function is given by influencing the effect of ADH (Iglesias et al. 2017).

The thyroid gland is controlled by higher-level centres in the hypothalamus and pituitary gland and by feedback mechanisms. In the hypothalamus, thyrotropin-releasing hormone (TRH) is produced in the event of an increased energy requirement, such as stress, cold, hypoglycaemia or catecholamine action. Corticoids, on the other hand, inhibit TRH synthesis. TRH is transported via the portal vein between the hypothalamus and the pituitary gland to its anterior lobe. There it acts via a G-protein coupled receptor and induces the synthesis and release of TSH. This, in turn, is transported via the blood to the thyroid gland where it binds to thyrocyte receptors and induces the formation and release of thyroid hormones T3 and T4. The increase in serum T4 concentration has a negative effect on the release of TRH and TSH via a feedback mechanism.

The breakdown of thyroid hormones is initiated via deiodination catalysed by a deiodase. Thyroid hormones can also be conjugated in the liver and then excreted in the bile.

General Consequences of the Malfunction

Thyroid function can be affected by hyperthyroidism or hypothyroidism. Both clinical pictures occur in dogs and cats, whereby dogs suffer more frequently from hypothyroidism and cats from hyperthyroidism. Both forms of the disease show extensive clinical and clinicopathological changes, which are discussed in Chapters 43.3.2 and 43.3.3. Overall, however, the clear alterations of the metabolism are in the foreground. These are summarised in Table 43.3.1.2.

References

van Hoek, I. and Daminet, S. (2009). Interactions between thyroid and kidney function in pathological conditions of these organ systems: a review. *General and Comparative Endocrinology* 160 (3): 205–215. https://doi.org/10.1016/j.ygcen.2008.12.008.

Iglesias, P., Bajo, M.A., Selgas, R., and Díez, J.J. (2017). Thyroid dysfunction and kidney disease: an update. *Reviews in Endocrine & Metabolic Disorders* 18 (1): 131–144. https://doi.org/10.1007/s11154-016-9395-7.

Schairer, B., Jungreithmayr, V., Schuster, M. et al. (2020). Effect of thyroid hormones on kidney function in patients after kidney transplantation. *Scientific Reports* 10 (1): 2156. https://doi.org/10.1038/s41598-020-59178-x.

Further Reading

Khan, Y.S. and Farhana, A. (2022). Histology, thyroid gland. In: *StatPearls*. StatPearls Publishing.

43.3.2

Hyperthyroidism

Definition

Hyperthyroidism is defined as a disease in which increased concentrations of thyroid hormones are present in the organism.

Aetiology

The disease is more common in the cat and is usually caused by a benign adenoma or hyperplasia of the thyroid tissue. The changes can be unilateral or bilateral. Bilateral occurrences are more common, accounting for 70% of cases. Hormonally active adenocarcinomas are rarely described in the cat. In dogs, adenocarcinomas account for the highest proportion of thyroid tumours, although most are not hormonally active. In addition, hyperthyroidism occurs in the dog due to increased supplementation of thyroid hormones in the diet.

Predisposing factors in cats are older age (>8 years) and female sex. Theoretically, a distinction can be made between hyperthyroidism caused primarily in the thyroid gland, secondarily in the pituitary gland and tertiarily in the hypothalamus. However, the last two causes are particularly rare in dogs and cats.

Thyroid tumours	alimentary
Adenoma (C)	(D)
Adenocarcinoma (D)	

D – Dog, C – Cat

Pathogenesis

The neoplastic causalities secrete increased thyroid hormones and thereby cause the clinical symptoms and laboratory diagnostic changes. The main function of thyroid hormones is to promote the activity of cells, especially in the organs of the brain, heart and kidney. After uptake of the thyroid hormones into the target cell, the actual effect is initiated via the intracellular formation of a receptor-hormone complex. This can bind to the DNA and influence the transcription of genes. This primarily stimulates the synthesis of enzymes, receptors, transport and structural proteins.

In the nervous system, this influences the formation of synapses, myelin sheaths, axons and dendrites. In the area of metabolism, carbohydrate breakdown and lipolysis are increased, as well as the breakdown of fats and the conversion of cholesterol. The increased energy consumption, in turn, leads to vasodilation with increased heart rate and cardiac output, thus influencing circulation and blood pressure. In the kidneys, renal blood flow and thus the glomerular filtration rate are increased. Overall, the thyroid hormones increase energy consumption in many parts of the body, which increases the basal metabolic rate and heat production.

Textbook of Small Animal Pathophysiology, First Edition. Stephan Neumann.
© 2025 John Wiley & Sons Ltd. Published 2025 by John Wiley & Sons Ltd.

Diagnostics

Clinical signs	Clinical pathology	Imaging	Histopathology	Microbiology
Non-specific	**T4, fT4**	**Ultrasonography** morphological thyroid changes	Not necessary in cats Cytology in dogs with thyroid tumour	Not necessary

Pathophysiologic Consequences

In accordance with the physiological effects of thyroid hormones, one finds numerous pathophysiologic consequences in hyperthyroidism. These result from the hormone excess. The mass in the thyroid gland itself usually has no consequences. Only malignant neoplasms tend to metastasise to the regional lymph nodes and the lungs.

Influenced organ systems	Clinical symptoms	Clinical pathological alterations
Cardiovascular system	Weight loss	Increased PCV
Gastrointestinal system	Polyphagia	Increased liver enzymes (ALT, AST)
Neuromuscular system	Hyperactivity	Increased ALP
Skin	PU/PD	Azotaemia
Systemic	Tachycardia	
	Vomiting	
	Diarrhoea	

Source: Peterson et al. (1983).

In the summary of the pathophysiologic consequences, an increase in heart activity, muscle metabolism, digestion and growth can be observed organically. Functionally, this is supported by increases in carbohydrate and fat metabolism.

The **weight loss** results from an overall increased metabolism in which energy reserves in the body are used up. One mechanism in this process is the increase of the ubiquinone-proteasome pathway. This mechanism is involved in the degradation of proteins and is activated in hyperthyroidism (Ciechanover and Schwartz 1998; Lino et al. 2019).

Polyphagia is considered a compensatory mechanism for the catabolic metabolic state. However, decreased leptin and increased ghrelin serum concentrations have been found in hyperthyroidism. Both hormones influence food intake by affecting the satiety centre. In principle, increased leptin concentrations lower the feeling of hunger, while increased ghrelin concentrations stimulate appetite (Havel 2002; Riis et al. 2003).

The causalities for **hyperactivity** are not fully understood. Various factors of influence of thyroid hormones on the central nervous system are discussed in humans and could also have an influence in cats. For example, some brain regions that influence behaviour, such as the limbic system (especially the amygdala and hippocampus), express T3 receptors and are thus directly influenced by thyroid hormones. In addition, hyperthyroidism leads to increased production of neurotransmitters, such as serotonin or dopamine. The modulation of the β-adrenergic receptor response to catecholamines is also influenced by thyroid hormones. This seems to be due to the molecular similarity of catecholamines and thyroid hormones (Lee et al. 2013).

The influence of thyroid hormones on the kidney leads to the symptom complex of **PU/PD**. The influence of thyroid hormones on cardiac activity and blood pressure leads to increased glomerular filtration, thus increasing the primary urine. At the same time, the expression of aquaporins in the collecting tube is reduced, which hinders water reabsorption. In combination, this leads to polyuria with low specific gravity. Polydipsia is considered a compensatory mechanism.

The influence on the heart and circulation is another effect of thyroid hormones and is altered in hyperthyroidism. The **tachycardia** seems to be due to increased sympathetic and decreased parasympathetic activity. This also increases the ejection capacity of the heart and thus the blood pressure.

Further clinical symptoms are **vomiting and diarrhoea**. Influencing factors of hyperthyroidism on intestinal activity are thought to be responsible as mechanisms for both symptoms. Hyperthyroidism leads to a shortened intestinal transit time postprandially due to an increase in smooth muscle contractions (Karaus et al. 1989; Papasouliotis et al. 1993).

Table 43.3.2.1 Influences on the metabolism of erythrocytes in hyperthyroidism.

System	Influence
Na^+-K^+-ATPase activity	Increase
Ca^{2+}-ATPase activity	Increase
Glucose metabolism	Increase
Catalase activity	Increase

Source: Adapted from Ford and Carter (1988).

The increase in **PCV** is attributed to stimulation of erythropoietin synthesis by thyroid hormones. The erythrocytes often show Heinz bodies, which are eccentric protrusions on the erythrocytes caused by oxidised haemoglobin. Numerous other influences on the metabolism of erythrocytes have been described in hyperthyroidism (Table 43.3.2.1).

The cause of the **elevated liver enzymes** is probably damage to the hepatocytes caused by hypoxia. The hypoxia is caused by an increase in the overall metabolism in hyperthyroidism with a locally reduced oxygen supply. This disturbs the membrane function of the hepatocytes and increases the release of liver enzymes. In addition, in hyperthyroidism, microthrombi in the sinusoids may be responsible for local hypoxia. Finally, direct 'toxic' effects of T4 on hepatocytes are discussed (Berent et al. 2007).

Increased **ALP serum activity** is predominantly due to the bone isoenzyme. This reflects an increasing influence of hyperthyroidism on bone metabolism. Hyperthyroidism is associated with an increase in osteocalcin concentration, which may be a mediator of thyroid hormone action on bone. Osteocalcin is predominantly synthesised by osteoblasts. It shows a matrix-building function in bone through calcium binding (Ferron et al. 2008).

Another influence of the thyroid gland on bone metabolism is through the inhibitory influence of TSH on bone resorption. In the case of hyperthyroidism, however, TSH secretion is suppressed by negative feedback, which can stimulate bone resorption (Abe et al. 2003).

The **azotaemia** may be a consequence of increased glomerular filtration. This leads to hyperfiltration and thus proteinuria. Proteinuria causes destruction of the mesangial cells and glomerulosclerosis; this in turn reduces the number of intact glomeruli. This can reduce the overall filtration capacity of the kidney and cause azotaemia to develop. This is predominantly caused by an increased urea concentration, as creatinine is present in the serum at a lower level due to muscle catabolism (Figure 43.3.2.1).

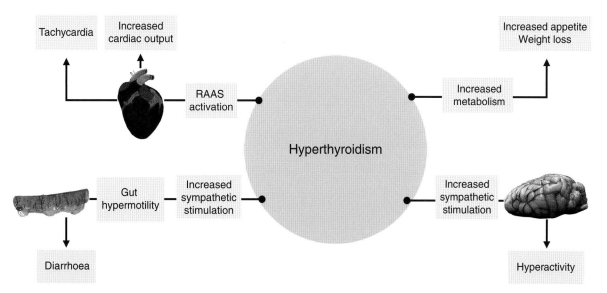

Figure 43.3.2.1 Pathophysiologic consequences of hyperthyroidism.

Therapy

Symptom	Therapy
Reduction of thyroid hormone concentration	Thyroid peroxidase inhibitors (e.g. Methimazole, Carbimazole)
	Radioiodine therapy
	Surgery

References

Abe, E., Marians, R.C., Yu, W. et al. (2003). TSH is a negative regulator of skeletal remodelling. *Cell* 115 (2): 151–162. https://doi.org/10.1016/s0092-8674(03)00771-2.

Berent, A.C., Drobatz, K.J., Ziemer, L. et al. (2007). Liver function in cats with hyperthyroidism before and after 131I therapy. *Journal of Veterinary Internal Medicine* 21 (6): 1217–1223. https://doi.org/10.1892/07-022.1.

Ciechanover, A. and Schwartz, A.L. (1998). The ubiquitin–proteasome pathway: the complexity and myriad functions of proteins death. *Proceedings of the National Academy of Sciences of the United States of America* 95 (6): 2727–2730. https://doi.org/10.1073/pnas.95.6.2727.

Ferron, M., Hinoi, E., Karsenty, G., and Ducy, P. (2008). Osteocalcin differentially regulates beta cell and adipocyte gene expression and affects the development of metabolic diseases in wild-type mice. *Proceedings of the National Academy of Sciences of the United States of America* 105 (13): 5266–5270. https://doi.org/10.1073/pnas.0711119105.

Ford, H.C. and Carter, J.M. (1988). The haematology of hyperthyroidism: abnormalities of erythrocytes, leucocytes, thrombocytes and haemostasis. *Postgraduate Medical Journal* 64 (756): 735–742. https://doi.org/10.1136/pgmj.64.756.735.

Havel, P.J. (2002). Control of energy homeostasis and insulin action by adipocyte hormones: leptin, acylation stimulating protein, and adiponectin. *Current Opinion in Lipidology* 13 (1): 51–59. https://doi.org/10.1097/00041433-200202000-00008.

Karaus, M., Wienbeck, M., Grussendorf, M. et al. (1989). Intestinal motor activity in experimental hyperthyroidism in conscious dogs. *Gastroenterology* 97 (4): 911–919. https://doi.org/10.1016/0016-5085(89)91497-2.

Lee, K.A., Park, K.T., Yu, H.M. et al. (2013). Subacute thyroiditis presenting as acute psychosis: a case report and literature review. *The Korean Journal of Internal Medicine* 28 (2): 242–246. https://doi.org/10.3904/kjim.2013.28.2.242.

Lino, C.A., Demasi, M., and Barreto-Chaves, M.L. (2019). Ubiquitin proteasome system (UPS) activation in the cardiac hypertrophy of hyperthyroidism. *Molecular and Cellular Endocrinology* 493: 110451. https://doi.org/10.1016/j.mce.2019.110451.

Papasouliotis, K., Muir, P., Gruffydd-Jones, T.J. et al. (1993). Decreased orocaecal transit time, as measured by the exhalation of hydrogen, in hyperthyroid cats. *Research in Veterinary Science* 55 (1): 115–118. https://doi.org/10.1016/0034-5288(93)90044-g.

Peterson, M.E., Kintzer, P.P., Cavanagh, P.G. et al. (1983). Feline hyperthyroidism: pretreatment clinical and laboratory evaluation of 131 cases. *Journal of the American Veterinary Medical Association* 183 (1): 103–110.

Riis, A.L., Hansen, T.K., Møller, N. et al. (2003). Hyperthyroidism is associated with suppressed circulating ghrelin levels. *The Journal of Clinical Endocrinology and Metabolism* 88 (2): 853–857. https://doi.org/10.1210/jc.2002-021302.

Further Reading

Looney, A. and Wakshlag, J. (2017). Dietary management of hyperthyroidism in a dog. *Journal of the American Animal Hospital Association* 53 (2): 111–118.

Köhler, B., Stengel, C., and Neiger, R. (2012). Dietary hyperthyroidism in dogs. *The Journal of Small Animal Practice* 53 (3): 182–184.

Kooistra, H.S. (2014). Feline hyperthyroidism: a common disorder with unknown pathogenesis. *The Veterinary Record* 175 (18): 456–457.

Mooney, C.T. (2002). Pathogenesis of feline hyperthyroidism. *Journal of Feline Medicine and Surgery* 4 (3): 167–169.

Peterson, M.E. and Ward, C.R. (2007). Etiopathologic findings of hyperthyroidism in cats. *The Veterinary Clinics of North America. Small Animal Practice* 37 (4): 633–645.

43.3.3

Hypothyroidism

Definition

Hypothyroidism is defined as a condition of underactive thyroid gland with insufficient production and secretion of thyroid hormones.

Aetiology

In hypothyroidism, a distinction is made between a primary (thyroid gland), a secondary (pituitary gland) and a tertiary form (hypothalamus) depending on the localisation of the causality. Hypothyroidism is much more common in the dog than in the cat and predominantly develops as a primary or secondary form. The primary form is the consequence of lymphoplasmacytic thyroiditis or idiopathic atrophy of the thyroid follicles. The causes of the secondary form are considered to be a pituitary tumour, a congenital pituitary malformation and, as the most frequent cause of secondary hypothyroidism, a suppression of pituitary secretion by corticoids (Figure 43.3.3.1, Table 43.3.3.1).

Pathogenesis

Lymphoplasmacytic thyroiditis is characterised by the infiltration of lymphocytes, plasma cells and macrophages into the thyroid parenchyma. Fibrosis develops as the disease progresses. At the same time, the follicles atrophy. Follicular destruction of more than 80% leads to clinical symptoms. The course of the disease is divided into four different stages, depending on the clinical symptoms and laboratory diagnostic changes. The latter refer to the concentration of thyroid hormones (T3, T4) of those of TSH and the presence of antibodies against thyroglobulin. In stage I, there are still no clinical findings, the thyroid hormones and TSH are still in the reference range, but thyroglobulin antibodies are already detectable, which indicate the autoimmune process. In stage II, there is also an increase in the serum concentration of TSH. This appears before a drop in T3 and T4. In stage III, the clinical picture and laboratory changes show the typical changes to be expected. Symptoms are present, serum thyroid hormone concentration is reduced and TSH concentration is increased. Thyroglobulin antibodies are also present. Finally, stage IV shows comparable changes to stage III, except for negative detection of thyroglobulin antibodies, suggesting morphological remodelling in the thyroid parenchyma with reduction of inflammation and presence of fibrosis and follicular atrophy (Graham et al. 2007).

Secondary hypothyroidism results from a malfunction of the pituitary gland. Tumorous changes are usually classified as adenomas. Pituitary tumours in dogs and cats are rare (Sanders et al. 2021).

Secondary hypothyroidism in dogs and cats therefore develops predominantly through suppression of TSH secretion. Corticoids, for example, inhibit the formation of TRH mRNA in the hypothalamus, thereby inhibiting the secretion of TSH in the pituitary gland (Alkemade et al. 2005).

Textbook of Small Animal Pathophysiology, First Edition. Stephan Neumann.
© 2025 John Wiley & Sons Ltd. Published 2025 by John Wiley & Sons Ltd.

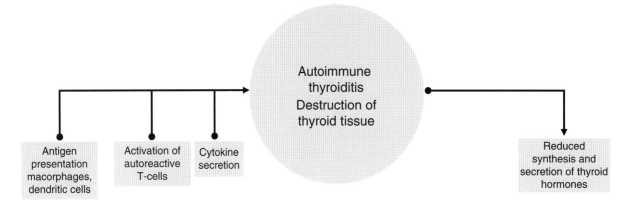

Figure 43.3.3.1   Development of autoimmune thyroiditis.

Table 43.3.3.1   Common causes of hypothyroidism.

Inflammation	Suppression
Lymphoplasma cellular thyroiditis (D)	Corticoid steroids (D)

D-dog

Diagnostics

Clinical signs	Clinical pathology	Imaging	Histopathology	Microbiology
Non-specific	**T4, fT4, TSH,** **TSH stimulation test**	CT/MRI Imaging of pituitary tumours	Not necessary	Not necessary

Pathophysiologic Consequences

The pathophysiologic consequences are metabolically associated and primarily affect behaviour and skin.

Influenced organ systems	Clinical symptoms	Clinical pathological alterations
Skin	Alopecia	Anaemia
Cardiovascular system	Obesity	Hypercholesterolaemia
Neuromuscular system	Lethargy	Hypertriglyceridaemia
Central nervous system	Weakness	
Bones, joints	Neuropathy	
Muscles	Infertility	
Reproduction	Bradycardia	

The **dermatological** changes in hypothyroidism include bilateral symmetrical non-itching hair loss, and also dry skin, seborrhoea and hyperkeratosis. The reason for this is the effect of thyroid hormones on hair and skin metabolism.

Thyroid hormones are essential for hair growth. If they are missing, the hair changes from the anagen growth phase to the telogen rest phase. Since this is not inflammatory, there is no itching.

The development of **obesity**, as well as the general **weakness**, result from a reduced metabolism. Different functions of the thyroid hormones on metabolism have been described. In most cases, the hormones have a positive metabolic effect and stimulate metabolism. The consequences of a hormone deficiency are a general reduction in metabolic performance. The metabolic effect of thyroid hormones will be illustrated using the example of heat production. Thyroid hormones maintain the physiological body temperature or increase a decreased body temperature through receptor-mediated action on the temperature regulation centre in the hypothalamus. In addition, they act on the musculature and on white, as well as brown adipose tissue. In brown adipose tissue, heat is generated by uncoupling glycolysis and the respiratory chain. Fatty acids are the starting material for energy production in brown adipose tissue. These are released by a hormone-sensitive lipase, which is activated by noradrenalin via cAMP as a second messenger. β-oxidation produces acetyl-CoA from the fatty acids, which in turn is the starting material for the citric acid cycle and the respiratory chain and thus serves for ATP synthesis. Thyroid hormones activate the protein (thermogenin) in the mitochondrial membrane. Thermogenin is able to stop the conversion of energy into ATP at the end of the respiratory chain and thus convert the energy into heat (Sentis et al. 2021).

Neurological changes in hypothyroidism can vary. Peripheral nerve paralyses are described, as are vestibular disorders; megaoesophagus is also associated with hypothyroidism, as are various myopathies. The effects of thyroid hormones on the nervous system are illustrated in hyperthyroidism. Another mechanism associated with peripheral neuropathies, in particular, could be immune-related neuropathy, as the underlying disease in the primary form of hypothyroidism is immune-related thyroiditis. Myopathies in hypothyroidism occur because thyroid hormone deficiency leads to reduced glycogenolysis and mitochondrial energy production. This leads, in particular, to atrophy of the type 2 muscle fibres (fast fibres), thus slowing down muscle contraction. In some cases, glucosaminoglycans are deposited in the affected muscle fibres. Lameness sometimes observed in dogs with hypothyroidism is due to fluid deposits in the tendon sheaths in the form of oedema, causing compression or irritation of the tendon.

Influences of hypothyroidism on **reproduction** exist in male and female dogs. In males, reduced libido, testicular atrophy and oligospermia are observed. In females, prolonged interoestrus, as well as reduced birth weight and increased mortality in the pups (Panciera et al. 2012). The causes are not fully understood but are thought to be related to a direct effect of thyroid hormones. Thyroxine receptors have been detected in the uterus. A further effect is seen due to the influence of thyroid hormones on various growth factors (epidermal growth factor, vascular endothelial growth factor) (Crocker et al. 2001).

The effects of hypothyroidism on cardiac activity are reduced cardiac output due to prolonged cardiac ejection time, increased left ventricular diameter and reduced left ventricular systolic wall thickness. This is accompanied by **sinus bradycardia** or grade I-II AV block (Satpathy et al. 2013).

The laboratory parameters show a normochromic, normocytic non-regenerative **anaemia**. The reason for this is probably the reduction of erythropoietin synthesis in hypothyroidism.

The increase in blood lipids is particularly noticeable in hypothyroidism. This concerns **cholesterol** and **triglycerides**. The lipid metabolism is influenced both by a lowered thyroid hormone concentration and by an increased TSH concentration. Thyroid hormones influence lipid absorption in the intestine and lipid uptake in the liver, as well as cholesterol synthesis and lipolysis. In the case of a reduced thyroid hormone concentration, the hepatogenic uptake of cholesterol from the blood is reduced. At the same time, the reduction of thyroid hormones increases the absorption of cholesterol in the intestine. This is explained by a positive influence on the Niemann-Pick-C1 protein, which is expressed as a transport protein on the apical membrane of the enterocytes and enables enteric cholesterol and lipid absorption. Another effect is inhibition of a lipoprotein lipase in hypothyroidism; this enzyme is involved in the degradation of circulating triglycerides. Another mechanism is through the influence of thyroid hormones on bile acids. Bile acids lower cholesterol stored in the liver by biliary removal. This allows hepatocytes to reabsorb cholesterol from the blood. Thyroid hormones influence the formation of bile acids. In the case of hypothyroidism, this influence is suppressed, thus reducing the removal of cholesterol and thus the uptake of cholesterol by hepatocytes, which causes its serum concentration to rise.

Finally, an increased TSH concentration stimulates cholesterol synthesis and lipolysis, which increases the serum concentration of fats (Duntas and Brenta 2018; Liu and Peng 2022) (Figure 43.3.3.2).

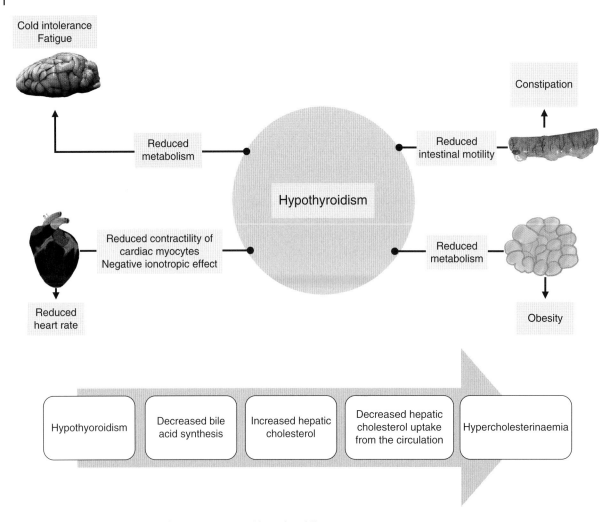

Figure 43.3.3.2 Pathophysiologic consequences of hypothyroidism.

Therapy

Symptom	Therapy
Hypothyroidism	Thyroid hormone (Levothyroxine)

References

Alkemade, A., Unmehopa, U.A., Wiersinga, W.M. et al. (2005). Glucocorticoids decrease thyrotropin-releasing hormone messenger ribonucleic acid expression in the paraventricular nucleus of the human hypothalamus. *The Journal of Clinical Endocrinology and Metabolism* 90 (1): 323–327. https://doi.org/10.1210/jc.2004-1430.

Crocker, I.P., Strachan, B.K., Lash, G.E. et al. (2001). Vascular endothelial growth factor but not placental growth factor promotes trophoblast syncytialization in vitro. *Journal of the Society for Gynecologic Investigation* 8 (6): 341–346.

Duntas, L.H. and Brenta, G. (2018). A renewed focus on the association between thyroid hormones and lipid metabolism. *Frontiers in Endocrinology* 9: 511. https://doi.org/10.3389/fendo.2018.00511.

Graham, P.A., Refsal, K.R., and Nachreiner, R.F. (2007). Etiopathologic findings of canine hypothyroidism. *The Veterinary Clinics of North America. Small Animal Practice* 37 (4): 617. -v. https://doi.org/10.1016/j.cvsm.2007.05.002.

Liu, H. and Peng, D. (2022). Update on dyslipidemia in hypothyroidism: the mechanism of dyslipidemia in hypothyroidism. *Endocrine Connections* 11 (2): e210002. https://doi.org/10.1530/EC-21-0002.

Panciera, D.L., Purswell, B.J., Kolster, K.A. et al. (2012). Reproductive effects of prolonged experimentally induced hypothyroidism in bitches. *Journal of Veterinary Internal Medicine* 26 (2): 326–333. https://doi.org/10.1111/j.1939-1676.2011.00872.x.

Sanders, K., Galac, S., and Meij, B.P. (2021). Pituitary tumour types in dogs and cats. *Veterinary Journal (London, England: 1997)* 270: 105623. https://doi.org/10.1016/j.tvjl.2021.105623.

Satpathy, P.K., Diggikar, P.M., Sachdeva, V. et al. (2013). Lipid profile and electrocardiographic changes in thyroid dysfunction. *Medical Journal of Dr. DY Patil University* 6: 250–253.

Sentis, S.C., Oelkrug, R., and Mittag, J. (2021). Thyroid hormones in the regulation of brown adipose tissue thermogenesis. *Endocrine Connections* 10 (2): R106–R115. https://doi.org/10.1530/EC-20-0562.

Further Reading

Bojanic, K., Acke, E., and Jones, B.R. (2011). Congenital hypothyroidism of dogs and cats: a review. *New Zealand Veterinary Journal* 59 (3): 115–122.

Mooney, C.T. (2011). Canine hypothyroidism: a review of aetiology and diagnosis. *New Zealand Veterinary Journal* 59 (3): 105–114.

Panciera, D.L. (2001). Conditions associated with canine hypothyroidism. *The Veterinary Clinics of North America. Small Animal Practice* 31 (5): 935–950.

43.4

Parathyroid Gland

Physiology

The parathyroid gland is a small endocrine gland (2–5 mm × 1 mm in dogs) located at the cranial pole of the thyroid gland. Starting from a connective tissue capsule, septa extend into the gland parenchyma and surround the hormone-producing epithelial cells. The blood supply of the parathyroid gland is closely connected to the thyroid gland. The essential function of the parathyroid gland consists of the regulation of calcium metabolism through the secretion of parathormone.

Calcium is an important element in the organism. It has structural and biochemical functions. The functions include the participation of calcium in the morphogenesis of bones and teeth. Half of the bone substance consists of calcium phosphate. In addition, calcium is involved in muscle contraction, blood clotting and heart function. These functions are fulfilled because calcium is involved in membrane potential and can activate enzymes. Calcium must be available to fulfil all functions. In blood serum, calcium is present bound to albumin. This is the biologically inactive form. Biologically active calcium is unbound. The concentration of calcium in the blood serum is maintained in a narrow physiological concentration range of approximately 2.3–3.0 mmol/l.

The calcium serum concentration is influenced by the enteral absorption of calcium supplied via food. In addition, calcium can be mobilised from body reserves, essentially the bones. Calcium excretion via the kidneys can also contribute to the maintenance of serum concentration. Three hormones are involved in the regulation of calcium metabolism – calcitonin, calcitriol and parathyroid hormone (PTH). Calcitonin is a peptide hormone produced by C-cells in the thyroid parenchyma. The function of **calcitonin** is to lower the serum calcium concentration. This is achieved by calcitonin-inhibiting osteoclast function via a receptor with cAMP as a second messenger. Osteoclasts induce bone resorption and promote the release of calcium from bone. In addition, calcitonin reduces calcium reabsorption in the renal tubules, which results in increased renal calcium excretion and lowers serum concentrations. Calcitonin is secreted when the serum calcium concentration increases. **Calcitriol** is the active form of vitamin D its essential function is to increase serum calcium concentration. In the intestine, calcitriol promotes calcium resorption and in the kidney its reabsorption. Calcitriol binds to intracellular receptors and induces the expression of proteins, such as calbindin. This binds intracellular calcium and thus lowers the intracellular calcium concentration, which creates a gradient for calcium and induces influx into the cells, whereby the serum concentration is initially lowered and calcium absorption is thereby increased.

The third hormone involved in calcium metabolism is PTH.

Parathyroid hormone is the secretion product of the parathyroid gland. It is a polypeptide that is secreted as an inactive precursor. The activation of parathormone occurs primarily in the liver. The hormone synthesis is controlled by the serum calcium concentration. A falling serum level promotes PTH secretion. High or normal serum calcium concentrations act via calcium receptors on the hormone-producing epithelial cells. Calcium binding leads to the release of intracellular calcium ions via a mechanism coupled to G-protein. These inhibit the secretion of PTH precursors by preventing fusion with the vesicles and the cell membrane.

The effects of PTH lead to an increase in serum concentration. In addition, PTH increases calcium mobilisation from the bone. High PTH concentrations have a stimulating effect on osteoclasts via the secretion of prostaglandins. In addition, PTH activates the calcitriol function at the proximal tubule and promotes calcium reabsorption there (Figure 43.4.1).

Thus, disorders of the PTH are accompanied by disorders in calcium metabolism. This can occur as hyperparathyroidism and hypoparathyroidism.

Textbook of Small Animal Pathophysiology, First Edition. Stephan Neumann.
© 2025 John Wiley & Sons Ltd. Published 2025 by John Wiley & Sons Ltd.

Figure 43.4.1 Calcium metabolism.

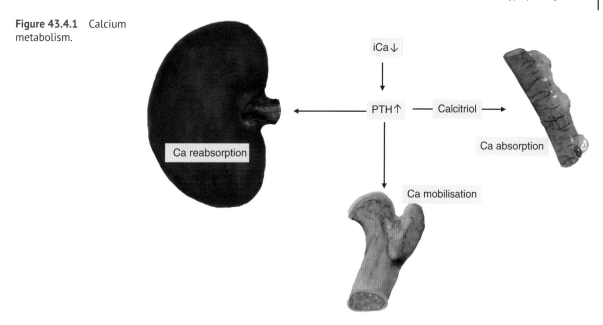

Hyperparathyroidism

Aetiology and Pathogenesis

Primary and Secondary Hyperparathyroidism

Primary hyperparathyroidism is defined as increased autonomous PTH production triggered by an adenoma or, more rarely, a carcinoma of the parathyroid gland. Dogs and cats are affected, although the clinical picture is rare. The secondary form is more common. This is secondary to chronic kidney failure. The consequences of chronic kidney failure are a reduced conversion of calcidiol to calcitriol. This means that less biological calcitriol is available, which reduces its functions. The result is reduced calcium absorption in the intestine, which can lead to hypocalcaemia. At the same time, in chronic kidney failure, reduced glomerular filtration leads to reduced phosphate excretion or hyperphosphataemia. Phosphorus binds free calcium in the serum and thus promotes hypocalcaemia. Both increase PTH secretion. Another secondary form of hyperparathyroidism is the nutritional form, which occurs as a result of reduced calcium absorption from the intestine (Figure 43.4.2).

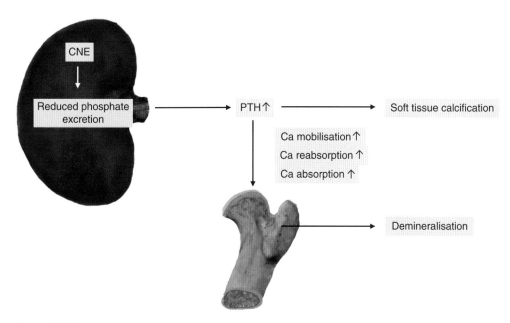

Figure 43.4.2 Aetiology of hyperparathyroidism.

Diagnostics

Clinical signs	Clinical pathology	Imaging	Histopathology	Microbiology
Non-specific	Ca serum concentration, parathyroid hormone serum concentration	**Ultrasonography** Tumour of parathyroid gland	Not necessary	Not necessary

Pathophysiologic Consequences

The pathophysiologic consequences are primarily based on the imbalances of calcium and phosphorus.

Influenced organ systems	Clinical symptoms	Clinical pathological alterations
Cardiovascular system	Lethargy	Hypercalcaemia
Gastrointestinal system	Weakness	Hypophosphataemia (primary)
Urinary tract	Anorexia	Hyperphosphataemia (secondary renal)
Neuromuscular system	Vomiting	
Bones	PU/PD	
	Uroliths	
	Rubber jaw	

The general symptomatology with lethargy, weakness and anorexia is attributed to disturbances of the membrane potential in hypercalcaemia. Electrophysiologically, the depolarisation is caused by an increased Na^+-influx followed by a Ca^{2+}-influx. The latter produces a plateau phase and thus prolongs the depolarisation. In the case of hypercalcaemia, the plateau phase is shortened due to increased calcium influx, and at the same time the opening of the sodium channels slows down. This leads to a weaker and shortened depolarisation. This is thought to be responsible for the symptoms of **weakness** and **lethargy**. In the intestine, this leads to reduced motility. Consequences can be **vomiting** and **inappetence**. Furthermore, hypercalcaemia can cause an intracellular increase in calcium concentration. This, in turn, can induce a release of neurotransmitters in emetic receptors in the gastrointestinal tract (enterochromaffin cells) or in the central vomiting centre, causing vomiting. Pancreatitis triggered by hypercalcaemia would be another cause of vomiting and inappetence (Frick et al. 1995; Mithöfer et al. 1995).

A major influence of hypercalcaemia on the kidneys is the inhibition of the incorporation of aquaporins in the distal tubule and the collecting tube. The result is reduced water reabsorption and thus **polyuria**. Simultaneous **polydipsia** results from a reduction in blood volume with activation of the RAAS.

The increased excretion of calcium phosphates leads to the formation of **uroliths** in the bladder.

A particular clinical manifestation of secondary renal hyperparathyroidism is renal osteodystrophy. This can present clinically as decalcification of the bone, primarily the jaw bones, and lead to a **rubber jaw**. The mechanism is not fully understood. A connection with the increased concentration of FGF-23 is being discussed. FGF-23 is a growth factor that is produced by osteocytes and osteoblasts. Its essential function is the reduction of phosphate, for example, by inhibiting its reabsorption in the proximal tubule. FGF-23 is considered an inhibitor of bone mineralisation. In dogs with chronic renal failure, the serum concentration of FGF-23 is increased. This could be responsible for the increased bone resorption and rubber jaw (Guo and Yuan 2015) (Figure 43.4.3).

Therapy

Symptom	Therapy
Secondary renal form	Therapy of chronic renal insufficiency
Primary form	Surgery

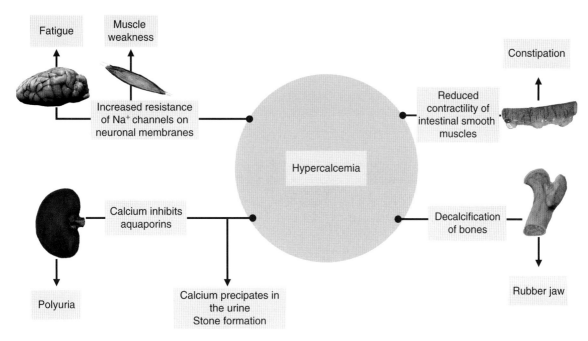

Figure 43.4.3 Pathophysiologic consequences of hypercalcaemia.

Hypoparathyroidism

Hypoparathyroidism is clinically less common than hyperparathyroidism. In addition to an idiopathic cause, thyroid surgery in particular can lead iatrogenically to damage of the parathyroid gland with the consequence of reduced parathormone secretion.

The pathophysiologic consequences result from hypocalcaemia. This leads to a limited depolarisation, since in the plateau phase of the depolarisation, calcium influx from the extracellular level is not possible due to the low calcium concentration. The consequence is a reduction in nervous activity and muscle contraction.

Diagnostics

Clinical signs	Clinical pathology	Imaging	Histopathology	Microbiology
Non-specific	Calcium serum concentration Parathormone serum concentration	Not necessary	Not necessary	Not necessary

Pathophysiologic Consequences

Influenced organ systems	Clinical symptoms	Clinical pathological alterations
Cardiovascular system	Syncope	Hypocalcaemia
Neuromuscular system (Figure 43.4.4)	Weakness	

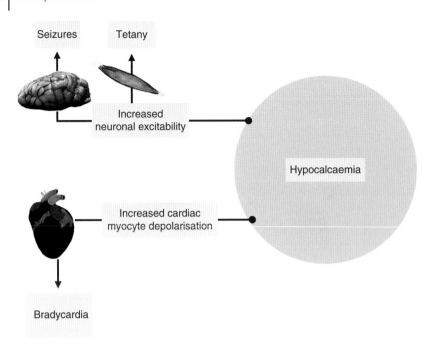

Figure 43.4.4 Pathophysiologic consequences of hypocalcaemia.

Therapy

Symptom	Therapy
Acute	Calcium infusion
Long-term therapy	Calcitriol

References

Frick, T.W., Mithöfer, K., Fernández-del Castillo, C. et al. (1995). Hypercalcemia causes acute pancreatitis by pancreatic secretory block, intracellular zymogen accumulation, and acinar cell injury. *American Journal of Surgery* 169 (1): 167–172. https://doi.org/10.1016/s0002-9610(99)80127-5.

Guo, Y.C. and Yuan, Q. (2015). Fibroblast growth factor 23 and bone mineralisation. *International Journal of Oral Science* 7 (1): 8–13. https://doi.org/10.1038/ijos.2015.1.

Mithöfer, K., Fernández-del Castillo, C., Frick, T.W. et al. (1995). Acute hypercalcemia causes acute pancreatitis and ectopic trypsinogen activation in the rat. *Gastroenterology* 109 (1): 239–246. https://doi.org/10.1016/0016-5085(95)90290-2.

Further Reading

Daniels, E. and Sakakeeny, C. (2015). Hypercalcemia: pathophysiology, clinical signs, and emergent treatment. *Journal of the American Animal Hospital Association* 51 (5): 291–299. https://doi.org/10.5326/JAAHA-MS-6297.

de Brito Galvão, J.F., Schenck, P.A., and Chew, D.J. (2017). A quick reference on hypercalcemia. *The Veterinary Clinics of North America. Small Animal Practice* 47 (2): 241–248. https://doi.org/10.1016/j.cvsm.2016.10.016.

Greco, D.S. (2012). Endocrine causes of calcium disorders. *Topics in Companion Animal Medicine* 27 (4): 150–155. https://doi.org/10.1053/j.tcam.2012.11.001.

Groman, R.P. (2012). Acute management of calcium disorders. *Topics in Companion Animal Medicine* 27 (4): 167–171. https://doi.org/10.1053/j.tcam.2012.11.002.

Holowaychuk, M.K. (2013). Hypocalcemia of critical illness in dogs and cats. *The Veterinary Clinics of North America. Small Animal Practice* 43 (6): 1299. -vii. https://doi.org/10.1016/j.cvsm.2013.07.008.

43.5

Endocrine Pancreas

43.5.1

Physiology of Endocrine Pancreas

Functions

Embryonically, the pancreas adjacent to the proximal small intestine develops from the endoderm. This has an exocrine part, which is described in Chapter 40.1, and an endocrine part. The development of both parts occurs simultaneously. The endocrine part of the pancreas is approximately 2% of the organ mass and is concentrated in local spots, the islets of Langerhans. Surrounded by a capillary network, different cell types with different endocrine functions are localised in the islets. The A (alpha) cells synthesise glucagon, the B (beta) cells insulin, the D (delta) cells gastrin and somatostatin and the F cells pancreatic polypeptide (Figure 43.5.1.1).

Glucagon is a peptide hormone. Glucagon is not only produced in the A cells of the pancreas, but also in other tissues, for example, as enteroglucagon in the intestine. In the endocrine active cells, the hormone is initially present in the inactive precursor preproglucagon in granules. For activation, the active hormone is formed from the precursor by hydrolytic cleavage and released from the A cells via exocytosis. In the blood, glucagon is present unbound and is transported to the target cells. These are primarily hepatocytes and adipocytes.

The essential function of glucagon is catabolic, to generate energy for stress situations in this way. Therefore, the release of glucagon is also stimulated by sympathetic activity, catecholamines and glucocorticoids. Another essential trigger is hypoglycaemia.

At the target cells, glucagon acts via a G-protein-coupled receptor, which activates adenylate cyclase after receptor binding and forms cAMP as a second messenger. The second messenger activates intracellular enzymes. These induce the following effects of glucagon.

In the hepatocytes, glycogen synthetase is inhibited and glycogen phosphorylase is stimulated. This stimulates glycogenolysis. Furthermore, there is an additional increase in gluconeogenesis from amino acids, which promotes the synthesis of urea. In adipocytes, glucagon activates a hormone-dependent lipase and thereby promotes the degradation of trialkylglycerides to fatty acids, as well as their β-oxidation.

Insulin is a peptide hormone produced in the βcells of the islets of Langerhans. The first precursor, preproinsulin, is synthesised in the rough endoplasmic reticulum and converted into proinsulin on its way to the Golgi apparatus. There, hormonally active insulin is formed from proinsulin via hydrolysis. This is released via exocytosis into the intercellular area and then into the blood. The release is stimulated by an increase in blood glucose. The glucose is taken up by the β cells where it undergoes glycolysis with synthesis of ATP. Increased intracellular ATP concentration leads to closure of potassium channels, which in turn leads to depolarisation of the cell membrane and opening of calcium channels. Ca^{2+} ions induce the transport of insulin vesicles along microtubules to the cell membrane in β cells and their fusion, which leads to exocytosis and thus to the release of insulin.

The essential function of insulin is anabolic, acting on carbohydrate, fat and protein metabolism. The main target organs are the liver, adipose tissue and muscles. Insulin acts on the target cells via a receptor that activates a tyrosine kinase. Through signal transduction, different cellular protein complexes are formed, which have different metabolic functions.

Insulin promotes the uptake of glucose into cells through the increased expression of glucose transport proteins in the cell membrane. Within the cells, insulin promotes glucose consumption, for example, via induced glycolysis or glycogen synthesis. At the same time, glucose-forming mechanisms are inhibited, such as glycogenolysis or gluconeogenesis.

Textbook of Small Animal Pathophysiology, First Edition. Stephan Neumann.
© 2025 John Wiley & Sons Ltd. Published 2025 by John Wiley & Sons Ltd.

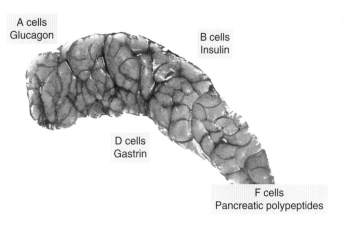

A cells
Glucagon

B cells
Insulin

D cells
Gastrin

F cells
Pancreatic polypeptides

Figure 43.5.1.1 Endocrine areas in the pancreas.

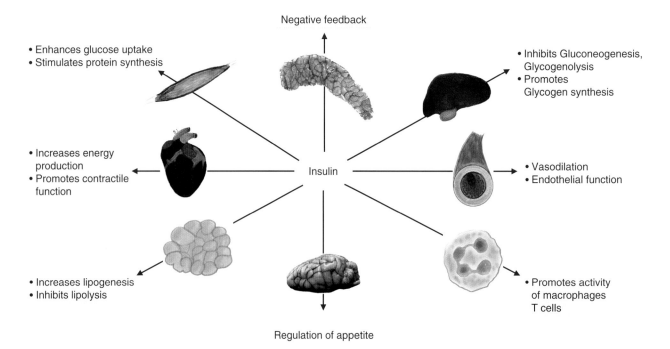

Negative feedback

• Enhances glucose uptake
• Stimulates protein synthesis

• Inhibits Gluconeogenesis,
  Glycogenolysis
• Promotes
  Glycogen synthesis

• Increases energy
  production
• Promotes contractile
  function

Insulin

• Vasodilation
• Endothelial function

• Increases lipogenesis
• Inhibits lipolysis

• Promotes activity
  of macrophages
  T cells

Regulation of appetite

Figure 43.5.1.2 Overview of insulin functions.

The effect of insulin on fat metabolism involves the promotion of fatty acid and triglyceride synthesis. The starting product of fatty acid synthesis acetyl-CoA is provided by insulin-induced glycolysis.

Finally, insulin shows a stimulating effect on protein synthesis by activating transcription and translation.

Insulin is degraded in different organs, especially in the liver. For this purpose, insulin is bound intra-sinusoidally to insulin receptors of the hepatocyte membrane after binding to an insulin-degrading enzyme. The complex is taken up intracellularly by lysosomes and while the insulin is degraded, the receptor is recycled and transported back to the hepatocyte membrane (Figure 43.5.1.2).

Gastrin and **somatostatin** are synthesised in the D cells of the islets of Langerhans. The former is described in Chapter 38. Somatostatin is also produced in other organs besides the pancreas, for example, the hypothalamus. It is also a peptide hormone. It acts via a G-protein-coupled receptor with cAMP as a second messenger. The main functions of somatostatin are inhibitory. It suppresses the synthesis of GH, insulin, glucagon, gastrin, secretin and thyroid hormones. Another inhibitory hormone from the pancreas is pancreatic polypeptide, which is produced in the F cells. It inhibits the secretion of somatostatin, pancreatic enzymes and bile.

Further Reading

Engelking, L.R. (1997). Physiology of the endocrine pancreas. *Seminars in Veterinary Medicine and Surgery (Small Animal)* 12 (4): 224–229. https://doi.org/10.1016/s1096-2867(97)80013-8.

Porte, D. Jr., Woods, S.C., Chen, M. et al. (1975). Central factors in the control of insulin and glucagon secretion. *Pharmacology, Biochemistry, and Behaviour* 3 (1 Suppl): 127–133.

Ruggere, M.D. and Patel, Y.C. (1984). Somatostatin, glucagon, and insulin secretion from perfused pancreas of BB rats. *The American Journal of Physiology* 247 (2 Pt 1): E221–E227. https://doi.org/10.1152/ajpendo.1984.247.2.E221.

Sutter, B.C. (1982). Régulation hormonale de la sécrétion de l'insuline [Hormonal regulation of insulin secretion]. *Journal de Physiologie* 78 (1): 119–130.

Unger, R.H., Dobbs, R.E., and Orci, L. (1978). Insulin, glucagon, and somatostatin secretion in the regulation of metabolism. *Annual Review of Physiology* 40: 307–343. https://doi.org/10.1146/annurev.ph.40.030178.001515.

43.5.2

Diabetes Mellitus

Definition

Diabetes mellitus is defined as a disease with persistent hyperglycaemia and glucosuria, based on reduced insulin secretion or response.

Aetiology

Different types of diabetes mellitus are distinguished. In **type I** or insulin-dependent type, there is permanent hypoinsulinaemia and insufficient secretion of insulin in the case of hyperglycaemia. The cause is presumably a multifactorial process. Genetic predispositions play a role. An autoimmune lymphoplasma cellular infiltration into the endocrine pancreatic tissue with fibrosis is another aetiology. The consequences of the different aetiologies are a reduction of the islets of Langerhans, the β cells or their vacuolisation and associated dysfunction of the βcells.

In **type II**, the insulin-independent type, insulin synthesis is reduced or there is an insufficient response of the target organs to insulin. The causes can be β-cell destruction due to amyloid deposits, which occurs particularly in cats. In addition, glucose uptake by liver, fat and muscle cells is reduced in type II. Both lead to a long-term increased glucose concentration with the consequence of a further desensitisation of the β cells, their reduced insulin synthesis and, in the advanced stage, their apoptosis.

Hormone-dependent forms of diabetes mellitus develop due to the insulin-antagonistic effect of, for example, progesterone and glucocorticoids.

Diabetes mellitus occurs in dogs and cats. Dogs are more frequently affected by type I diabetes. Female animals in the age range of 4–14 years are more frequently affected. Cats are more often affected by type II diabetes, and males are more likely to be affected. Often the affected cats are obese (Gilor et al. 2016).

Pathogenesis

The pathogenesis of autoimmune diabetes mellitus **type I** is associated with lymphoplasma cellular infiltration in the islet of Langerhans. The T cells and antibodies from the plasma cells attack the β cells, destroy them and lead to atrophy of the islet tissue. The reaction follows the principle of other autoimmune diseases. There is a genetic predisposition based on mutations of leukocyte antigens. These are glycoproteins embedded in the cell membrane, which are counted as immunoglobulins and are important for differentiating between the body's own and foreign structures. Through mutation, this function of the leukocyte antigens can be lost with the consequence of a reduced tolerance to molecular structures of the β cells. These are now regarded as foreign to the body and destroyed by the formation of antibodies. Another mechanism of the autoimmune reaction to β cells is based on the mimicry hypothesis. Here, foreign antigen showed molecular mimicry to the body's own cell structures. Through an immunological reaction to the foreign antigen, T lymphocytes and plasma cells can be sensitised to β cells.

Textbook of Small Animal Pathophysiology, First Edition. Stephan Neumann.
© 2025 John Wiley & Sons Ltd. Published 2025 by John Wiley & Sons Ltd.

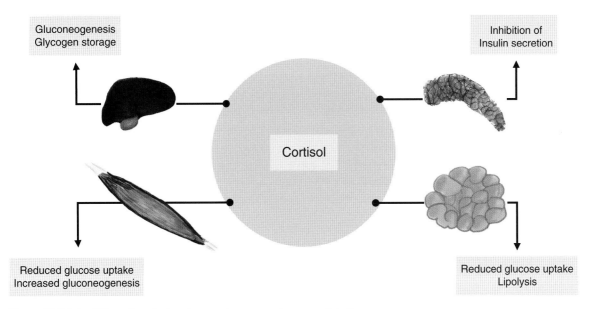

Figure 43.5.2.1   Effect of cortisol and progesterone on glucose metabolism.

The pathogenesis of **type II** diabetes mellitus is more complex. Here, the focus is on the reduced reaction of insulin to hyperglycaemia and its reduced effect on the target cells.

Obesity is an important trigger of type II diabetes mellitus.

On the one hand, obesity causes an increased presence of fatty acids in the blood. These accumulate in muscle cells and hepatocytes. This produces more diacylglycerol, which increases the activity of protein kinase C isoenzymes. These cause a reduction in the phosphorylation of tyrosine, the second messenger of the activated insulin receptor, at the insulin receptor. The consequence is a reduced insulin effect on the cell, resulting in insulin resistance (Boden 2011). This lowers glucose utilisation in the hepatocytes and muscle cells and leads to hyperglycaemia, which in turn leads to increased insulin secretion. Sustained elevated insulin concentrations reduce receptor density on target cells, resulting in decreased insulin sensitivity. In addition, sustained hyperglycaemia has a direct cytotoxic effect on βcells and reduces their density.

Other possible mechanisms are based on the knowledge that obesity is an inflammatory condition with an increased concentration of proinflammatory cytokines. Fatty acids or diacylglycerols have an activating effect on the transcription factor NF-κB, either directly or via protein kinase C isozymes. This, in turn, leads to an increased expression of proinflammatory cytokines, such as TNF-α, IL-1 and IL-6, which can interact with the insulin receptor and negatively influence the formation of the second messenger (Gao et al. 2004; Lebrun and Van Obberghen 2008).

The influence of glucocorticoids and progesterones on the development of diabetes mellitus results from their glycoplastic effect. Both hormones induce the formation of glucose via gluconeogenesis and glycogenolysis in the liver. At the same time, insulin action at the receptor is blocked with the consequence of reduced cellular glucose uptake. This leads to hyperglycaemia, which in turn stimulates insulin secretion. Increased insulin leads to a receptor reduction at the target cells and thus to a further hyperglycaemic effect (Figures 43.5.2.1 and 43.5.2.2).

Diagnostics

Clinical signs	Clinical pathology	Imaging	Histopathology	Microbiology
PU/PD	Glucose Fructosamine serum concentrations HbA1c serum concentration	Not necessary	Not necessary	Not necessary

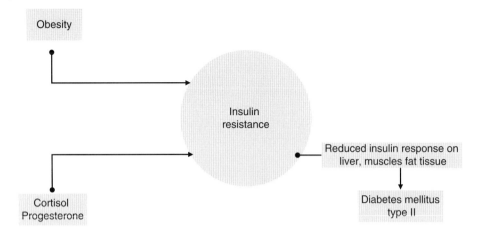

Figure 43.5.2.2 Pathogenesis of type II diabetes mellitus.

Pathophysiologic Consequences

The pathophysiologic consequences of diabetes mellitus are essentially based on the persistently high glucose serum concentration.

Influenced organ systems	Clinical symptoms	Clinical pathological alterations
Gastrointestinal system	PU/PD	Hyperglycaemia
Hepatobiliary system	Dehydration	Increased fructosamine, HbA1c
Urinary Tract	Polyphagia	Increased liver enzymes
Ophthalmic system	Weight loss	Increased cholesterol and fatty acids
Nerves	Cataract	Glucosuria
	Neuropathy	

Source: Behrend et al. (2018).

The symptom complex of **PU/PD** is explained by the osmotic diuresis that develops as a result of the increased glucose serum concentration. The renal threshold for glucose is reached at a serum concentration above 180–220 mg/dl in dogs and 200–280 mg/dl in cats. At higher concentrations, glucose is excreted in the urine in increased concentrations, thereby also exceeding the capacities of tubular glucose reabsorption. The glucose localised in the tubule builds up an osmotic gradient and reduces water reabsorption. The result is diuresis. This leads to **dehydration** due to the increased excretion of water. The consequence of dehydration is an increase in plasma osmolality, which is perceived by receptors in the brain. In humans, these are the subfornical organ and the organum vasculosum in the lamina terminalis. Receptor activation produces thirst. At the same time, dehydration reduces blood pressure. This, in turn, is registered by baroreceptors in the blood vessels and heart and can produce thirst. Both lead to compensatory **polydipsia** (Leib et al. 2016).

Polyphagia is thought to be caused by a mechanism originating from the satiety centre in the brain. The absorption of glucose controlled by insulin produces a feeling of satiety. In the case of diabetes mellitus (type I), however, the insulin concentration is reduced so that less glucose can be absorbed by the cells of the satiety centre and thus the feeling of hunger arises. The reduced cellular glucose uptake puts the organism into a catabolic metabolic state, which eventually results in **weight loss** (Barrett 2012).

The genesis of **cataracts,** which are predominantly observed in dogs, is due to an increased concentration of sorbitol in the lens of dogs with diabetes mellitus. Sorbitol is produced from glucose catalysed by the enzyme aldolase. Sorbitol builds up a higher osmotic pressure and there is increased water retention in the lens, which affects light refraction and leads to lens opacification. The higher the blood glucose concentration, the more sorbitol is synthesised. Furthermore, in the lens of dogs with diabetogenic cataract, there is increased connective tissue synthesis through TGF action, which affects light refraction (Neumann et al. 2017).

Cats, more than dogs, with diabetes mellitus show a plantigrade gait caused by **neuropathy**. The mechanism is thought to be a disturbance in the axon due to increased tubulin aggregation as a result of hyperglycaemia. Hyperglycaemia leads

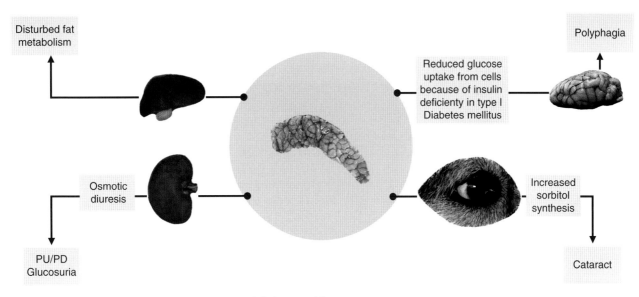

Figure 43.5.2.3 Pathophysiologic consequences of diabetes mellitus.

to glycolisation of cytoskeletal components, causing them to lose their functionality, which interferes with nerve cell transmission (King 2001).

In addition, the increased incidence of infections, especially in the urinary tract, is observed in animals with diabetes mellitus. A reduced T-cell response or a reduced function of the neutrophilic granulocytes is assumed to be the cause (Geerlings and Hoepelman 1999).

Prolonged hyperglycaemia leads to the glycolisation of numerous molecules in the organism. **Fructosamines** are glycolised serum proteins that are formed when hyperglycaemia lasts more than three weeks. The same applies to glycolised haemoglobin as **HbA1c**, which indicates hyperglycaemia over a period of three months. Both are based on the half-life of the respective molecules. Consequently, glycolised molecules can be used as indicators of the duration of hyperglycaemia.

Diabetes mellitus is associated with increased lipolysis. This has various consequences. On the one hand, the concentrations of **fats** in the blood increase in diabetes mellitus patients. On the other hand, the increased mobilisation of fatty acids leads to an overload of the fatty acid metabolism in the liver. This leads to disturbances in the area of hepatic cell integrity, which results in increased activity of **transaminases** in the blood (Figure 43.5.2.3).

Therapy

Symptom	Therapy
Diabetic hyperglycaemia	Insulin

References

Barrett, K.E. (2012). *Endocrine Function of Pancreas. Ganong's Review of Medical Physiology*, 24e, 423–441. McGraw-Hill Lange.

Behrend, E., Holford, A., Lathan, P. et al. (2018). 2018 AAHA diabetes management guidelines for dogs and cats. *Journal of the American Animal Hospital Association* 54 (1): 1–21. https://doi.org/10.5326/JAAHA-MS-6822.

Boden, G. (2011). Obesity, insulin resistance and free fatty acids. *Current Opinion in Endocrinology, Diabetes, and Obesity* 18 (2): 139–143. https://doi.org/10.1097/MED.0b013e3283444b09.

Gao, Z., Zhang, X., Zuberi, A. et al. (2004). Inhibition of insulin sensitivity by free fatty acids requires activation of multiple serine kinases in 3T3-L1 adipocytes. *Molecular endocrinology (Baltimore, Md.)* 18 (8): 2024–2034. https://doi.org/10.1210/me.2003-0383.

Geerlings, S.E. and Hoepelman, A.I. (1999). Immune dysfunction in patients with diabetes mellitus (DM). *FEMS Immunology and Medical Microbiology* 26 (3–4): 259–265. https://doi.org/10.1111/j.1574-695X.1999.tb01397.x.

Gilor, C., Niessen, S.J., Furrow, E., and DiBartola, S.P. (2016). What's in a name? Classification of diabetes mellitus in veterinary medicine and why it matters. *Journal of Veterinary Internal Medicine* 30 (4): 927–940. https://doi.org/10.1111/jvim.14357.

King, R.H. (2001). The role of glycation in the pathogenesis of diabetic polyneuropathy. *Molecular Pathology: MP* 54 (6): 400–408.

Lebrun, P. and Van Obberghen, E. (2008). SOCS proteins causing trouble in insulin action. *Acta Physiologica (Oxford, England)* 192 (1): 29–36. https://doi.org/10.1111/j.1748-1716.2007.01782.x.

Leib, D.E., Zimmerman, C.A., and Knight, Z.A. (2016). Thirst. *Current Biology: CB* 26 (24): R1260–R1265. https://doi.org/10.1016/j.cub.2016.11.019.

Neumann, S., Linek, J., Loesenbeck, G. et al. (2017). TGF-β1 serum concentrations and receptor expressions in the lens capsular of dogs with diabetes mellitus. *Open Veterinary Journal* 7 (1): 12–15. https://doi.org/10.4314/ovj.v7i1.2.

Further Reading

Davison, L.J. (2015). Diabetes mellitus and pancreatitis—cause or effect? *The Journal of Small Animal Practice* 56 (1): 50–59.

Gilor, C., Rudinsky, A.J., and Hall, M.J. (2016). New approaches to feline diabetes mellitus: glucagon-like peptide-1 analogs. *Journal of Feline Medicine and Surgery* 18 (9): 733–743.

Jouvion, G., Abadie, J., Bach, J.M. et al. (2006). Lymphocytic insulitis in a juvenile dog with diabetes mellitus. *Endocrine Pathology* 17 (3): 283–290.

Nelson, R.W. and Reusch, C.E. (2014). Animal models of disease: classification and etiology of diabetes in dogs and cats. *The Journal of Endocrinology* 222 (3): 1–9.

Rios, L. and Ward, C. (2008). Feline diabetes mellitus: diagnosis, treatment, and monitoring. *Compendium (Yardley, PA)* 30 (12): 626–640.

43.5.3

Diabetic Ketoacidosis

Definition

Ketoacidosis is a severe metabolic disorder caused by insulin deficiency.

Aetiology

The cause of ketoacidosis is the increased synthesis of ketone bodies during metabolic alteration due to insulin deficiency. Ketoacidosis can develop in dogs and cats.

Pathogenesis

In type I diabetes, there is an absolute lack of insulin. As a result, the intravascular glucose concentration is increased. However, there is no or only insufficient glucose uptake by the cells. Accordingly, there is a lack of glucose intracellularly. To maintain the intracellular energy metabolism, fatty acids are degraded via β-oxidation to acetyl-CoA and $NADH/H^+$. Further degradation in the citrate cycle is limited by the high concentration of acetyl-CoA produced and inhibition of the citrate cycle by $NADH/H^+$. The acetyl-CoA produced is alternatively used for ketogenesis and cholesterol synthesis. This results in a high concentration of ketone bodies (acetoacetate and β-hydroxybutyrate). The ketone bodies act as weak acids and release protons. Bicarbonate is consumed to buffer the protons. This leads to a shift between cations and anions, the anion gap.

The anion gap describes the ratio between cations and anions in the serum. This is balanced in terms of electroneutrality and depends on the concentrations of essential cations and anions (Table 43.5.3.1).

If one parameter is reduced, another parameter is compensated for in the sense of electroneutrality. If there is a lack of bicarbonate, this can be compensated by increasing organic acids, such as lactate.

These are stronger acids than ketone bodies and can lead to metabolic acidosis if synthesis is increased (Figure 43.5.3.1).

Diagnostics

Clinical signs	Clinical pathology	Imaging	Histopathology	Microbiology
Strongly disturbed general condition	Glucose serum concentration Serum pH	Not necessary	Not necessary	Not necessary

Textbook of Small Animal Pathophysiology, First Edition. Stephan Neumann.
© 2025 John Wiley & Sons Ltd. Published 2025 by John Wiley & Sons Ltd.

Table 43.5.3.1 Major cations and anions in serum.

Cations	Anions
Na^+	Cl^-
K^+	HCO_3^-
Ca^{2+}	Proteins
Mg^{2+}	Organic acids
H^+	PO_4^-
	SO_4^-

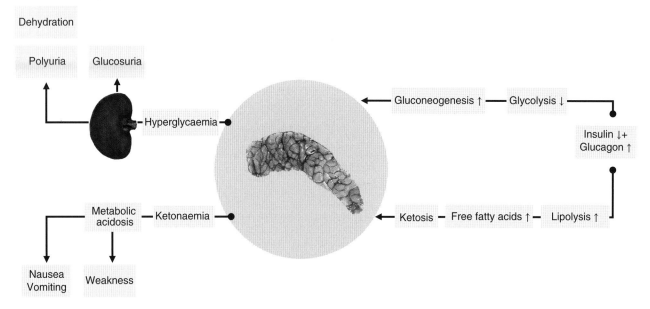

Figure 43.5.3.1 Pathogenesis and pathophysiologic consequences of ketoacidosis.

Pathophysiologic Consequences

The pathophysiologic consequences of ketoacidosis are closely related to hyperglycaemia and the resulting acidosis.

Influenced organ systems	Clinical symptoms	Clinical pathological alterations
Respiratory system	Shock	Metabolic acidosis
Gastrointestinal system	Weakness	Azotaemia
Endocrine system	PU/PD	Hypocalcaemia
Central nervous system	Dehydration	Hyponatraemia
Haematological system	Tachypnoea	Hyperglycaemia
Systemic		Glucosuria
		Increased liver enzymes

The **shock** results from a volume deficiency. Due to the hyperglycaemia, an osmotic diuresis develops. This leads to **polyuria** and a loss of **electrolytes** through the urine. The developing volume deficiency leads first to **dehydration** and progressively to shock. **Polydipsia** is the result of the volume deficiency, which leads to increased secretion of ADH. This in turn increases the feeling of thirst and increases the intake of water. The volume deficiency activates the RAAS and the action of aldosterone implies sodium reabsorption at the distal tubule. In the context of ketoacidosis, these mechanisms are not sufficient to compensate for the loss. On the contrary, aldosterone action increases urinary potassium excretion. Although at the same time the existing acidosis leads to hyperkalaemia. Under the influence of acidosis, protons are exchanged with intracellular potassium via various processes, such as influencing Na^+-K^+-ATPase. As a result, the serum potassium concentration increases, but this is overcompensated by the renal loss in ketoacidosis.

The electrolyte shifts are responsible for disturbances in nervous function by affecting the membrane potentials; this has neurogenic consequences, such as **weakness**.

Tachypnoea is seen as respiratory compensation for metabolic acidosis. The increased proton concentration stimulates breathing via central chemoreceptors (Kussmaul breathing).

Metabolic acidosis, in turn, can influence shock through a negative inotropic effect on the heart associated with peripheral vasodilation and increased capillary permeability. Renal blood flow is reduced and pre-renal renal failure with **azotaemia** may develop.

The increased **liver enzymes** are the consequence of the altered metabolic activity in the hepatocytes in ketoacidosis. The increased lipolysis can influence the hepatocyte function and lead to enzyme leakage. At the same time, there is an influence on the hepatocyte membrane via the acidosis with a leakage.

Therapy

Symptom	Therapy
Insulin deficiency	Insulin
Shock	Infusion
Acidosis	Bicarbonate infusion
Electrolyte deficiency	Infusion
Azotaemia	Infusion

Further Reading

Charfen, M.A. and Fernández-Frackelton, M. (2005). Diabetic ketoacidosis. *Emergency Medicine Clinics of North America* 23 (3): 609–vii. https://doi.org/10.1016/j.emc.2005.03.009.

Dhatariya, K.K., Glaser, N.S., Codner, E., and Umpierrez, G.E. (2020). Diabetic Ketoacidosis. *Nature Reviews. Disease Primers* 6 (1): 40. https://doi.org/10.1038/s41572-020-0165-1.

Misra, S. and Oliver, N.S. (2015). Diabetic ketoacidosis in adults. *BMJ (Clinical Research Ed.)* 351: h5660. https://doi.org/10.1136/bmj.h5660.

Thomovsky, E. (2017). Fluid and electrolyte therapy in diabetic ketoacidosis. *The Veterinary Clinics of North America. Small Animal Practice* 47 (2): 491–503. https://doi.org/10.1016/j.cvsm.2016.09.012.

43.5.4

Insulinoma

Definition

An *insulinoma* is an insulin-producing tumour of the pancreas.

Aetiology and Pathogenesis

Insulinoma is a neoplasm arising from the β cells of the pancreas. The entity is predominantly malignant with a tendency to metastasise to regional organs, such as lymph nodes, liver or spleen. The tumour is hormonally active and can synthesise other hormones besides insulin, such as GH, IGF-1, glucagon, somatostatin. Insulin synthesis is largely independent of the regulatory mechanisms of glucose balance, which leads to a lack of suppression of insulin synthesis during hypoglycaemia. Insulinomas occur in dogs and cats. They are rare overall, but more common in dogs than in cats.

The consequence of insulin production by the neoplasia is increased glucose uptake by glucose-sensitive cells, such as muscle or fat cells. At the same time, glucose release in the liver is inhibited. This results from an inhibition of glycogenolysis or gluconeogenesis by insulin. The result is an insufficient presence of glucose in the serum.

Due to the severity of the clinical picture, the organism tries to compensate for the hypoglycaemia through numerous mechanisms. Controlled by peripheral and central sensors, hypoglycaemia causes increased activity of the sympathetic nervous system. This can induce the intake of carbohydrates by increasing appetite. At the same time, the production of catecholamines is increased in the adrenal medulla. These reduce the glucose uptake of muscle and fat cells and, together with increased glucagon secretion, activate glycogenolysis and gluconeogenesis in hypoglycaemia.

Diagnostics

Clinical signs	Clinical pathology	Imaging	Histopathology	Microbiology
Weakness Syncope	**Glucose serum concentration Insulin serum concentration**	Ultrasonography CT/MRI Imaging of the insulinoma	Not necessary	Not necessary

Pathophysiologic Consequences

The pathophysiologic consequences result predominantly from the persistent hypoglycaemia. In the advanced stage, consequences can also result from metastatic events.

Influenced organ systems	Clinical symptoms	Clinical pathological alterations
Urinary tract	Weakness	Hypoglycaemia
Endocrine system	Seizures	
Neuromuscular system	Tremor	
Central nervous system	Ataxia	
Muscles		

Glucose, the organism's main source of energy, is not sufficiently available in insulinoma. Since the CNS only has small reserves of glucose, the glucose deficit here leads very quickly to a failure of nerve function. Glucose is needed to generate ATP for the functioning of Na^+-K^+-ATPase. This in turn is essential for the maintenance of membrane potentials and the formation of nerve impulses through action potentials. Depending on the severity, the symptoms are **weakness** and **ataxia** with **tremor,** followed by **seizures** and **coma** (Figure 43.5.4.1).

Therapy

Symptom	Therapy
Acute hypoglycaemia	Glucose infusion
Long-term therapy	Prednisolone
Inhibition of insulin release	Diazoxid
Tumour treatment	Surgery

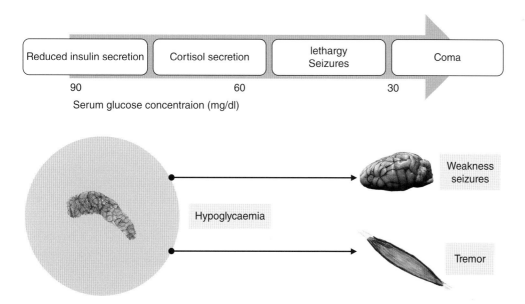

Figure 43.5.4.1 Relationship between blood glucose concentration and symptoms and pathophysiologic consequences of insulinoma.

Further Reading

Arya, V.B., Mohammed, Z., Blankenstein, O. et al. (2014). Hyperinsulinaemic hypoglycaemia. *Hormones and Metabolic Research = Hormones et metabololisme* 46 (3): 157–170. https://doi.org/10.1055/s-0034-1367063.

Greene, S.N. and Bright, R.M. (2008). Insulinoma in a cat. *The Journal of Small Animal Practice* 49 (1): 38–40. https://doi.org/10.1111/j.1748-5827.2007.00404.x.

Lurye, J.C. and Behrend, E.N. (2001). Endocrine tumors. *The Veterinary Clinics of North America. Small Animal Practice* 31 (5): 1083-x. https://doi.org/10.1016/s0195-5616(01)50014-5.

Veytsman, S., Amsellem, P., Husbands, B.D. et al. (2023). Retrospective study of 20 cats surgically treated for insulinoma. *Veterinary Surgery: VS* 52 (1): 42–50. https://doi.org/10.1111/vsu.13892.

43.6

Adrenal Gland

43.6.1

Physiology of the Adrenal Gland

Functions

The adrenal glands are a diverse hormonally active organ. They regulate numerous mechanisms in the body. Histologically, the adrenal glands can be divided into different zones. In the centre lies the adrenal medulla, which emerged embryonically from the ectoderm and is functionally connected to the autonomic nervous system. In contrast, the adrenal cortex arises from the mesoderm. While the adrenal medulla is histologically uniform, the cortex can be differentiated from the outside inwards into the zona glomerulosa, zona fasciculata and zona reticularis. Each zone has specific hormonal functions. While aldosterone synthesis is localised in the zona glomerulosa, cortisol is produced in the zona fasciculata and testosterone and oestrogen in the zona reticularis. The starting product for the different hormones is the steroid cholesterol. This is formed from acetoacetate. Most of the cholesterol needed is produced in the adrenal gland itself. A smaller part is supplied to the adrenal glands via the blood. The hormonally active target molecule is formed from the original molecule via various intermediate stages (Figure 43.6.1.1).

The hormones synthesised in the adrenal gland intervene in numerous control mechanisms.

The mineralocorticoid aldosterone is formed in the **zona glomerulosa.** Aldosterone influences the electrolyte balance of sodium and potassium and also influences the fluid balance, blood volume and blood pressure. In addition, aldosterone has a direct vascular effect by inducing contraction of vascular smooth muscle cells, presumably by regulating Na^+-K^+-ATPase activity.

The release of aldosterone is promoted by the RAAS and an increased potassium plasma concentration. Other promoting factors are ACTH, serotonin and catecholamines. Inhibitors of aldosterone release include atrial natriuretic peptide (ANP) and dopamine.

In the blood, aldosterone is transported to the target cells in approximately equal parts freely and bound to transport proteins, for example, transcortin. The main site of action of aldosterone is the distal part of the nephron. After diffusion through the cell membrane, aldosterone binds to receptors located in the cytoplasm or the nucleus. The binding separates a protein (heat shock protein) from the receptor. This leads to a conformational change, whereby the steroid-receptor complex can enter the cell nucleus and induce gene transcription by attaching to a specific promoter region. The formed mRNA migrates to the ribosomes, where proteins are synthesised in the course of translation. Their function, for example, as an enzyme or structural protein, corresponds to the steroid effect.

In the distal nephron and collecting duct, aldosterone action induces the expression of Na^+ channels in the apical membrane and Na^+-K^+-ATPase in the basolateral membrane.

The result is increased reabsorption of Na^+ from the filtrate. An increased sodium concentration within the cells triggers the exchange of sodium for potassium and hydrogen ions through specific transport proteins. This process leads to an increased excretion of potassium. Water is reabsorbed with Na^+, which results in an increase in blood volume and thus blood pressure.

Steroids, such as aldosterone, have a half-life in the organism of a few days. Excretion begins with the conjugation of the hormones in the liver. Conjugated steroids are then excreted to a smaller extent via the bile into the intestine. Of this, a portion is also reabsorbed via the entero-hepatic circulation. The larger part of the conjugated steroids is excreted via the urine.

Textbook of Small Animal Pathophysiology, First Edition. Stephan Neumann.
© 2025 John Wiley & Sons Ltd. Published 2025 by John Wiley & Sons Ltd.

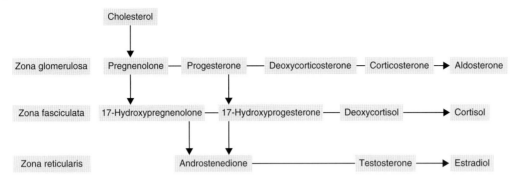

Figure 43.6.1.1 Synthesis of steroid hormones from cholesterol.

The glucocorticoid cortisol is produced in the **zona fasciculata.** The functions of glucocorticoids essentially relate to metabolism, in that they have a catabolic effect, and to the immune system, in that glucocorticoids have an anti-inflammatory and immunosuppressive effect.

The release of glucocorticoids in the adrenal gland is controlled by different hormones. An ACTH-dependent and an independent regulation are described. The former form originates from the hypothalamus. Under the influence of numerous triggers, such as proinflammatory cytokines, corticotropin-releasing hormone (CRH) is secreted in the hypothalamus and is transported via a portal venous system to the pituitary gland, where CRH induces the release of ACTH by cleaving ACTH from an ACTH precursor molecule proopiomelanocortin (POMC). In addition, CRH also stimulates the new synthesis of ACTH. ACTH reaches the adrenal gland via the blood and stimulates the formation of cortisol in the zona fasciculata. Through a negative feedback mechanism, released cortisol inhibits the release of ACTH.

The ACTH-independent release of corticoids in the zona fasciculata is influenced by direct nervous effects in the adrenal gland, as well as by neurotransmitters and growth factors. For example, TGF-ß inhibits ACTH-stimulated cortisone synthesis. This makes pathophysiologic sense, as TGF-ß is an important growth factor in the synthesis of connective tissue, while cortisone inhibits the function of fibroblasts.

After synthesis, glucocorticoids are usually transported in the blood bound to transport proteins, such as albumin or transcortin.

The mechanism by which mineral and glucocorticoids act on cells is receptor-associated. Corticoid receptors are usually located in the cytoplasm. For this purpose, the corticoids diffuse through the cell membrane and bind to the respective receptor. The glucocorticoid binding induces a conformational change by separating the protein (heat shock protein) from the receptor. After translocation into the cell nucleus, the activated receptor binds to specific promoter sequences of the target genes and regulates their transcription.

The effects of glucocorticoids are manifold, but are primarily concentrated on the metabolism, in which they have a catabolic effect. In addition, they have a general anti-inflammatory effect by preventing the formation of inflammatory metabolites at different levels (Table 43.6.1.1).

Glucocorticoids are eliminated via the liver by being conjugated in hepatocytes and then excreted either via bile or urine.

Table 43.6.1.1 Functions of glucocorticoids.

Metabolic effect	Mechanism
Catabolism	Degradation of structural proteins to generate glucoplastic amino acids
Gluconeogenesis	Increased gluconeogenesis from amino acids
Lipolysis	Increasing the lipolytic effect of glucagon
Inflammatory effect	**Mechanism**
Arachidonic acid	Inhibition of the synthesis of arachidonic acid metabolites (prostaglandins, leukotrienes)
Proinflammatory cytokines	Inhibition of TGF, IL-1, IL-2

Finally, the sex hormones are synthesised in the **zona reticularis.**

Their synthesis is subject to the influence of the hypothalamic hormone GnRH and the pituitary hormones FSH and LH. The latter reach the adrenal gland via the blood and induce the synthesis of the sex hormones androstenedione and androstenediol from cholesterol. These are converted into testosterone and oestradiol in the sex glands. The function of the hormones is sex-specific and metabolic. Oestrogens serve the expression of female sexual characteristics. In addition, they affect bone metabolism by exerting a promoting effect on osteoblasts and an inhibiting effect on osteoclasts. Consequently, oestrogens prevent bone resorption. Testosterone also affects the expression of male sexual characteristics, but also metabolism. For example, testosterone promotes bone and muscle formation, as well as erythropoiesis.

The catecholamines, adrenaline and noradrenaline are formed in the **adrenal medulla.** The source molecules are the amino acids phenylalanine and tyrosine.

The function of catecholamines focuses on controlling the organism in a state of emergency. To this end, they act on the metabolism and the cardiovascular system. The metabolic function focuses on the provision of energy; for this purpose, source molecules of cellular energy production, such as fatty acids and glucose, are released from the depot. The cardiovascular effect serves to increase cardiac activity, vasoconstriction and pulmonary vasodilation, thus enabling the organism to be better controlled in an emergency situation in the sense of the 'fight or flight' principle. Cardiovascular function is controlled by receptors.

A higher-level function of the adrenal gland is the stress response.

Selye (1946) was the first to recognise the similarity in the body's response to the effects of certain stimuli. He called this non-specific reaction of the body a 'general adaptation syndrome', which takes place in three phases, the alarm phase, the resistance phase and the exhaustion phase. He called the stimuli 'stressors', the reactions of the organism 'stress response' and the overall situation the 'stress system'.

The stress system is localised in the central and peripheral nervous system. Central components of the stress system, for example, the neurons that synthesise CRH, are located in the hypothalamus.

The release and new production of ACTH is induced by the binding of CRH to specific receptors in the anterior pituitary lobe. This hypothalamic-pituitary-adrenal axis together with the sympathetic-adrenomedullary axis (SAM axis) are peripheral components of the stress system. In order for the organism to react quickly to danger, this system is activated in stressful situations.

Reference

Selye, H. (1946). The general adaptation syndrome and the diseases of adaptation. *The Journal of Clinical Endocrinology and Metabolism* 6: 117–230. https://doi.org/10.1210/jcem-6-2-117.

Further Reading

Kanczkowski, W., Sue, M., and Bornstein, S.R. (2017). The adrenal gland microenvironment in health, disease and during regeneration. *Hormones (Athens, Greece)* 16 (3): 251–265. https://doi.org/10.14310/horm.2002.1744.

Keegan, C.E. and Hammer, G.D. (2002). Recent insights into organogenesis of the adrenal cortex. *Trends in Endocrinology and Metabolism: TEM* 13 (5): 200–208. https://doi.org/10.1016/s1043-2760(02)00602-1.

Koos, R.D. (2011). Minireview: putting physiology back into estrogens' mechanism of action. *Endocrinology* 152 (12): 4481–4488. https://doi.org/10.1210/en.2011-1449.

Le Roy, C., Li, J.Y., Stocco, D.M. et al. (2000). Regulation by adrenocorticotropin (ACTH), angiotensin II, transforming growth factor-beta, and insulin-like growth factor I of bovine adrenal cell steroidogenic capacity and expression of ACTH receptor, steroidogenic acute regulatory protein, cytochrome P450c17, and 3beta-hydroxysteroid dehydrogenase. *Endocrinology* 141 (5): 1599–1607. https://doi.org/10.1210/endo.141.5.7457.

Lightman, S.L., Windle, R.J., Ma, X.M. et al. (2002). Hypothalamic-pituitary-adrenal function. *Archives of Physiology and Biochemistry* 110 (1–2): 90–93. https://doi.org/10.1076/apab.110.1.90.899.

Matthews, S.G. (2002). Early programming of the hypothalamo-pituitary-adrenal axis. *Trends in Endocrinology and Metabolism: TEM* 13 (9): 373–380. https://doi.org/10.1016/s1043-2760(02)00690-2.

Sapolsky, R.M., Romero, L.M., and Munck, A.U. (2000). How do glucocorticoids influence stress responses? Integrating permissive, suppressive, stimulatory, and preparative actions. *Endocrine Reviews* 21 (1): 55–89. https://doi.org/10.1210/edrv.21.1.0389.

Simpson, E.R., Misso, M., Hewitt, K.N. et al. (2005). Estrogen—the good, the bad, and the unexpected. *Endocrine Reviews* 26 (3): 322–330. https://doi.org/10.1210/er.2004-0020.

Snyder, P.J., Peachey, H., Berlin, J.A. et al. (2000). Effects of testosterone replacement in hypogonadal men. *The Journal of Clinical Endocrinology and Metabolism* 85 (8): 2670–2677. https://doi.org/10.1210/jcem.85.8.6731.

Weber, K.T. (2003). A neuroendocrine-immune interface. The immunostimulatory state of aldosteronism. *Heart* 28 (8): 692–701. https://doi.org/10.1007/s00059-003-2511-y.

43.6.2

Hyperadrenocorticism

Definition

Hyperadrenocorticism is an adrenal cortex hyperfunction with clinical and biochemical changes in the organism that develop as a result of increased glucocorticoid concentration. The disease was first described in humans in 1990 by the American neurosurgeon Harvey Williams Cushing and is also known as 'Cushing's disease'.

Aetiology

The disease is more common in dogs than in cats. The cause may be a hormone-producing tumour in the adrenal or pituitary glands, or the disease may be the result of long-term increased iatrogenic cortisone therapy. The central or pituitary-dependent form is usually due to an ACTH-producing adenoma. This is called a 'microadenoma' if the diameter is <10 mm. If the tumour is larger in diameter, it is called a 'macroadenoma'. Adenocarcinomas of the pituitary gland as a causality are very rare. In the peripheral or adrenal form, there is autonomous cortisone production due to an adenoma or adenocarcinoma of the adrenal cortex. The neoplasia is usually unilateral. Rarely, an ectopic form of Cushing's disease has also been described, in which an ACTH-acting molecule is produced in the sense of a paraneoplastic syndrome. In dogs, carcinomas in the liver and pancreas are possible causes.

In the iatrogenic form, Cushing's disease develops after long-term external cortisone application. The following criteria apply:

Symptoms of hyperadrenocorticism due to exogenous cortisone administration:

Minimum four weeks
Long acting worse than short acting
Kristal and -acetate worse than -succinate
Also possible with topical corticoids
Recovery approximately six weeks after weaning

Source: Huang et al. (1999).

Neoplastic	Iatrogenic
Adenoma pituitary gland, adrenal gland (D, C)	Long-term corticoid administration

D-dog, C-cat

Pathogenesis

The pathogenesis of Cushing's disease results from the effects of glucocorticoids. Other hormones of the adrenal glands are not excessively active in this clinical picture.

Diagnostics

Clinical signs	Clinical pathology	Imaging	Histopathology	Microbiology
Non-specific PU/PD	**Dexamethasone suppression test** **ACTH Stimulation test** **Urine cortisol creatinine ratio**	**Ultrasonography, CT, MRI** Imaging of adrenocortical tumour or pituitary tumour	Not necessary	Not necessary

Pathophysiologic Consequences

The pathophysiologic consequences are predominantly a consequence of cortisol excess and to a lesser extent dependent on local neoplastic growth.

Influenced organ systems	Clinical symptoms	Clinical pathological alterations
Cardiovascular system	PU/PD	Stress leukogram
Gastrointestinal system	Polyphagia	Increased ALT
Hepatobiliary system	Hepatomegaly	Increased ALP
Urinary tract	Muscle weakness	Hypercholesterinaemia
Endocrine system	Lethargy	Hypertriglyceridaemia
Haematological system	Alopecia	Hyperglycaemia
Bones, joints	Hyperpigmentation	Proteinuria
Muscles	Thin skin	
Skin		

Source: Adapted from Behrend et al. (2012).

The **PU/PD** results from an increase in glomerular filtration under the influence of the corticoids, this can also lead to **proteinuria.** At the same time, the ADH effect at the collecting tube decreases, as corticoids negatively influence the expression of aquaporins. Loss of body water decreases blood volume and blood pressure. This leads to increased ADH secretion, the renal function of which is inhibited, but the central function of the 'feeling of thirst' is maintained. Accordingly, polydipsia occurs (Joles et al. 1980).

Polyphagia, which is more pronounced in dogs than in cats, may be a consequence of the general catabolic metabolic state and may represent a compensatory mechanism. However, there is also a direct stimulating effect of cortisol on the feeding centre. This can take place via the increased production of active ghrelin. Ghrelin is a peptide hormone that is produced as a prohormone in chromaffin cells of the stomach wall and other organs, such as the intestine, pancreas, kidney and brain. Stress or corticoids can have a positive effect on the formation of ghrelin. Activated ghrelin reaches the brain via the blood and activates appetite in the feeding centre of the hypothalamus (Kageyama et al. 2012; Bouillon-Minois et al. 2021).

Dogs with clinically manifest Cushing's disease show **abdominal enlargement.** This may be a consequence of an enlarged liver. Corticoids act via hepatocyte glucocorticoid receptors and induce hepatic gluconeogenesis and glycogen synthesis (Petrescu et al. 2018). An exaggerated effect leads to an accumulation of glycogen in the hepatocytes and their enlargement. Another effect that explains the abdominal enlargement and especially the hanging belly is the **muscle atrophy** that happens under the influence of cortisone excess. This is due to protein degradation in the muscle fibres under the influence of corticosteroid excess. This makes glucoplastic amino acids available for increased gluconeogenesis.

Gluconeogenesis occurs predominantly in the liver and partly in the kidney. Hepatogenic gluconeogenesis is realised under the influence of 'stress hormones', such as catecholamines and corticoids. At the same time, these hormones inhibit glycolysis by inhibiting pyruvate kinase. Lactate, glycerol, fatty acids and glucogenic amino acids from muscle protein breakdown are used as starting products for gluconeogenesis.

Glucogenic amino acids:

Alanine
Arginine
Aspartate
Cysteine
Glutamine
Glutamate
Glycine
Histidine
Methionine
Proline
Serine
Valine

Further metabolic consequences of glucocorticoid excess are increased lipolysis. This increases the concentration of **serum cholesterol** and **triglycerides.** Lipolysis is regulated by insulin and the antagonistically acting catecholamines and corticoids. Adrenalin, for example, activates a protein kinase via cAMP as a second messenger in the fat cells, which in turn activates the hormone-sensitive lipase, which cleaves triglycerides and cholesterol esters. The influence of corticoids consists of an increase in lipolysis and a reduction in lipogenesis through insulin antagonism (Djurhuus et al. 2002; Gathercole et al. 2011).

The increased hepatogenic metabolism under the influence of glucocorticoids leads to histological changes in the sense of a 'steroid hepatopathy'. This leads to an accumulation of glycogen and fat in the hepatocytes. Morphologically, the hepatocytes change their size, they swell and change the internal structure by displacing the organelles through the vacuoles into the cell periphery. The consequences are disturbances in hepatic metabolism, such as energy production. This, in turn, can lead to loss of cell membrane integrity. This leads to a leakage of primarily cytosolic enzymes, such as **ALT** or **AST** into the serum (Fittschen and Bellamy 1984).

ALP is a hydrolase that is synthesised in various organs. The activity of the enzyme measured in serum results mainly from the liver-, bone- and cortisol-induced isoenzymes, as these have a half-life of several days. The cortisol-induced form of ALP is found only in dogs and is expressed by hepatocytes under the influence of corticoids. Dogs with hyperadrenocorticism show an increase in cortisol- and liver-specific ALP.

The effects on the **immune system** result from suppression of the activity of the transcription factors Activator protein-1 (AP-1) and Nuclear factor-κB (NF-κB). Another mechanism involved in the regulation of the immune response is the induction of apoptosis of immune cells. In addition, glucocorticoids inhibit T and B cell proliferation, natural killer cell activity and macrophage differentiation. For this reason, immune responses and inflammatory reactions are suppressed under the influence of corticoids. This also affects wound healing, in which the inflammatory response is involved.

There are also **cardiovascular consequences** of glucocorticoid excess. Corticoids cause an increase in blood pressure. This is due to the fact that glucocorticoids can also have a mineralocorticoid effect. In addition, there is an increased expression of Ca^{2+}-dependent ion channels on the vascular wall muscles and an increased expression of α and β receptors, which increases the effect of vasoactive substances (Chrousos 2015).

The skin changes in Cushing's disease are extensive, consisting of **alopecia** due to hair follicle atrophy. The thin **skin** is the result of reduced collagen formation under the influence of glucocorticoids on the fibroblasts. The **hyperpigmentation** is attributed to an increased secretion of melanocyte stimulating hormone (MSH) from the pituitary gland (Figure 43.6.2.1).

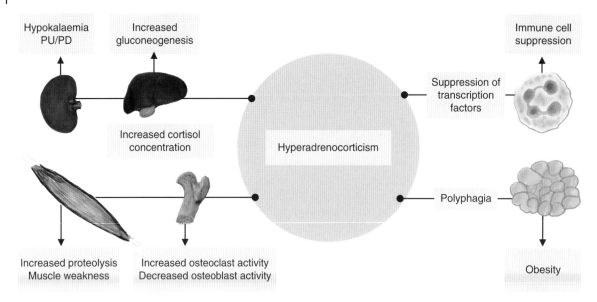

Figure 43.6.2.1 Pathophysiologic consequences of hyperadrenocorticism.

Therapy

Symptom	Therapy
Hyperadrenocorticism	Reduction of cortisol formation (e.g. Trilostane, Mitotane)

References

Behrend, E.N., Kooistra, H.S., Nelson, R. et al. (2013). Diagnosis of spontaneous canine hyperadrenocorticism: 2012 ACVIM consensus statement (small animal). *Journal of Veterinary Internal Medicine* 27 (6): 1292–1304. https://doi.org/10.1111/jvim.12192.

Bouillon-Minois, J. B., Trousselard, M., Thivel, D., Gordon, B. A., Schmidt, J., Moustafa, F., Oris, C., & Dutheil, F. (2021). Ghrelin as a biomarker of stress: a systematic review and meta-analysis. *Nutrients*, 13(3), 784. https://doi.org/10.3390/nu13030784

Chrousos, G.P. (2015, Chapter 99). Glucocorticoid action: physiology. In: *Endocrinology Adult and Pediatric*, 7e (ed. J.L. Jameson, L.J. De Groot, D.M. de Kretser, et al.), 1727–1740. Saunders.

Djurhuus, C.B., Gravholt, C.H., Nielsen, S. et al. (2002). Effects of cortisol on lipolysis and regional interstitial glycerol levels in humans. *American Journal of Physiology. Endocrinology and Metabolism* 283 (1): E172–E177. https://doi.org/10.1152/ajpendo.00544.2001.

Fittschen, C. and Bellamy, J.E. (1984). Prednisone-induced morphologic and chemical changes in the liver of dogs. *Veterinary Pathology* 21 (4): 399–406. https://doi.org/10.1177/030098588402100406.

Gathercole, L.L., Morgan, S.A., Bujalska, I.J. et al. (2011). Regulation of lipogenesis by glucocorticoids and insulin in human adipose tissue. *PLoS One* 6 (10): e26223. https://doi.org/10.1371/journal.pone.0026223.

Huang, Y.S., Rousseau, K., Sbaihi, M. et al. (1999). Cortisol selectively stimulates pituitary gonadotropin beta-subunit in a primitive teleost, *Anguilla anguilla*. *Endocrinology* 140 (3): 1228–1235. https://doi.org/10.1210/endo.140.3.6598.

Joles, J.A., Rijnberk, A., van den Brom, W.E., and Dogterom, J. (1980). Studies on the mechanism of polyuria induced by cortisol excess in the dog. *Tijdschrift voor Diergeneeskunde* 105 (20): 199–205.

Kageyama, K., Akimoto, K., Yamagata, S. et al. (2012). Dexamethasone stimulates the expression of ghrelin and its receptor in rat hypothalamic 4B cells. *Regulatory Peptides* 174 (1–3): 12–17. https://doi.org/10.1016/j.regpep.2011.11.003.

Petrescu, A.D., Kain, J., Liere, V. et al. (2018). Hypothalamic-pituitary-adrenal dysfunction in cholestatic liver disease. *Frontiers in Endocrinology* 9: 660. https://doi.org/10.3389/fendo.2018.00660.

Further Reading

Bennaim, M., Shiel, R.E., and Mooney, C.T. (2019). Diagnosis of spontaneous hyperadrenocorticism in dogs. Part 1: pathophysiology, aetiology, clinical and clinicopathological features. *Veterinary Journal (London, England: 1997)* 252: 105342. https://doi.org/10.1016/j.tvjl.2019.105342.

Braddock, J.A. (2003). Diagnosis of hyperadrenocorticism in the dog. *Australian Veterinary Journal* 81 (1–2): 25–27. https://doi.org/10.1111/j.1751-0813.2003.tb11413.x.

Hoenig, M. (2002). Feline hyperadrenocorticism—where are we now? *Journal of Feline Medicine and Surgery* 4 (3): 171–174. https://doi.org/10.1053/jfms.2002.0178.

Lien, Y. H., Huang, H. P., & Chang, P. H. (2006). Iatrogenic hyperadrenocorticism in 12 cats. *Journal of the American Animal Hospital Association*, 42(6), 414–423. https://doi.org/10.5326/0420414

43.6.3

Hypoadrenocorticism

Definition

Hypoadrenocorticism is characterised by reduced production of glucocorticoids and mineralocorticoids. The clinical picture is also described as Addison's disease, named after the English physician Thomas Addison, who in 1855 was able to assign the clinical picture of the adrenal insufficiency.

Aetiology

Different forms with different aetiologies are distinguished in hypoadrenocorticism. The most common primary form develops after atrophy of the adrenal cortex, which in turn can be the result of lymphoplasma cellular inflammation or amyloid deposition. A distinction must be made between this and the secondary form, which can be attributed to reduced ACTH secretion caused by various processes in the pituitary gland, such as neoplasia. Addison's disease occurs in dogs and very rarely in cats.

Primary, adrenal	Secondary, pituitary
Autoimmune (D/C)	Neoplasia (D)
Neoplasia (D/C)	Trauma (D)
Amyloid (D)	Inflammation (D)
Coagulopathy (D)	
Cushing therapy (D)	

D – Dog, C – Cat

Pathogenesis

The most common form of hypoadrenocorticism is the primary form resulting from adrenal destruction due to autoimmune lymphoplasma cellular infiltration into the adrenal tissue with apoptosis of the functional adrenal cells and fibrotic replacement of the functional tissue. The process is more pronounced in the zona glomerulosa than in the zona fasciculata. Thus, the mineralocorticoid insufficiency is usually more pronounced than the glucocorticoid form. The reason for this seems to be the high concentration of glucocorticoids in the zona fasciculata. This in turn has a local anti-inflammatory effect, as corticoids suppress the lymphocytes (Pearce et al. 2021).

Textbook of Small Animal Pathophysiology, First Edition. Stephan Neumann.
© 2025 John Wiley & Sons Ltd. Published 2025 by John Wiley & Sons Ltd.

Diagnostics

Clinical signs	Clinical pathology	Imaging	Histopathology	Microbiology
Non-specific	Basal cortisol serum concentration **ACTH stimulation test**	Ultrasonography Maybe reduced adrenal gland volume	Not necessary	Not necessary

Pathophysiologic Consequences

The pathophysiologic consequences of adrenal insufficiency result essentially from the deficiency of mineralocorticoids and glucocorticoids.

Influenced organ systems	Clinical symptoms	Clinical pathological alterations
Cardiovascular system	Shock	Leucocyte abnormalities
Gastrointestinal system	Lethargy	Anaemia
Urinary tract	Vomitus	Hyponatraemia
Muscles	Diarrhoea	Hypercalcaemia
		Hypoglycaemia
		Hypercalcaemia
		Pre-renal azotaemia

The lack of mineralocorticoids leads to a reduced Na^+ reabsorption combined with reduced water reabsorption. As a consequence, the blood volume and thus the blood pressure decrease. Both lead to **shock symptoms** and **pre-renal renal failure,** which is a consequence of shock. This process is supported by the discontinuation of direct cardiovascular effects of glucocorticoids (vasoconstriction). Reduced blood flow to the kidney reduces the filtration pressure in the glomerulum, resulting in a reduced GFR. As a result, urinary substances, such as urea and creatinine are filtered less. Since urea is reabsorbed from the primary filtration in contrast to creatinine in the proximal tubule, there is an altered urea-creatinine ratio in the blood, urea increases more markedly than creatinine. If the ratio is $>43:1$, this indicates pre-renal renal failure.

The **lethargy** in hypoadrenocorticism results from disturbances of the cardiovascular system and metabolism. The former results from the lowered blood pressure when the mineralocorticoid effect ceases. The second may be associated with **hypoglycaemia.** The reduced corticoid concentration inhibits gluconeogenesis, and at the same time insulin sensitivity is increased. Both lead to a reduced provision of glucose for energy production, a reduction of the alternative pathway 'gluconeogenesis'.

The cause of **vomiting** and **diarrhoea** in animals with hypoadrenocorticism is seen in the glucocorticoid deficiency, which reduces the peristalsis of the intestinal wall. At the same time, under the influence of hypovolaemia, blood stasis develops in the intestinal wall, resulting in inflammation or ulceration. Both effects cause the clinical symptoms.

The electrolyte changes, **hyperkalaemia** and **hyponatraemia** are due to the lack of mineral corticoids. Meanwhile, the mostly **non-regenerative anaemia** and the changes in leucocytes (**eosinophilia and lymphocytosis**) are explained by the reduction of glucocorticoids. Glucocorticoids cause apoptosis in eosinophil granulocytes and lymphocytes. In addition, they reduce the receptor activity on T lymphocytes. If this influence is absent, **eosinophilia** and **lymphocytosis** occur.

The same applies to **hypercalcaemia**. Glucocorticoids reduce plasma calcium levels by reducing calcium absorption in the intestine and Ca^{2+} reabsorption in the tubule (Figure 43.6.3.1).

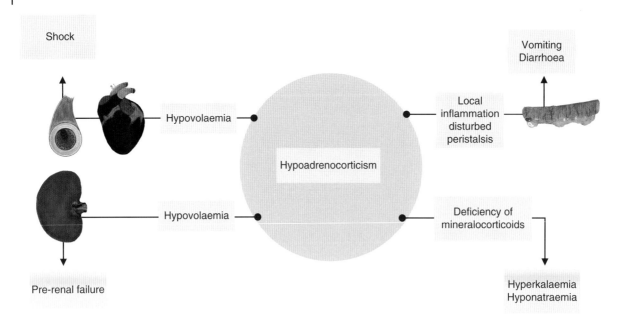

Figure 43.6.3.1 Pathophysiologic consequences of hypoadrenocorticism.

Therapy

Symptom	Therapy
Mineralocorticoid deficiency	Fludrocortisone, deoxycortone pivalate
Glucocorticoid deficiency	Prednisolone, hydrocortisone

Reference

Pearce, S., Gan, E.H., and Napier, C. (2021). Management of Endocrine Disease: residual adrenal function in Addison's disease. *European Journal of Endocrinology* 184 (2): R61–R67. https://doi.org/10.1530/EJE-20-0894.

Further Reading

Lathan, P. and Thompson, A.L. (2018). Management of hypoadrenocorticism (Addison's disease) in dogs. *Veterinary Medicine (Auckland, N.Z.)* 9: 1–10. https://doi.org/10.2147/VMRR.S125617.

Stonehewer, J. and Tasker, S. (2001). Hypoadrenocorticism in a cat. *The Journal of Small Animal Practice* 42 (4): 186–190. https://doi.org/10.1111/j.1748-5827.2001.tb01800.x.

Van Lanen, K. and Sande, A. (2014). Canine hypoadrenocorticism: pathogenesis, diagnosis, and treatment. *Topics in Companion Animal Medicine* 29 (4): 88–95. https://doi.org/10.1053/j.tcam.2014.10.001.

43.6.4

Hyperaldosteronism

Definition

Hyperaldosteronism is characterised by an increased concentration of aldosterone in the blood.

Aetiology

The causalities of hyperaldosteronism are an autonomous secretion of aldosterone from the adrenal gland (primary hyperaldosteronism = PHA) or a disease of other organs affecting its synthesis or degradation (secondary hyperaldosteronism). The disease occurs in both forms in dogs and cats. Overall, it is a rare disease, with the cat being more commonly affected than the dog.

Primary hyperaldosteronism is due to a benign or malignant (adenoma, adenocarcinoma) tumour of the zona glomerulosa of the adrenal glands.

The secondary form is a consequence of disease processes that cause increased aldosterone synthesis via chronic activation of the RAAS.

Primary	Secondary
Idiopathic (D/C)	Heart failure (D)
Adrenocortical tumour (D/C)	Chronic renal failure (D/C)
	Hyperthyroidism (C)

D – Dog, C – Cat

Pathogenesis

Primary hyperaldosteronism results from a permanent autonomous synthesis of aldosterone. In this way, aldosterone synthesis evades the feedback control mechanism of angiotensin II. After initiation of the RAAS, aldosterone causes sodium and water reabsorption in the distal tubule. As a result, blood volume and blood pressure increase. This reduces renin secretion, resulting in reduced angiotensinogen synthesis in the liver, which leads to reduced concentrations of angiotensin I and II. The latter has a depressive effect on aldosterone synthesis, but is suppressed in the case of autonomous synthesis by an adrenal tumour.

The heart influences aldosterone through its own synthesis in the heart muscle cells. This synthesis is subject to the regulatory mechanisms of the RAAS. In the case of heart disease, synthesis may be altered. Dogs with dilated cardiomyopathy synthesise more aldosterone in the heart cells than healthy dogs (Reynoso-Palomar et al. 2017). In addition, heart disease exerts a negative influence on blood pressure. This in turn activates the RAAS in a physiological way. Due to the persistence

Textbook of Small Animal Pathophysiology, First Edition. Stephan Neumann.
© 2025 John Wiley & Sons Ltd. Published 2025 by John Wiley & Sons Ltd.

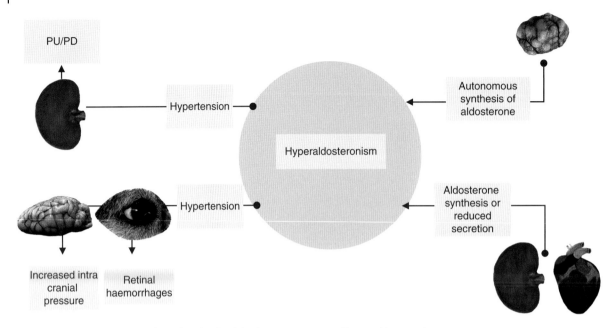

Figure 43.6.4.1 Pathogenesis and pathophysiologic consequences of hyperaldosteronism.

of heart failure, there is a long-term increased concentration of aldosterone. Finally, if heart disease is present, peripheral perfusion may be impaired. If the liver is affected, aldosterone metabolism may be affected, impairing its excretion (Hostetter and Ibrahim 2003).

Renal hyperaldosteronism could be a consequence of decreased renal excretion of aldosterone. Furthermore, in chronic kidney disease, due to morphological remodelling processes, renin synthesis, as well as sodium and water reabsorption are affected, which would lead to an inadequate response to RAAS activation. This could cause permanent activation with hyperaldosteronism (Hené et al. 1982; Ibrahim and Hostetter 2003) (Figure 43.6.4.1).

Diagnostics

Clinical signs	Clinical pathology	Imaging	Histopathology	Microbiology
Non-specific, Hypertension	Hypokalaemia **Aldosterone serum concentration** Aldosterone-renin ratio	Ultrasonography adrenal gland with evidence of neoplasia	Not necessary	Not necessary

Pathophysiologic Consequences

The main consequences of hyperaldosteronism result from increased sodium and water reabsorption and the associated increase in blood pressure, as well as increased potassium excretion resulting in hypokalaemia.

Influenced organ systems	Clinical symptoms	Clinical pathological alterations
Central nervous system	Hypertension	Hypernatraemia
Cardiovascular system	Seizures	Hypokalaemia
Urinary tract	Ocular haemorrhage	Increased CK
Ophthalmic system	Polymyopathy	Increased urea and creatinine
	PU/PD	Proteinuria

Table 43.6.4.1 Categories of hypertension in dogs and cats.

Category	Blood pressure systolic/diastolic (mmHg)
I	150/95
II	150–159/95–99
III	160–179/100–119
IV	>180/120

Source: Adapted from Brown et al. (2007).

A primary causality for the pathophysiologic consequences of hyperaldosteronism is arterial **hypertension.** Hypertension in dogs and cats is classified into categories I–IV depending on the extent (Table 43.6.4.1).

Central nervous consequence of high blood pressure can be a stroke. This is rare in dogs and cats. Hypertensive encephalopathy would be another consequence of central nervous elevated blood pressure. Central nervous blood pressure is kept constant within narrow limits by adaptive vasoconstriction and vasodilation, largely independent of systemic blood pressure. However, a significant increase in systemic blood pressure can overcome the regulatory mechanism.

This can increase the hydrostatic pressure of the cerebral vessels and cause fluid leakage into the nervous tissue with cerebral oedema and increased intracranial pressure. Both can affect vision and also cause **seizures** (Potter and Schaefer 2022).

Independently of this, the eye is directly affected by the increased arterial blood pressure. **Retinal haemorrhages** or oedema formation are possible and correspond to the principle of increasing vascular permeability with an increase in blood pressure.

Polymyopathy is a consequence of hypokalaemia. Potassium ions play an important role in maintaining the membrane potential as they are involved in the regulation of the resting potential. Low potassium levels can lead to less K^+ being taken up into the cells, resulting in a positive shift in the resting potential. This means that the cells become less negative and thus less excitable. The result is hypokalaemic paralysis. This can lead to an increase in the activity of **creatine kinase** in the blood through destruction of the muscles.

The symptom complex of **PU/PD** associated with **azotaemia** and **proteinuria** reflects the renal consequences of hyperaldosteronism. These are partly a consequence of a profibrotic property of aldosterone. Mesangial cells or vascular smooth muscle cells express aldosterone receptors. The result is increased synthesis of collagens and thus parenchymal fibrosis. In the case of glomerular fibrosis, there is a reduction of functional glomeruli. In the remaining glomeruli, this leads to glomerular hyperfiltration to maintain renal function. This in turn increases proteinuria (Wakisaka et al. 1994; Kornel 1994).

Therapy

Symptom	Therapy
Aldosterone-producing tumour	Surgery
Idiopathic hyperaldosteronism	Spironolactone
Hypokalaemia	Potassium gluconate
Hypertension	Calcium channel blocker (e.g. Amlodipine)

References

Brown, S., Atkins, C., Bagley, R. et al. (2007). Guidelines for the identification, evaluation, and management of systemic hypertension in dogs and cats. *Journal of Veterinary Internal Medicine* 21 (3): 542–558. https://doi.org/10.1892/0891-6640 (2007)21[542:gftiea]2.0.co;2.

Hené, R.J., Boer, P., Koomans, H.A., and Mees, E.J. (1982). Plasma aldosterone concentrations in chronic renal disease. *Kidney International* 21 (1): 98–101. https://doi.org/10.1038/ki.1982.14.

Hostetter, T.H. and Ibrahim, H.N. (2003). Aldosterone in chronic kidney and cardiac disease. *Journal of the American Society of Nephrology: JASN* 14 (9): 2395–2401. https://doi.org/10.1097/01.asn.0000086472.65806.73.

Ibrahim, H.N. and Hostetter, T.H. (2003). Aldosterone in renal disease. *Current Opinion in Nephrology and Hypertension* 12 (2): 159–164. https://doi.org/10.1097/00041552-200303000-00006.

Kornel, L. (1994). Colocalization of 11 beta-hydroxysteroid dehydrogenase and mineralocorticoid receptors in cultured vascular smooth muscle cells. *American Journal of Hypertension* 7 (1): 100–103. https://doi.org/10.1093/ajh/7.1.100.

Potter, T. and Schaefer, T. J. (2022). *Hypertensive Encephalopathy*. StatPearls. StatPearls Publishing.

Reynoso-Palomar, A., Mena-Aguilar, G., Cruz-García, M. et al. (2017). Production of aldosterone in cardiac tissues of healthy dogs and with dilated myocardiopathy. *Veterinary World* 10 (11): 1329–1332. https://doi.org/10.14202/vetworld.2017.1329-1332.

Wakisaka, M., Spiro, M.J., and Spiro, R.G. (1994). Synthesis of type VI collagen by cultured glomerular cells and comparison of its regulation by glucose and other factors with that of type IV collagen. *Diabetes* 43 (1): 95–103. https://doi.org/10.2337/diab.43.1.95.

43.6.5

Pheochromocytoma

Definition

Pheochromocytoma is a hormone-producing tumour of the adrenal medulla.

Aetiology

The disease rarely occurs in dogs and very rarely in cats. The neoplasia affects the chromaffin cells in the adrenal medulla. Rarely, extra-adrenal tumours of the chromaffin cells have also been described.

Pathogenesis

Although the neoplastic process is largely concentrated in the adrenal gland, regional metastases do occur. However, the endocrine activity of the tumour is prominent. This originates from the chromaffin adrenal cells. The name comes from their staining behaviour in histology. The chromaffin cells are modified sympathetic postganglionic neurons. They are differentiated into two types with different granules. Type I cells contain large-volume granules that store adrenaline (epinephrine) and make up about 80% of the chromaffin cells. Type II cells with small-volume granules and stored noradrenaline (norepinephrine) are differentiated from these. These make up about 20% of the chromaffin cells. Both cell types synthesise catecholamines from tyrosine.

L-tyrosine >> L-dopa >> Dopamine >> L-norepinephrine >> L-epinephrine

    The catecholamines are synthesised and stored in the chromaffin cells. The catecholamines produced control their own synthesis via a negative feedback mechanism. The release of catecholamines is controlled by the sympathetic nervous system. Dogs secrete more epinephrines, and cats secrete more norepinephrines. Due to the good vascularisation of the adrenal medulla, the catecholamines quickly enter the systemic circulation. Catecholamines act on the cardiovascular apparatus and the smooth muscles of other organs (Table 43.6.5.1).

    The degradation of catecholamines takes place via the enzyme systems monoaminooxidase (MAO) catechyl-O-methyltansferase (COMT) in various neuronal and extraneuronal tissues. The degradation product of the catecholamines, vanillin mandelic acid, is excreted via the kidneys.

    Pheochromocytomas are particularly conspicuous because of their complex symptoms, which result from the diverse functions of the catecholamines.

Textbook of Small Animal Pathophysiology, First Edition. Stephan Neumann.
© 2025 John Wiley & Sons Ltd. Published 2025 by John Wiley & Sons Ltd.

Table 43.6.5.1 Target organs and selected effects of catecholamines.

Organ	Receptor	Effect
Heart	β-1	Increased heart rate, contractility, conduction velocity
Arterioles	α-1, β-2	Constriction, dilatation
Systemic veins	α-1	Constriction
Bronchial smooth muscle	β-2	Relaxation
Urinary bladder	Detrusor β-2	Relaxation
	Sphincter α	Contraction
Stomach	α, β-2	Decreased motility
Intestine	α, β-2	Decreased motility

Source: Adapted from Feldmann E.C. and Nelson R.W. (1996).

Diagnostics

Clinical signs	Clinical pathology	Imaging	Histopathology	Microbiology
Hypertension	Non-specific	**Ultrasonography/MRI** Imaging of adrenal gland, tumour	Not necessary	Not necessary

Pathophysiologic Consequences

The pathophysiologic consequences are primarily due to the catechol effects. In addition, consequences arise from the locally expansive tumour growth in the adrenal glands.

Influenced organ systems	Clinical symptoms	Clinical pathological alterations
Central nervous system Cardiovascular system	Weakness	Mild non-regenerative anaemia
Respiratory system	Anorexia	Leucocytosis
Urinary tract Gastrointestinal system	Weight loss	Mild azotaemia
	Collapse	Proteinuria
	Epistaxis/ocular bleeding	Increased liver enzymes
	Tachycardia	
	Tachypnoea	
	PU/PD	
	Vomiting	

Adapted from Feldmann E.C. and Nelson R.W. (1996).

Pheochromocytoma is characterised by its hormone activity. Accordingly, numerous symptoms develop as a consequence of the increased hormone secretion. The adrenal medullary hormones epinephrine and norepinephrine are considered stress hormones. Accordingly, the symptoms are comparable to those of a massive stress reaction.

Under stress, the organism organises itself according to the premise of fight or flight. This has a positive influence on heart activity, lung activity, energy metabolism and muscle function. Other organ functions, such as gastrointestinal activity or kidney function, are negatively influenced. Due to the reduction of food absorption, the symptoms of **anorexia** and consequently **weight loss** or **weakness** may develop. Overall, however, the endogenous provision of energy sources is increased. Another explanation for the weakness that occurs could be direct effects of the catecholamines on the central nervous system. Cerebral ischaemia due to catecholamine-induced vasospasm would be possible (Rupala et al. 2017).

Elevated blood pressure occurs regularly in pheochromocytoma patients and can be mildly to severely elevated. Symptoms, such as **collapse** or **epistaxis** may result from these hypertensive phases. Long-term hypertension can cause endothelial dysfunction of the vessel wall cells. This is often accompanied by increased oxidative stress in the endothelial cells. As a result, the integrity of the vessel wall can be disrupted, tight-junctions are broken and haemorrhage can develop.

The following symptoms are attributed to the increased catecholamine concentration.

Catecholamines act on β receptors in the heart and lead to accelerated cardiac activity through a positive chronotropic and positive ionotropic effect. This leads to **tachycardia**. The effect of catecholamines on the bronchi occur via the β-2 receptor, the excitation of which leads to a relaxation of the smooth muscle cells, resulting in bronchodilation. At the same time, catecholamines act on the respiratory centre and induce **tachypnoea**.

Vomiting is thought to occur in patients with pheochromocytoma via direct stimulation of the vomiting centre by circulating catecholamines (King et al. 2010).

More common haematological changes in patients with pheochromocytoma are non-regenerative anaemia and leukocytosis. The anaemia is interpreted as **anaemia** of chronic disease. The **leukocytosis** is accompanied by eosinopenia and lymphopenia and can therefore be interpreted as a stress leukogram.

Renal symptoms in pheochromocytoma consist of PU/PD, azotaemia and proteinuria. **PU/PD** develops from polyuria, which is due to the inhibitory effect of catecholamines on ADH secretion. This leads to reduced water reabsorption in the distal tubule and collecting tube. Urine is formed iso- or hypostenuric and in greater volume. The loss of fluid reduces the blood volume, which produces centrally controlled thirst.

One explanation for the **mild azotaemia** is attributed to the vasoconstrictor effect of catecholamines via α receptors, which can result in reduced renal blood flow with ischaemia-induced damage to the glomerula. This is also seen as the cause of **proteinuria.**

The mild increase in **liver enzymes** is a consequence of the influence of catecholamines. On the one hand, the liver is supplied by nerve fibres of the autonomic nervous system. These induce, for example, communication between the liver and the central centres in the hypothalamus by metabolites or cytokines generating receptor impulses that reach the hypothalamus via sympathetic afferents. Secondly, catecholamines induce numerous liver functions, such as increased glycogenolysis and gluconeogenesis. Finally, Kupffer cells, resident macrophages in the liver parenchyma, secrete proinflammatory cytokines such as TNF-α, IL-1 and IL-6 under the influence of catecholamines. The increase in liver synthesis activity and the increased local concentration of proinflammatory cytokines contribute to hepatocyte dysfunction with an increased release of liver enzymes (Yang et al. 2000; Lelou et al. 2022) (Figure 43.6.5.1).

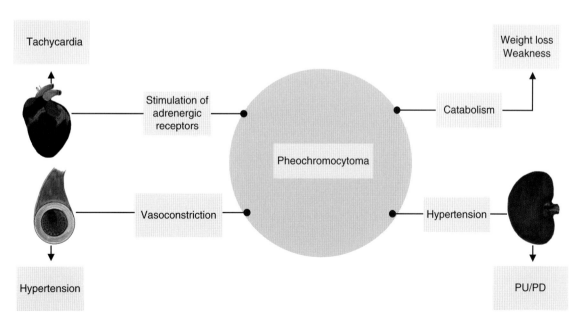

Figure 43.6.5.1 Pathophysiologic consequences of pheochromocytoma.

Therapy

Symptom	Therapy
Tumour	Surgery
β-antagonists	Atenolol (preparation for surgery)

References

Feldmann, E.C. and Nelson, R.W. (1996). *Canine and Feline Endocrinology and Reproduction*, 2e, 308. Saunders.

King, K.S., Darmani, N.A., Hughes, M.S. et al. (2010). Exercise-induced nausea and vomiting: another sign and symptom of pheochromocytoma and paraganglioma. *Endocrine* 37 (3): 403–407. https://doi.org/10.1007/s12020-010-9319-3.

Lelou, E., Corlu, A., Nesseler, N. et al. (2022). The role of catecholamines in pathophysiological liver processes. *Cell* 11 (6): 1021. https://doi.org/10.3390/cells11061021.

Rupala, K., Mittal, V., Gupta, R., and Yadav, R. (2017). Atypical presentation of pheochromocytoma: central nervous system pseudovasculitis. *Indian Journal of Urology: IJU: Journal of the Urological Society of India* 33 (1): 82–84. https://doi.org/10.4103/0970-1591.195760.

Yang, S., Koo, D.J., Zhou, M. et al. (2000). Gut-derived norepinephrine plays a critical role in producing hepatocellular dysfunction during early sepsis. *American Journal of Physiology. Gastrointestinal and Liver Physiology* 279 (6): G1274–G1281. https://doi.org/10.1152/ajpgi.2000.279.6.G1274.

Further Reading

Maher, E.R. Jr. and McNiel, E.A. (1997). Pheochromocytoma in dogs and cats. *The Veterinary Clinics of North America. Small Animal Practice* 27 (2): 359–380. https://doi.org/10.1016/s0195-5616(97)50037-4.

Reusch, C., Feldmann, E.C., Nelson, R.W. et al. (2015). *Canine and Feline Endocrinology*, 4e, 529. Elsevier.

44

Reproduction System

44.1

Pyometra

Definition

Pyometra is a purulent inflammation of the uterus.

Aetiology

The following causes are possible for the development of pyometra:

– Primary bacterial infection of the uterus in metoestrus
– Nidation prevention with oestrogen preparations
– Suppression of heat by means of progestogens
– Ovarian tumours (with hormonal activity)

However, hormonal dysregulation due to prolonged progesterone action without pregnancy and bacterial infection, usually by *Escherichia coli, are* seen as the most common causal factors. Dogs are clearly more frequently affected than cats, where the disease is rare (Table 44.1.1).

In metoestrus, there is initially an increase in the progesterone concentration. This induces hyperplasia of the endometrial glands and increased synthesis of glandular secretions, which collect in the uterine lumen. Since at the same time, under the influence of progesterone, the contractility of the myometrium is suspended, the secretion can remain in the lumen; in addition, the leucocytic reaction in the uterus is reduced (Dhaliwal et al. 1997; De Bosschere et al. 2002).

Pathogenesis

Due to the formation of an optimal environment in the uterus, bacterial infection can easily develop, usually with *E. coli*. The pathogens reach the uterus either haematogenously or as an ascending infection. The latter sometimes develops from bacterial cystitis (Wadås et al. 1996; Stone et al. 1988).

The pathogens bind to receptors of the brush border membrane of the endometrium (Johnson 1989). The infection that then develops, proceeds according to the usual rules of an infectious disease. A large amount of purulent secretion may form in the uterus (Figure 44.1.1).

Textbook of Small Animal Pathophysiology, First Edition. Stephan Neumann.
© 2025 John Wiley & Sons Ltd. Published 2025 by John Wiley & Sons Ltd.

Table 44.1.1 Bacteria detected in pyometra.

E. coli

Staphylococcus

Streptococcus

Klebsiella

Pasteurella

Pseudomonas

Proteus

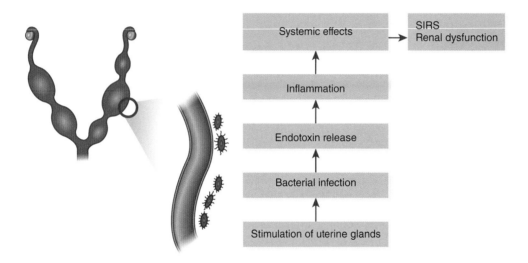

Figure 44.1.1 Pathogenesis of pyometra.

Diagnostics

Clinical signs	Clinical pathology	Imaging	Histopathology	Microbiology
PU/PD	Leucocytosis	**Ultrasonography** Dilated uterus	Not necessary	Pathogen detection for antibiosis
Vaginal discharge	Increased acute-phase proteins	Radiology		
		Increased uterus diameter		

Pathophysiologic Consequences

The pathophysiologic consequences of pyometra can be local or systemic.

Influenced organ systems	Clinical symptoms	Clinical pathological alterations
Systemic	Lethargy	Leucocytosis
Reproduction	Anorexia	Increased CRP (D), SAA (C)
	Fever	Hypoalbuminaemia
	PU/PD	Anaemia
	Vomiting	Increased liver enzymes
	Vulvar discharge	Proteinuria

The general symptoms of uterine inflammation **lethargy**, **anorexia** and **fever** can be attributed to the endotoxin action of the pathogen. Endotoxin is a lipopolysaccharide of the bacterial wall; it induces an inflammatory reaction with the synthesis of numerous, proinflammatory cytokines. These act via the autonomic nervous system or, after crossing the blood-brain barrier, directly on the nervous structures of the central nervous system (CNS). There, the microglia can also be activated to produce cytokines. The result is the non-specific symptoms, such as lethargy and anorexia (Lasselin et al. 2021).

The prominent symptom of **PU/PD** in patients with pyometra is primary polyuria with secondary polydipsia. The mechanisms described are disturbances in glomerular and tubular function. These influence the amount and composition of the primary filtrate. An important influencing factor is the reduced renal response to ADH. This physiologically induces the expression of aquaporins in the distal tubule and the collecting tubes and thus promotes the reabsorption of water. ADH acts via a receptor. Changes in receptor density or receptor response can cause primary polyuria in patients with pyometra.

Vomiting can occur as a result of central endotoxin action when the vomiting centre in the brain is activated. A second cause is peritonitis, which develops during uterine inflammation. Even before a rupture of the uterine wall, a translocation of bacteria into the abdominal cavity can occur. The inflammation of the uterine wall leads to a structural destruction of the epithelial cell structures with loss of the tight-junctions.

Changes in the laboratory parameters are primarily characterised by an intense inflammatory reaction. This is characterised by **leucocytosis with a left shift** or, in the case of a chronic inflammation of the uterus, a degenerative left shift can also develop.

In an inflammatory reaction, there is an increase in neutrophilic granulocytes in the blood. These partly originate from the granulocyte stores in the bone marrow. There, the neutrophilic granulocytes are present as a "juvenile" band neutrophils. Activation leads to the increased release of these cells into the blood, a left shift is present. If the inflammation is very pronounced, the number of band neutrophils is higher than that of the mature segmented neutrophils, in such a case a degenerative left shift is present.

The increase of positive acute-phase proteins (**CRP dog, SAA cat**) is also typical change and indicator of the inflammatory reaction. **Hypoalbuminaemia,** which is sometimes observed, can be evaluated as a negative acute phase. In contrast to the acute-phase proteins CRP or SAA, the concentration of albumin in the blood decreases during acute inflammation. Albumin is, therefore, referred to as a negative acute-phase protein. In the acute inflammatory phase, there is a reduced concentration of albumin in the blood. Possibly, the inflammatory reaction leads to an increase in the permeability of the capillary walls, which results in the leakage of fluid and proteins from the blood vessels. This results in a decrease in circulating blood volume and an increase in interstitial volume.

The **anaemia** in pyometra is usually moderate and represents anaemia of chronic inflammation. This develops as a result of cytokine action on the bone marrow.

Finally, the elevation of **liver enzymes** ALT and AST, which is moderate, based on endotoxin action on hepatocytes.

The **proteinuria** based on a glomerulopathy, which in turn may be a consequence of the massive inflammatory response, or, more likely, from an associated infection of the urinary tract organs.

Therapy

Symptom	Therapy
Infection	Antibiotics
Pyogenic process	Surgery, hormone therapy (e.g. Aglepristone)

References

De Bosschere, H., Ducatelle, R., Vermeirsch, H. et al. (2002). Estrogen-alpha and progesterone receptor expression in cystic endometrial hyperplasia and pyometra in the bitch. *Animal Reproduction Science* 70 (3–4): 251–259. https://doi.org/10.1016/s0378-4320(02)00013-1.

Dhaliwal, G.K., England, G.C., and Noakes, D.E. (1997). Immunocytochemical localization of estrogen and progesterone receptors in the uterus of the normal bitch during oestrus and metoestrus. *Journal of Reproduction and Fertility. Supplement* 51: 167–176.

Johnson, C. (1989). Uterine diseases. In: *Textbook of Veterinary Internal Medicine*, 3e (ed. S. Ettinger), 1797–1805. Philadelphia: WB Saunders.

Lasselin, J., Lekander, M., Benson, S. et al. (2021). Sick for science: experimental endotoxemia as a translational tool to develop and test new therapies for inflammation-associated depression. *Molecular Psychiatry* 26 (8): 3672–3683. https://doi.org/10.1038/s41380-020-00869-2.

Stone, E.A., Littman, M.P., Robertson, J.L., and Bovée, K.C. (1988). Renal dysfunction in dogs with pyometra. *Journal of the American Veterinary Medical Association* 193 (4): 457–464.

Wadås, B., Kühn, I., Lagerstedt, A.S., and Jonsson, P. (1996). Biochemical phenotypes of *Escherichia coli* in dogs: comparison of isolates isolated from bitches suffering from pyometra and urinary tract infection with isolates from faeces of healthy dogs. *Veterinary Microbiology* 52 (3–4): 293–300. https://doi.org/10.1016/s0378-1135(96)00067-3.

Further Reading

Hanh, N. D. (2009). On pyometra in dogs – A literature study and the presentation of two learning cases created with the Casus-System. Diss Munich.

44.2

Prostate Diseases

Aetiology and Pathogenesis

Prostate diseases occur as non-inflammatory benign prostatic hyperplasia or prostatic cysts. Prostatitis and prostate abscesses are inflammatory changes and finally prostate carcinoma is a malignant neoplasia of the organ.

A distinction is made between causalities:

Benign prostatic enlargement is hormone-dependent and occurs only in the intact male. An increase in the oestrogen-testosterone ratio results in the expression of more androgen receptors, which increase the effect of testosterone (Barsanti and Finco 1986).

Prostatitis is an inflammatory change of the prostate caused by a bacterial infection, usually with *Escherichia coli*. Other pathogens that occur in prostatitis are *Proteus, Staphylococcus, Streptococcus, Pseudomonas, Pasteurella* and *Brucella*. The inflammation can be diffuse or organised as a prostate abscess. The pathogens reach the prostate haematogenously or ascending via the urinary tract.

Prostate cysts occur intra-prostatically and para-prostatically. The intra-prostatic cysts can develop as a result of inflammatory or hyperplastic prostate disease. The prostatic remodelling processes can lead to a disturbance of the tissue architecture, resulting in obstructions of prostatic ducts that hinder the flow of secretions. This can lead to cystic dilatation. The causality of paraprostatic cysts is not fully understood. A dilatation of embryonic structures, such as the Wolffian duct (ductus mesonephricus) is discussed.

Prostate tumours are usually hormone-independent carcinomas with a high metastasis rate.

Diagnostics

Clinical signs	Clinical pathology	Imaging	Histopathology	Microbiology
Defaecation complaints Haematuria Pain	Non-specific	**Ultrasonography** Prostate enlargement, Parenchymal destruction **Radiology** Prostate enlargement	For diagnosis of carcinoma	Detection in prostatitis for antibiosis

Pathophysiologic Consequences

The consequences of prostate diseases are related to the respective genesis.

Textbook of Small Animal Pathophysiology, First Edition. Stephan Neumann.

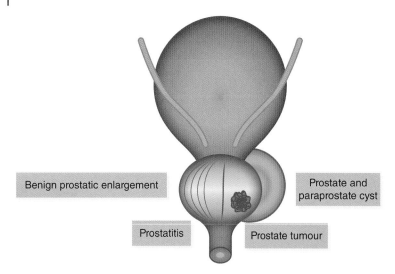

Figure 44.2.1 Overview of prostate diseases.

Influenced organ systems	Clinical symptoms
Urinary tract	Constipation
Bones, joints	Dysuria
	Haematuria
	Pain
	Paralysis

Constipation and **dysuria** are consequences of the enlargement of the prostate. In particular, the rectum is displaced dorsally by the enlarged prostate. The narrowing of the intestinal canal restricts defaecation. Affected dogs press on faeces and defaecate deformed faeces. Increased pressure during defaecation may cause rupture of small rectal vessels, resulting in haematochezia.

Obstruction of the cranial urethra or bladder neck may lead to dysuria. **Haematuria** may result either from leakage of inflamed prostatic secretions into the urethra or from rupture of small urethral vessels due to dysuria.

Both constipation and dysuria cause **pain** due to delayed bowel or bladder emptying or difficult defaecation or micturition. Prostate cancer tends to metastasise to the ventral lumbar vertebral bodies. Metastatic destruction of the vertebral bodies or invasion of the vertebral canal can cause **paralysis** due to compression of the spinal cord or cauda equina (Figure 44.2.1).

Therapy

Symptom	Therapy
Constipation, dysuria	Anti-androgens (e.g. Delmadinone, Osaterone)
Prostatitis	Antibiotics, pain killer (e.g. Morphine)
Prostate cysts, prostate abscess	Surgery

Reference

Barsanti, J.A. and Finco, D.R. (1986). Canine prostatic diseases. *The Veterinary Clinics of North America. Small Animal Practice* 16 (3): 587–599. https://doi.org/10.1016/s0195-5616(86)50063-2.

Further Reading

Palmieri, C., Fonseca-Alves, C.E., and Laufer-Amorim, R. (2022). A review on canine and feline prostate pathology. *Frontiers in Veterinary Science* 9: 881232. https://doi.org/10.3389/fvets.2022.881232.

45

Nerve System

45.1

Brain Tumours

Definition

Brain tumours are neoplasms that can arise from all histological structures of the central nervous system (CNS).

Aetiology

The genesis of brain tumours is mostly unknown. Primary and secondary tumours can be distinguished. A common intracranial tumour is a neoplasia of the pituitary gland; this is discussed in the specific clinical picture of Cushing's disease (Table 45.1.1).

Pathogenesis

The intracranial tumours grow expansively or infiltratively and can thus directly lead to compression of the nerve substance. Perineoplastic inflammation with oedema formation, intracranial haemorrhage and drainage disorders of the cerebrospinal fluid (CSF) with the formation of hydrocephalus are secondary consequences of growing brain tumours, which in turn cause compression of nerve substance.

Compensatory mechanisms of the CNS are a reduced CSF synthesis or a shift of the CSF towards the spinal subarachnoid space. Slow-growing tumours, such as meningiomas, can expand over long periods of time without noticeable clinical symptoms.

Further expansion of the tumour tissue leads to compression of intracranial vessels. This results in reduced perfusion of the nerve substance. This reacts promptly to a reduced supply, as considerable amounts of energy in the form of ATP are required for nervous function (Figure 45.1.1).

Diagnostics

Clinical signs	Clinical pathology	Imaging	Histopathology	Microbiology
Behavioural changes Involuntary movements Seizures	Non-specific	**CT/MRI** Presentation of the neoplasia	Is not usually carried out	Not necessary

Table 45.1.1 Brain tumours in dogs and cats in descending frequency.

Dog	Cat
Meningioma	Meningioma
Glioma	Ependymoma
Ependymoma	Astrocytoma
Haemangiosarcoma	Lymphoma
Lymphoma	Metastatic carcinoma
Metastatic carcinoma	Haemangiosarcoma

Source: Troxel et al. (2003) and Moore et al. (1996).

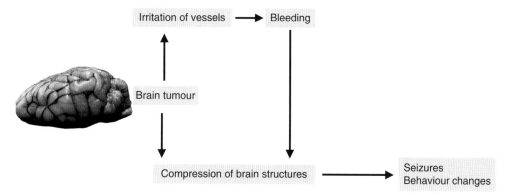

Figure 45.1.1 Pathogenesis of intracranial tumours.

Pathophysiologic Consequences

The pathophysiologic consequences are essentially based on the impaired function of different brain areas.

Influenced organ systems	Clinical symptoms
Central nervous system	Seizures
	Lethargy
	Head tilt
	Diminished vision
	Head pressing

The primary consequence of brain tumours is the compression and displacement of normal brain tissue. This can lead to a range of neurological symptoms, such as **seizures**, behavioural changes like **lethargy** and motor dysfunction. More specific symptoms are, for example, head tilt in cases of tumours in the vestibular apparatus. As the tumour grows and expands, it can cause increased pressure within the skull, leading to a condition known as 'intracranial hypertension', which can further exacerbate these symptoms. Brain tumours can also disrupt normal neuronal signalling and communication within the brain. As the tumour cells grow and divide, they can interfere with the normal connectivity and function of neurons, leading to cognitive deficits, memory impairment and other neurological symptoms. In addition, brain tumours can cause changes in the surrounding microenvironment, such as alterations in blood flow and oxygen delivery to the brain tissue. This can lead to tissue hypoxia, inflammation and the release of cytotoxic factors that can further damage surrounding brain tissue.

Therapy

Symptom	Therapy
Causal treatment	Radiation, chemotherapy, surgery
Symptoms	Antiepileptic drugs (e.g. Phenobarbital)

References

Moore, M.P., Bagley, R.S., Harrington, M.L., and Gavin, P.R. (1996). Intracranial tumors. *The Veterinary Clinics of North America. Small Animal Practice* 26 (4): 759–777. https://doi.org/10.1016/s0195-5616(96)50104-x.

Troxel, M.T., Vite, C.H., Van Winkle, T.J. et al. (2003). Feline intracranial neoplasia: retrospective review of 160 cases (1985–2001). *Journal of Veterinary Internal Medicine* 17 (6): 850–859. https://doi.org/10.1111/j.1939-1676.2003.tb02525.x.

Further Reading

Miller, A.D., Miller, C.R., and Rossmeisl, J.H. (2019). Canine primary intracranial cancer: aclinicopathologic and comparative review of glioma, meningioma, and choroid plexus Tumours. *Frontiers in Oncology* 9: 1151. http://dx.doi.org/10.3389/fonc.2019.01151.

45.2

Idiopathic Epilepsy

Definition/Aetiology

Idiopathic epilepsy is a seizure disorder that has central nervous causes but whose causality is unknown. It is characterised by short-term, seizure-like dysfunctions of the brain, which are due to excessive nervous discharges.

The disease is more common in the first three years of life and is typical in dogs. Certain breeds are predisposed, which makes a genetic cause likely (Table 45.2.1).

Pathogenesis

Although *idiopathic epilepsy* is by definition a disease of unknown aetiology, some alterations are associated with the clinical picture. Congenital disorders of ion channels are considered a possible causality. The ion channels themselves, or the transmitter receptors, seem to play a role. GABA transmitters, Na^+-K^+ and Ca^{2+} channels are therefore involved in epilepsy.

Controlled by calcium channels in the presynaptic area, an increased release of glutamate into the synaptic cleft can occur. This leads to overexcitation at the postsynaptic membrane, associated with an increased influx of sodium ions and the increasing formation of action potentials. At the same time, a reduction in the effect of GABA-dependent inhibitory neurons takes place (Figure 45.2.1).

Diagnostics

Clinical signs	Clinical pathology	Imaging	Histopathology	Microbiology
Seizures as petit male or grand male or status epilepticus	Non-specific	Non-specific	Is not usually carried out	Not necessary

Pathophysiologic Consequences

The pathophysiologic consequences are essentially based on the impaired function of different brain areas

Influenced organ systems	Clinical symptoms	Clinical pathology
Central Nervous System	Seizures	Increased enzymes CK, AST

Table 45.2.1 Breeds with predisposition to epilepsy.

Beagles

Bernese mountain dogs

Border collies

Boxers

Cocker spaniels

Dachshunds

Retriever

Shepherds

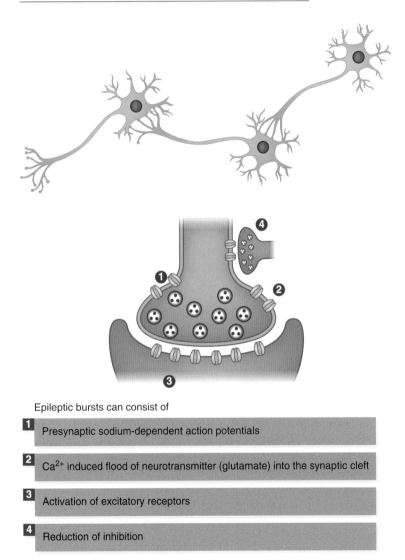

Epileptic bursts can consist of

1 Presynaptic sodium-dependent action potentials

2 Ca^{2+} induced flood of neurotransmitter (glutamate) into the synaptic cleft

3 Activation of excitatory receptors

4 Reduction of inhibition

Figure 45.2.1 Pathogenesis of idiopathic epilepsy.

The genesis of seizures in idiopathic epilepsy is already described in the pathogenesis. In the seizure state, the animals show a more or less distinct tonic-clonic convulsiveness.

Canine and feline idiopathic epilepsy can have significant pathophysiologic consequences that affect multiple organ systems and can lead to a range of clinical symptoms. The pathophysiology of idiopathic epilepsy is complex and multifactorial, involving the dysregulation of various cellular and molecular processes within the brain.

One of the primary pathophysiologic consequences of idiopathic epilepsy is the development of recurrent seizures. Seizures can lead to alterations in brain function, cognitive impairment and motor dysfunction. Repeated seizures can also lead to neuronal damage and loss, particularly in regions of the brain that are involved in seizure generation and propagation. In addition to the direct effects of seizures on brain function, idiopathic epilepsy can also have indirect effects on other organ systems. For example, prolonged or frequent seizures can lead to metabolic disturbances, such as hypoglycaemia, hypoxia and acidosis. These metabolic changes can cause additional neuronal damage and contribute to the development of further seizures. Idiopathic epilepsy can also lead to changes in behaviour and affective state. Seizures can be frightening and distressing for animals, leading to anxiety, fear and changes in personality.

Therapy

Symptom	Therapy
Seizures	Antiepileptic drugs (e.g. phenobarbital, potassium bromide, imepition, levetiracetam, diazepam)

Further Reading

Ekenstedt, K.J. and Oberbauer, A.M. (2013). Inherited epilepsy in dogs. *Topics in Companion Animal Medicine* 28 (2): 51–58. https://doi.org/10.1053/j.tcam.2013.07.001.

Forsgård, J.A., Metsähonkala, L., Kiviranta, A.M. et al. (2019). Seizure-precipitating factors in dogs with idiopathic epilepsy. *Journal of Veterinary Internal Medicine* 33 (2): 701–707. https://doi.org/10.1111/jvim.15402.

Podell, M., Volk, H.A., Berendt, M. et al. (2016). 2015 ACVIM small animal consensus statement on seizure management in dogs. *Journal of Veterinary Internal Medicine* 30 (2): 477–490. https://doi.org/10.1111/jvim.13841.

Watson, F., Packer, R.M.A., Rusbridge, C., and Volk, H.A. (2020). Behavioural changes in dogs with idiopathic epilepsy. *The Veterinary Record* 186 (3): 93. https://doi.org/10.1136/vr.105222.

45.3

Intervertebral Disc Disease

Definition

A *discopathy* is a degeneration of the disc material with a displacement of parts of the nucleus pulposus into the spinal canal.

Aetiology

Different diseases can lead to protrusion of the disc material. This article focuses on the breed-specific incidents of type Hansen I in chondrodystrophic dog breeds and type Hansen II in non-chondrodystrophic dog breeds. The fact that the diseases accumulate in certain dog breeds makes a genetic predisposition likely. Short-legged dog breeds, namely dachshunds, are frequently affected by Hansen I. Here, chondrodystrophy is seen as a causal factor. This is characterised by a metaplasia of cartilage material with a subsequent loss of stability. Different gene mutations are suspected of causing chondrodystrophy. For example, mutations in the fibroblast growth factor (FGF) gene have been found in chondrodystrophic dog breeds. FGF genes are involved in a number of embryological developmental processes; they have a proliferative effect and can control cell differentiation and migration. FGF binds to tyrosine kinase-type receptors and indexes protein expression via secondary signal transduction. Discopathy also occurs in cats, but much less frequently (Lu et al. 2006; Dailey et al. 2005; Brown et al. 2017).

Pathogenesis

Degeneration of the disc material is the essential pathogenetic step that precedes disc herniation. The degeneration process extends to the nucleus pulposus and the annulus fibrosus. The former lies as a bean-shaped structure in the centre of the disc. The nucleus pulposus consists of an osmotically active basic structure consisting of collagens (collagen-2), proteoglycans, and glucosamine glycans, predominantly as chondroitin-6-sulphate and keratin sulphate. The structures are synthesised by notochord cells and show high osmotic activity. This leads to the fact that the nucleus pulposus consists of almost 90% water.

The annulus fibrosis surrounds the nucleus pulposus and is composed of chondrocytes and collagen (collagen-1) forming fibrocytes. The water content in the annulus fibrosus is lower than in the nucleus and is about 60% (Johnson et al. 2010).

During disc degeneration, the notochordal cells of the nucleus pulposus are replaced by chondrocytes, which cause fibrocartilage metaplasia with the loss of proteoglycans and thus the loss of water as well as their replacement by collagen, mostly type I. The result is metaplastic calcification of the nucleus pulposus associated with cell necrosis. Parallel to the degeneration of the nucleus pulposus, degeneration of the annulus fibrosus can occur. This changes the lamellar collagen structure of the annulus and reduces its resistance.

Minimal trauma can cause the annulus fibrosus to tear and nucleus material to penetrate into the spinal canal (Hansen type I). If there is only a partial rupture of the annulus and thus a protrusion into the spinal canal, this is called 'Hansen type II' (Figure 45.3.1).

Textbook of Small Animal Pathophysiology, First Edition. Stephan Neumann.
© 2025 John Wiley & Sons Ltd. Published 2025 by John Wiley & Sons Ltd.

Figure 45.3.1 Hansen type I and Hansen type II.

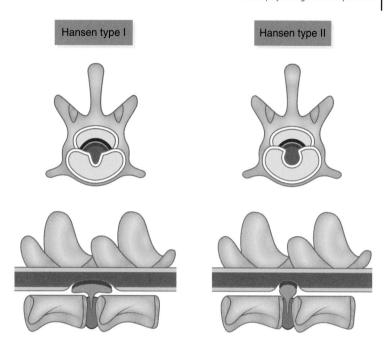

Diagnostics

Clinical signs	Clinical pathology	Imaging	Histopathology	Microbiology
Paresis	Non-specific	Radiology/**CT/MRI**	Not necessary	Not necessary
Paralysis		Prolapse detection		
Pain				
Faecal and urinary problems				

Pathophysiologic Consequences

The consequences of a herniated disc focus primarily on locomotion. Paresis or paralysis leads to movement disorders. Another component is pain.

Influenced organ systems	Clinical symptoms
Systemic	Paresis/paralysis
Central nervous system	Pain
Urinary tract	Kidney failure
	Cystitis

Prolapsed disc material compresses the nerve cord, the local vessels and causes inflammation. These factors explain the clinical consequences of a herniated disc.

Nerve fibre degeneration develops due to direct compression or compression of the supplying vessels with restriction of microcirculation and ischaemia. This is accompanied by nerve cell apoptosis and secondary inflammation. Both lead to dysfunction and cause **paralysis**.

The **pain** of a herniated disc is caused by irritation of free nerve endings of the A-δ fibres and C-fibres. They normally have a high mechanical stimulus threshold, but this is lowered under pathological conditions, such as inflammation.

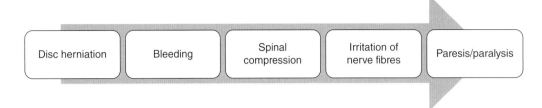

Figure 45.3.2 Consequences of the herniated disc.

In addition, local inflammation causes a pain response via the various inflammatory mediators, such as bradykinin, serotonin, histamines and prostaglandins. For example, phospholipase A2 induces arachidonic acid to synthesise eicosanoids (leukotrienes and prostaglandins) from cell membrane lipids, both of which are important mediators of pain and inflammation.

Both paralysis and pain affect the emptying of the bladder. Increased amounts of residual urine can cause bacterial colonisation and thus cystitis. Accordingly, patients with herniated discs should be monitored with regard to their urine output. If large amounts of urine remain in the bladder, or if urine output is disturbed overall, post-renal failure can develop from a herniated disc (Akter et al. 2020) (Figure 45.3.2).

Therapy

Symptom	Therapy
Pain	Analgesics (e.g. Morphine)
Neurological deficits/pain	Surgery
Neurological deficits	Physiotherapy

References

Akter, F., Yu, X., Qin, X. et al. (2020). The pathophysiology of degenerative cervical myelopathy and the physiology of recovery following decompression. *Frontiers in Neuroscience* 14: 138. https://doi.org/10.3389/fnins.2020.00138.

Brown, E.A., Dickinson, P.J., Mansour, T. et al. (2017). FGF4 retrogene on CFA12 is responsible for chondrodystrophy and intervertebral disc disease in dogs. *Proceedings of the National Academy of Sciences of the United States of America* 114 (43): 11476–11481. https://doi.org/10.1073/pnas.1709082114.

Dailey, L., Ambrosetti, D., Mansukhani, A., and Basilico, C. (2005). Mechanisms underlying differential responses to FGF signalling. *Cytokine & Growth Factor Reviews* 16 (2): 233–247. https://doi.org/10.1016/j.cytogfr.2005.01.007.

Johnson, J.A., da Costa, R.C., and Allen, M.J. (2010). Micromorphometry and cellular characteristics of the canine cervical intervertebral discs. *Journal of Veterinary Internal Medicine* 24 (6): 1343–1349. https://doi.org/10.1111/j.1939-1676.2010.0613.x.

Lu, P., Minowada, G., and Martin, G.R. (2006). Increasing Fgf4 expression in the mouse limb bud causes polysyndactyly and rescues the skeletal defects that result from loss of Fgf8 function. *Development (Cambridge, England)* 133 (1): 33–42. https://doi.org/10.1242/dev.02172.

Further Reading

Fenn, J., Olby, N.J., and Canine Spinal Cord Injury Consortium (CANSORT-SCI) (2020). Classification of intervertebral disc disease. *Frontiers in Veterinary Science* 7: 579025. https://doi.org/10.3389/fvets.2020.579025.

Stigen, O. (1991). Calcification of intervertebral discs in the dachshund. A radiographic study of 327 young dogs. *Acta Veterinaria Scandinavica* 32 (2): 197–203. http://dx.doi.org/10.1186/BF03546981.

45.4

Peripheral Neuropathy

Definition

Neuropathies are diseases of the peripheral nerves. These can develop as a result of different causalities.

Aetiology

The causes of neuropathies can be divided into congenital, toxic, metabolic, inflammatory, vascular and idiopathic forms. The diseases are more common in dogs than in cats.

Genetic (e.g.)	Toxic	Metabolic	Inflammatory	Vascular
Boxer	Aminoglycosides	Diabetic	Acute polyradiculoneuritis	Ischaemic neuropathy
Progressive Axonopathy	Heavy metals	Hypothyroid		
Norwegian Forest Cat	Lead	Uraemic		
Sphingomyelinosis	Mercury			
West Highland White Terrier	Organophosphates			
Globoid leukodystrophy				

Pathogenesis

In principle, neuropathies are differentiated according to their occurrence in mono- and polyneuropathies and according to their respective function in sensitive, motor or autonomous.

Based on the primary disease some secondary neuropathies can be differentiated.

Diabetic neuropathy results from vascular and metabolic consequences for the peripheral nerve. Due to the reduction in peripheral blood flow caused by vasculitis triggered by diabetes, axonal atrophy develops, resulting in a reduction in nerve conduction velocity with a functional neuropathy. At the same time, due to the hyperglycaemia, the sorbitol concentration in the nerve cell increases via the polyol pathway. This results in a reduction of the myo-inositol concentration, which negatively affects the activity of Na^+-K^+-ATPase. The formation of ROS simultaneously increases the oxidative stress within the nerve cells.

Uraemic neuropathy leads to nerve cell degeneration characterised by axonal atrophy and demyelination. The influence of various uraemic toxins on the nerve cell is considered to be the cause. One candidate is guanidine. Guanidines are arginine metabolites; arginine is a component of the urea cycle. In the case of an increased urea concentration, azotaemia, an altered conversion of arginine to ornithine occurs via guanidines, so these are present in increased concentrations in uraemia. They have an inhibitory effect on GABA receptors and an activating effect on N-methyl-D-aspartate (NMDA) receptors at the nerve cell (Franch et al. 2008).

Further influences can result from inhibition of Na^+-K^+-ATPase and thus a dysfunction of the transmembrane Na^+ pump. Inhibition of Na^+ efflux reduces the resting membrane potential (Nielsen 1973; Welt et al. 1964).

Finally, the mechanism of neuropathy in **hypothyroidism** will be explained. Atrophies of the axon also develop in connection with this endocrinopathy. A possible explanation is seen in the general metabolic performance of the thyroid hormones. Their deficiency has an influence on mitochondrial function and can lead to reduced ATP provision. Consequences of the energy deficiency are disturbances in ion transport, especially of Na^+ through a reduction in the activity of the Na^+-K^+-ATPase (Sidenius et al. 1987).

Diagnostics

Clinical signs	Clinical pathology	Imaging	Histopathology	Microbiology
Pain	Non-specific	Mostly non-specific	Maybe diagnostic	Not necessary
Neurological deficits		MRI for nerve sheath tumours		

Pathophysiologic Consequences

The consequences of neuropathies depend very much on the damaged nerve. Disturbances in locomotion, sensation or even pain can develop.

Influenced organ systems	Clinical symptoms
Neuromuscular system	Lameness
	Pain

Therapy

Symptom	Therapy
Pain	Painkillers (e.g. morphines, NSAID)
Paralysis	Physiotherapy

References

Franch, H.A., McClellan, W.C., and Mitch, W.E. (2008). Chronic kidney disease: pathophysiology and influence of dietary protein. In: *Seldin and Giebisch's the Kidney*, Physiology and Pathophysiology, 4e, vol. 2 (ed. R.J. Alpern and S.C. Hebert), 2615–2669.

Nielsen, V.K. (1973). The peripheral nerve function in chronic renal failure. V. Sensory and motor conduction velocity. *Acta Medica Scandinavica* 194 (5): 445–454. https://doi.org/10.1111/j.0954-6820.1973.tb19470.x.

Sidenius, P., Nagel, P., Larsen, J.R. et al. (1987). Axonal transport of slow component a in sciatic nerves of hypo- and hyperthyroid rats. *Journal of Neurochemistry* 49 (6): 1790–1795. https://doi.org/10.1111/j.1471-4159.1987.tb02437.x.

Welt, L.G., Sachs, J.R., and McManus, T.J. (1964). An ion transport defect in erythrocytes from uremic patients. *Transactions of the Association of American Physicians* 77: 169–181.

Further Reading

Wolff, B. (2004). *Morphological Studies on Endocrine and Metabolic Neuropathies in Dogs, Cats and Horses*. Diss Munich.

46

Joints

46.1

Arthritis

Definition

Arthritis is defined as inflammation of one or more joints.

Aetiology

Causes of arthritis are often based on infectious or immunological causalities. Depending on the extent of the joint damage, they are further divided into erosive and non-erosive forms. A further classification is made according to the duration of the disease into acute or chronic. Finally, arthritis can occur as monoarthritis or polyarthritis. Arthritis occur more frequently in dogs than in cats.

	Erosive	Non-erosive
Infectious	Bacterial infection (*Staphylococci*, *Streptococci*) (D/C) Leishmaniasis (D)	Borreliosis (D) Anaplasmosis (D)
Non-infectious	Rheumatoid (D)	Immunological (SLE, polyarthritis-myositis, polyarthritis-meningitis) (D) Reactive (D)

D – Dog, C – Cat

Pathogenesis

The pathogenesis of the different forms of arthritis may differ. First, the pathogenesis of **infectious arthritis** will be presented. The invasion of bacteria into the joint can occur directly through trauma, such as a bite wound. Alternatively, bacteria may be moved from an infection in the organism to one or more joints by bacteraemia. In this case, the bacteria enter the circulation freely or are bound to defence cells due to the increased blood flow caused by the inflammation. The bacteria are distributed with the blood, and in areas of low blood flow velocity, the bacteria can enter the tissue from the blood. In the joint area, the bacteria migrate from the synovial capillaries into the joint space. There, the bacteria multiply and invade the joint cartilage and the joint capsule. Due to the inflammatory cell infiltration, the joint capsule thickens and, in the chronic course, fibrosis occur. Intra-articular pressure increases in the joint due to the inflammation, leading to obstruction and thrombosis in the synovial capillaries with the consequence of ischaemia and reduced supply to the articular cartilage. This can lead to destruction of the articular cartilage. The articular inflammatory cell infiltration also destroys the articular cartilage through mediators.

Textbook of Small Animal Pathophysiology, First Edition. Stephan Neumann.
© 2025 John Wiley & Sons Ltd. Published 2025 by John Wiley & Sons Ltd.

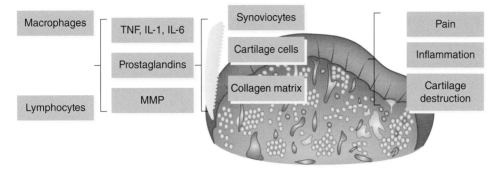

Figure 46.1.1 Mechanism of arthritis.

The pathogenesis of **immunological arthritis** will be presented using the example of rheumatoid arthritis. Triggered by different causes in the sense of an autoimmune reaction, CD4+ T lymphocytes are activated. These activate B lymphocytes into plasma cells which synthesise immunoglobulins. As a result, immune complexes are formed which can be deposited in various tissues, such as the joints. This in turn induces an inflammatory response. On the other hand, CD4+ T lymphocytes activate mononuclear inflammatory cells and synovial fibroblasts to secrete proinflammatory cytokines. These induce an inflammatory response with IL-8 induced angiogenesis via activation of endothelial cells. At the same time, osteoclasts are activated and induce destruction of the subchondral bone, from which chondrocyte degeneration may develop, as regeneration of articular cartilage occurs through the subchondral bone. Suppression of matrix metalloproteinase (MMP) inhibitors promotes destruction of articular cartilage. The morphological consequences of this immunologically triggered arthritis are hyperplasia of the synovium, formation of granulation tissue leading to pannus formation. The result is erosive destruction of the joint structures.

There are different types of immune-mediated and reactive arthritis. Vaccine-associated reactive arthritis (VARA) is one type of reactive arthritis that has been associated with certain vaccines in dogs and should be explained. The molecular mechanisms underlying VARA are not fully understood, but it is believed that the vaccine components may trigger an immune response that leads to the development of arthritis symptoms. This response may be mediated by immune cells, such as T-cells and B-cells, as well as cytokines and other signalling molecules. In dogs with VARA, the immune response is directed against the joint tissue, causing inflammation and damage. This response may be triggered by the presence of certain vaccine components, such as adjuvants, which are substances that are added to vaccines to enhance the immune response. The development of VARA may also be influenced by other factors, such as the dog's genetics, age and overall health status. Certain breeds may be more susceptible to developing VARA than others, and older dogs or those with pre-existing joint disease may be at a higher risk (Figure 46.1.1).

Diagnostics

Clinical signs	Clinical pathology	Imaging	Histopathology	Microbiology
Lameness	Cytology	**Radiology/CT**	Rarely necessary	Mandatory in infectious arthritis
Pain	Synovia, leucocytes	Erosive arthritis		
Swollen joints	Immunological tests			
	Serum ANA-titre			
	Rheumatoid factors			

Pathophysiologic Consequences

The arthritis may be local events or become systemic, especially if they are septic in nature.

Influenced organ systems	Clinical symptoms
Bones, joints	Lameness
Muscles	Weakness
Systemic	Anorexia
	Fever

Infectious arthritis develops from local or systemic infections. Common pathogens in dogs and cats are *Staphylococci* and *Streptococci* as causative agents of erosive infectious arthritis. Leishmaniasis can cause erosive or non-erosive arthritis. Lyme disease and anaplasmosis are systemic infections with joint involvement in which non-erosive arthritis usually develops (both diseases are detailed in Chapter 48.3.1 and Chapter 48.4.3.).

Rheumatoid arthritis is predominantly polyarthritic in the distal joints of the extremities (carpus). There, lympho-plasma cellular synovitis and destruction of the articular cartilage and subchondral bone develops. This leads to the clinical symptoms of lameness and joint pain. Due to the immunological reaction, specific immunoglobulins, rheumatoid factors can be detected elevated in the blood at times.

Finally, so-called 'reactive arthritis', which have an immunological cause and are seen in connection with infections in the gastrointestinal tract, neoplasia or after vaccinations, lead to mono- or polyarthritis, especially of the distal limb joints. A peripheral inflammatory reaction recognisable by leukocytosis and an increased CRP concentration may be present.

Therapy

Symptom	Therapy
Infectious arthritis	Antibiosis after resistance test
Non-infectious arthritis	Immunosuppressants (e.g. prednisolone, cyclosporine, cyclophosphamide, azathioprine)

Further Reading

García-Arias, M., Balsa, A., and Mola, E.M. (2011). Septic arthritis. Best practice & research. *Clinical Rheumatology* 25 (3): 407–421. https://doi.org/10.1016/j.berh.2011.02.001.

Lee, D.M. and Weinblatt, M.E. (2001). Rheumatoid arthritis. *Lancet (London, England)* 358 (9285): 903–911. https://doi.org/10.1016/S0140-6736(01)06075-5.

Mathews, C.J., Weston, V.C., Jones, A. et al. (2010). Bacterial septic arthritis in adults. *Lancet (London, England)* 375 (9717): 846–855. https://doi.org/10.1016/S0140-6736(09)61595-6.

Schmitt, S.K. (2017). Reactive arthritis. *Infectious Disease Clinics of North America* 31 (2): 265–277. https://doi.org/10.1016/j.idc.2017.01.002.

Scott, D.L., Wolfe, F., and Huizinga, T.W. (2010). Rheumatoid arthritis. *Lancet (London, England)* 376 (9746): 1094–1108. https://doi.org/10.1016/S0140-6736(10)60826-4.

46.2

Osteoarthritis

Definition

Osteoarthritis is a chronic progressive degenerative joint disease.

Aetiology

Different aetiologies are seen as reasons of joint arthrosis. These can be direct diseases of the joint. These include congenital deformities or trauma. Systemic influencing factors, such as weight, which lead to degeneration of the joint structures over a lifetime, must be distinguished from these. Arthrosis occurs in dogs and cats, although dogs are more frequently affected.

Local causes	Systemic causes
Congenital deformities	Obesity (D/C)
Hip dysplasie (D)	Age
Elbow dysplasia (D)	Race (D)
Osteochondrosis (D)	
Trauma (D/C)	
Infection (D/C)	

D – Dog, C – Cat

Pathogenesis

Osteoarthritis can be differentiated as primary or secondary form. The primary form is diagnosed when pathogenetic factors are unknown. In contrast, secondary osteoarthritis is caused either by congenital disorders or is acquired.

Osteoarthritis affects all joint structures, i.e. bone, synovial membrane, muscles, tendons and ligaments. The disease is triggered by synovitis, cartilage degradation, subchondral bone remodelling and osteophyte formation. This process continues until the joint progressively stiffens and ankylosis begins.

The synovial inflammation is carried by the synovial cells and macrophages which secrete proinflammatory cytokines, such as interleukin-1-β (IL-1 β), IL-6, IL-17, tumour necrosis factor-α (TNF-α), TGF-β. The synovial membrane thickens, and the synovia produced shows loss of function through reduction of viscosity.

The involvement of cartilage cells in osteoarthritis begins with the destruction of the cells by fissures and mechanical stress. There is secretion of cytokines, such as IL-1-β, IL-6, TNF-α and proteinases (mainly matrix metalloproteinases [MMPs] such as MMP-1), which lead to matrix degradation. Instead of collagen II and aggrecan, more type X collagen is produced. In addition, pathological calcification takes place. These factors are responsible for the degradation of cartilage.

Textbook of Small Animal Pathophysiology, First Edition. Stephan Neumann.
© 2025 John Wiley & Sons Ltd. Published 2025 by John Wiley & Sons Ltd.

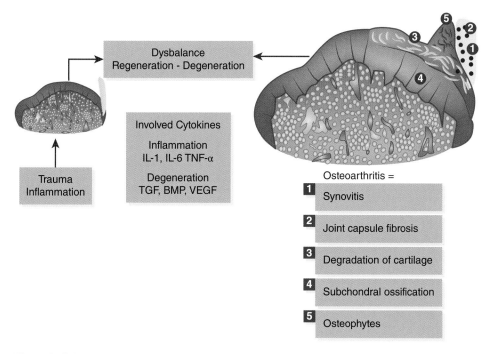

Figure 46.2.1 Pathogenesis of the development of osteoarthritis.

Mechanisms of endochondral ossification take place in the subchondral bone. Osteoblasts and osteoclasts are activated and begin increased bone turnover. This bone turnover leads to a thickened subchondral bone mass of inferior quality, as the new bone is less mineralised. Growth factors, such as vascular endothelial growth factor (VEGF) initiate vascular infiltration and neoangiogenesis towards cartilage. In addition, osteophytes are built up at predisposed positions and subchondral cysts develop. Histologically, microfractures are seen in areas of cartilage damage. As subchondral bone is strongly innervated, an important pain generation in osteoarthritis could be localised here (Figure 46.2.1).

Diagnostics

Clinical signs	Clinical pathology	Imaging	Histopathology	Microbiology
Restricted range of motion of the joints Pain Lameness	Non-specific	**Radiology/CT** Articular remodelling processes	Usually not necessary maybe to exclude neoplasia	Not necessary

Pathophysiologic Consequences

The consequences of osteoarthritis are localised to the joints.

Influenced organ systems	Clinical symptoms
Bones, joints	Lameness
Muscles	Pain

Pain and limited range of motion are the main reasons for lameness in osteoarthritis. The limited mobility is essentially due to capsular fibrosis. After the resting phase, the fibrosis must first be stretched, which explains the initial lameness. In addition, associated muscles of arthritic joints also show fibrotic remodelling, which also leads to a restricted 'range of motion'.

Therapy

Symptom	Therapy
Pain	Analgesics, NSAID
Limited range of motion	Physiotherapy

Further Reading

Bruecker, K.A., Benjamino, K., Vezzoni, A. et al. (2021). Canine elbow dysplasia: medial compartment disease and osteoarthritis. *The Veterinary Clinics of North America. Small Animal Practice* 51 (2): 475–515. https://doi.org/10.1016/j.cvsm.2020.12.008.

McCoy, A.M. (2015). Animal models of osteoarthritis: comparisons and key considerations. *Veterinary Pathology* 52 (5): 803–818. https://doi.org/10.1177/0300985815588611.

Mehana, E.E., Khafaga, A.F., and El-Blehi, S.S. (2019). The role of matrix metalloproteinases in osteoarthritis pathogenesis: an updated review. *Life Sciences* 234: 116786. https://doi.org/10.1016/j.lfs.2019.116786.

Sanderson, R.O., Beata, C., Flipo, R.M. et al. (2009). Systematic review of the management of canine osteoarthritis. *The Veterinary Record* 164 (14): 418–424. https://doi.org/10.1136/vr.164.14.418.

47

Haematology

47.1

Physiological Functions of Red Blood Cells

Functions

Erythrocytes are the most common type of cell in the blood. Their number is approximately 6.2 million/µl in dogs and approximately 7.2 million/µl in cats. Erythrocytes in mammals are nucleus-free and have a diameter of 6.3 µm in the cat and 7.3 µm in the dog. Their thickness is 2 µm. Erythrocytes are flexible and can therefore pass through even the smallest capillaries. The erythrocyte consists mainly of water (65–68%). The structural part of the erythrocyte consists mainly of haemoglobin (approximately 90% of the dry mass). The essential function of the erythrocyte is the transport of oxygen. The transport of bicarbonate also takes place to a smaller extent via the erythrocytes. Thus, they are also involved in the acid-base balance.

The formation of new erythrocytes (haematopoiesis) is in the bone marrow after birth. There, blood cells emerge from totipotent stem cells. These are localised in niches of the red bone marrow, which are particularly pronounced in the large tubular bones, the pelvic bones, the vertebrae and the ribs.

Stem cells are able to proliferate and then differentiate into red blood cell progenitors. Differentiation takes place under the influence of cytokines, essentially colony-stimulating factors. Numerous growth factors are involved in erythropoiesis (Table 47.1.1).

During the differentiation process, nucleated proerythroblasts develop first, and then they lose numerous cell components including the nucleus during further differentiation. This reduces the cell size and the cell structure. In particular, the concave cell shape of the erythrocyte is a consequence of the loss of internal structures. The enucleation of the erythrocyte occurs around the middle of the approximately seven-day differentiation period. It consists of condensation and subsequent peripheral enucleation. The latter is achieved by actin filaments of the cytoskeleton which, under the influence of GTPases, move the cell nucleus from the cell centre to the cell membrane. There, the cell nucleus is enucleated in the form of a vesicle formation surrounded by cell membrane. This causes the erythrocyte to shrink. The erythrocyte change including enucleation leads to the erythrocytes becoming more flexible. In addition, the maturation process leads to less energy being consumed in the erythrocyte itself (Figure 47.1.1).

The entire development time of an erythrocyte takes about seven days. In humans, approximately 2.5 million erythrocytes are formed per second. At the end of the differentiation process, the nucleus-less erythrocytes are released into the blood system.

An important regulator of erythropoiesis is erythropoietin.

Erythropoietin is a polypeptide consisting of 165 amino acids. It has a structure composed of four α-helices. Erythropoietin is predominantly formed in peritubular fibroblasts of the kidney. Erythropoietin reaches the bone marrow via the blood. There it binds via an erythropoietin receptor to the erythrocyte surface of the Erythroid Burst Forming Unit (BFU-E) type progenitor cells. Tyrosine kinases mediate signal transduction. Subsequently, the cell differentiates into the more mature progenitor cell type Erythroid Colony Forming Unit (CFU-E) and finally into the erythrocyte. The stimulus for the production of erythropoietin is a reduced oxygen saturation of the renal arteries. The consequence is an intracellular shift of a 'hypoxia-induced factor' (HIF) from the cytoplasm to the nucleus, which leads to the expression of erythropoietin.

Erythrocytes have a lifespan of 70–100 days. Due to their loss of mitochondria, they are only capable of synthesising ATP via anaerobic glycolysis, which only allows a small amount of ATP formation. The consequence is an age-related further reduction of energy formation in the erythrocyte. This eventually leads to disturbances in membrane function and

Table 47.1.1   Growth factors and cytokines in haematopoiesis.

Growth factor	Function
Erythropoietin	Differentiation, proliferation
Granulocyte macrophage colony-stimulating factor	White blood cell growth factor
IL-3	Differentiation and proliferation of myeloid progenitor cells
Stem cell factor	Regulates haematopoietic stem cells in the bone marrow
Granulocyte colony-stimulating factor	Inducer of haematopoietic stem cell mobilisation from the bone marrow into the bloodstream
IGF	Inhibits apoptosis in haematopoietic progenitor cells

Source: Adapted from Singh et al. (2014).

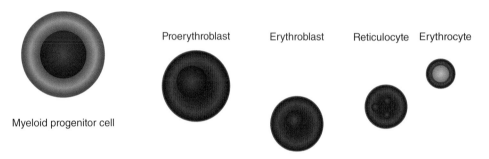

Figure 47.1.1   Development of the erythrocytes.

membrane structure. The latter is characterised by a change in the phospholipid layer and is recognised by macrophages, which eliminate the ageing erythrocytes.

The process is located in the spleen or liver.

Haemoglobin Formation

Haemoglobin is the most abundant protein in the erythrocyte and occupies about 90% of the dry mass of the erythrocyte cell. Structurally, a haemoglobin molecule is composed of two α polypeptides and two β polypeptides, and four porphyrin ring systems are embedded in the protein structure as haem per haemoglobin molecule. The latter are formed in the mitochondria. One molecule of oxygen can be bound per haem molecule, i.e. a total of four molecules of oxygen per haemoglobin molecule. Oxygen binds to an iron ion, which is located in the centre of the porphyrin ring. This iron ion is 2+ charged in order to be able to bind oxygen. The binding of oxygen oxidises the iron molecule to Fe^{3+}. In this state, the molecule is called 'oxyhaemoglobin'. Oxidised iron can no longer take up oxygen, so that after the release of oxygen the iron ion must be reduced again. The presence of haemoglobin increases the oxygen capacity of the blood a hundredfold, underlining the usefulness of the molecule.

The degradation of haemoglobin is located in the mononuclear phagocyte system (MPS).

In the process, the haem molecule is broken down by haemoxygenase to biliverdin, from which bilirubin is formed by reduction. Bound to albumin, bilirubin is transported to the liver. The bilirubin bound to albumin is also called 'indirect bilirubin'. Via a transporter for organic anions (OATPs), bilirubin is taken up into the hepatocytes where it is conjugated by uridine diphosphate (UDP)-glucuronyltransferase (UGT) to bilirubin mono- or diglucuronide. The conjugated bilirubin diglucuronide is also known as 'direct bilirubin' or 'conjugated bilirubin' and is secreted into the bile by active transport via the multidrug-resistance-related protein 2 (MRP2) transporter and, to a lesser extent, into the blood via MRP3 transporters and eliminated renally. In the colon, the conjugated bilirubin is deglucuronised by bacterial enzymes and finally degraded in several reductions to stercobilin and urobilin, which are responsible for the characteristic dark colour of the faeces.

Iron Metabolism

The importance of iron for oxygen transport means that the majority of iron in the organism is bound in haemoglobin. Another iron-binding molecule is myoglobin. About one-third of the body's iron is stored in liver cells or bound in macrophages of the MPS. Since iron ions react cytotoxically, iron is usually bound to proteins. Ferritin is the essential intracellular iron storage protein. Unbound ferritin is called 'apoferritin'.

Iron is supplied through the diet. The iron ions are usually absorbed as Fe^{2+} in the duodenum and jejunum through transcellular transport. In the blood, iron binds to the transport protein apotransferrin, from which transferrin is formed. This transports the iron ions into the bone marrow, where it binds to transferrin receptors of the erythroblasts. These are also found in body cells, but the receptor density is particularly high on the erythroblasts. After transferrin binds to the protein-receptor binding, the iron ion is released and transferrin is again available for iron transport as apotransferrin. The iron ion is transported intracellularly into the mitochondria, where the ion is incorporated into the porphyrin ring system under the influence of haem synthetase and haem is formed. Iron not used for the synthesis of haemoglobin is stored as ferritin or haemosiderin.

The regulation of iron metabolism is controlled by the hormone 'hepcidin'. Hepcidin is synthesised in the liver; triggers are the iron concentration in the organism, erythropoiesis and oxygen saturation. Hepcidin influences the expression of ferroportin, a transmembrane iron transport protein, which is expressed in many cells, but especially in enterocytes.

During erythrocyte degradation, iron is released during the degradation of porphyrin in the macrophages of the MPS and is again available for metabolism (Figure 47.1.2).

Extramedullary haematopoiesis is the formation of blood cells outside the bone marrow in response to reduced haematopoiesis in the bone marrow. Causes of reduced haematopoiesis are infections or myeloproliferative changes in the bone marrow.

Histologically, erythroblast nests are found outside the bone marrow in the tissue. Common sites for the development of extramedullary haematopoiesis are the liver and the spleen. Different theories exist on the origin of extramedullary haematopoiesis. One of these is that haematopoietic stem cells are translocated from the bone marrow to other tissues and induce haematopoiesis there. Another theory is that sessile haematopoietic stem cells are activated outside the bone marrow when medullary haematopoiesis is reduced and lead to haematopoiesis (Schütz 2009) (Figure 47.1.3).

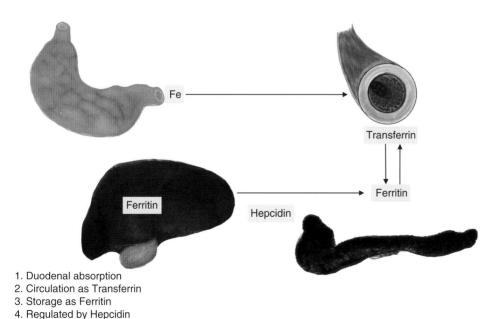

1. Duodenal absorption
2. Circulation as Transferrin
3. Storage as Ferritin
4. Regulated by Hepcidin

Figure 47.1.2 Iron metabolism.

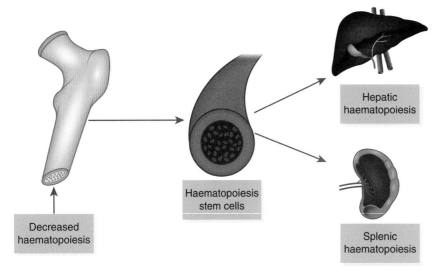

Figure 47.1.3 Extramedullary haematopoiesis.

References

Schütz, K. (2009). Morphological picture, frequency and localisation of extramedullary haematopoiesis Literature review and retrospective study. Dissertation Berlin.

Singh, V.K., Saini, A., and Chandra, R. (2014). Role of erythropoietin and other growth factors in ex vivo erythropoiesis. *Advances in Regenerative Medicine* https://doi.org/10.1155/2014/426520.

47.2

Erythrocytosis

Definition

Erythrocytosis is defined as an abnormal increase in the red blood cell (RBC) mass. Polycythaemia vera, a myeloproliferative disease with an increase in all bone marrow cells, must be differentiated from this.

Aetiology

Besides the primary erythropoietin-independent form, the secondary erythropoietin-dependent form plays the more important role clinically. Erythrocytosis occurs equally in dogs and cats.

Cardiovascular	Respiratory	Metabolic	Renal diseases
Right-to-left-shunt (D/C)	Feline asthma (C)	Hyperthyroidism (C)	Renal neoplasia (D/C)
Atrial septal defect (D)	Lung fibrosis (D)	Hyperadrenocorticism (D)	
Ventricular septum defect (D)	Lung tumour (D/C)		

D – Dog, C – Cat

Pathogenesis

In polycythaemia vera, there is a mutation that causes clonal proliferation of erythrocytes. The mutation causes an activation of JAK/STAT signal transduction, which leads to erythropoiesis. Due to the autonomous cell proliferation, polycythaemia vera is not associated with an increased concentration of serum erythropoietin (EPO) (Archana et al. 2021; Regimbeau et al. 2022).

In erythrocytosis as secondary form, there is an underlying causality that initiates the proliferation of the erythroid progenitor cells. In principle, this includes diseases that are accompanied by hypoxia. Essentially, these are diseases of the respiratory tract and the heart. In the former case, oxygen uptake by the RBCs is reduced and in the latter, oxygen supply to the periphery is limited. Both lead to tissue hypoxia and thus to the stimulation of erythropoiesis. To be distinguished from this are diseases that stimulate the metabolism and thus cause an increased oxygen demand. And finally, neoplastic processes of the kidney can be caused by an increased synthesis of erythropoietin (Figure 47.2.1).

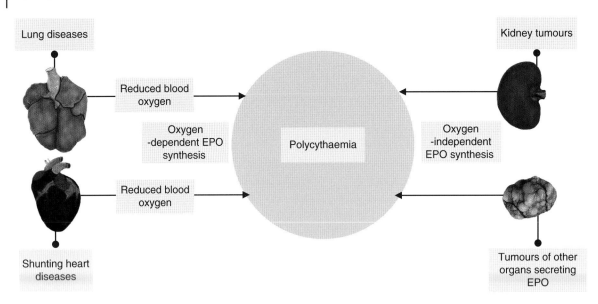

Figure 47.2.1 Mechanisms of secondary polycythaemia.

Diagnostics

Clinical signs	Clinical pathology	Imaging	Histopathology	Microbiology
Lethargy	Increased PCV	Ultrasound/Radiology	Not necessary	Not necessary
Headache		Detect the underlying disease (heart/lung) in the secondary form.		
Reddened mucous membranes				

Pathophysiologic Consequences

The clinical consequences of erythrocytosis are primarily based on the lack of oxygen supply in the periphery due to the underlying disease or the altered flow properties of the blood with an increase in the erythrocyte mass. These increase the probability of thrombus formation or lead to vascular ruptures.

Influenced organ systems	Clinical symptoms	Clinical pathological alterations
Cardiovascular system	Depression	High PCV
Respiratory system	Anorexia	Leucocytosis
Central nervous system	Weakness	
Haematological system	Blindness	
Ophthalmic system		

The main clinical changes are due to the altered flow properties of the blood. Symptoms include **depression**, **weakness**, **anorexia** or **blindness**.

The altered flow properties lead to hypoxia, as the blood cannot flow sufficiently through the blood vessels. As a result, organs are not sufficiently supplied with oxygen.

The increased viscosity of the blood can put a strain on the cardiovascular system, as the heart has to generate more force to pump the 'viscous' blood through the blood vessels. This can lead to symptoms, such as high blood pressure and an increased heart rate.

The neurological symptoms are based on a reduced supply of oxygen to the brain due to blockage of capillaries, and the same applies to the kidneys and other organs.

The observed **PU/PD** may be a consequence of reduced ADH secretion due to the increasing viscosity of the blood (van Vonderen et al. 1997).

Therapy

Symptom	Therapy
Reduction of the erythrocyte mass	Phlebotomy, infusion
Polycythaemia vera	Hydroxyurea, chlorambucil

References

Archana, A., Ramamoorthy, J.G., Ranjith Kumar, V. et al. (2021). JAK2V617F Exon-14 mutation driven polycythemia vera. *Indian Journal of Pediatrics* 88 (4): 402–403. https://doi.org/10.1007/s12098-020-03579-3.

Regimbeau, M., Mary, R., Hermetet, F., and Girodon, F. (2022). Genetic background of polycythemia vera. *Genes* 13 (4): 637. https://doi.org/10.3390/genes13040637.

van Vonderen, I.K., Meyer, H.P., Kraus, J.S., and Kooistra, H.S. (1997). Polyuria and polydipsia and disturbed vasopressin release in 2 dogs with secondary polycythemia. *Journal of Veterinary Internal Medicine* 11 (5): 300–303. https://doi.org/10.1111/j.1939-1676.1997.tb00469.x.

Further Reading

Hocking, W.G. and Golde, D.W. (1989). Polycythemia: evaluation and management. *Blood Reviews* 3 (1): 59–65. https://doi.org/10.1016/0268-960x(89)90026-x.

Hodges, V.M., Rainey, S., Lappin, T.R., and Maxwell, A.P. (2007). Pathophysiology of anemia and erythrocytosis. *Critical Reviews in Oncology/Hematology* 64 (2): 139–158. http://dx.doi.org/10.1016/j.critrevonc.2007.06.006.

47.3

Anaemia

Definition

Anaemia is a medical condition characterised by a decrease in the number of red blood cells (RBCs) or a decrease in the amount of haemoglobin in the blood.

Aetiology

Anaemia can be divided into a non-regenerative and a regenerative form. The latter is further differentiated into haemorrhagic and haemolytic. Depending on the type, different causalities come into question. The non-regenerative form is based on a reduced production of erythrocytes from the precursor cells in the bone marrow. This in turn can be further differentiated into a reduced number of precursors or insufficient activation by erythropoietin.

The regenerative forms of anaemia result from a loss of erythrocytes during bleeding, which can be the consequence of trauma or vascular erosion in neoplasia. A second cause is the destruction or shortened life span of the erythrocytes, which is usually immunologically triggered. Anaemia occurs equally in dogs and cats.

Non-regenerative	Haemorrhagic	Haemolytic
Anaemia of chronic disease (D/C)	Bleeding	Congenital red cell defects (D/C)
Bone marrow depression	Trauma (D/C)	Immune-mediated (D/C)
Medication	Tumour (D/C)	Mechanical destruction (D/C)
Oestrogen	Coagulopathy (D/C)	
Infection		
Neoplasia (D/C)		
Erythropoietin deficiency (D/C)		

D – Dog, C – Cat

Pathogenesis

Non-regenerative Anaemia

This form of anaemia occurs less frequently in dogs and cats than regenerative anaemia. The cause may be a disturbance in the formation of erythrocytes at the level of haematopoietic stem cells. This is often associated with a disturbance of the entire formation of blood cells from the bone marrow and is accompanied by pancytopenia, which also suppresses the leucocyte and platelet count.

The causalities are genetic diseases, but more often secondary destruction of the stem cells by radiation, drugs, such as chemotherapeutics or displacement of the bone marrow by neoplastic processes.

An isolated form of suppression of only erythroid proliferation can also be caused by congenital defects, infections and neoplasia, but it also arises secondarily as a result of disorders of proliferation by influencing haemoglobin synthesis or iron deficiency.

Other forms of non-regenerative anaemia develop in chronic diseases of different genesis. Non-regenerative anaemias have been described together with chronic liver and kidney diseases, chronic inflammations and chronic infections. The mechanisms described are the influence of inflammatory cytokines on erythropoietin synthesis. According to this, the proinflammatory cytokines IL-1, IL-6 and TNF-α in particular have a depressive effect on erythropoietin synthesis (Frede et al. 1997).

In addition, the increase in oxidative stress and the formation of ROS in chronic inflammation is seen as a trigger of non-regenerative anaemia. ROS directly damage the precursor cells of erythropoiesis. In the process, ROS act on different molecules. Lipids are peroxidised and thus structurally altered. The same applies to proteins and DNA.

Another mechanism appears to be the influence of proinflammatory cytokines, such as IL-6, on hepcidin levels. IL-6 can upregulate the production of hepcidin in the liver. Higher hepcidin levels result in decreased iron absorption or absorbed iron is sequestered for storage in the reticuloendothelial system, resulting in decreased iron availability for haemoglobin production in maturing erythrocytes. Hepcidin may contribute to the anaemia of chronic inflammation by reducing the responsiveness of bone marrow erythroid cells to low erythropoietin levels.

A common form of non-regenerative anaemia arises in connection with renal failure; it is more frequent in chronic renal failure and is attributed to the structural remodelling of the renal parenchyma, with reduction of renal erythropoietin production. In addition to erythropoietin deficiency, there is also an impact of chronic renal failure through uraemic inhibitors that negatively affect erythropoiesis (Mikhail et al. 2017; Weiss et al. 2019; Chikazawa and Dunning 2016; Pagani et al. 2019) (Figure 47.3.1).

The **regenerative anaemias** can be differentiated into haemorrhagic anaemia and haemolytic anaemia based on their causalities. Haemorrhage is considered to be the cause of haemorrhagic anaemia. Clinically, acute bleeding into the body cavities or to the outside is in the foreground. These are usually due to tumour bleeding or trauma. Various factors play a role here. On the one hand, tumours can promote the formation of blood vessels via angiogenic growth factors, such as VEGF, which means that tumour tissue is in principle well supplied with blood. In the case of strong tumour proliferation, necrosis of the tumour tissue increases because supplying blood vessels cannot keep up with the proliferation. Necrotic changes in the tumour also erode blood vessels, resulting in haemorrhage (Zhou et al. 2014). In addition, metastasising tumour cells are able to destroy the tight-junctions of the endothelial cells and thus generate a leakage of tumour cells but also blood cells.

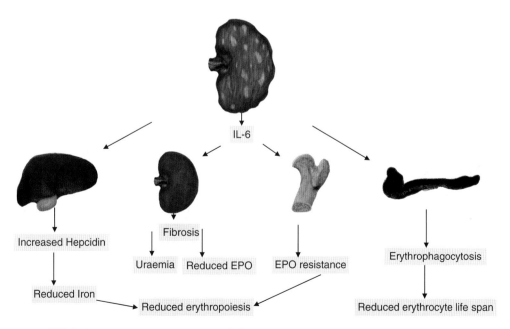

Figure 47.3.1 Non-regenerative anaemia in CKD.

Bleeding anaemia is initially non-regenerative for a few days. Immediately after blood loss, the PCV and serum protein are not altered as both are equally lost. Overall, however, the blood volume decreases, which induces a movement of extracellular fluid into the intravascular space to expand the volume. The fluid shift dilutes the plasma and PCV and total protein decrease. EPO production is directly stimulated when tissue hypoxia is present, but it takes about two to three days for the first reticulocytes to be seen in the blood (Figure 47.3.2).

The second form of regenerative anaemia is haemolytic anaemia. This is often immune-mediated and leads to a shortened life span of the erythrocytes or their lysis. This can take place intravascularly or extravascularly in cells of the mononuclear phagocyte system.

In immune-haemolytic anaemia, antibodies develop against molecules on the surface of the erythrocytes. The cause is, according to the 'mimicry hypothesis', a cross-reaction between molecular structures of the organism and foreign proteins. In this form, the organism forms antibodies against the foreign antigen, which cross-react with the erythrocyte structures.

The induction of the autoimmune response begins with the presentation of foreign antigen by antigen-presenting cells. Subsequently, first T lymphocytes and then B lymphocytes are activated. The reaction is finally carried by antibody-forming plasma cells. The antibodies bind to the erythrocyte surface and can destroy complement-supported erythrocyte membranes. Usually IgM antibody-loaded erythrocytes lead to their intravascular haemolysis. If the erythrocytes react with IgG, they are phagocytosed extravascularly by macrophages in the spleen and liver.

Another causality for immune haemolysis is the alteration of the erythrocyte surface due to structural alterations. These in turn are due to infections of the erythrocytes or mechanical damage due to flow turbulence in the vascular system. These erythrocytes are also attacked and eliminated by the immune system.

The following primary diseases have been described in connection with immune- haemolytic anaemia:

Infectious agents	Inflammations	Neoplasia	Immunological diseases	Medicines
Anaplasmosis	Pancreatitis	Lymphoma	Systemic lupus erythematosus	Trimethoprim–sulphonamide
Ehrlichiosis	Prostatitis	Carcinoma	Vaccinations	Penicillins
Haemoplasmosis	Pyometra	Sarcoma		Tetracyclines
Leptospirosis				
Babesiosis				
Dirofilariasis				

Source: Day (1999); Day (2010); Day (2012a, b).

Figure 47.3.2   Mechanism of bleeding anaemia.

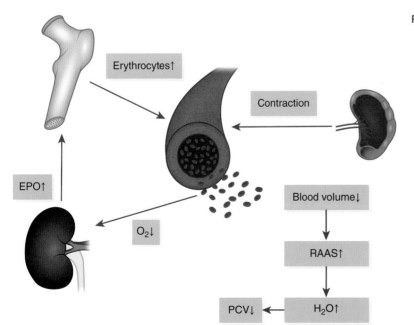

Diagnostics

Clinical signs	Clinical pathology	Imaging	Histopathology	Microbiology
Weakness	Reduced PCV, Reduced erythrocyte count	**Ultrasonography/Radiology** Detect bleeding into the body cavities	Not necessary	Not necessary
Pale mucous membranes	Changed erythrocyte indices			
Tachypnoea	Reduced TP in case of bleeding			
Visible bleeding				

Pathophysiologic Consequences

The pathophysiologic consequences of anaemia are based on the underlying disease or the consequences of insufficient oxygen supply to the organism.

Influenced organ systems	Clinical symptoms	Clinical pathological alterations
Cardiovascular system	Weakness	Thrombocytopenia
Respiratory system	Tachycardia	Prolonged PT, aPTT
Hepatobiliary system	Heart murmur	Leucocytosis
Haematological system	Tachypnoea	Decreased PCV
	Hepato-splenomegaly	Increased liver enzymes
	Fever	Bilirubinaemia
	jaundice	Bilirubinuria

The severity of symptoms in anaemia is related to the extent of the anaemia and the speed of its development. Most clinical symptoms of anaemia are due to hypoxia. This manifests itself in general **weakness** and lethargy. Due to the lack of oxygen, cellular energy production is permanently disturbed. Overall, the various organ functions are restricted as a result. This induces **tachycardia** in the heart as a compensation mechanism for the insufficient oxygen supply. In moderate and severe anaemia, a **heart murmur** can increasingly be heard, which is caused by flow turbulence of the blood that has changed its flow properties due to the anaemia.

Tachypnoea is a compensation mechanism for the lack of oxygen; dyspnoea can also be the result of an embolism due to disseminated intravascular coagulopathy (DIC). This can also lead to systemic inflammation and multiple organ failure. Laboratory diagnosis shows **thrombocytopenia** and prolonged **PT** and **aPTT**. The mechanism by which immune-haemolytic anaemia can lead to DIC is explained by endothelial damage and complement activation due to the active immunological response in IMHA. As a result, microthrombi may form, leading to consumption of coagulation factors and factors of the fibrinolytic system. Since immunohaemolytic anaemia is associated with a marked inflammatory reaction, **hepato-splenomegaly** as a sign of the immunological reaction and leukocytosis with nuclear left shift, as well as an increase in acute-phase proteins and proinflammatory cytokines are clinically evident. This in turn can trigger **fever.**

Elevated liver enzymes in the case of IMHA are due to hypoxia. Centrilobular hepatocytes, in particular, are sensitive to a reduction in oxygen, as they are already subject to a low oxygen concentration under physiological conditions. The strong increase in the degradation products of haemoglobin, which are glucuronidated in the liver, can also influence the activity of the hepatocytes and lead to an increase in liver enzymes. The latter also leads to **bilirubinaemia**, **bilirubinuria** and clinically visible **jaundice** (Figure 47.3.3).

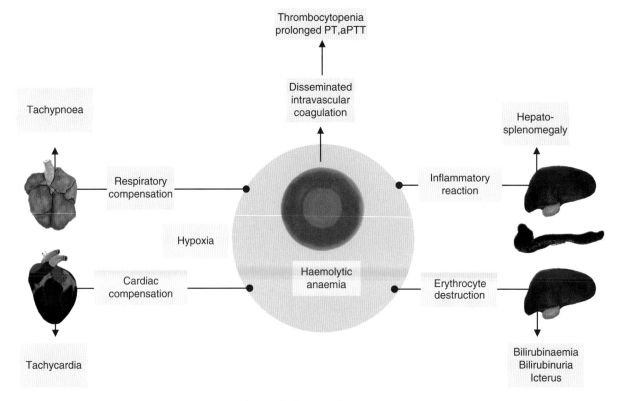

Figure 47.3.3 Pathophysiologic consequences of haemolytic anaemia.

Therapy

Symptom	Therapy
Non-regenerative anaemia	Erythropoietin
Acute anaemia	Transfusion
Thromboembolism	Heparin, platelet aggregation inhibitors (e.g. Acetylsalicylic acid, Clopidogrel)
Immune mediation	Immunosuppressive drugs (e.g. Corticosteroids, Cyclosporine, Azathioprine)

References

Chikazawa, S. and Dunning, M.D. (2016). A review of anaemia of inflammatory disease in dogs and cats. *The Journal of Small Animal Practice* 57 (7): 348–353. https://doi.org/10.1111/jsap.12498.

Day, M.J. (1999). Antigen specificity in canine autoimmune haemolytic anaemia. *Veterinary Immunology and Immunopathology* 69 (2–4, 224): 215. https://doi.org/10.1016/s0165-2427(99)00055-0.

Day, M.J. (2010). Immune-mediated anemias in the dog. In: *Schalm's Veterinary Hematology*, 6e (ed. D.J. Weiss and K.J. Wardrop), 216–225. Wiley Blackwell.

Day, M.J. (2012a). The basis of immune-mediated disease. In: *Clinical Immunology of the Dog and Cat*, 2e (ed. M.J. Day), 75–93. Manson Publishing Ltd.

Day, M.J. (2012b). Immune-mediated haemolytic anemia in the dog. In: *Clinical Immunology of the Dog and Cat*, 2e (ed. M.J. Day), 94–106. Manson Publishing Ltd.

Frede, S., Fandrey, J., Pagel, H. et al. (1997). Erythropoietin gene expression is suppressed after lipopolysaccharide or interleukin-1 beta injections in rats. *The American Journal of Physiology* 273 (3 Pt 2): R1067–R1071. https://doi.org/10.1152/ajpregu.1997.273.3.R1067.

Mikhail, A., Brown, C., Williams, J.A. et al. (2017). Renal association clinical practice guideline on Anaemia of chronic kidney disease. *BMC Nephrology* 18 (1): 345. https://doi.org/10.1186/s12882-017-0688-1.

Pagani, A., Nai, A., Silvestri, L., and Camaschella, C. (2019). Hepcidin and anemia: a tight relationship. *Frontiers in Physiology* 10: 1294. https://doi.org/10.3389/fphys.2019.01294.

Weiss, G., Ganz, T., and Goodnough, L.T. (2019). Anemia of inflammation. *Blood* 133 (1): 40–50. https://doi.org/10.1182/blood-2018-06-856500.

Zhou, W., Fong, M.Y., Min, Y. et al. (2014). Cancer-secreted miR-105 destroys vascular endothelial barriers to promote metastasis. *Cancer Cell* 25 (4): 501–515. https://doi.org/10.1016/j.ccr.2014.03.007.

47.4

Coagulation Disorders

Definition

Coagulation disorder is the term used to describe the disturbed process of blood clotting.

Physiological Basics

Blood coagulation is composed of primary and secondary haemostasis. During primary haemostasis, platelet aggregation produces a provisional, still unstable platelet plug, which is to be transformed into a stable fibrin thrombus during secondary haemostasis. Various coagulation factors are involved in this transformation, which are thereby assigned to an intrinsic and extrinsic system. The coagulation factors are initially inactive and are activated one after the other in a kind of signalling cascade. Most coagulation factors are synthesised in the liver. Vitamin K1 is necessary for the synthesis of factors II, VII, IX and X (Figure 47.4.1).

Aetiology

A distinction is made between diseases of the blood platelets or changes in the plasmatic coagulation system as the cause of a blood coagulation disorder. Diseases of the coagulation system occur in dogs and cats.

Platelets	Plasmatic coagulation	Miscellaneous
Thrombocytopathy (D)	Von Willebrand disease (D)	DIC (D/C)
Thrombocytopenia (D/C)	Congenital clotting factor deficiency (D)	
Bone marrow	Anticoagulant toxicity (D)	
Drugs		
Infections		
Immune mediated		
Sequestration		

D – Dog, C – Cat

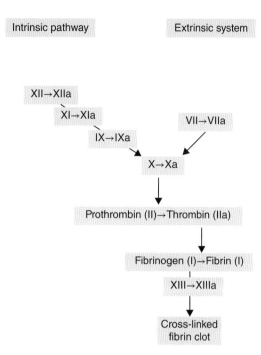

Figure 47.4.1 The coagulation cascade.

Pathogenesis

The coagulation disorders that originate from **platelets** are clinically primarily due to thrombocytopenia. Different causes come into question. This can be primarily idiopathic without an identifiable cause. In the secondary form, there is a destruction of the platelets due to an antibody reaction. Autoantibodies bind to the platelet surface, whereupon they are phagocytosed by macrophages.

Disorders of plasmatic blood coagulation occur as congenital haemophilia. Von Willebrand disease can also be seen as a disorder of the plasmatic coagulation system, as von Willebrand factor is a cofactor of factor VIII. Clinically, however, disorders of plasmatic coagulation are predominantly seen due to poisoning with anticoagulants.

Deficiency of Clotting Factors

Besides the congenital deficiency of coagulation factors, which is most frequently observed as factor VIII deficiency (haemophilia A) and factor IX deficiency (haemophilia B), clinical coagulopathies caused by intoxications are in the foreground. In Central Europe, coumarin is most frequently used in the control of rodents.

Coumarin derivatives influence secondary haemostasis by interfering with the vitamin K1-dependent synthesis of coagulation factors. During the synthesis of the factors, vitamin K1 is 'consumed' by being converted into vitamin K1 epoxide by oxidation. The reactivation from the epoxide back to the original vitamin K1 takes place with the help of the enzyme vitamin K1 epoxide reductase. This enzyme is inhibited by coumarin derivatives, which means that once the endogenous vitamin K store has been used up, no further synthesis of factors II, VII, IX and X is possible.

Disseminated intravascular coagulation (DIC) is an acquired syndrome characterised by intravascular coagulation activation. Excessive intravascular coagulation leads to microthromboses in organs. The consumption of platelets and coagulation factors together with active fibrinolysis results in a bleeding tendency.

An essential triggering mechanism is the activation of platelets by endothelial damage with the exposure of subendothelial collagens. If massive endothelial damage is present, then there is a pronounced accumulation of platelets and a marked

Table 47.4.1 Causes and mechanism of DIC.

Cause	Mechanism
Sepsis	Cytokine release
	Endotoxin
Trauma	Cytokine release
	Cell component release
Shock	Cytokine release
	Influenced circulation of coagulation factors
Neoplasia	Cytokine release
	Neoplastic molecules with properties in blood coagulation
Liver and spleen diseases	Influencing the synthesis and degradation of factors of the coagulation system and the fibrinolytic system

consumption of coagulation factors. Simultaneously with the thrombosis, the fibrinolytic system is activated. Due to the massive activation of both systems, there is a deficiency of factors and bleeding occurs. The combination of microthrombi and bleeding, eventually, leads to organ failure. Since DIC is the consequence of a massive pathomechanism, it occurs as an accompanying syndrome in numerous severe diseases (Table 47.4.1).

Diagnostics

Clinical signs	Clinical pathology	Imaging	Histopathology	Microbiology
External bleeding, Mucosal bleeding	**Platelet count**	Ultrasonography/Radiology	Not necessary	Not necessary
Bleeding into the body cavities	**Platelet function**	Detect bleeding inside the body		
	PT			
	aPTT			
	Factor determination			

Pathophysiologic Consequences

Coagulopathies show themselves clinically and laboratory-diagnostically primarily through a bleeding tendency. This then gives rise to the subsequent symptoms, which are based, on the one hand, on the undersupply of the organs with oxygen. In addition, acute bleeding leads to fluid loss and hypovolaemia. This can lead to shock.

Influenced organ systems	Clinical symptoms	Clinical pathological alterations
Systemic	Bleeding	Decreased platelets
	Lethargy	Increased PT, aPTT
	Seizures	
	Haematuria	
	Melena	
	Haematochezia	
	Dyspnoea	
	Tachypnoea	

In addition to the obvious or obscure bleeding, the haemorrhage leads to clinical symptoms via reduced perfusion of tissue or organs. These can be caused by the blood loss itself or by the obstruction of vessels due to the formation of micro-thrombi. If the blood loss or reduced perfusion occurs acutely, systemic symptoms, such as **lethargy** and **seizures** may result. Bleeding into different organs develops its own symptoms. **Haematuria** occurs with bleeding into the bladder or lower hand. **Melena** or **haematochezia** are consequences of bleeding into the intestinal area. Melena tends to indicate bleeding in the proximal bowel and haematochezia indicates bleeding in the distal bowel. Finally, bleeding into the lungs may be accompanied by symptoms of **dyspnoea** or **tachypnoea**.

The bleeding tendency, as well as the respective type of disorder, can be recognised from the clinically pathological parameters of the platelet count, its function, as well as the parameters of the extrinsic system (PT) and the intrinsic system (aPTT).

Therapy

Symptom	Therapy
Vitamin K intoxication	Vitamin K over several weeks as an injection and orally
Acute bleeding	Blood transfusion

Further Reading

Brooks, M.B. and Catalfamo, J.L. (2013). Current diagnostic trends in coagulation disorders among dogs and cats. *The Veterinary Clinics of North America. Small Animal Practice* 43 (6): 1349-vii. https://doi.org/10.1016/j.cvsm.2013.07.003.

Bruchim, Y., Aroch, I., Saragusty, J., and Waner, T. (2008). Disseminated intravascular coagulation. *Compendium (Yardley, PA)* 30 (10): E3.

Ralph, A.G. and Brainard, B.M. (2012). Update on disseminated intravascular coagulation: when to consider it, when to expect it, when to treat it. *Topics in Companion Animal Medicine* 27 (2): 65–72. https://doi.org/10.1053/j.tcam.2012.06.004.

Webster, C.R. (2017). Hemostatic disorders associated with hepatobiliary disease. *The Veterinary Clinics of North America. Small Animal Practice* 47 (3): 601–615. https://doi.org/10.1016/j.cvsm.2016.11.009.

47.5

Hypercoagulability

Definition

Hypercoagulability describes a condition of increased tendency to clot.

Aetiology

The causes of the condition of hypercoagulability are diverse and can be divided into disturbances of blood flow, damage to the vascular endothelium and increased activity of coagulation factors. The diseases occur in dogs and cats.

Abnormal blood flow	Vascular endothelial damage	Increased activity of the coagulation factors
Heart failure (D/C)	Heart failure (D/C)	Inflammation (D/C)
Neoplasia (D/C)	Neoplasia (D/C)	Neoplasia (D/C)
Trauma (D/C)	Trauma (D/C)	Endocrinopathy (D/C)
Operation (D/C)	Operation (D/C)	Protein-loss syndrome (D/C)
	Inflammation (D/C)	Hepatopathy (D/C)
		Heart failure (D/C)

D – Dog, C – Cat

Pathogenesis

Normal endothelium is physiologically non-thrombogenic and responsible for normal blood flow. Endothelial cells influence platelet regulation through endothelial ADP and nitric oxide inhibiting platelet aggregation. At the same time, prostacyclin released by platelets inhibits platelet adhesion and aggregation.

Abnormalities in blood flow due to turbulence and blood stasis can lead to hypoxia of the endothelial cells, which stimulates the secretion of an activating factor of the factor X.. In this way, there may be an increased tendency to coagulate due to hypercoagulability. In vessel wall injury, endothelial cells release endothelin-1 and platelet activating factor, increase the production of vWF, PAI-1 and factor V. In this way, platelet aggregation and thrombus formation are initiated.

Some diseases can cause hypercoagulability secondarily. One of these is sepsis. This is characterised by an increased formation of proinflammatory cytokines. These include IL-6, which in turn can trigger the coagulation cascade via the tissue factor, and IL-6 also promotes fibrin formation. TNF-α, on the other hand, reduces fibrinolysis through reduced concentrations of protein C and antithrombin III (de Laforcade et al. 2003).

In addition, local inflammation can irritate the vascular endothelium, which results in an invasion of leukocytes. This leads to increased expression of leukocyte adhesion molecules and inhibition of the protein C system. Through this release of further mediators and formation of molecular networks, platelets are activated and can initiate further thrombosis through 'self-catalysis'.

Textbook of Small Animal Pathophysiology, First Edition. Stephan Neumann.
© 2025 John Wiley & Sons Ltd. Published 2025 by John Wiley & Sons Ltd.

Antiphospholipid antibodies are also important in the genesis of hypercoagulability or thrombosis. These are a heterogeneous group of antibodies directed against the phospholipids of the cell membrane (Shapiro 1996; Levine et al. 2002).

Neoplastic diseases can cause a state of hypercoagulability through local compression and invasion of the vessel wall, expression of tissue factor on the tumour cell surface and increased fibrinogen concentration with simultaneously reduced concentration of factors of the fibrinolytic system (Hisada and Mackman 2019; Stokol et al. 2011).

Of the endocrinopathies, Cushing's disease in particular is associated with hypercoagulability. Increased activity of coagulation factors combined with an increased concentration of fibrinogen and an increased platelet count are seen as promoting factors of hypercoagulability. At the same time, there is a reduced concentration of factors of the fibrinolytic system and endothelial damage may occur due to dyslipidaemia (Boscaro et al. 2002).

Protein-loss diseases increase the tendency to clot by losing factors of the fibrinolytic system. This includes antithrombin III, which has a comparable molecular size to albumin and is therefore also excreted in cases where albumin is lost via the kidneys or intestines (Goodwin et al. 2011).

The liver's influence on blood coagulation and thus also on an increased tendency to clot is manifold; this is promoted in particular by the reduced synthesis of anticoagulants (Kavanagh et al. 2011).

Diagnostics

Clinical signs	Clinical pathology	Imaging	Histopathology	Microbiology
Consequences of thrombosis	**Thrombelastography**	**Ultrasonography**	Not necessary	Not necessary
Dyspnoea (pulmonary emboli)	**Measurement of Antithrombin III**	Detection of thrombi		
Paresis and paralysis (arterial thromboemboli)	**D-dimer**	**Radiology**		
		Detection of pulmonary emboli		

Pathophysiologic Consequences

The pathophysiologic consequences of hypercoagulability usually result from the formation of thrombi, which may be arterial or venous in location. Depending on the localisation, different symptoms result.

Influenced organ systems	Clinical symptoms	Clinical pathological alterations
Systemic	Dyspnoea	
	Tachypnoea	
	Paresis/Paralysis	
	Ascites	

Emboli to the lungs, in particular, can lead to life-threatening consequences of hypercoagulability. The associated symptoms are **tachypnoea** and **dyspnoea**. The formation of a pulmonary emboli leads to reduced gas exchange in the affected areas of the lungs. The result can be a reduced oxygen concentration and an increased concentration of CO_2. Triggered by sensitive chemoreceptors, this causes an increased respiratory rate to compensate for the lack of oxygen. The reduced lung perfusion distal to the embolus can lead to necrosis of the lung parenchyma, producing a pleural reaction with pleuritis, which causes painful breathing, dyspnoea, due to irritation of pain receptors in the pleura (Figure 47.5.1).

Emboli in the arterial system are more frequently observed in the area of the aortic branch or the spinal vessels. Both lead to symptoms of **paresis** or **paralysis**. The cause is a reduced supply of oxygen to the cells in the arterial target area. This produces hypoxic tissue necrosis and thus limited functionality. If the nervous system is affected, paresis or paralysis develops.

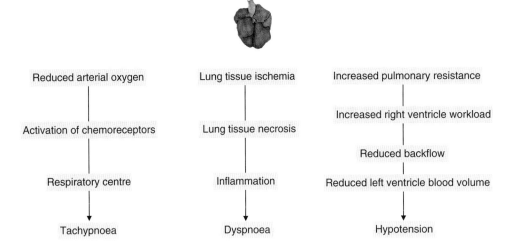

Figure 47.5.1 Consequences of pulmonary emboli.

Therapy

Symptom	Therapy
Anti-coagulation therapy	Heparin, Clopidogrel, Acetylsalicylic acid
Thrombolysis	Urokinase

References

Boscaro, M., Sonino, N., Scarda, A. et al. (2002). Anticoagulant prophylaxis markedly reduces thromboembolic complications in Cushing's syndrome. *The Journal of Clinical Endocrinology and Metabolism* 87 (8): 3662–3666. https://doi.org/10.1210/jcem.87.8.8703.

Goodwin, L.V., Goggs, R., Chan, D.L., and Allenspach, K. (2011). Hypercoagulability in dogs with protein-losing enteropathy. *Journal of Veterinary Internal Medicine* 25 (2): 273–277. https://doi.org/10.1111/j.1939-1676.2011.0683.x.

Hisada, Y. and Mackman, N. (2019). Tissue factor and cancer: regulation, tumor growth, and metastasis. *Seminars in Thrombosis and Hemostasis* 45 (4): 385–395. https://doi.org/10.1055/s-0039-1687894.

Kavanagh, C., Shaw, S., and Webster, C.R. (2011). Coagulation in hepatobiliary disease. *Journal of Veterinary Emergency and Critical Care (San Antonio, Tex.: 2001)* 21 (6): 589–604. https://doi.org/10.1111/j.1476-4431.2011.00691.x.

de Laforcade, A.M., Freeman, L.M., Shaw, S.P. et al. (2003). Hemostatic changes in dogs with naturally occurring sepsis. *Journal of Veterinary Internal Medicine* 17 (5): 674–679. https://doi.org/10.1111/j.1939-1676.2003.tb02499.x.

Levine, J.S., Branch, D.W., and Rauch, J. (2002). The antiphospholipid syndrome. *The New England Journal of Medicine* 346 (10): 752–763. https://doi.org/10.1056/NEJMra002974.

Shapiro, S.S. (1996). The lupus anticoagulant/antiphospholipid syndrome. *Annual Review of Medicine* 47: 533–553. https://doi.org/10.1146/annurev.med.47.1.533.

Stokol, T., Daddona, J.L., Mubayed, L.S. et al. (2011). Evaluation of tissue factor expression in canine tumor cells. *American Journal of Veterinary Research* 72 (8): 1097–1106. https://doi.org/10.2460/ajvr.72.8.1097.

48

Infectious Diseases

48.1

Feline

48.1.1

Feline Leukaemia Virus Infection

Aetiology

The feline leukaemia virus (FeLV) is an enveloped RNA virus. It belongs to the retrovirus family. Its structure contains a single-stranded RNA surrounded by a capsid and an envelope. Different subtypes are present in the cat, which can cause different diseases. There is a tropism to bone marrow cells.

Pathogenesis

Excretion of the virus happens to a large extent via saliva. Urine and faeces are of lesser importance for virus excretion. Horizontal transmission to a recipient occurs through direct contact, such as licking, use of shared feedings bowls, but also through bites. Transmission through fleas is discussed. In addition, there is vertical transmission to the unborn puppies.

After ingestion, virus multiplication occurs in lymphocytes and macrophages of the regional lymphoid tissue. The further course of the disease is determined, in particular, by immunological factors of the cat. The following courses are possible:

With sufficient immunity, the ingested virus can be eliminated and the cat does not become ill. Immunity in these regressively infected cats is based on virus-neutralising antibodies and cytotoxic T cells (Flynn et al. 2000).

If immunity is insufficient, viraemia occurs based on virus distribution via monocytes and lymphocytes. Target organs are initially lymphatic organs, such as the thymus, spleen and lymph nodes or the salivary glands. Later, infection of the bone marrow occurs. In this phase, the cats excrete virus material mostly via the salivary glands. If the immune system is able to stop the infection by eliminating the virus in this phase, it is called 'transient viraemia'. If this is not successful, the cats become persistently viraemic (Figure 48.1.1.1).

While transiently viraemic cats develop only mild disease symptoms, such as fever or lymphadenopathy, persistently viraemic cats have the typical clinical symptoms, which depend on the respective target organ in the viraemia. The damaging mechanism of the disease is based on cell damage of infected cells by the replication mechanism. This is composed of the phases – absorption, penetration, uncoating, transcription, integration, transcription, translation, assembly and budding.

Absorption occurs after reaction with cellular surface molecules, the virus receptors and viral surface molecules (e.g. gp70). Fusion of the viral envelope with the cell membrane leads to **penetration** of the virus through the cell membrane and uptake of the 'uncovered' virus into the cytoplasm. There, the RNA is released from the capsid by **uncoating**. Two complexes, the 'reserve-transcription complex' and the 'pre-integration complex' are formed. These use subcellular structures of the cytoskeleton, such as microtubules, as a transport path to the cell nucleus. On the way to the cell nucleus, viral RNA is transcribed into DNA by reverse transcription. Together with viral and cellular proteins, the 'pre-integration complex' is formed. This reaches the cell nucleus, where the viral DNA is **integrated** into the cellular DNA by virus-encoded integrase. The choice of the integration locus is not random.

Textbook of Small Animal Pathophysiology, First Edition. Stephan Neumann.
© 2025 John Wiley & Sons Ltd. Published 2025 by John Wiley & Sons Ltd.

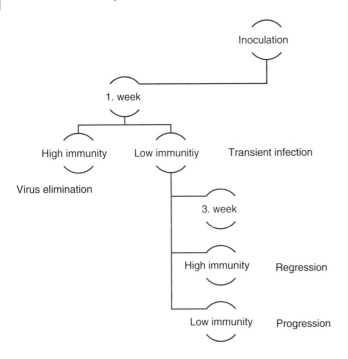

Figure 48.1.1.1 Infection mode of FeLV.

The viral genome integrated into the cell DNA is called a 'provirus'. A viral mRNA is formed by transcription of viral DNA; this migrates to the ribosomes where viral proteins are formed by the process of **translation**. The proteins are generated as precursor proteins and, in the case of the *Gag* and *Pol proteins,* are cleaved into the individual components by a viral protease, and in the case of the *Env proteins,* by a cellular protease, in the sense of maturing into the infectious virus particle. The precursor proteins are also involved in the formation of matrix proteins, which are important for capsid formation and **assembly**. Assembly of the virion occurs at the plasma membrane. Triggered by the attachment of the Gag precursor protein, the virion is **budded**. After budding, the virion undergoes a maturation process that turns it into a virus (Goff 2001; Nisole and Saïb 2004).

The mechanism of cell damage by FeLV infection is based, among other things, on agglutination and apoptosis of the infected cells (Rojko et al. 1996).

Diagnostics

Clinical signs	Clinical pathology	Imaging	Histopathology	Microbiology
Non-specific	Antigen ELISA Point-of-care test PCR	Not necessary	Not necessary	Not necessary

Pathophysiologic Consequences

The main clinical manifestations of FeLV infection are tumours as lymphomas, myelosuppression as pancytopenia or anaemia, thrombocytopenia and granulocytopenia or immune complex deposition as glomerulonephritis.

Influenced organ systems	Clinical symptoms	Clinical pathological alterations
Urinary tract	Lymphoma	Anaemia
Central nervous system	Anaemia	Leucopenia
Haematological system	Glomerulopathy	Thrombocytopenia
Reproductive system		

Tumours resulting from FeLV infection occur as alimentary, central nervous, renal or ocular **lymphomas.** The alimentary lymphomas are T cell lymphomas or B cell lymphomas. The former are more likely to occur in the mid-small intestine, and the latter in the caudal small intestine or stomach (Moore et al. 2012). Other tumours, such as fibrosarcomas are sometimes associated with leukaemia virus infection, where FeLV is thought to play a helper role by recombination of FeLV genes and cellular oncogenes to form feline sarcoma virus. Central nervous symptoms develop depending on the regional localisation of the tumour tissue and lead to ataxia, paresis or Horner's syndrome.

Anaemia is another common clinical symptom of FeLV infection. When it is a consequence of bone marrow infection by the virus with corresponding apoptosis of the erythrocytic stem cells, it occurs as a **non-regenerative anaemia** called 'pure red cell aplasia'.

Also non-regenerative is the anaemia of chronic inflammation, which can be caused by FeLV infection. Various causal mechanisms are possible. The influence of proinflammatory cytokines can influence iron metabolism, erythropoiesis directly and their stimulation by erythropoietin. IL-6 can reduce intestinal iron absorption via increased hepatic synthesis of hepcidin. Hepcidin is a peptide that inhibits the iron transport protein, ferroportin, by promoting its metabolism. Ferroportin is involved in iron absorption and its release from the reticuloendothelial system. The result is an iron deficiency for erythrocyte synthesis.

Another effect of IL-6 is the downregulation of genes of haemoglobin synthesis as well as a reduction of mitochondrial function. Both lead to a direct disturbance in erythropoiesis (Nemeth et al. 2003; Raj 2009).

Finally, in the anaemia of chronic inflammation, there is a relative erythropoietin deficiency, recognisable by inadequate erythropoietin synthesis (de Lurdes Agostinho Cabrita et al. 2011) (Table 48.1.1.1).

Another causality for anaemia due to FeLV infection can develop from bleeding due to **thrombocytopenia.** These are surface bleedings of the mucous membranes (gastrointestinal, bladder) or prolonged bleedings after trauma. Initially, bleeding anaemias are non-regenerative but become regenerative after a few days.

Another form of FeLV-induced anaemia is regenerative immune-haemolytic anaemia. In this form, the haemolysis is the result of a hypersensitivity reaction. Infections lead to the expression of atypical proteins on the erythrocyte surface, whereby these antibodies bind. Associated complement binding opens transmembrane channels on the erythrocyte surface and an osmotic gradient allows water to enter the cell, destroying it (Tuomari et al. 1984). It is not fully understood whether and how FeLV damages red blood cells, causing haemolysis.

The immunosuppression caused by **pancytopenia** allows opportunistic pathogens to form a co-infection with the FeLV infection. Co-infections with feline immunodeficiency virus, feline coronavirus, mycoplasma or dermatophytes occur. Myelosuppression is the result of an inhibition of the function of different lymphocyte forms and is caused by different virally expressed proteins, for example, from the viral envelope (Haraguchi et al. 2008).

Another group of diseases develops when FeLV break down into antigenically active protein complexes by lysis. This produces a specific antibody reaction. The resulting antigen–antibody complexes are deposited in the glomerula, for example, and lead to glomerulopathy (Hardy 1982).

Reproductive problems in the form of infertility occur in female cats. The cause is a vertical viral infection. The infection of the puppies can lead to fruit resorption or abortion. In addition, bacterial infections can develop in the uterus, promoted by the pancytopenia caused by FeLV. Altogether, this can lead to infertility of the queen (Figure 48.1.1.2).

Table 48.1.1.1 Influence of cytokines on erythropoiesis.

Cytokines	Effect
TNF-α	Inhibition of erythropoietin synthesis
	Stimulation of erythrocyte phagocytosis and/or apoptosis
INF-γ	Inhibition of erythropoietin synthesis
IL-6	Inhibition of erythrocyte progenitor cells

Source: Adapted from Madu and Ughasoro (2017).

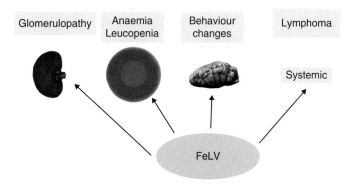

Figure 48.1.1.2 Pathophysiology of FeLV infection.

Therapy

Symptom	Therapy
Antiviral therapy	Interferon
Antibiotic therapy co-infection	Doxycycline, Amoxycillin
Non-regenerative anaemia	Erythropoietin
Prevention	Vaccination

References

De Lurdes Agostinho Cabrita, A., Pinho, A., Malho, A. et al. (2011). Risk factors for high erythropoiesis stimulating agent resistance index in pre-dialysis chronic kidney disease patients, stages 4 and 5. *International Urology and Nephrology* 43 (3): 835–840. https://doi.org/10.1007/s11255-010-9805-9.

Flynn, J.N., Hanlon, L., and Jarrett, O. (2000). Feline leukaemia virus: protective immunity is mediated by virus-specific cytotoxic T lymphocytes. *Immunology* 101 (1): 120–125. https://doi.org/10.1046/j.1365-2567.2000.00089.x.

Goff, S.P. (2001). Intracellular trafficking of retroviral genomes during the early phase of infection: viral exploitation of cellular pathways. *The Journal of Gene Medicine* 3 (6): 517–528. https://doi.org/10.1002/1521-2254(200111)3:6<517::AID-JGM234>3.0.CO;2-E.

Haraguchi, S., Good, R.A., and Day-Good, N.K. (2008). A potent immunosuppressive retroviral peptide: cytokine patterns and signalling pathways. *Immunologic Research* 41 (1): 46–55. https://doi.org/10.1007/s12026-007-0039-6.

Hardy, W.D. Jr. (1982). Immunopathology induced by the feline leukemia virus. *Springer Seminars in Immunopathology* 5 (1): 75–106. https://doi.org/10.1007/BF00201958.

Madu, A.J. and Ughasoro, M.D. (2017). Anaemia of chronic disease: an in-depth review. *Medical Principles and Practice: International Journal of the Kuwait University, Health Science Centre* 26 (1): 1–9. https://doi.org/10.1159/000452104.

Moore, P.F., Rodriguez-Bertos, A., and Kass, P.H. (2012). Feline gastrointestinal lymphoma: mucosal architecture, immunophenotype, and molecular clonality. *Veterinary Pathology* 49 (4): 658–668. https://doi.org/10.1177/0300985811404712.

Nemeth, E., Valore, E.V., Territo, M. et al. (2003). Hepcidin, a putative mediator of anemia of inflammation, is a type II acute-phase protein. *Blood* 101 (7): 2461–2463. https://doi.org/10.1182/blood-2002-10-3235.

Nisole, S. and Saïb, A. (2004). Early steps of retrovirus replicative cycle. *Retrovirology* 1: 9. https://doi.org/10.1186/1742-4690-1-9.

Raj, D.S. (2009). Role of interleukin-6 in the anemia of chronic disease. *Seminars in Arthritis and Rheumatism* 38 (5): 382–388. https://doi.org/10.1016/j.semarthrit.2008.01.006.

Rojko, J.L., Hartke, J.R., Cheney, C.M. et al. (1996). Cytopathic feline leukemia viruses cause apoptosis in hemolymphoid cells. *Progress in Molecular and Subcellular Biology* 16: 13–43. https://doi.org/10.1007/978-3-642-79850-4_2.

Tuomari, D.L., Olsen, R.G., Singh, V.K., and Kraut, E.H. (1984). Detection of circulating immune complexes by a Clq/protein A ELISA during the preneoplastic stages of feline leukemia virus infection. *Veterinary Immunology and Immunopathology* 7 (3–4): 227–238. https://doi.org/10.1016/0165-2427(84)90081-3.

Further Reading

Sykes, J. E., & Hartmann, K. (2014). Feline leukemia virus infection. *Canine and Feline Infectious Diseases*, 224–238. https://doi.org/10.1016/B978-1-4377-0795-3.00022-3

48.1.2

Feline Infectious Peritonitis

Aetiology

The causative agent of feline infectious peritonitis (FIP) is an enveloped RNA virus and belongs to the coronavirus family. Two types of coronaviruses are described in the cat, with type II causing more than two-thirds of infections in the cat. The morphology of the coronavirus is characterised by the spike proteins of the 'corona', the envelope, the capsid and the RNA.

Pathogenesis

The infection cycle of the coronavirus infection of the cat begins with the oro-nasal uptake of the pathogen. Regionally, the virus first multiplies in the epithelial cells of the oral cavity and lymphoid tissues, e.g. the tonsils. Subsequently, an infection of the enterocytes develops. Virus multiplication includes the following steps in viral infections:

Adsorption
Penetration
Uncoating
Integration
Transcription
Translation
Assembly
Budding

Adsorption takes place via a cellular membrane protein, aminopeptidase N, which is primarily expressed by enterocytes (Tresnan et al. 1996).

There, aminopeptidase N is involved in protein digestion and amino acid absorption. Further functions are involvement in angiogenesis and the cleavage of peptides presented as antigen.

After ingestion, multiplication and release of the virus, the enterocytes are damaged via the mechanism of caspase-driven apoptosis. The consequence is villus atrophy of the mucosa. This, in turn, leads to reduced absorption and secretion. The consequence is osmotic-secretory diarrhoea. However, many infections with the feline coronavirus are clinically inconspicuous (Pedersen et al. 1984; Le Poder 2011).

The more pathogenic virus of FIP compared to the enteric corona virus arises from mutations of the enteric corona virus. These occur particularly when there is a high level of virus replication due to immunosuppression caused by age, nutritional status, competing diseases, glucocorticoids, etc. (Foley et al. 1997). Mutations in different viral genes have been described, e.g. gene 3c or the spike protein gene (Bank-Wolf et al. 2014; Tekes and Thiel 2016). The consequence of the mutation is that the mutated coronavirus, when phagocytosed by macrophages, causes massive viral replication on the ribosomes.

Textbook of Small Animal Pathophysiology, First Edition. Stephan Neumann.
© 2025 John Wiley & Sons Ltd. Published 2025 by John Wiley & Sons Ltd.

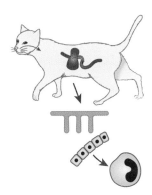

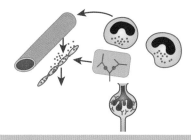

1. Oral uptake of FCoV	1. Distribution of viruses by macrophages
2. Colonisation of enterocytes	2. Lysis of infected endothelial cells
3. Mutation prevents enterocyte colonisation	3. Effusion
4. Uptake of mutant viruses by macrophages	4. Deposition of immune complexes
	5. Consumptive coagulopathy

Figure 48.1.2.1 Course of coronavirus infection.

The virus is distributed systemically by the macrophages. Antibodies against the infected macrophages that bind complement cause pyogranulomatous inflammation. Accordingly, the clinical symptoms are not a direct consequence of the viral infection but of the immune response to the infected macrophages. The usual immunological response to viral infection by the cellular and humoral immune responses is altered in FIP-infected macrophages. On the one hand, the reduced synthesis of interferon-γ by FIP-infected cells seems to reduce the cellular immune response and prevent an adequate immune response with lysis of the infected cells. On the other hand, there is a marked reaction of the humoral immune response as a result of FIP infection, but this does not lead to lysis of the infected cells because the FIP virus prevents complement-assisted cell lysis. As a result, in the case of FIP virus infection, the cellular immune response is reduced, while the humoral immune response is increased. The latter, however, does not lead to virus elimination, but to the formation of immune complexes. These are related to the subsequent increased vascular permeability, which leads to the effusion form of FIP virus infection (Olsen 1993; Felten and Hartmann 2019).

The consequences of FIP virus infection are systemic pyogranulomatous inflammatory lesions and systemic vasculitis. These are possible in all organs. Vasculitis is associated with perivascular infiltration with macrophages, lymphocytes, plasma cells and polymorphonuclear neutrophilic granulocytes (Figure 48.1.2.1).

The FIP virus-infected macrophages release proinflammatory cytokines, such as IL-1, IL-6 and TNF-α. IL-6 induces the synthesis of acute-phase proteins in hepatocytes and the proliferation of B lymphocytes into antibody-forming plasma cells. IL-1 triggers the synthesis of matrix metalloproteins. These, in turn, can degrade parts of the extracellular matrix and thus cause an increase in the permeability of the vessels.

Diagnostics

Clinical signs	Clinical pathology	Imaging	Histopathology	Microbiology
Non-specific	PCR Effusion, tissue EDTA-blood	Not necessary	Not necessary	Not necessary

Pathophysiologic Consequences

The clinically inconspicuous enteric coronavirus infection will not be considered further in the following. Instead, the focus is on the pathophysiology of FIP disease.

Influenced organ systems	Clinical symptoms	Clinical pathological alterations
Hepatobiliary system	Fever	Neutrophilia
Central nervous system	Weight loss	Lymphopenia
Ophthalmic system	Icterus	Hyperglobulinaemia
Systemic	Effusion	Hyperbilirubinaemia

As a systemic disease, FIP can affect numerous organ systems and trigger corresponding symptoms. Non-specific symptoms include fever or weight loss. Further symptoms can be assigned to the two basic clinical forms of the so-called 'wet form' with body cavity effusions and the 'dry form' with only pyogranulomatous inflammatory foci. However, there is also a mixed form of wet and dry FIP.

Fever is caused by a setpoint shift in viral infections. The infection process leads to the release of proinflammatory and, at the same time, pyogenic cytokines (IL-1, IL-6, TNF-α). These induce the release of prostaglandin E2 in the temperature regulation centre by activating cyclooxigenase 2. Prostaglandin, in turn, binds to receptors of the hypothalamus and leads to a shift in the physiological body temperature. This setpoint shift increases the body temperature and fever develops. At the same time, mechanisms are activated that reduce the body's heat loss, for example through peripheral vasoconstriction (Young and Saxena 2014).

Weight loss with its clinical consequences, such as lethargy is explained by the virus-induced cytokine-mediated change in metabolism towards a catabolic metabolic state. Different factors play a role in the metabolic change. These include CD8+ T-cell-mediated lipolysis of fat cells. This leads to interferon-mediated downregulation of anabolic metabolic pathways in adipocytes (Baazim et al. 2019).

Icterus is the clinical symptom of bilirubin elevation. The mechanism leading to **hyperbilirubinaemia** and jaundice is based on the histological changes that develop in the liver as a result of pyogranuloma formation. Cats with FIP show liver changes in terms of fibrinous hepatitis or pyogranulomatous foci. Both can lead to necrosis of the hepatocytes and thus to increased serum activity of transaminase, or to hyperbilirubinaemia. The latter is not exclusively due to cholestatic changes but can also result from hepatocyte destruction intrahepatically (Giordano et al. 2005).

A very important change in cats suffering from FIP is **effusion**. Although the disease occurs in dry, without effusion, and wet, with effusion, forms, wet FIP is the classic clinical presentation. Effusion may occur thoracically and abdominally in the form of an exudate with a protein concentration >3.5 g/dl. Effusion is a consequence of peritonitis or pleuritis. Peritonitis is the result of the reaction to the virus-carrying macrophages. The release of vasoactive mediators, such as histamine or prostaglandins leads to vascular dilatation and increased vascular permeability with exudation of fibrin-containing blood plasma. Under the influence of tissue thromboplastin, prothrombin is activated to thrombin, which polymerises the fibrin. At the same time, the fibrinolytic system is suppressed in peritonitis by inhibition of plasminogen. Both lead to the formation of fibrinous deposits, which are detectable abdominally or thoracically in FIP (Hall et al. 1998).

The dry form of FIP is not clinically conspicuous by effusion, but by numerous organ dysfunctions that develop due to the pyogranulomas and vasculitides.

Affected organs can be: liver, spleen, kidneys, pancreas, intestines, eyes, central nervous system (CNS) and lungs.

Pyogranulomas are focal inflammatory lesions composed of a necrotic core, multiple layers of macrophages or lymphocytes, and a connective tissue capsule.

Vasculitides are characterised by infiltration with macrophages and, to a lesser extent, lymphocytes, plasma cells and neutrophilic granulocytes. In FIP, they are visible in the smallest vessels. The result of the inflammation is endothelial swelling and cell necrosis, which in turn induces blood stasis with thrombus formation or ischaemia in the local tissue.

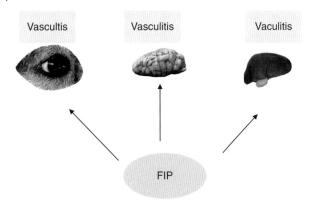

Figure 48.1.2.2 Pathophysiology of FIP.

The main haematological changes in FIP-affected cats are **neutrophilia** and **lymphopenia**. Neutrophilia is often associated with a nuclear left shift, which can be interpreted as an inflammatory response to the infection, or immunological response. In cases where there is no nuclear left shift, a stress reaction would be a causal factor. In the course of the disease, both mechanisms are possible. Lymphopenia may be a consequence of the infectious-inflammatory process in FIP or may reflect a depletion of lymphocytes in the inflammatory changes.

The main laboratory diagnostic change in FIP is **hyperproteinaemia** with **polyclonal hypergammaglobulinaemia.** This is the result of an activation of plasma cell clones with the synthesis and secretion of different globulins. The trigger for the secretion of globulins in FIP can be activation by IL-6.

IL-6 as a proinflammatory cytokine fulfils numerous functions within the inflammatory process. It induces antibody production by plasma cells, directly or via activation of CD4+ T helper cells, which in turn activate the plasma cells for antibody synthesis (Dienz et al. 2009) (Figure 48.1.2.2).

Therapy

Symptom	Therapy
Infection	Antiviral therapy (e.g. Remdesivir)
Vasculitis	Anti-inflammatory therapy (e.g. Prednisolone, interferon)

References

Baazim, H., Schweiger, M., Moschinger, M. et al. (2019). CD8[+] T cells induce cachexia during chronic viral infection. *Nature Immunology* 20 (6): 701–710. https://doi.org/10.1038/s41590-019-0397-y.

Bank-Wolf, B.R., Stallkamp, I., Wiese, S. et al. (2014). Mutations of 3c and spike protein genes correlate with the occurrence of feline infectious peritonitis. *Veterinary Microbiology* 173 (3-4): 177–188. https://doi.org/10.1016/j.vetmic.2014.07.020.

Dienz, O., Eaton, S.M., Bond, J.P. et al. (2009). The induction of antibody production by IL-6 is indirectly mediated by IL-21 produced by CD4+ T cells. *The Journal of Experimental Medicine* 206 (1): 69–78. https://doi.org/10.1084/jem.20081571.

Felten, S. and Hartmann, K. (2019). Diagnosis of feline infectious peritonitis: a review of the current literature. *Viruses* 11 (11): 1068. https://doi.org/10.3390/v11111068.

Foley, J.E., Poland, A., Carlson, J., and Pedersen, N.C. (1997). Risk factors for feline infectious peritonitis among cats in multiple-cat environments with endemic feline enteric coronavirus. *Journal of the American Veterinary Medical Association* 210 (9): 1313–1318.

Giordano, A., Paltrinieri, S., Bertazzolo, W. et al. (2005). Sensitivity of Tru-cut and fine needle aspiration biopsies of liver and kidney for diagnosis of feline infectious peritonitis. *Veterinary Clinical Pathology* 34 (4): 368–374. https://doi.org/10.1111/j.1939-165x.2005.tb00063.x.

Hall, J.C., Heel, K.A., Papadimitriou, J.M., and Platell, C. (1998). The pathobiology of peritonitis. *Gastroenterology* 114 (1): 185–196. https://doi.org/10.1016/s0016-5085(98)70646-8.

Le Poder, S. (2011). Feline and canine coronaviruses: common genetic and pathobiological features. *Advances in Virology* 2011: 609465. https://doi.org/10.1155/2011/609465.

Olsen, C.W. (1993). A review of feline infectious peritonitis virus: molecular biology, immunopathogenesis, clinical aspects, and vaccination. *Veterinary Microbiology* 36 (1–2): 1–37. https://doi.org/10.1016/0378-1135(93)90126-r.

Pedersen, N.C., Black, J.W., Boyle, J.F. et al. (1984). Pathogenic differences between various feline coronavirus isolates. *Advances in Experimental Medicine and Biology* 173: 365–380. https://doi.org/10.1007/978-1-4615-9373-7_36.

Tekes, G. and Thiel, H.J. (2016). Feline coronaviruses: pathogenesis of feline infectious peritonitis. *Advances in Virus Research* 96: 193–218. https://doi.org/10.1016/bs.aivir.2016.08.002.

Tresnan, D.B., Levis, R., and Holmes, K.V. (1996). Feline aminopeptidase N serves as a receptor for feline, canine, porcine, and human coronaviruses in serogroup I. *Journal of Virology* 70 (12): 8669–8674. https://doi.org/10.1128/JVI.70.12.8669-8674.1996.

Young, P.J. and Saxena, M. (2014). Fever management in intensive care patients with infections. *Critical Care (London, England)* 18 (2): 206. https://doi.org/10.1186/cc13773.

48.1.3

Feline Immunodeficiency Virus Infection

Aetiology

The feline immunodeficiency virus (FIV) is an enveloped RNA virus. This occurs in various subtypes worldwide. The pathogen belongs to the group of lentiviruses.

Pathogenesis

The excretion of the virus occurs via saliva. Since the virus is predominantly cell-bound, the presence of virus-bearing inflammatory cells in the saliva is advantageous for transmission. These cells originate, for example, from oral inflammatory lesions and ulcers that occur in connection with an FIV infection. In this case, the virus is transmitted cell-associated to other cats through bites.

Other transmission mechanisms, such as during sexual contact or vertical transmission to the kittens, are possible but of secondary importance. After transmission, the virus is taken up by lymphocytes (CD4+; CD8+) or macrophages. Through these, the virus is spread in the organism.

The cell cycle of FIV infection follows the sequence described in Chapters 9.1. The described process generates various defence mechanisms in the body cells, which are controlled by interferon. The TRIM protein can inhibit the uncoating process of the virus from the capsid. Inhibition of reverse transcription and transport into the nucleus occurs through APOBEC3 and SAMDH1 and the tetherin protein prevents virus release (Doyle et al. 2015). If the defence mechanisms are overcome, disease symptoms can develop due to impaired function of the infected defence cells (Figure 48.1.3.1).

Diagnostics

Clinical signs	Clinical pathology	Imaging	Histopathology	Microbiology
Non-specific	ELISA	Not necessary	Not necessary	Not necessary
	Point-of-care test			
	Antibody			
	Antigen			
	PCR			

Textbook of Small Animal Pathophysiology, First Edition. Stephan Neumann.
© 2025 John Wiley & Sons Ltd. Published 2025 by John Wiley & Sons Ltd.

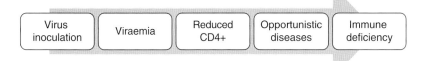

Figure 48.1.3.1   Course of an FIV infection.

Pathophysiologic Consequences

The course of an FIV infection is divided into four phases. In the first phase, which lasts a few weeks after transmission, symptoms such as fever, lymphadenopathy or gastrointestinal and respiratory symptoms develop. This phase is followed by the second phase, which can last for months to years. In this stage, the animals show no clinical signs. In the third phase, the cats show clinical symptoms in the sense of fever, swelling of the lymph nodes, stomatitis and behavioural changes. Laboratory diagnostics show leukopenia and anaemia. Finally, the fourth phase, the 'FAIDS', follows in which the cats increasingly develop symptoms due to progressive immunodeficiency. Here, neurological symptoms also occur, but also symptoms depending on the localisation of an opportunistic infection.

Influenced organ systems	Clinical symptoms	Clinical pathological alterations
Respiratory system	Inappetence	Leucopenia
Gastrointestinal system	Weight loss	Anaemia
Central nervous system	Fever	Polyclonal gammopathy
Haematological system	Changed behaviour	
Systemic	Enlarged lymph nodes	
Ophthalmic system	Stomatitis	
Reproduction	Pneumonia	
	Cystitis	
	Uveitis	

The general symptoms of **inappetence** and **weight loss** follow the general mechanisms of infectious diseases or are carried by reduced feed intake due to stomatitis. In this case, the weight loss would be secondary to the reduced feed intake. Independently of this, the symptoms are induced by central cytokine effects. Inappetence may be a consequence of TNF-α effects on the hypothalamus. In addition, the proinflammatory cytokines induce the release of leptin from fat cells, which also suppresses the feeling of hunger via an effect on the hypothalamus (Francesconi et al. 2016; Aviello et al. 2021).

Fever is the result of a setpoint change in the hypothalamus. Under the influence of proinflammatory cytokines, prostaglandin is released which binds to specific receptors in the hypothalamus. The consequence of fever is an increase in the immune defence in the organism. Lymphocyte migration and adhesion, as well as the activity of killer cells, is increased at elevated body temperature (Lin et al. 2019; Umar et al. 2020).

The **neurological consequences** of an FIV infection develop through virus-infected monocytes that pass the blood-brain barrier and accumulate in the microglia. There they release neurotoxic effective factors that lead to calcium accumulation in the nerve cells via a disturbance of the Na^+-Ca^{2+} exchanger. Calcium activates enzymes, such as calpain, which lead to actin destruction. Disruption of the cytoskeleton disrupts transmembrane transport processes and eventually leads to cell swelling and dysfunction (Meeker and Hudson 2017) (Figure 48.1.3.2).

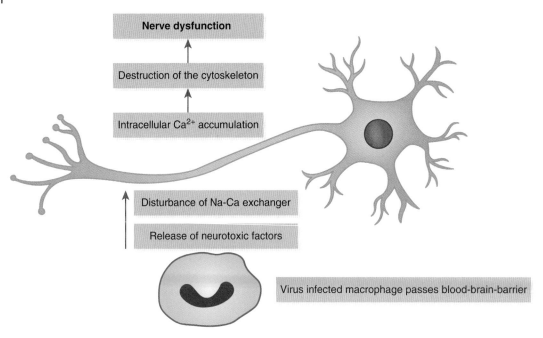

Figure 48.1.3.2 Mechanisms of neuropathic dysfunction due to FIV.

Stomatitis is a common clinical consequence of FIV infection. Histologically, lymphoplasma cellular infiltration is in the foreground. Bacterial secondary infections to the causal FIV infection would probably result in more neutrophilic infiltrates. However, secondary infections with caliciviruses are possible, influencing the expression of stomatitis.

Inflammations in other organs, such as **cystitis, pneumonia, gastroenteritis** are attributed to secondary infections. The described uveitis can be accompanied by toxoplasmosis. Common competing infections to an FIV infection are:

Viral	Bacterial	Protozoal	Mycologic
Feline leukaemia virus	*Mycoplasma* spp.	*Toxoplasma*	Dermatophytes
Calicivirus		Babesia	
		Hepatozoon	

Significant laboratory diagnostic changes in FIV infection relate to haematology. Here, depressive changes in the sense of a reduction in the number of white and red blood cells are in the foreground. **Leucopenias** mainly occur during the acute phases of the disease and reflect the extent of the disease. Lymphopenias are seen in connection with a reduction of CD4+ helper cells infected by the FIV virus. Neutropenias are due to apoptosis or a reduction in colony forming units (CFU) (Linenberger et al. 1995; Sprague et al. 2010).

The **anaemia** of FIV infection is predominantly non-regenerative and is often seen in association with secondary infections, such as mycoplasma (Grimes and Fry 2015).

Polyclonal hypergammaglobulinaemia is the regularly occurring laboratory diagnostic change in cats with FIV. Competing infections do not fully explain the occurrence of this change. Increased activity of B lymphocytes in response to viral antigen is thought to be another mechanism (Gleich and Hartmann 2009) (Figure 48.1.3.3).

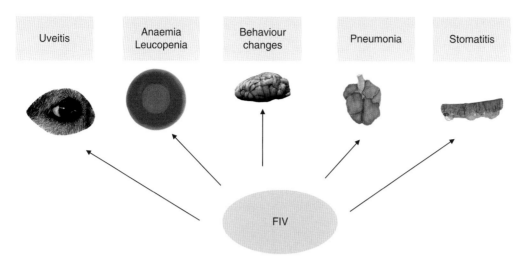

Figure 48.1.3.3 Pathophysiology of FIV infection.

Therapy

Symptom	Therapy
Antiviral therapy	Interferon
Antibiotics, if co-infection	e.g. Amoxycillin
Antimycotics, if co-infection	e.g. Miconazole

References

Aviello, G., Cristiano, C., Luckman, S.M., and D'Agostino, G. (2021). Brain control of appetite during sickness. *British Journal of Pharmacology* 178 (10): 2096–2110. https://doi.org/10.1111/bph.15189.

Doyle, T., Goujon, C., and Malim, M.H. (2015). HIV-1 and interferons: who's interfering with whom? *Nature Reviews. Microbiology* 13 (7): 403–413. https://doi.org/10.1038/nrmicro3449.

Francesconi, W., Sánchez-Alavez, M., Berton, F. et al. (2016). The proinflammatory cytokine interleukin 18 regulates feeding by acting on the bed nucleus of the Stria terminalis. *The Journal of Neuroscience: The Official Journal of the Society for Neuroscience* 36 (18): 5170–5180. https://doi.org/10.1523/jneurosci.3919-15.2016.

Gleich, S. and Hartmann, K. (2009). Hematology and serum biochemistry of feline immunodeficiency virus-infected and feline leukemia virus-infected cats. *Journal of Veterinary Internal Medicine* 23 (3): 552–558. https://doi.org/10.1111/j.1939-1676.2009.0303.x.

Grimes, C.N. and Fry, M.M. (2015). Nonregenerative anemia: mechanisms of decreased or ineffective erythropoiesis. *Veterinary Pathology* 52 (2): 298–311. https://doi.org/10.1177/0300985814529315.

Lin, C., Zhang, Y., Zhang, K. et al. (2019). Fever promotes T lymphocyte trafficking via a thermal sensory pathway involving heat shock protein 90 and α4 integrins. *Immunity* 50 (1): 137–151.e6. https://doi.org/10.1016/j.immuni.2018.11.013.

Linenberger, M.L., Beebe, A.M., Pedersen, N.C. et al. (1995). Marrow accessory cell infection and alterations in hematopoiesis accompany severe neutropenia during experimental acute infection with feline immunodeficiency virus. *Blood* 85 (4): 941–951.

Meeker, R.B. and Hudson, L. (2017). Feline immunodeficiency virus neuropathogenesis: a model for HIV-induced CNS inflammation and neurodegeneration. *Veterinary Sciences* 4 (1): 14. https://doi.org/10.3390/vetsci4010014.

Sprague, W.S., TerWee, J.A., and VandeWoude, S. (2010). Temporal association of large granular lymphocytosis, neutropenia, proviral load, and FasL mRNA in cats with acute feline immunodeficiency virus infection. *Veterinary Immunology and Immunopathology* 134 (1–2): 115–121. https://doi.org/10.1016/j.vetimm.2009.10.016.

Umar, D., Das, A., Gupta, S. et al. (2020). Febrile temperature change modulates CD4 T cell differentiation via a TRPV channel-regulated notch-dependent pathway. *Proceedings of the National Academy of Sciences of the United States of America* 117 (36): 22357–22366. https://doi.org/10.1073/pnas.1922683117.

Further Reading

Krapić, M., Kavazović, I., and Wensveen, F.M. (2021). Immunological mechanisms of sickness behavior in viral infection. *Viruses* 13 (11): 2245. https://doi.org/10.3390/v13112245.

48.2

Canine

48.2.1

Distemper

Aetiology

The causative agent of canine distemper belongs to the family of paramyxoviruses and the genus *Morbillivirus*. The structure is an enveloped RNA virus. The pathogen occurs worldwide and infects members of the order Carnivora.

The virus structure contains numerous molecules that play a pathogenetic or diagnostic role (Table 48.2.1.1).

Pathogenesis

The virus is transferred aerogenically and reaches the tissues of the respiratory tract. There, the viruses are taken up by epithelial cells or defence cells, such as macrophages and dendritic cells. Canine distemper viruses can infect cells via two different receptors. The SLAM receptor is predominantly expressed in the membrane of defence cells such as lymphocytes, macrophages or dendritic cells. The nectin receptor, on the other hand, is expressed by epithelial cells and central nervous endothelial cells (Pratakpiriya et al. 2012).

Infected lymphocytes carry the virus into the regional lymphoid organs, where primary viraemia occurs through infection of the sessile lymphoid cells via SLAM receptor in the first two days post infection. Drainage of the lymphoid organs distributes the distemper virus bound to lymphocytes via the blood to the secondary target organs. This process takes place between four and seven days post infection. In the secondary target organs, the resident epithelial cells are infected via nectin receptors. Nerve cells of the brain are infected after passage of the blood-brain barrier. The histopathological changes in the target organs are interstitial bronchopneumonia with proliferation of alveolar cells and thickening of the alveolar septa, haemorrhagic enteritis and meningoencephalitis. The latter can also occur protracted and probably has an immune-mediated genesis (Summers and Appel 1994).

Diagnostics

Clinical signs	Clinical pathology	Imaging	Histopathology	Microbiology
Non-specific	Immunofluorescence smear conjunctive, tonsils PCR blood, Cerebrospinal fluid (CSF)	Not necessary	Not necessary	Not necessary

Table 48.2.1.1   Molecules of the canine distemper virus.

Localisation	Name	Function
Capsid	Nucleocapsid protein (N), Phosphoprotein (P), L protein, Matrix protein (M), Haemagglutinin protein (H) Fusion protein (F)	Structural proteins
Envelope	Surface glycoproteins F and H	

Source: Kalbermatter et al. (2023).

Pathophysiologic Consequences

The pathophysiologic consequences of the distemper virus infection are characterised by insufficiencies of the secondary target organs of the respiratory tract, the gastrointestinal tract and the central nervous system. Hyperkeratosis on the pads and on the nose are further symptoms.

Influenced organ systems	Clinical symptoms	Clinical pathological alterations
Respiratory system	Anorexia	Lymphopenia
Gastrointestinal system	Lethargy	Thrombocytopenia
Central nervous system	Fever	
Haematological System	Dyspnoea	
Skin	Cough	
	Vomiting	
	Diarrhoea	
	Ataxia	
	Hard pad	
	Nasal and ocular discharge	

The development of **anorexia, lethargy** and **fever** follows the usual mechanisms of a viral infection.

The symptomatology of infections of the organs of the respiratory tract and the gastrointestinal tract is based on a viral infection of the epithelial cells and their dysfunction. The inflammations are often complicated by secondary bacterial infections. These are due, among other things, to the immunosuppression caused by a distemper infection. The distemper virus proteins, V protein and C protein, lead to rapid viral replication in T lymphocytes and antagonise proinflammatory cytokines, such as IL-2, IL-6, TNF-α and interferons. The result is a secondary infection with various pathogens. Known are *Bordetella*, *Salmonella*, *Nocardia*, *Toxoplasma* etc. (von Messling et al. 2006; Zhao et al. 2020).

This results in symptoms that indicate inflammation in the respiratory tract, such as **dyspnoea** or **cough.** In the gastrointestinal tract, the inflammation can cause **vomiting** and **diarrhoea**. In addition to virus-induced symptoms, consequences of immune-mediated dysfunction are also seen in this manifestation.

The distemper infection of the central nervous system may affect the grey or white matter, less frequently polioencephalitis occurs. Cellularly, demyelination develops associated with low or moderate lymphocytic infiltration. In demyelination, the myelin sheaths are destroyed. These are formed centrally by oligodendrocytes and surround the axon. Myelination leads to saltatory conduction of the action potential between Ranvier's constrictions. Demyelination decreases the electrical resistance along the axon and results in a delayed or precipitated action potential. This, in turn, causes the various nerve function failures, the symptomatology of which depends on the affected region. The symptoms that occur can be tonic-clonic spasms (cerebrum), tremors and ataxias (cerebellum).

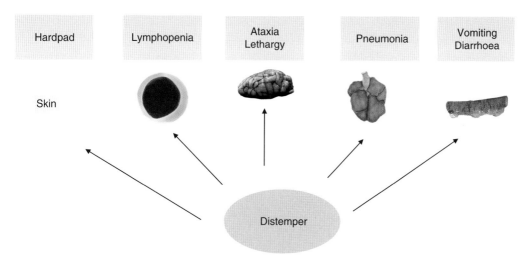

Figure 48.2.1.1 Pathophysiology of distemper infection.

Hyperkeratosis in the area of the pads or on the nose leather are further symptoms of distemper observed in the chronic course. Histologically, orthokeratotic hyperkeratosis, acanthosis and mild mononuclear cell infiltrates are found. Infection of the cells of the stratum spinosum and granulosum is considered to be the cause (Koutinas et al. 2004).

In laboratory diagnostics, suppression of white blood cells or platelets is seen in distemper infections. A direct infection of the **lymphocytes** with their destruction through apoptosis but also an infection-independent destruction is seen as a mechanism (Schobesberger et al. 2005) (Figure 48.2.1.1).

Therapy

Symptom	Therapy
Secondary infection	Antibiotics (e.g. Ampicillin)
Seizures	Anticonvulsants (e.g. Phenobarbital, Potassium-bromide)
Prevention	Vaccination

References

Kalbermatter, D., Jeckelmann, J.M., Wyss, M. et al. (2023). Structure and supramolecular organization of the canine distemper virus attachment glycoprotein. *Proceedings of the National Academy of Sciences of the USA* 120 (6): e2208866120. https://doi.org/10.1073/pnas.2208866120.

Koutinas, A.F., Baumgärtner, W., Tontis, D. et al. (2004). Histopathology and immunohistochemistry of canine distemper virus-induced footpad hyperkeratosis (hard pad disease) in dogs with natural canine distemper. *Veterinary Pathology* 41 (1): 2–9. https://doi.org/10.1354/vp.41-1-2.

von Messling, V., Svitek, N., and Cattaneo, R. (2006). Receptor (SLAM [CD150]) recognition and the V protein sustain swift lymphocyte-based invasion of mucosal tissue and lymphatic organs by a morbillivirus. *Journal of Virology* 80 (12): 6084–6092. https://doi.org/10.1128/JVI.00357-06.

Pratakpiriya, W., Seki, F., Otsuki, N. et al. (2012). Nectin4 is an epithelial cell receptor for canine distemper virus and involved in neurovirulence. *Journal of Virology* 86 (18): 10207–10210. https://doi.org/10.1128/JVI.00824-12.

Schobesberger, M., Summerfield, A., Doherr, M.G. et al. (2005). Canine distemper virus-induced depletion of uninfected lymphocytes is associated with apoptosis. *Veterinary Immunology and Immunopathology* 104 (1–2): 33–44. https://doi.org/10.1016/j.vetimm.2004.09.032.

Summers, B.A. and Appel, M.J. (1994). Aspects of canine distemper virus and measles virus encephalomyelitis. *Neuropathology and Applied Neurobiology* 20 (6): 525–534. https://doi.org/10.1111/j.1365-2990.1994.tb01006.x.

Zhao, J., Ren, Y., Chen, J. et al. (2020). Viral pathogenesis, recombinant vaccines, and oncolytic virotherapy: applications of the canine distemper virus reverse genetics system. *Viruses* 12 (3): 339. https://doi.org/10.3390/v12030339.

Further Reading

Klotz, D. (2019). The importance of the type I interferon signalling pathway in dogs with special reference to canine distemper virus infection. Dissertation Hanover.

48.2.2

Canine Parvovirus

Aetiology

The Parvoviridae family is divided into two subfamilies. The canine parvoviruses belong to the subfamily Parvovirinae. The genus *Parvovirus* includes the clinically significant variant canine parvovirus-2 (CPV-2). Canine parvovirus-1 is of lesser clinical importance. Feline panleukopenia viruses also belong to the parvoviruses, but are not identical to CPV-2. CPV-2 is a non-enveloped DNA virus. It occurs worldwide and causes an infectious disease in dogs, usually of younger age. This is characterised by symptoms resulting from destruction of mitotically active cells, for example, of the gastrointestinal tract. The virus can remain infectious outside the organism for up to 12 months. Accordingly, clusters of infections have been observed in dogs during months of high outdoor activity (Houston et al. 1996).

Pathogenesis

Canine parvovirus-2 is transmitted via faecal-oral transmission. After excretion of the virus particles via vomit or diarrhoea, the viruses can be ingested orally. Initially, the virus multiplies in the local lymphatic organs of the mouth and throat region for about one to three days. Virus uptake by lymphocytes corresponds to the usual path of virus replication (Table 48.2.2.1).

The cellular uptake of canine parvovirus occurs via a transferrin receptor. After binding, the complex is taken up by an invagination of the cell membrane and is cut off from the cell membrane as an endosome. Within the endosome, the viral capsid remains bound to the receptor for several hours. Afterwards, the capsids enter the nucleus via nuclear pores for replication (Hueffer et al. 2004).

After the first local multiplication phase in the lymphatic tissue, viraemia follows three to five days post infection, during which the parvoviruses are distributed haematogenously. In this process, the viruses are distributed freely or via the lymphocytes into other body organs (Meunier et al. 1985).

The target organs for virus distribution are organs with a high mitotic rate, including the thymus, bone marrow, mesenteric lymph nodes, spleen, Peyer's patches and intestinal epithelium. In young dogs, cardiac muscle cells are also involved. In the target organs, cellular multiplication of the viruses occurs according to the principle described above. The target cells are destroyed in the process. The histological changes of affected organs are characterised by necrosis. In the small intestine, necrosis of the epithelium of the intestinal crypts, loss of the enterocyte villi and collapse of the intestinal villi are found in dogs with parvovirus infection. Necrosis and atrophy of the intestinal-associated lymphatic system are also prominent. The same applies to extraintestinal lymphoid organs, such as the spleen or thymus. In dogs suffering from a cardiac form of parvovirus infection, pathohistologically a myocarditis with necrosis of the cardiomyocytes is found. The mechanism of cell death is probably initially due to induced apoptosis. Infected cells show structural changes, condensation on cellular DNA, mitochondrial membrane depolarisation and increased caspase activity. As a result, the cells go into apoptosis. However, histological changes often show necrosis in the affected organs. It was concluded that apoptosis is not completed in canine parvovirus infection, but that secondary necrosis occurs as a result of activated phagocytosis of the 'apoptotic bodies' (Nykky et al. 2010) (Figure 48.2.2.1).

Textbook of Small Animal Pathophysiology, First Edition. Stephan Neumann.
© 2025 John Wiley & Sons Ltd. Published 2025 by John Wiley & Sons Ltd.

Table 48.2.2.1 Mechanisms of virus replication.

Phase	Mechanism
Absorption	Attachment of the virus to a membranous receptor
Penetration	Invagination of the virus-receptor complex in an endosome
Uncoating	Release of viral nucleic acids from the endosome
Replication	Integration of viral nucleic acids into cellular genetic information
Translation	Formation of viral proteins
Assembly	Synthesis of viruses
Elution	Release of the viruses from the host cell

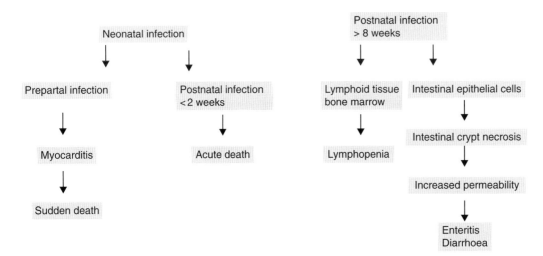

Figure 48.2.2.1 Pathogenesis of parvovirus infection in dogs.

Diagnostics

Clinical signs	Clinical pathology	Imaging	Histopathology	Microbiology
Non-specific	ELISA point-of-care test antigen detection faeces	Not necessary	Not necessary	Not necessary

Pathophysiologic Consequences

The pathophysiologic consequences of a parvovirus infection become clinically noticeable after the incubation period of 7–14 days.

Influenced organ systems	Clinical symptoms	Clinical pathological alterations
Cardiovascular system	Anorexia (71%)	Leucopenia (35%)
Gastrointestinal system	Lethargy (71%)	Lymphopenia (61%)
Haematological system	Fever (33%)	Panhypoproteinaemia (27%)
Systemic	Diarrhoea (69%)	Hyponatraemia (56%)
	Vomiting (66%)	
	Dehydration (64%)	
	Sudden death	

Source: Mylonakis et al. 2016

Anorexia due to CPV-2 infection probably follows the general mechanisms of anorexia in infectious diseases. A direct induction of anorexia can occur through molecules of the pathogen when these act on the feeding centre in the hypothalamus. Another mechanism is an indirect effect via the inflammatory response. Proinflammatory cytokines, such as IL-1, IL-6 and TNF-α play a role here. On the one hand, the cytokines can induce a peripheral mechanism, for example, by inducing the leptin synthesis of the fat cells. Leptin is a peptide hormone synthesised by adipocytes. It can cross the blood-brain barrier, and acts on structures of the hypothalamus. There it promotes the synthesis of anorexigenic hormones (e.g. neurotensin, serotonin) and reduces the synthesis of orexigenic hormones (e.g. neuropeptide Y). The result is a reduced feeling of hunger. In addition to this peripheral effect, the proinflammatory cytokines can also act directly on the central nervous system. After passage across the blood-brain barrier, the cytokines bind to endothelial receptors and induce the synthesis of mediators, such as eicosanoids, which in turn act on the neuronal structures of the hypothalamus (Langhans 2000).

Lethargy is related to anorexia. By reducing the feed intake, the organism changes into a catabolic metabolic state. This depletes the body's energy reserves and leads to lethargy. **Fever** as a result of the infectious process, triggered by pyrogens through the inflammatory process, can also affect the general condition and thus cause lethargy.

The central clinical symptoms of parvovirus infection are **vomiting** and **diarrhoea**. Mostly, vomiting occurs clinically first, followed by sometimes bloody diarrhoea. The mechanisms are essentially based on the destruction of the mucous membrane of the small intestine. There, a reduction of the absorption surface develops due to atrophy and collapse of the intestinal villi. This causes osmotically active molecules to remain in the intestine and induces osmotic diarrhoea by actively inducing a water shift through the intestinal wall into the intestinal lumen. Another mechanism is that the destruction of the villous structure increases the permeability of the intestinal vessels, leading to bleeding into the intestinal lumen with loss of plasma and blood cells. The enzymatic digestion of enterocytes and blood cells results in the typical odour of dogs with parvovirus enteritis.

The consequence of massive diarrhoea is dehydration. This has its own pathophysiologic consequences. With a loss of extracellular fluidity >5%, the haematocrit rises into areas where the altered blood viscosity changes the flow behaviour of the blood and can induce thrombogenesis. The latter is associated with reduced mobility, which is evident in critically ill patients. In addition, water loss reduces blood volume and blood pressure. This activates the RAAS, leading to tachycardia and vasoconstriction of the splanchnic vessels. This, in turn, reduces renal blood flow and can lead to pre-renal renal failure. The consequences are sometimes **shock** and **death**. Sudden death in dogs with parvovirus infection is from myocarditis. This is particularly seen in puppies in the first few weeks of life. In these animals, the cardiomyocytes are still markedly proliferative and are among the target cells of the parvoviruses. The infection results in cardiomyocyte necrosis, infiltration with macrophages, lymphocytes, plasma cells and neutrophilic granulocytes. In some cases, tissue fibrosis is also observed (Ford et al. 2017).

An essential laboratory diagnostic change is the reduction of blood cells. This affects the erythrocytes less than the leucocytes, and especially the lymphocytes. The mechanism is not completely clear, but could correspond to the generally assumed mechanism in viral infections. In this case, lymphopenia develops from direct apoptosis or necrosis of the lymphocytes; in addition, the viral infection can inhibit lymphopoiesis in a cytokine-mediated manner. Stress associated with infection causes glucocortcoid release. Increased glucocorticoids in turn induce lymphopenia by inhibiting lymphopoiesis and inhibiting the release of lymphocytes from lymphoid organs. Finally, sequestration of lymphocytes can cause peripheral lymphopenia. In addition, direct suppressive effects on the bone marrow are possible (Guo et al. 2021) (Figures 48.2.2.2 and 48.2.2.3).

Figure 48.2.2.2 Influence of viral infection on lymphocyte count.

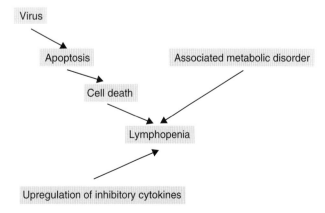

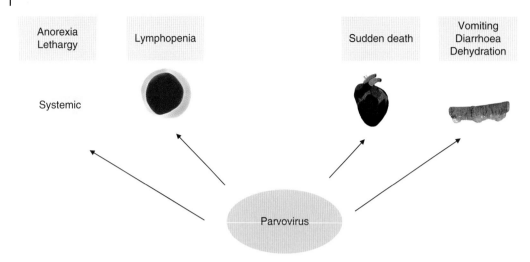

Figure 48.2.2.3 Pathophysiologic consequences of canine parvovirus infection.

Therapy

Symptom	Therapy
Shock	Infusion therapy
Vomiting	Antiemetics (e.g. Ondansetron, Maropitant)
Sepsis	Antibiotics (e.g. Ampicillin)
Prevention	Vaccination

References

Ford, J., McEndaffer, L., Renshaw, R. et al. (2017). Parvovirus infection is associated with myocarditis and myocardial fibrosis in young dogs. *Veterinary Pathology* 54 (6): 964–971. https://doi.org/10.1177/0300985817725387.

Guo, Z., Zhang, Z., Prajapati, M., and Li, Y. (2021). Lymphopenia caused by virus infections and the mechanisms beyond. *Viruses* 13 (9): 1876. https://doi.org/10.3390/v13091876.

Houston, D.M., Ribble, C.S., and Head, L.L. (1996). Risk factors associated with parvovirus enteritis in dogs: 283 cases (1982–1991). *Journal of the American Veterinary Medical Association* 208 (4): 542–546.

Hueffer, K., Palermo, L.M., and Parrish, C.R. (2004). Parvovirus infection of cells by using variants of the feline transferrin receptor altering clathrin-mediated endocytosis, membrane domain localization, and capsid-binding domains. *Journal of Virology* 78 (11): 5601–5611. https://doi.org/10.1128/JVI.78.11.5601-5611.2004.

Langhans, W. (2000). Anorexia of infection: current prospects. *Nutrition (Burbank, Los Angeles County, Calif.)* 16 (10): 996–1005. https://doi.org/10.1016/s0899-9007(00)00421-4.

Meunier, P.C., Cooper, B.J., Appel, M.J., and Slauson, D.O. (1985). Pathogenesis of canine parvovirus enteritis: the importance of viremia. *Veterinary Pathology* 22 (1): 60–71. https://doi.org/10.1177/030098588502200110.

Mylonakis, M.E., Kalli, I., and Rallis, T.S. (2016). Canine parvoviral enteritis: an update on the clinical diagnosis, treatment, and prevention. *Veterinary Medicine (Auckland, N.Z.)* 7: 91–100. https://doi.org/10.2147/VMRR.S80971.

Nykky, J., Tuusa, J.E., Kirjavainen, S. et al. (2010). Mechanisms of cell death in canine parvovirus-infected cells provide intuitive insights to developing nanotools for medicine. *International Journal of Nanomedicine* 5: 417–428. https://doi.org/10.2147/ijn.s10579.

Further Reading

Engelbrecht, M., Botha, W.J., Pazzi, P. et al. (2022). Serum cobalamin concentrations in dogs infected with canine parvoviral enteritis. *Journal of the American Veterinary Medical Association* 260 (7): 1–8. https://doi.org/10.2460/javma.21.05.0240.

Mazzaferro, E.M. (2020). Update on canine parvoviral enteritis. *The Veterinary Clinics of North America. Small Animal Practice* 50 (6): 1307–1325. https://doi.org/10.1016/j.cvsm.2020.07.008.

Park, J.S., Guevarra, R.B., Kim, B.R. et al. (2019). Intestinal microbial dysbiosis in beagles naturally infected with canine parvovirus. *Journal of Microbiology and Biotechnology* 29 (9): 1391–1400. https://doi.org/10.4014/jmb.1901.01047.

Rueckert, N. (2007). Characterisation of canine and feline parvoviruses in archived organ material from the years 1970 to 1978. Dissertation, Leipzig.

480

48.3

Bacterial Diseases

48.3.1

Anaplasmosis

Aetiology

Canine anaplasmosis belongs to the vector-borne diseases and is caused by *Anaplasma platys* or *Anaplasma phagocytophilum*. Both are gram-negative obligate intracellular bacteria of the Anaplasmataceae family. Wild animals that belong to the rodents, such as various mouse species, are considered to be the reservoir. Wild ruminants or birds can also be reservoirs. It is transmitted by the tick as a vector. *Ixodes ricinus* is the transmitter of *A. phagocytophilum* and *Rhipicephalus sanguineus* of *A. platys*. Accordingly, the respective form of anaplasmosis occurs depending on the distribution of the vector. *I. ricinus* the vector of *A. phagocytophilum* begins its life cycle with the laying of eggs by the female tick. Larvae hatch from the eggs. These live in the low vegetation layers, where they can infest small rodents and become infected with *A. phagocytophilum* by ingesting blood. After the blood meal, the larva sheds its skin and becomes a nymph. This requires another blood meal for metamorphosis into an adult. Infected nymphs can transmit *Anaplasma* during this process. Non-infected nymphs can ingest pathogens during this meal. After moulting to become an adult, the female tick takes another blood meal after mating before laying eggs. This can lead to further transmission of *A. phagocytophilum*. A similar life cycle with blood meals before each moult is also found in the brown dog tick. Anaplasmosis appears clinically primarily in dogs.

Pathogenesis

The pathogenesis of the disease begins with the ingestion of the pathogens by the vector. During the sucking act by the tick, the *Anaplasma* are ingested and enter the midgut of the tick. Replication of the *Anaplasma* is located in the epithelial cells of the midgut. The *Anaplasma* migrate into haemocytes and through these into the salivary glands of the tick, where they remain until they are transmitted during the next blood meal. The uptake of the blood by the tick is carried out by two different mechanisms. Firstly, the tick can destroy the superficial skin layers with its mouthparts, which erodes superficial blood vessels and causes bleeding. More important for the pathogenesis is the absorption of blood from deeper blood vessels. To do this, the tick bites its biting apparatus into the skin and injects saliva. This contains, among other things, proteins that are anticoagulant and prevent platelet aggregation. In this way, the sucking act can take place over several days without blood clotting preventing the absorption of blood (Figure 48.3.1.1).

The transfer of the *Anaplasma* to the respective target cells occurs in steps. In general, *A. phagocytophilum* shows tropism for granulocytes and leads to granulocytic anaplasmosis, while *A. platys* has tropism for platelets and causes canine cyclic thrombocytopenia. For *A. phagocytophilum*, the infection cycle presumably begins initially with infection of endothelial cells. This induces the increased expression of adhesion molecules (e.g. ICAM-1). Subsequently, granulocytes bind to the endothelial cells, resulting in pathogen transmission. The mechanism is supported by an induction of the release of IL-8 by infected granulocytes. IL-8, in turn, is a chemotactic cytokine and implies the immigration of neutrophilic granulocytes, which increases the rate of infection. At the same time, infected granulocytes show a reduced diapedesis and therefore remain in the vascular system for a longer time (Figure 48.3.1.2).

The pathogens are transmitted by receptor-mediated endocytosis. In the neutrophilic granulocytes, *A. phagocytophilum* multiplies in membrane-bound vesicles and forms so-called 'morulae'. Increased synthesis can lead to rupture of the cell

Textbook of Small Animal Pathophysiology, First Edition. Stephan Neumann.
© 2025 John Wiley & Sons Ltd. Published 2025 by John Wiley & Sons Ltd.

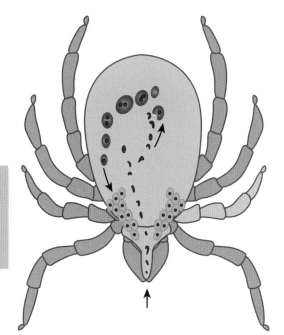

1. Ingestion of the pathogens
2. Replication of the anaplasmas in the epithelial cells of the midgut
3. Migrate into haemocytes
4. Transport of haemocytes to salivary glands
5. Transmission during the next blood meal.

Figure 48.3.1.1 Pathogen uptake in the tick.

membrane of the neutrophilic granulocytes, releasing *A. phagocytophilum*. Within the granulocytes, *A. phagocytophilum* can prevent its own elimination by, for example, inhibiting the synthesis of superoxides. In addition, the pathogen can prevent granulocytic apoptosis and thus ensure its survival by prolonging granulocytic lifespan (Severo et al. 2012).

The target cell of *A. platys* is the platelet. Here, too, there is invasion by the pathogens, multiplication and finally destruction of the target cell as the degree of multiplication increases.

Diagnostics

Clinical signs	Clinical pathology	Imaging	Histopathology	Microbiology
Non-specific	Anaplasmosis antibodies Serum, ELISA Anaplasmosis antigen EDTA-blood, PCR	Not necessary	Not necessary	Not necessary

Pathophysiologic Consequences

Influenced organ systems	Clinical symptoms	Clinical pathological alterations
Haematological system Bones, joints	Lethargy Fever Inappetence Surface bleeding Lameness	Thrombocytopenia Leukopenia Anaemia Increased liver enzymes

Lethargy, fever, inappetence follow the general mechanisms of infectious disease.

The lethargy that often accompanies infections is closely linked to the body's immune response. The activation of the immune system involves various cells, such as macrophages and T cells, which release proinflammatory cytokines, such as

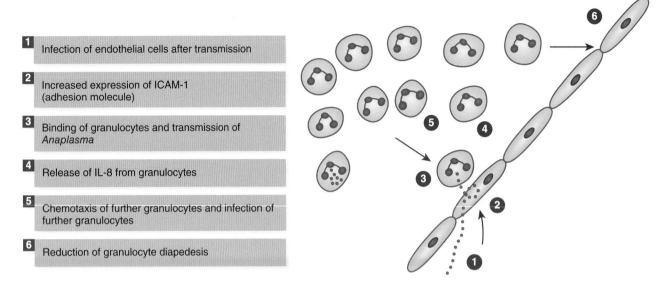

1 Infection of endothelial cells after transmission

2 Increased expression of ICAM-1 (adhesion molecule)

3 Binding of granulocytes and transmission of *Anaplasma*

4 Release of IL-8 from granulocytes

5 Chemotaxis of further granulocytes and infection of further granulocytes

6 Reduction of granulocyte diapedesis

Figure 48.3.1.2 Infection of granulocytes by *A. phagocytophilum*.

IL-1, IL-6 and TNF-α. These cytokines play a central role in coordinating immune defence against pathogens. They also affect the central nervous system by crossing the blood-brain barrier or stimulating peripheral nerves.

In the brain, these cytokines interact with microglia, the immune cells of the central nervous system. This interaction triggers a cascade of events involving the production of other inflammatory mediators, such as prostaglandins and reactive oxygen species. As a result, these molecules alter the balance of neurotransmitters, particularly serotonin, dopamine and glutamate, affecting mood, motivation and energy levels. Dysregulation of these neurotransmitters is associated with symptoms, such as lethargy and depression during infection.

In addition, anorexia during infection can be attributed to several biochemical mechanisms. Cytokines released during the immune response not only affect the brain, but also target specific hypothalamic nuclei responsible for regulating appetite and satiety. These cytokines disrupt the balance of neuropeptides, such as neuropeptide Y (NPY) and suppress the action of appetite-stimulating hormones, such as ghrelin, while promoting anorexigenic signals, such as corticotropin-releasing hormone (CRH) and leptin.

In addition, the shift in metabolic priorities from digestion to immune defence influences hormonal signalling related to hunger and satiety. The body's redirection of energy resources to fight infection reduces the production of gastrointestinal hormones involved in appetite regulation, thereby reducing the desire to eat.

Bleeding can occur in anaplasmosis due to **thrombocytopenia.** Although the tropism with regard to thrombocytes is given by *A. platys*, infections with *A. phagocytophilum* also lead to thrombocytopenia. The mechanism is based, on the one hand, on an infection of the megakaryocytes, which reduces the formation of thrombocytes. Another mechanism is based on an immune-mediated thrombocytopenia caused by the presence of anti-platelet antibodies (Kohn et al. 2008).

Mild non-regenerative anaemia, which occurs in anaplasmosis, could be a consequence of the effect of the *Anaplasma* on the bone marrow or a consequence of an immune-mediated reaction. The anaemia, in turn, could cause mild hypoxia leading to elevation of **liver enzymes.**

Lameness in dogs with anaplasmosis develops as a result of immune-mediated non-erosive arthritis.

Therapy

Symptom	Therapy
Antibiotics	Doxycycline

References

Kohn, B., Galke, D., Beelitz, P., and Pfister, K. (2008). Clinical features of canine granulocytic anaplasmosis in 18 naturally infected dogs. *Journal of Veterinary Internal Medicine* 22 (6): 1289–1295. https://doi.org/10.1111/j.1939-1676.2008.0180.x.

Severo, M.S., Stephens, K.D., Kotsyfakis, M., and Pedra, J.H. (2012). Anaplasma phagocytophilum: deceptively simple or simply deceptive? *Future Microbiology* 7 (6): 719–731. https://doi.org/10.2217/fmb.12.45.

Further Reading

Atif, F.A., Mehnaz, S., Qamar, M.F. et al. (2021). Epidemiology, diagnosis, and control of canine infectious cyclic thrombocytopenia and granulocytic anaplasmosis: emerging diseases of veterinary and public health significance. *Veterinary Sciences* 8 (12): 312. https://doi.org/10.3390/vetsci8120312.

Carrade, D.D., Foley, J.E., Borjesson, D.L., and Sykes, J.E. (2009). Canine granulocytic anaplasmosis: a review. *Journal of Veterinary Internal Medicine* 23 (6): 1129–1141. https://doi.org/10.1111/j.1939-1676.2009.0384.x.

Chirek, A., Silaghi, C., Pfister, K., and Kohn, B. (2018). Granulocytic anaplasmosis in 63 dogs: clinical signs, laboratory results, therapy and course of disease. *The Journal of Small Animal Practice* 59 (2): 112–120. https://doi.org/10.1111/jsap.12787.

Diniz, P.P.V.P. and Moura de Aguiar, D. (2022). Ehrlichiosis and anaplasmosis: an update. *The Veterinary Clinics of North America. Small Animal Practice* 52 (6): 1225–1266. http://dx.doi.org/10.1016/j.cvsm.2022.07.002.

48.3.2

Borreliosis

Aetiology

Lyme borreliosis is an infectious disease that occurs predominantly in dogs. The pathogen belongs to the Spirochaetaceae family and the genus *Borrelia*. The clinically relevant genospecies belong to the *B. burgdorferi* sensu lato complex. They occur worldwide and have different reservoirs. *B. burgdorferi* sensu stricto has rodents in the larvae and nymphs or wild animals, such as deer, in the adults as reservoirs. *B. garinii* has birds as reservoirs, and *B. afzelii* and *B. spielmanii* rodents.

The pathogen is a spirally coiled, motile bacterium with a length of 8–30 μm and a width of 0.18–0.25 μm. The motility is made possible by 7–11 periplasmic endoflagellae located in the cell membrane.

Lyme borreliosis belongs to the vector-borne diseases. The vector is *Ixodes ricinus*, which have a life cycle of two to four years with the developmental stages: egg, larva, nymph and adult. In each developmental stage, there is a blood meal. This takes two to four days for larvae and nymphs, and five to seven days for adults.

Pathogenesis

The pathogenesis of Lyme borreliosis begins with the uptake of the *Borrelia* by the ticks. This takes place during the sucking act in animals of the reservoir. In the ticks, the *Borrelia* lives in the midgut after ingestion. During another blood meal before the next moult, transmission of the *Borrelia* occurs. In the preliminary phase of transmission, the *Borrelia* bacteria are inactive in the midgut. This can be recognised by an increased expression of a surface protein A. After ingestion of blood, the expression of surface protein A is downregulated and there is increased expression of surface protein C. This altered structure of the bacterial surface allows translocation of the *Borrelia* into the salivary glands of the ticks. The *Borrelia* is transmitted from these. Since activation and translocation take some time, there is a delay of about 24 hours after a tick bite before the *Borrelia* bacteria is transmitted. The *Borrelia* species with which the vectors are infected also seems to influence the speed of transmission. Thus, *I. ricinus* transmits *B. afzelii* faster than *B. burdorferi* sensu stricto (Crippa et al. 2002).

After transmission, there is a multiplication of *Borrelia* at the site of entry. This leads to an invasion and activation of defence cells, such as dendritic cells, macrophages and T and B lymphocytes. *Borrelia* with surface protein A, if transmitted, is eliminated by the body's own defences. The expression of surface protein C, on the other hand, protects the *Borrelia* from intervention by the immune system. A second protective factor is the tick salivary protein 15, which covers the *Borrelia* and protects it against the immune system, as well as the surface lipoprotein VlsE. The body's own defence system can inactivate *Borrelia* by phagocytosis and the formation of oxygen radicals. *Borrelia* that has survived this initial defences spreads throughout the organism. Dissemination via the blood with migration into target organs is discussed. These are preferentially rich in connective tissue; especially N-acetyl-glucosamine seems to be an important factor for the survival of the *Borrelia*. Another migration discussed is movement along connective tissue structures, such as fasciae (Figure 48.3.2.1).

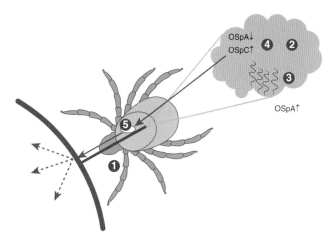

1 Uptake of the *Borrelia* by the ticks

2 In the ticks, the *Borrelia* live in the midgut after ingestion

3 In the preliminary phase of transmission, the *Borrelia* is inactive in the midgut. This can be recognised by an increased expression of a surface protein A

4 After ingestion of blood, the expression of surface protein A is down-regulated and there is increased expression of surface protein C

5 This altered structure of the bacterial surface allows translocation of the *Borrelia* into the salivary glands of the ticks. The *Borrelia* is transmitted from these

Figure 48.3.2.1 Mechanism of transmission of *Borrelia* by *Ixodes*.

Diagnostics

Clinical signs	Clinical pathology	Imaging	Histopathology	Microbiology
Non-specific	PCR skin or tick *Borrelia* antibodies (C6) Serum	Not necessary	Not necessary	Not necessary

Pathophysiologic Consequences

The clinical symptoms of Lyme borreliosis can be systemic in the acute phase or local in the joints and kidneys due to immune-mediated processes.

Influenced organ systems	Clinical symptoms	Clinical pathological alterations
Urinary tract	Fever	Thrombocytopenia
Bones, joints	Lymph node swelling	Non- regenerative Anaemia
	Anorexia	Azotaemia
	Lameness	Hypoalbuminaemia
	Joint swelling	Proteinuria
	PU/PD	

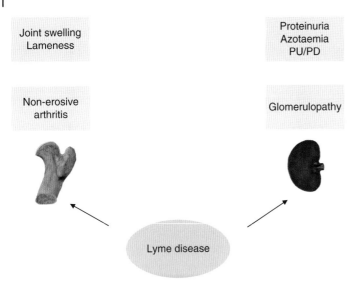

Figure 48.3.2.2 Pathophysiology of Lyme borreliosis.

In the acute infection phase, Lyme disease may be accompanied by **fever** and **swelling of the lymph nodes** as signs of active infection.

Clinically, dogs suffering from joint or kidney manifestations are presented more frequently.

The **lameness** is a consequence of mono- or polyarthritis, which occurs a few months (two to four months) post infection. The arthritis may be associated with systemic symptoms, such as fever or lethargy. Locally, there is an increase in synovial fluid and an accumulation of leucocytes in the form of neutrophilic granulocytes in the synovium. The mechanism could be based on a joint infection with *Borrelia*, but an immune-mediated genesis is also possible. According to this, the immune system would be sensitised to surface proteins of the *Borrelia* and, in accordance with the mimicry hypothesis, autoantibodies would be formed against joint structures, which leads to arthritis (Steere and Glickstein 2004; Nardelli et al. 2008).

Nephropathy is a consequence of immune-complex associated with tubulopathy and is more common in some dog breeds, such as retrievers. In addition to necrosis in the renal parenchyma, signs of regeneration or repair processes (fibrosis) are recognisable, accompanied by lymphoplasma cellular interstitial nephritis. The changes lead to increased protein secretion via the glomerula and thus to proteinuria and hypoalbuminuria. (Littman 2013) (Figure 48.3.2.2).

Therapy

Symptom	Therapy
Antibiotics	Amoxycillin, Doxycycline
Glomerulopathy	ACE inhibitors, acetylsalicylic acid

References

Crippa, M., Rais, O., and Gern, L. (2002). Investigations on the mode and dynamics of transmission and infectivity of *Borrelia burgdorferi* sensu stricto and *Borrelia afzelii* in *Ixodes ricinus* ticks. *Vector Borne and Zoonotic Diseases (Larchmont, N.Y.)* 2 (1): 3–9. https://doi.org/10.1089/153036602760260724.

Littman, M.P. (2013). Lyme nephritis. *Journal of Veterinary Emergency and Critical Care (San Antonio, Tex.: 2001)* 23 (2): 163–173. https://doi.org/10.1111/vec.12026.

Nardelli, D.T., Callister, S.M., and Schell, R.F. (2008). Lyme arthritis: current concepts and a change in paradigm. *Clinical and Vaccine Immunology: CVI* 15 (1): 21–34. https://doi.org/10.1128/CVI.00330-07.

Steere, A.C. and Glickstein, L. (2004). Elucidation of Lyme arthritis. *Nature Reviews. Immunology* 4 (2): 143–152. https://doi.org/10.1038/nri1267.

Further Reading

Donta, S.T., States, L.J., Adams, W.A. et al. (2021). Report of the pathogenesis and pathophysiology of Lyme disease subcommittee of the HHS Tick Borne Disease Working Group. *Frontiers in Medicine* 8: 643235. https://doi.org/10.3389/fmed.2021.643235.

Krupka, I. and Straubinger, R.K. (2010). Lyme borreliosis in dogs and cats: background, diagnosis, treatment and prevention of infections with Borrelia burgdorferi sensu stricto. *The Veterinary Clinics of North America. Small Animal Practice* 40 (6): 1103–1119. https://doi.org/10.1016/j.cvsm.2010.07.011.

Littman, M.P., Gerber, B., Goldstein, R.E. et al. (2018). ACVIM consensus update on Lyme borreliosis in dogs and cats. *Journal of Veterinary Internal Medicine* 32 (3): 887–903. https://doi.org/10.1111/jvim.15085.

Lochhead, R. B., Strle, K., Arvikar, S. L., Weis, J. J., & Steere, A. C. (2021). Lyme arthritis: linking infection, inflammation and autoimmunity. *Nature Reviews. Rheumatology*, 17(8), 449-461. https://doi.org/10.1038/s41584-021-00648-5

48.3.3

Ehrlichiosis

Aetiology

Ehrlichia are gram-negative, obligate intracellular bacteria. They belong to the family Anaplasmataceae and the order Rickettsiales. The pathogen is transmitted by ticks and canines are considered the reservoir. The disease occurs in dogs and cats, but is more common in dogs. *E. canis*, *E. chaffeensis* and *E. ewingii* are of veterinary importance.

Pathogenesis

The pathogenesis of ehrlichiosis begins with the ingestion of the pathogens by the vector. These are ticks, primarily *Rhipicephalus sanguineus* is considered the vector for the transmission of ehrlichiosis. The uptake of the pathogens takes place during the blood meal by the tick, which is before each moult. Larvae and nymphs are susceptible and can transmit the pathogens to the next stage before moulting. Transmission is possible after only a few hours. After transmission, the *Ehrlichia* bind to glycoproteins expressed by monocytes. After binding, the *Ehrlichia* are taken up into the cell by an invagination of the monocyte membrane. This results in the formation of a so-called 'endosome'. Endosomes are eliminated under physiological conditions by fusion with lysosomes. The latter contain numerous hydrolytic enzymes, such as proteases, nucleases and lipases. *Ehrlichia* prevent the fusion of the endosome with the lysosome. Thus, the pathogens escape elimination in the monocytes and can be transported with them via the blood flow. Within the monocytes, the *Ehrlichia* form a morula by division. This can rupture after the *Ehrlichia* have proliferated and the *Ehrlichia* can be released by cell destruction and infect further monocytes. The resulting clinical picture is monocytic ehrlichiosis. In addition, granulomatous ehrlichiosis has also been described after infection of neutrophilic granulocytes. In the case of infection with *E. canis*, the incubation period is two to three weeks. Clinically manifest ehrlichiosis can take an acute course lasting two to four weeks. Subacute and chronic infections have also been described. The latter forms develop through persistence of the pathogens in cells of the spleen and bone marrow (Figure 48.3.3.1).

Diagnostics

Clinical signs	Clinical pathology	Imaging	Histopathology	Microbiology
Non-specific	PCR EDTA-blood Antibodies Serum	Not necessary	Not necessary	Not necessary

Pathophysiologic Consequences

Antibodies against *E. canis* are detectable from about 15 days post infection in experimental studies. Furthermore, the formation of high, non-protective antibody titres, polyclonal or monoclonal hypergammaglobulinaemia with hyperviscosity,

Textbook of Small Animal Pathophysiology, First Edition. Stephan Neumann.
© 2025 John Wiley & Sons Ltd. Published 2025 by John Wiley & Sons Ltd.

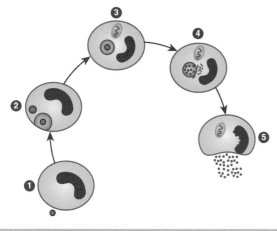

1 *Ehrlichia* bind to glycoproteins expressed by monocytes

2 After binding, the *Ehrlichia* are taken up into the cell by an invagination of the monocyte membrane

3 This results in the formation of a so-called endosome. Endosomes are eliminated under physiological conditions by fusion with lysosomes. The latter contain numerous hydrolytic enzymes, such as proteases, nucleases and lipases. *Ehrlichia* prevent the fusion of the endosome with the lysosome. Thus, the pathogens escape elimination in the monocytes and can be washed away with them via the blood flow.

4 Within the monocytes, the *Ehrlichia* form a morula by division.

5 This can rupture after the *Ehrlichia* have proliferated and the *Ehrlichia* can be released by cell destruction and infect further monocytes.

Figure 48.3.3.1 Mechanism of infection of monocytes.

and immunopathology with circulating immune complexes and formation of autoantibodies play an important role in the pathogenesis (Day 2011).

Clinically manifest ehrlichiosis shows a variety of organ dysfunctions.

Influenced organ systems	Clinical symptoms	Clinical pathological alterations
Respiratory system	Weight loss	Thrombocytopenia
Hepatobiliary system	Anorexia	Pancytopenia (chronic cases)
Central nervous system	Lethargy	Non-regenerative anaemia
Haematological system	Fever	Polyclonal gammopathy
Ophthalmic system	Nasal discharge	Hypoalbuminaemia
	Petechiae	Proteinuria
	Splenomegaly	Autoagglutination
	Lymphadenopathy	Positive Coombs test
	Eye changes	
	Conjunctivitis	
	Uveitis	
	Corneal oedema	
	Neurological symptoms	
	Seizures	
	Ataxia	
	Paresis	

Weight loss, anorexia, lethargy, fever are typical generalised symptoms of the infectious process (see Anaplasmosis or Babesiosis which is described in Chapter 48.3.1. in detail).

Splenomegaly and **lymphadenopathy** are consequences of the activation of the defence system. As a result of the infection, **thrombocytopenia** also occurs due to minor synthesis, aggregation or sequestration. This in turn disturbs blood coagulation and can explain manifestations, such as petechiae or neurological deficits or ocular changes as a consequence of bleeding. Other symptoms such as **proteinuria, hypoalbuminaemia,** but also **anaemia** can be immune-mediated. This is underlined by the massive synthesis of globulins after an infection with *Ehrlichia*. This is reflected in a polyclonal gammopathy. The synthesis of non-protective antibodies in high concentrations can lead to hyperviscosity in the blood and to the formation and deposition of immune complexes in various organs, for example the kidneys, with the development of glomerulonephritis.

Different **ocular symptoms** are common in ehrlichiosis. One mechanism is that *E. canis* induces an inflammatory response in the body, which can cause damage to the blood vessels in the eyes. When *E. canis* infects white blood cells, it triggers the production of cytokines. The cytokines can cause inflammation and damage to the blood vessels, leading to a reduction in blood flow to the eyes. Reduced blood flow can cause different ocular symptoms, including uveitis, retinal haemorrhage and vision disturbances. Another mechanism is that *E. canis* directly invades the cells of the eyes, including the cornea, iris and retina, and triggers an immune response that leads to inflammation and damage to these structures. Finally, *E. canis* can cause ocular changes through the formation of immune complexes. When the body produces antibodies against the bacteria, the antibodies can form immune complexes that can deposit in the blood vessels and tissues of the eyes. The immune complexes can trigger an immune response and cause inflammation and damage to the eye tissues.

Therapy

Symptom	Therapy
Antibiotics	Doxycycline

Reference

Day, M.J. (2011). The immunopathology of canine vector-borne diseases. *Parasites & Vectors* 4: 48. https://doi.org/10.1186/1756-3305-4-48.

Further Reading

Crivellenti, L.Z., Cintra, C.A., Maia, S.R. et al. (2021). Glomerulotubular pathology in dogs with subclinical ehrlichiosis. *PLoS One* 16 (12): e0260702. https://doi.org/10.1371/journal.pone.0260702.

Diniz, P.P.V.P. and Moura de Aguiar, D. (2022). Ehrlichiosis and anaplasmosis: an update. *The Veterinary Clinics of North America. Small Animal Practice* 52 (6): 1225–1266. https://doi.org/10.1016/j.cvsm.2022.07.002.

Little, S.E. (2010). Ehrlichiosis and anaplasmosis in dogs and cats. *The Veterinary Clinics of North America. Small Animal Practice* 40 (6): 1121–1140. https://doi.org/10.1016/j.cvsm.2010.07.004.

Mylonakis, M.E., Harrus, S., and Breitschwerdt, E.B. (2019). An update on the treatment of canine monocytic ehrlichiosis (*Ehrlichia canis*). *Veterinary Journal (London, England: 1997)* 246: 45–53. https://doi.org/10.1016/j.tvjl.2019.01.015.

Neer, T.M., Breitschwerdt, E.B., Greene, R.T., and Lappin, M.R. (2002). Consensus statement on ehrlichial disease of small animals from the infectious disease study group of the ACVIM. American College of Veterinary Internal Medicine. *Journal of Veterinary Internal Medicine* 16 (3): 309–315. https://doi.org/10.1892/0891-6640(2002)016<0309:csoedo>2.3.co;2.

48.3.4

Leptospirosis

Aetiology

Leptospirosis is a bacterial infectious disease caused by a gram-negative spiral-shaped bacterium belonging to the Spirochaetaceae family. A total of more than 250 serovars in different serogroups have been described. Of veterinary importance are the species *Leptospira interrogans* and *Leptospira kirschneri*. These can also be differentiated into different serogroups.

Leptospires are characterised by a curved cell body, which has a length of 20–24 μm and has a width of 0.1 μm. Leptospires are motile; motility results from rotation around their own axis. The disease occurs regularly in the dog. In the cat, infections have been described without clinical symptoms.

Pathogenesis

Numerous warm-blooded animals, such as rats, mice, dogs, horses and ruminants, are considered reservoirs for leptospirosis. The pathogens are excreted by infected animals via various body fluids. Particularly high pathogen concentrations are found in urine. In dogs, up to 10^5 leptospires/ml are detected in the first weeks of infection (Heath and Johnson 1994). Even clinically inconspicuous dogs can excrete leptospires (Rojas et al. 2010).

Outside the organism, the survival time of leptospires depends on the environmental conditions. Humid and cool months allow a survival time of several weeks.

The pathogens are transmitted directly through contact with infected urine or blood or indirectly through ingestion of the pathogens from infected waters or infected cadavers (Greene et al. 2006).

The leptospires can be absorbed through the intact mucous membrane, for example, of the mouth or the conjunctiva. Skin wounds are also considered entry points. After ingestion, the leptospires are spread haematogenously. The pathogens multiply significantly in the blood, especially if no antibodies have been formed yet. The leptospires protect themselves from intervention by the body's own defences through various mechanisms. Inhibitory influences on the complement system have been described, for example through the binding of plasmin on the bacterial surface, which inactivates complement (Barbosa and Isaac 2020). After haematogenous spread, organ colonisation occurs, which can begin as early as one day post infection. The target organs in a leptospirosis infection are:

Liver
Kidney
Lungs
Musculature
Eyes
Pancreas
Spleen

Of greater clinical relevance are the infections of the liver, kidneys and lungs.

The liver is the first parenchymatous organ to be colonised during haematogenous dissemination. Leptospires have been detected in liver tissue as early as 24 hours post infection. In the liver parenchyma, the leptospires cause acute hepatitis.

Textbook of Small Animal Pathophysiology, First Edition. Stephan Neumann.

Different bacterial proteases, such as phospholipases and collagenases cause damage to the hepatocyte membrane with cell necrosis (Schuller et al. 2015). Another mechanism is the downregulation of the expression of cadherins, which are involved in cell-to-cell contact of hepatocytes. This results in reduced intercellular communication and disruption of intercellular transport (De Brito et al. 2018).

Persistence of leptospires in the liver parenchyma can additionally destroy the liver tissue via fibrosis induction due to the persisting inflammation.

Invasion of the renal parenchyma begins approximately 72 hours post infection. The leptospires penetrate the renal capillaries and enter the renal interstitium and renal tubular epithelial cells, where they multiply (Greene et al. 2006). The invasion leads to capillary damage with ischaemia of the parenchyma. Consequently, reduced ATP formation develops, which in turn inhibits the activity of Na^+-K^+-ATPase, causing water to enter the cell following the osmotic gradient and inducing cell oedema with loss of cell function. This affects both glomerular filtration and tubule function. Reduced expression of aquaporins in the collecting tubule limits the retention of water in the kidneys.

In the lung parenchyma, leptospirosis causes interstitial pneumonia. The pathomechanism is multifaceted. If leptospirosis proceeds septically, pulmonary vasculitis can lead to lung damage. In addition, immune complex deposits in the alveoli have been described as triggers of pneumonia (Croda et al. 2010; Medeiros et al. 2010).

Experimental studies have demonstrated deposits of IgG, IgA and C3 along the alveolar basement membrane, leading to alveolar destruction (Nally et al. 2004). Leptospirosis-associated coagulopathies may also contribute to pulmonary vascular damage (Greene et al. 2006).

Diagnostics

Clinical signs	Clinical pathology	Imaging	Histopathology	Microbiology
Non-specific	Organ involvement liver – kidney	Not necessary	Not necessary	Microagglutination test (MAT-test) PCR blood, urine

Pathophysiologic Consequences

Influenced organ systems	Clinical symptoms	Clinical pathological alterations
Respiratory system	Anorexia	Regenerative anaemia
Hepatobiliary system	Lethargy	Leukocytosis> 40 000/microl
Urinary tract	Vomitus	Thrombocytopenia
Systemic	Fever	Creatinine
Haematological system	Diarrhoea	Urea
	PU/PD	ALT
	Muscle pain	ALP
	Uveitis	T-Bili

Source: Greene et al. (2006).

The non-specific symptoms of **anorexia** and **lethargy** result from mostly cytokine-driven mechanisms which are described in Chapter 48.3.1. in detail.

Mechanism of **diarrhoea** and **vomiting** in leptospirosis is complex; vomiting may result from gastritis or associated pancreatitis. Diarrhoea is the result of a disturbance of Na^+-K^+-ATPase induced by the leptospira. The disturbance leads to a reduced Na^+ resorption from the intestinal lumen, water also remains, in addition to a disturbed Cl^- resorption, even a secretion is possible, this further reduces the water resorption. Glucose is reabsorbed in cotransport with Na^+, which is also impaired. All this together leads to osmotic-secretory diarrhoea.

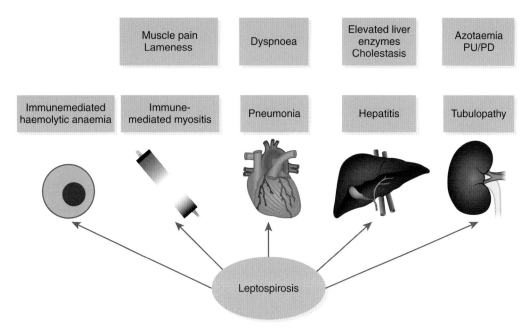

Figure 48.3.4.1 Pathophysiology of leptospirosis.

PU/PD is associated with renal damage caused by leptospires. Reduced glomerular filtration initially leads to oliguria and **azotaemia,** but as tubular damage progresses, renal water reabsorption along the nephron is reduced and by reducing aquaporin expression, leptospires also affect water reabsorption in the distal tubule and collecting duct. Thus, they produce functional peripheral diabetes insipidus (Etish et al. 2014). In addition, metabolic acidosis can result from renal bicarbonate loss.

The elevation of **liver enzymes** initially shows increased cellular disintegration due to hepatocyte necrosis; this causes an increase in the activity of ALT and AST. ALP and T-bilirubin, on the other hand, are consequences of **cholestasis** caused by leptospires. This is mainly caused by the destruction of the tight-junctions between the hepatocytes. This causes leakage of bile into the sinusoids (Miyahara et al. 2014).

Leptospirosis-associated **myositis** is accompanied by a marked increase in the muscle enzymes CK and AST, indicating destruction of the myocytes. Immune-complex-mediated destruction is suspected as the cause.

This mechanism is also responsible for the associated immune-mediated haemolytic **anaemia.** The mechanism of IMHA is based on a structural change of the erythrocyte surface due to leptospiral infection. This results in an antibody (AK) reaction with complement activation leading to intravascular haemolysis with haemoglobin release or extravascular haemolysis with activation of the MPS and spherocyte formation (Figure 48.3.4.1).

Therapy

Symptom	Therapy
Antibiotics against pathogen	Amoxycillin, Doxycycline
Vomitus	Antiemetic drugs (e.g. Ondansetron, Maropitant, Omeprazole)

References

Barbosa, A.S. and Isaac, L. (2020). Strategies used by Leptospira spirochetes to evade the host complement system. *FEBS Letters* 594 (16): 2633–2644. https://doi.org/10.1002/1873-3468.13768.

Croda, J., Neto, A.N., Brasil, R.A. et al. (2010). Leptospirosis pulmonary haemorrhage syndrome is associated with linear deposition of immunoglobulin and complement on the alveolar surface. *Clinical Microbiology and Infection: The Official Publication of the European Society of Clinical Microbiology and Infectious Diseases* 16 (6): 593–599. https://doi.org/10.1111/j.1469-0691.2009.02916.x.

De Brito, T., Silva, A.M.G.D., and Abreu, P.A.E. (2018). Pathology and pathogenesis of human leptospirosis: a commented review. *Revista do Instituto de Medicina Tropical de Sao Paulo* 60: e23. https://doi.org/10.1590/s1678-9946201860023.

Etish, J.L., Chapman, P.S., and Klag, A.R. (2014). Acquired nephrogenic diabetes insipidus in a dog with leptospirosis. *Irish Veterinary Journal* 67 (1): 7. https://doi.org/10.1186/2046-0481-67-7.

Greene, C.E., Sykes, J., Brown, C.A., and Hartmann, K. (2006). Leptospirosis. In: *Infectious Diseases of the Dog and Cat*, 3e (ed. C.E. Greene), 402–417. Philadelphia: WB Saunders.

Heath, S.E. and Johnson, R. (1994). Leptospirosis. *Journal of the American Veterinary Medical Association* 205 (11): 1518–1523.

Medeiros, F.d.R., Spichler, A., and Athanazio, D.A. (2010). Leptospirosis-associated disturbances of blood vessels, lungs and hemostasis. *Acta Tropica* 115 (1–2): 155–162. https://doi.org/10.1016/j.actatropica.2010.02.016.

Miyahara, S., Saito, M., Kanemaru, T. et al. (2014). Destruction of the hepatocyte junction by intercellular invasion of Leptospira causes jaundice in a hamster model of Weil's disease. *International Journal of Experimental Pathology* 95 (4): 271–281. https://doi.org/10.1111/iep.12085.

Nally, J.E., Chantranuwat, C., Wu, X.Y. et al. (2004). Alveolar septal deposition of immunoglobulin and complement parallels pulmonary hemorrhage in a Guinea pig model of severe pulmonary leptospirosis. *The American Journal of Pathology* 164 (3): 1115–1127. https://doi.org/10.1016/S0002-9440(10)63198-7.

Rojas, P., Monahan, A.M., Schuller, S. et al. (2010). Detection and quantification of leptospires in urine of dogs: a maintenance host for the zoonotic disease leptospirosis. *European Journal of Clinical Microbiology & Infectious Diseases: Official Publication of the European Society of Clinical Microbiology* 29 (10): 1305–1309. https://doi.org/10.1007/s10096-010-0991-2.

Schuller, S., Francey, T., Hartmann, K. et al. (2015). European consensus statement on leptospirosis in dogs and cats. *The Journal of Small Animal Practice* 56 (3): 159–179. https://doi.org/10.1111/jsap.12328.

Further Reading

Furlanello, T. and Reale, I. (2019). Leptospirosis and immune-mediated hemolytic anemia: a lethal association. *Veterinary Research Forum: An International Quarterly Journal* 10 (3): 261–265. https://doi.org/10.30466/vrf.2019.99876.2385.

Knöpfler, S. V. (2015).Clinical, laboratory diagnostic, radiological findings and course in 99 dogs with leptospirosis (2006-2013). Dissertation, Berlin.

Raj, J., Campbell, R., and Tappin, S. (2021). Clinical findings in dogs diagnosed with leptospirosis in England. *The Veterinary Record* 189 (7): e452. https://doi.org/10.1002/vetr.452.

Reagan, K.L. and Sykes, J.E. (2019). Diagnosis of canine leptospirosis. *The Veterinary Clinics of North America. Small Animal Practice* 49 (4): 719–731. https://doi.org/10.1016/j.cvsm.2019.02.008.

Zamagni, S., Troìa, R., Zaccheroni, F., Monari, E., Grisetti, C., Perissinotto, L., Balboni, A., & Dondi, F. (2020). Comparison of clinicopathological patterns of renal tubular damage in dogs with acute kidney injury caused by leptospirosis and other aetiologies. *Veterinary Journal (London, England: 1997)*, 266, 105573. https://doi.org/10.1016/j.tvjl.2020.105573.

48.4

Protozoal Infections

48.4.1

Babesiosis

Aetiology

The causative agent of babesiosis is a protozoan that parasitises in erythrocytes and is transmitted by vectors. Vectors include different tick species (*Dermacentor*, *Rhipicephalus*, *Ixodes*). Babesias are differentiated into small and large forms, which are also distinguished by different courses of disease. Babesiosis occurs in dogs and cats, but plays a greater role in dogs. Different wild and domestic animals are considered to be the reservoir for the babesia (Table 48.4.1.1).

Pathogenesis

Pathogenesis begins with the ingestion of the babesia by the vector. The babesias are ingested by the ticks during the blood meal before moulting and can thus be ingested by larvae and nymphs. Adult female ticks can also ingest the babesia and transmit it transovarially to the eggs and thus to the next generation. The merozoites are ingested by the ticks as products of the asexual reproduction of the babesia (merogony) in the erythrocytes. After ingestion, sexual reproduction (gamogony) takes place in the vector with the formation of a zygote in the intestinal cells of the ticks' midgut. From there, the ookinetes migrate as an intermediate form into the salivary glands of the tick and, after asexual reproduction, are transmitted as sporozoites during the sucking act. After transfer, the sporozoites, which are self-motile, penetrate through the membrane into the erythrocytes.

Within the erythrocytes, asexual reproduction then takes place as merogony (Figures 48.4.1.1 and 48.4.1.2).

Anti-erythrocytic antibodies develop, as well as increased macrophage activity and complement activation. This triggers intra- and extravascular haemolysis. After activation of the kallikrein-kinin system, vasodilation and increase of capillary permeability occur. Fibrinogen-like proteins are released, triggering increased adhesion of erythrocytes to capillary endothelia and thus clumping of erythrocytes. As a result, circulatory stasis and disseminated intravascular coagulopathy occur. The tissue hypoxia leads to the release of cytokines and organ damage in the kidneys, liver, lungs and central nervous system (Rafaj et al. 2009).

Diagnostics

Clinical signs	Clinical pathology	Imaging	Histopathology	Microbiology
Non-specific	Haemolytic anaemia Serum antibody detection EDTA-blood antigen detection by PCR	Not necessary	Not necessary	Not necessary

Textbook of Small Animal Pathophysiology, First Edition. Stephan Neumann.
© 2025 John Wiley & Sons Ltd. Published 2025 by John Wiley & Sons Ltd.

Table 48.4.1.1 Differentiation of some veterinary relevant babesias.

Pathogen	Vector	Degree of illness
B. canis	*Dermacentor reticularis*	Moderate to severe
B. vogeli	*Rhipicephalus sanguineus*	Low to moderate
B. gibsoni	*Rhipicephalus sanguineus*	Moderate to severe
B. vulpis	*Ixodes*	Moderate to severe

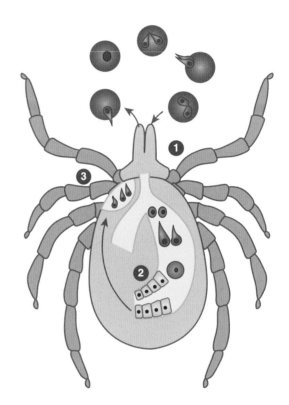

1 The Babesia are ingested by the ticks during the blood meal. The merozoites are ingested by the ticks as products of the asexual reproduction of the Babesia (merogony) in the erythrocytes

2 After ingestion, sexual reproduction (gamogony) takes place in the vector with the formation of a zygote in the intestinal cells of the ticks' midgut

3 From there, the kinetes migrate as an intermediate form into the salivary glands of the tick and, after asexual reproduction, are transmitted as sporozoites during the sucking act

Figure 48.4.1.1 Babesiosis cycle.

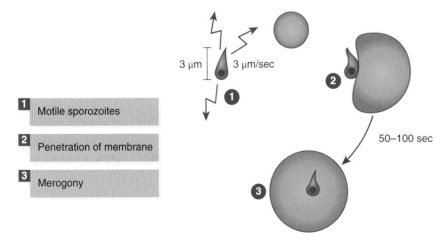

1 Motile sporozoites

2 Penetration of membrane

3 Merogony

Figure 48.4.1.2 Invasion of the erythrocytes and release of the parasites.

Pathophysiologic Consequences

The pathophysiologic consequences of babesiosis result from the destruction of the erythrocytes and the associated reduced oxygen supply. In addition, an immunological reaction against the erythrocytes can lead to immune-mediated reactions.

Influenced organ systems	Clinical symptoms	Clinical pathological alterations
Urinary tract	Generalised	Anaemia
Central nervous system	Lethargy	Thrombocytopenia
Haematological system	Depression	Autoagglutination
	Fever	Positive Coombs tests
	Pale mucous membranes	Elevated liver enzymes
	Icterus	Bilirubinaemia
	Brown urine	Increased
	Neurological Symptoms	urea and creatinine
	Seizures	
	Coma	

Lethargy, depression, fever are consequences of the infectious process or the inflammation triggered by it. The mechanisms are described in Chapter 48.3.1 in detail.

Lethargy, or a feeling of fatigue and lack of energy, can be caused by several factors during an infection. Firstly, the immune system's response requires a lot of energy, and this can make the body feel tired and sluggish. Additionally, the immune response can cause the release of cytokines, which are small signalling molecules that can cause fatigue and reduce the motivation to move or perform physical activity.

Inappetence, or a lack of appetite, is another common symptom of infection. This can also be caused by the release of cytokines, which can affect the brain and cause a feeling of nausea or loss of appetite. Additionally, during an infection, the body may divert its resources away from the digestive system to focus on the immune response, leading to a decreased desire to eat.

The anaemia is a regenerative, haemolytic **anaemia** and results, on the one hand, from the direct destruction of the erythrocyte membrane during eversion of the merozoites. Another mechanism is increased osmotic fragility of the erythrocytes, which reduces their resistance to haemolysis. Effects of babesia, which reduce membrane stability through enzymes, are suspected. In addition, an immunological reaction takes place by means of anti-erythrocytic antibodies.

All these mechanisms destroy erythrocytes. This produces the clinically visible symptoms of anaemia, such as **pale membranes,** etc. Due to haemolysis, more haemoglobin is released, this leads to haemoglobinaemia and **bilirubinaemia** and thus clinically to **icterus**. This is followed by haemoglobinuria. Acute renal failure may develop due to obstruction of the structures of the nephron. This is accompanied by **azotaemia.** In addition to pigmenturia in the form of haemoglobinuria, glomerulonephritis can also lead to renal failure due to the deposition of immune complexes. Increased liver enzyme activities can result from an increased release of enzymes from the hepatocytes when, due to hypoxia, the transport processes at the hepatocyte membrane are impeded and the hepatocytes absorb more water and become fragile.

The **neurological symptoms** are mainly caused by the destruction of red blood cells which lead to anaemia and as consequence a reduced oxygen supply of the central nervous system. Further, proinflammatory cytokines, like TNF-α, IL-1, IL-6 and INF can cause an increase in the levels of excitatory neurotransmitters, such as glutamate, which can lead to overstimulation of nerve cells and damage to the cells themselves. This overstimulation can cause seizures and other neurological symptoms. Additionally, the cytokines can cause a decrease in the levels of inhibitory neurotransmitters, such as GABA, which can lead to a reduction in the ability of nerve cells to regulate their activity. This reduction in regulation can lead to altered behaviour and disorientation (Figure 48.4.1.3).

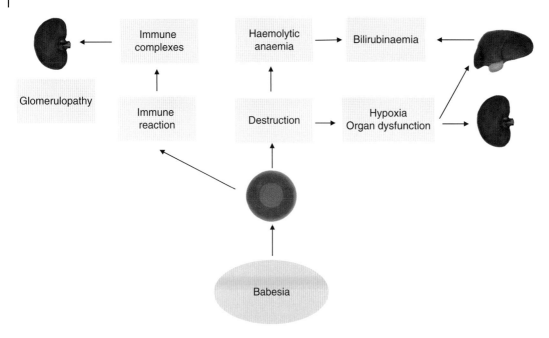

Figure 48.4.1.3 Pathophysiology of babesiosis.

Therapy

Symptom	Therapy
Large babesia	Imidocarb
Small babesia	Atovaquone + Azithromycin
Uncomplicated cases	Clindamycin + Metronidazole + Doxycycline

Reference

Rafaj, R.B., Matijatko, V., Kis, I. et al. (2009). Alterations in some blood coagulation parameters in naturally occurring cases of canine babesiosis. *Acta Veterinaria Hungarica.* 57 (2): 295–304. https://doi.org/10.1556/AVet.57.2009.2.10.

Further Reading

Esch, K.J. and Petersen, C.A. (2013). Transmission and epidemiology of zoonotic protozoal diseases of companion animals. *Clinical Microbiology Reviews* 26 (1): 58–85. https://doi.org/10.1128/CMR.00067-12.

MacWilliams, P.S. (1987). Erythrocytic rickettsia and protozoa of the dog and cat. *The Veterinary Clinics of North America. Small Animal Practice* 17 (6): 1443–1461. https://doi.org/10.1016/s0195-5616(87)50011-0.

48.4.2

Giardiasis

Aetiology

Giardiasis is caused by protozoa of the genus *Giardia*. *Giardia duodenalis* occurs in dogs and cats.

Pathogenesis

Giardia have a simple life cycle. In the environment, the *Giardia* are present in a roundish-oval cyst.

These are resistant survival forms with a rigid wall that protects against temperature and drying out.

This creates a resistance that leads to survival in the environment for several months. After oral ingestion of the cysts, two trophozoites are released from each cyst in the intestine by an excystation. The release is triggered by macro-organism factors, such as temperature, low pH and pancreatic enzymes. Internal mechanisms include the activation of proteases, such as cathepsin protease. After excystment, motile trophozoites (9–21 µm × 5–12 µm) are present in the intestine. These have an adhesion disc on their ventral side, which allows them to adhere to enterocytes of the small intestine. Adhesion is achieved by receptor binding of adhesins of the trophozoites. The dorsal side of the trophozoites can take up nutrients by pinocytosis. The expression of various surface proteins protects the trophozoites from the digestive enzymes of the intestine or pancreas. The multiplication is carried out by a simple division into two parts. Through intestinal peristalsis, the trophozoites reach the caudal region of the small intestine. There, the process of encystation happens in which the trophozoites are transformed into the resistant cyst. Bile salts or cholesterol deficiency in the caudal small intestine are discussed as triggers for encystation. The cholesterol deficiency causes a disruption of the membrane structure of the trophozoites, which triggers encystation. The cysts are subsequently released into the environment via faeces (Payne and Artzer 2009; Ryan and Zahedi 2019) (Figure 48.4.2.1).

The clinical consequence of giardiasis is diarrhoea. This is triggered by different mechanisms. On the one hand, trophozoites infected enterocytes induce the activity of caspases, which initiates apoptosis. At the same time, the release of apoptosis-inhibiting factors, e.g. Bcl-2, is inhibited. In addition, *Giardia* increase the permeability of the intestinal wall through caspase-induced destruction of the tight-junctions between the enterocytes. In this process, the proteins of the tight-junction are taken up intracellularly. By inhibiting the release of IL-8 by the enterocytes, the trophozoites are able to prevent the chemotaxis of neutrophilic granulocytes (Chin et al. 2002; Cotton et al. 2011).

Nevertheless, trophozoite infection induces an inflammatory response by allowing luminal antigens to pass through the intestinal wall.

The inflammatory reaction leads to morphological changes in the intestinal wall with a shortening of the villi length, thus reducing the absorption surface. Decreased secretion of disaccharidase prevents the cleavage of disaccharides, thus increasing the osmotic pressure in the intestinal lumen. Increased chloride secretion due to enterocyte destruction leads to secretory diarrhoea (Figure 48.4.2.2).

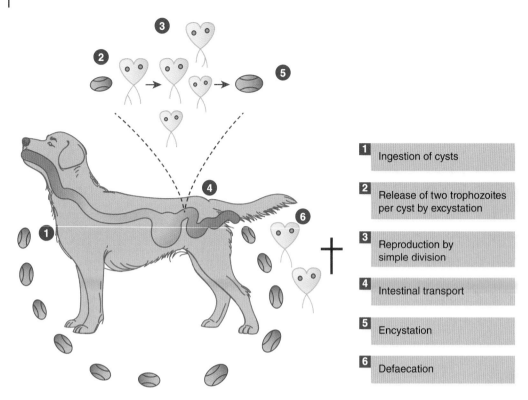

Figure 48.4.2.1   Cycle of giardiasis.

1	Ingestion of cysts
2	Release of two trophozoites per cyst by excystation
3	Reproduction by simple division
4	Intestinal transport
5	Encystation
6	Defaecation

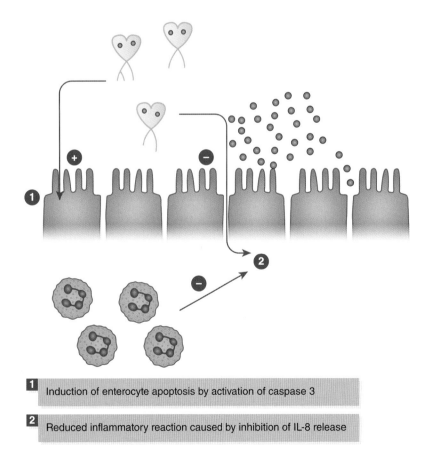

1	Induction of enterocyte apoptosis by activation of caspase 3
2	Reduced inflammatory reaction caused by inhibition of IL-8 release

Figure 48.4.2.2   Mechanism of interaction between giardiasis and enterocytes.

Diagnostics

Clinical signs	Clinical pathology	Imaging	Histopathology	Microbiology
Diarrhoea	Faeces	Not necessary	Not necessary	Not necessary
	Microscopic detection of trophozoites or cysts			
	Faeces			
	Point-of-care test Antigen detection			

Pathophysiologic Consequences

The pathophysiologic consequences of giardiasis are based on the destruction of the intestinal wall cells.

Influenced organ systems	Clinical symptoms	Clinical pathological alterations
Gastrointestinal system	Diarrhoea	

Diarrhoea is the main clinical symptom of giardiasis. However, this is accompanied by other symptoms. These include weight loss and dehydration. The former is the result of malabsorption, and the latter is due to enteral water loss. The faeces in giardiasis are mucous, greasy or even bloody (Tangtrongsup and Scorza 2010). The mechanism of greasy or fatty diarrhoea in giardiasis is due to the disruption of the normal absorption of fat in the small intestine. *Giardia duodenalis* attaches to the lining of the small intestine and interferes with the normal digestive and absorptive processes. Specifically, the parasite causes damage to the microvilli. The damaged microvilli cannot effectively absorb fat, which leads to the excretion of fatty acids and other lipids in the faeces, giving it a greasy appearance. This condition is known as 'steatorrhoea'.

Therapy

Symptom	Therapy
Therapy against *Giardia*	Fenbendazole, Metronidazole

References

Chin, A.C., Teoh, D.A., Scott, K.G. et al. (2002). Strain-dependent induction of enterocyte apoptosis by *Giardia lamblia* disrupts epithelial barrier function in a caspase-3-dependent manner. *Infection and Immunity* 70 (7): 3673–3680. https://doi.org/10.1128/IAI.70.7.3673-3680.2002.

Cotton, J.A., Beatty, J.K., and Buret, A.G. (2011). Host parasite interactions and pathophysiology in Giardia infections. *International Journal for Parasitology* 41 (9): 925–933. https://doi.org/10.1016/j.ijpara.2011.05.002.

Payne, P.A. and Artzer, M. (2009). The biology and control of Giardia spp and *Tritrichomonas foetus*. The Veterinary Clinics of *North America. Small Animal Practice* 39 (6): 993–v. https://doi.org/10.1016/j.cvsm.2009.06.007.

Ryan, U. and Zahedi, A. (2019). Molecular epidemiology of giardiasis from a veterinary perspective. *Advances in Parasitology* 106: 209–254. https://doi.org/10.1016/bs.apar.2019.07.002.

Tangtrongsup, S. and Scorza, V. (2010). Update on the diagnosis and management of Giardia spp infections in dogs and cats. *Topics in Companion Animal Medicine* 25 (3): 155–162. https://doi.org/10.1053/j.tcam.2010.07.003.

Further Reading

Gillin, F.D., Reiner, D.S., and McCaffery, J.M. (1996). Cell biology of the primitive eukaryote *Giardia lamblia*. *Annual Review of Microbiology* 50: 679–705.

Lujan, H.D., Mowatt, M.R., and Nash, T.E. (1997). Mechanisms of Giardia lamblia differentiation onto cysts. *Microbiology and Molecular Biology Review* 61: 294–304.

48.4.3

Leishmaniasis

Aetiology

The disease is caused by an obligate intracellular protozoan of the genus *Leishmania*. *Leishmania infantum* is of greatest veterinary importance. Leishmaniasis is a vector-borne disease and occurs in dogs and cats.

Pathogenesis

The infection cycle begins with the ingestion of the *Leishmania* by the vector. These belong to the genus of sandflies (*Phlebotomus*). Of the sandflies, only the females suck blood facultatively before laying eggs and thus serve as a vector. During the sucking act, the vector bites into the skin of the organism and absorbs wound secretions and blood from superficial skin vessels. In the process, amastigote *Leishmania* present in macrophages can be ingested. Within the midgut of the phlebotomes, the non-motile amastigote stage transforms into the motile promastigote stage. Triggers are thought to be temperature or pH changes following ingestion by the vector (Bates and Rogers 2004). Sexual reproduction of the promastigote stages is located in the midgut of the phlebotomes. The next time the sandfly sucks, the promastigote stages are transmitted. In the process, the parasites enter the blood and tissue of the macro-organism and are taken up there by phagocytosing macrophages. Within the cell, the phagosome fuses with lysosomes and the promastigote stage develops into the amastigote stage, which reproduces asexually. The multiplication destroys the macrophages and releases amastigote stages into the blood or tissue, which are then, in turn, taken up by other macrophages (Figure 48.4.3.1).

Diagnostics

Clinical signs	Clinical pathology	Imaging	Histopathology	Microbiology
Non-specific	Cytology	Not necessary	Bone marrow	Not necessary
Maybe skin lesions	Bone marrow		Lymph nodes	
	Lymph nodes			

Pathophysiologic Consequences

Leishmaniasis can show different clinical pictures. These range from severe multisystemic diseases to asymptomatic forms. The respective manifestation of the disease depends on the immune response of the organism. A distinction can be made between cellular and humoral responses. Presumably, cellular-based immunity (Th-1 and Th-2) is more effective in

Textbook of Small Animal Pathophysiology, First Edition. Stephan Neumann.

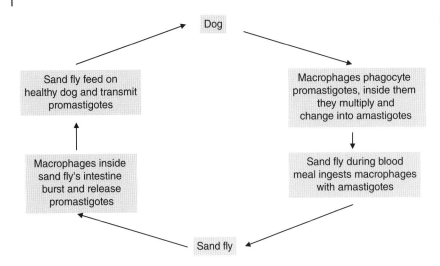

Figure 48.4.3.1 Leishmaniasis cycle.

suppressing infection than humoral-based responses. Another predisposing factor in dogs appears to be breed. Spaniels and German Shepherds are more frequently affected. No breed predispositions have been described in cats.

Influenced organ systems	Clinical symptoms Frequency (%)	Clinical pathological alterations
Hepatobiliary system	Lymphadenopathy (60–90%)	Hyperproteinaemia
Haematological system	Splenomegaly (10–50%)	Hypergammaglobulinaemia
Bones, joints	Skin lesions	Hypoalbuminaemia
Muscles	(Dermatitis, ulceration) (80–90%)	Elevated liver enzymes
Systemic	Eyes (Conjunctivitis, uveitis) (10–80%)	Non-regenerative anaemia
Ophthalmic system	Weight loss (10–48%)	Leukocytosis/Leukopenia
Skin	Epistaxis (10%)	Thrombocytopenia
		Proteinuria
		Azotaemia

Source: Baneth et al. (2008).

The clinical symptoms can be differentiated into a cutaneous and a visceral form of the disease.

The **lymphadenopathy** and **splenomegaly** are an expression of the permanent stimulation of the immune system. Histologically, the lymph nodes show hyperplasia of medullary macrophages (Lima et al. 2004). In the spleen, there is hyperplasia of plasma cells (Santana et al. 2008). The marked humoral response of the immune system is reflected in **hyperproteinaemia** and **hypergammaglobulinaemia.** The latter can be mono- or polyclonal. This reflects the complex immunological response to leishmaniasis. While the monoclonal form represents an increase in immunoglobulins, the polyclonal forms also include an increase in complement and other inflammation-associated proteins.

An essential symptomatology of leishmaniasis are the various **skin lesions**, which show a predilection for the head area and the limbs. Purulent and erosive forms may occur, and the mucocutaneous areas are also affected. Histologically, infiltrates with infected macrophages are evident. These also seem to be the main trigger of the skin changes. The exact pathomechanism is not fully understood.

A major visceral form of leishmaniasis is glomerulonephritis. This occurs in different histological variations, such as the membranoproliferative or mesangioproliferative form (Plevraki et al. 2006).

Glomerular deposits of immune complexes (Ig-G, Ig-M, C3), as well as lymphatic infiltrates (CD4+) are seen as the cause for the development of glomerulonephritis. This is followed by **proteinuria**. This can contribute to a marked loss of protein and cause **hypoalbuminaemia,** as well as **cachexia.** The latter symptom, however, is furthermore related to other energy-demanding processes in leishmaniasis, such as the activity of the immune system.

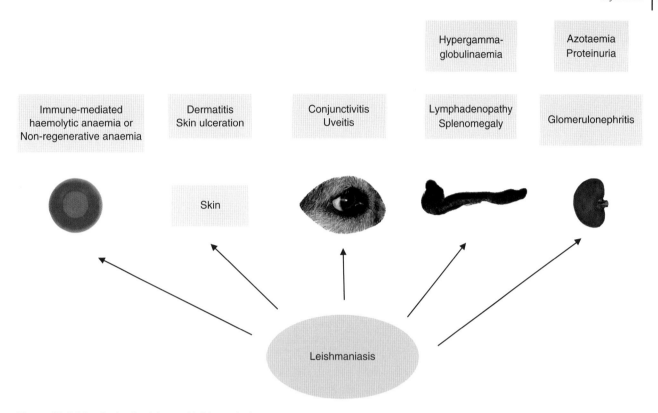

Figure 48.4.3.2 Pathophysiology of leishmaniasis.

Another consequence of proteinuria can be a nephrotic syndrome or **azotaemia**, which develops into uraemia. However, this is only immanent in advanced courses of the disease.

Leishmaniasis-associated **anaemia** can have different causes and is accordingly possible as a regenerative or non-regenerative form. The synthesis of erythrocytic autoantibodies causes immune-mediated haemolytic anaemia. Another cause of anaemia associated with leishmaniasis is found in dysplasia of the erythrocytic stem cell lineage. This in turn could be due to destruction of the bone marrow beginning with infiltration by macrophages and synthesis of proinflammatory cytokines. Finally, the morphological changes in the kidney also lead to a reduced synthesis of erythropoietin and thus cause a non-regenerative anaemia.

Finally, animals with leishmaniasis show an increased bleeding tendency due to vascular erosions and coagulation disorders. This results from thrombocytopenia, platelet dysfunction, and reduced plasmatic coagulation function (Ciaramella et al. 2005). Blood loss also contributes to the development of anaemia (Figure 48.4.3.2).

Therapy

Symptom	Therapy
Therapy against pathogen	Meglumine antimoniate, Miltefosine, Allopurinol
Prevention	Vector reduction

References

Baneth, G., Koutinas, A.F., Solano-Gallego, L. et al. (2008). Canine leishmaniosis – new concepts and insights on an expanding zoonosis: part one. *Trends in Parasitology* 24 (7): 324–330. https://doi.org/10.1016/j.pt.2008.04.001.

Bates, P.A. and Rogers, M.E. (2004). New insights into the developmental biology and transmission mechanisms of Leishmania. *Current Molecular Medicine* 4 (6): 601–609. https://doi.org/10.2174/1566524043360285.

Ciaramella, P., Pelagalli, A., Cortese, L. et al. (2005). Altered platelet aggregation and coagulation disorders related to clinical findings in 30 dogs naturally infected by *Leishmania infantum*. *Veterinary Journal (London, England: 1997)* 169 (3): 465–467. https://doi.org/10.1016/j.tvjl.2004.03.009.

Lima, W.G., Michalick, M.S., de Melo, M.N. et al. (2004). Canine visceral leishmaniasis: a histopathological study of lymph nodes. *Acta Tropica* 92 (1): 43–53. https://doi.org/10.1016/j.actatropica.2004.04.007.

Plevraki, K., Koutinas, A.F., Kaldrymidou, H. et al. (2006). Effects of allopurinol treatment on the progression of chronic nephritis in canine leishmaniosis (*Leishmania infantum*). *Journal of Veterinary Internal Medicine* 20 (2): 228–233. https://doi.org/10.1892/0891-6640(2006)20[228:eoatot]2.0.co;2.

Santana, C.C., Vassallo, J., de Freitas, L.A. et al. (2008). Inflammation and structural changes of splenic lymphoid tissue in visceral leishmaniasis: a study on naturally infected dogs. *Parasite Immunology* 30 (10): 515–524. https://doi.org/10.1111/j.1365-3024.2008.01051.x.

Further Reading

Geisweid, K. M. (2013). Investigation into the diagnosis and prognosis of canine leishmaniasis. Dissertation, Munich.

49

Common Immune-mediated Diseases

49.1

Autoimmunity

Definition

Autoimmunity is the reduction of an organism's self-tolerance. The consequence is an immunological reaction against the body's own structures.

Aetiology and Pathogenesis

The immune system is able to distinguish between the body's own antigen and foreign antigens. There is tolerance to the body's own antigen. This is maintained by eliminating autoaggressive lymphocytes. This happens through different mechanisms. In clonal deletion, autoaggressive T lymphocytes undergo apoptosis and are thus eliminated. The mechanism is controlled by the expression of apoptosis-promoting receptors (Fas receptor) or pro-apoptotic proteins in the lymphocytes. Another mechanism of maintaining self-tolerance is provided by the so-called 'co-stimulation', in which the activity of the lymphocytes depends on two signals. If the co-signal is missing, the lymphocytes are not activated.

A loss of self-tolerance promotes the autoimmune reaction. The development of an autoimmune reaction is based on different assumptions. On the one hand, the mechanisms of apoptosis described above may fail in autoaggressive lymphocytes. A cross-reaction between antigen peptides and physiological peptides is called the 'mimicry hypothesis' and can also lead to an autoimmune reaction. Finally, structural changes to the MHC proteins lead to an autoimmune response.

The Major Histocompatibility Complex (MHC) consists of transmembrane protein complexes that have a function in antigen presentation. MHC I and II complexes can be subdivided.

The MHC I proteins are expressed on almost all cell surfaces of the organism. They are activated by intracellular triggers, such as viruses or neoplastic molecules, and interact with cytotoxic T lymphocytes (CD 8+). The consequence of this interaction is the activation of the cytotoxic activity of the lymphocytes. Their cytotoxicity can cause cell lysis, in which the lymphocytes release perforin, which destroys the cell membrane. A second mechanism, mediated by granzymes, induces apoptosis in the target cell. A structural alteration of the MHC I complex can lead to a misdirected reaction of the lymphocytes.

The proteins of the MHC II are predominantly expressed by cells of the non-specific defence, such as macrophages or dendritic cells. They present extracellular antigens, which are broken down after phagocytosis, to the cells of the specific defence, mostly T helper cells (CD 4+).

The mode of antigen presentation is via proteolysis of the antigen by ubiquitin. The peptide fragments are first fixed into the wall structure of the endoplasmic reticulum. Then, triggered by transport proteins, such as tapasin, the transfer to MHC takes place. The complex of MHC and peptide reaches the cell membrane via the Golgi apparatus and finally via exocytosis, where it can present the antigen fragments to the lymphocytes. Here, too, structural alterations of the MCH II complex can lead to a malfunction (Figure 49.1.1).

Textbook of Small Animal Pathophysiology, First Edition. Stephan Neumann.
© 2025 John Wiley & Sons Ltd. Published 2025 by John Wiley & Sons Ltd.

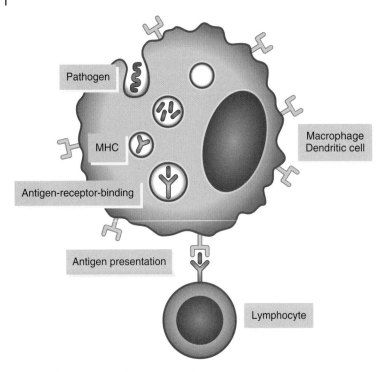

Figure 49.1.1   The antigen presentation pathway.

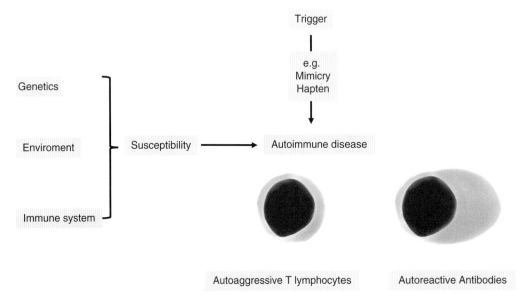

Figure 49.1.2   Induction of autoimmunity.

The consequence of the autoaggression that arises due to different mechanisms is the formation of autoreactive T lymphocytes and B lymphocytes, as well as the synthesis of antibodies against body cells.

Autoimmune diseases are divided into systemic and organ-specific diseases.

In the case of antibody formation, these can be directed against different cellular structures. These include components of the cell nucleus, such as histones, but also mitochondrial structures and components of the cell membrane. The respective disease mechanisms result from the immunological reaction (Figure 49.1.2).

Further Reading

Kamradt, T. and Mitchison, N.A. (2001). Tolerance and autoimmunity. *The New England Journal of Medicine* 344 (9): 655–664. https://doi.org/10.1056/NEJM200103013440907.

Rosenblum, M.D., Remedios, K.A., and Abbas, A.K. (2015). Mechanisms of human autoimmunity. *The Journal of Clinical Investigation* 125 (6): 2228–2233. https://doi.org/10.1172/JCI78088.

Theofilopoulos, A.N. and Kono, D.H. (1999). The genes of systemic autoimmunity. *Proceedings of the Association of American Physicians* 111 (3): 228–240. https://doi.org/10.1046/j.1525-1381.1999.99244.x.

Theofilopoulos, A.N., Kono, D.H., and Baccala, R. (2017). The multiple pathways to autoimmunity. *Nature Immunology* 18 (7): 716–724. https://doi.org/10.1038/ni.3731.

49.2

Lupus Erythematosus

Definition

Systemic lupus erythematosus is an autoimmune disease in which organ structures of the organism are destroyed by autoantibodies.

Aetiology

The exact causes of lupus erythematosus (LE) are not known. A mixture of a genetic predisposition with different triggers is assumed. The genetic predisposition results from mutations in the range of genes encoding complement factors, proteins of the MHC or proteins of signal transduction (STAT) (Selvaraja et al. 2022).

Hormones, environmental factors, stress and infections are described as triggers. The disease occurs more frequently in dogs than in cats. Male dogs are overrepresented (Table 49.2.1).

Pathogenesis

The pathogenesis of LE begins with the formation of autoreactive B cells, which secrete anti-DNA and other autoantibodies and thus form pathogenetically relevant immune complexes. These can activate cells of the immune system via nucleic acid-specific toll-like receptors (TLR).

In the process, transcription factors (NF-κB) are produced that induce the expression of proinflammatory mediators, such as interferons. The activation of proinflammatory mediators leads to a release of granulocytic nuclear material, which triggers a lymphocytic reaction as a self-antigen or mediates thrombosis or endothelial damage.

In the further course of the disease, a proliferation of T lymphocytes and a formation of antibodies by B lymphocytes develops, which are directed against structures of different body tissues (Tayem et al. 2022; Scheen et al. 2022).

The respective organ damage is based on the formation of autoantibody immune complexes and immune-mediated tissue damage. The skin, kidneys, joints, lymph nodes and erythrocytes are predominantly affected.

Morphological changes in the kidneys result from the deposition of immune complexes in the glomeruli and tubules, as well as interstitially (Figure 49.2.1).

Diagnostics

Clinical signs	Clinical pathology	Imaging	Histopathology	Microbiology
Lethargy	**ANA-titre**	Non-specific	Detection of immune complexes	Not necessary
Skin lesions	LE-cells			
Muco-cutaneous lesions	Proteinuria			
	Haemolytic anaemia, Coombs test positive			

Textbook of Small Animal Pathophysiology, First Edition. Stephan Neumann.
© 2025 John Wiley & Sons Ltd. Published 2025 by John Wiley & Sons Ltd.

Table 49.2.1 Triggers of systemic lupus erythematosus.

Trigger	Mechanism
Oestrogen	Stimulation of lymphocytes, macrophages
Drugs (e.g. Hydralazine)	Demethylation of DNA
Environment (ultraviolet light)	Cell apoptosis
Infection	Molecular mimicry

1. Antibody binds on glomerular basement membrane
2. Antigen-immunoglobulin complexes and complement damage mesangia cells
3. Antigen-immunoglobulin complexes and complement damage podocytes

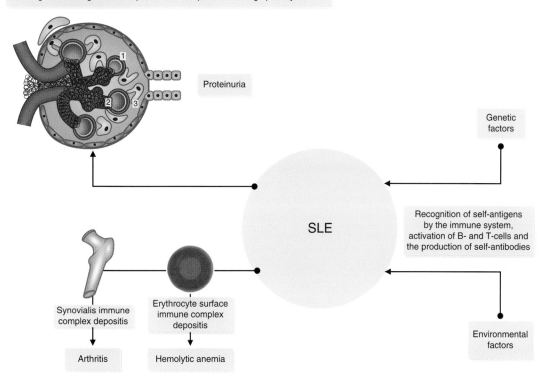

Figure 49.2.1 Pathogenesis of systemic LE.

Pathophysiologic Consequences

The pathophysiologic consequences are based on the symptoms resulting from the respective organ damage.

Influenced organ systems	Clinical symptoms	Clinical pathological alterations
Urinary tract	Lethargy	Anaemia
Haematological system	Skin lesions	Proteinuria
Bones, joints	Lameness	
Muscles	Lymphadenopathy	
Systemic	Fever	
Ophthalmic system		
Skin		

Lethargy may be a symptom of the intense immune response and a consequence of a cytokine-mediated central nervous response. **Skin lesions** develop as a result of inflammation and necrosis in the skin and mucocutaneous areas. In the skin in LE, deposits of immune complexes, perivascular infiltrates with mononuclear cells and tissue necrosis are found particularly at the epidermis–dermis junction.

The **lameness** is mostly a non-erosive arthritis in different joints. Distal joints seem to be affected more often. One of the key mechanisms involved in the development of lameness in LE is inflammation. Autoantibodies can form immune complexes with self-antigens in the joints, triggering an inflammatory response. This can lead to the activation of various immune cells, including neutrophils, macrophages and T-cells, which can produce proinflammatory cytokines, chemokines and reactive oxygen species that further exacerbate the inflammation. This chronic inflammation can damage the joint tissue and lead to pain and lameness. Another mechanism that can contribute to lameness in LE is antibody-mediated cytotoxicity. Autoantibodies can activate complement proteins, which can lead to the destruction of joint tissue. This can further exacerbate the inflammation and contribute to the development of joint pain and lameness. Furthermore, LE can also affect the structure and function of blood vessels in the joints, leading to vascular damage and ischaemia. This can further contribute to joint damage and pain.

Lymph nodes in LE are characterised by follicular hyperplasia, which is seen as a reactive change.

Fever is caused by an effect of cytokines on the temperature regulation centre. One of the key mechanisms involved in the development of fever in LE is the activation of the immune system. Autoantibodies produced by the immune system can target self-antigens, leading to the production of inflammatory cytokines, such as IL-1, IL-6 and TNF-α. These cytokines can act on the hypothalamus, a region in the brain that regulates body temperature, and trigger a fever response. Fever in LE may also be caused by the presence of immune complexes in the blood. These immune complexes can activate complement proteins, leading to the production of anaphylatoxins, such as C3a and C5a. These anaphylatoxins can also act on the hypothalamus and trigger a fever response (Timlin et al. 2018).

Patients with LE show haemolytic **anaemia** due to destruction of red cells by antiphospholipid antibodies. The mechanism involved in the development of haemolytic anaemia in LE is the production of autoantibodies that target red blood cells. These autoantibodies can form immune complexes with red blood cells, leading to their destruction by the complement system. Another mechanism that can contribute to haemolytic anaemia in LE is the production of cytokines, such as IL-1 and TNF-α, by immune cells. These cytokines can activate macrophages, which can engulf and destroy red blood cells. Finally, LE can also affect the structure and function of blood vessels, leading to vascular damage and ischaemia. This can further contribute to the destruction of red blood cells and the development of haemolytic anaemia.

Finally, **proteinuria** occurs as a result of glomerulonephritis in LE. One of the key mechanisms involved in the development of proteinuria in LE is the deposition of immune complexes in the kidneys. Autoantibodies produced by the immune system can target self-antigens, leading to the formation of immune complexes that can deposit in the kidneys and activate complement proteins. The activation of the complement system can lead to inflammation and damage to the glomeruli. This damage can cause the glomeruli to become leaky, allowing proteins to pass into the urine. LE can also cause inflammation, scarring and fibrosis, leading to damage to the glomeruli and proteinuria.

Therapy

Symptom	Therapy
Immunosuppression	Corticoids, Azathioprine, Chlorambucil, Cyclosporine

References

Scheen, M., Adedjouma, A., Esteve, E. et al. (2022). Kidney disease in antiphospholipid antibody syndrome: risk factors, pathophysiology and management. *Autoimmunity Reviews* 21 (5): 103072. https://doi.org/10.1016/j.autrev.2022.103072.

Selvaraja, M., Too, C.L., Tan, L.K. et al. (2022). Human leucocyte antigens profiling in Malay female patients with systemic lupus erythematosus: are we the same or different? *Lupus Science & Medicine* 9 (1): e000554. https://doi.org/10.1136/lupus-2021-000554.

Tayem, M.G., Shahin, L., Shook, J., and Kesselman, M.M. (2022). A review of cardiac manifestations in patients with systemic lupus erythematosus and antiphospholipid syndrome with focus on endocarditis. *Cureus* 14 (1): e21698. https://doi.org/10.7759/cureus.21698.

Timlin, H., Syed, A., Haque, U. et al. (2018). Fevers in adult lupus patients. *Cureus* 10 (1): e2098. https://doi.org/10.7759/cureus.2098.

Further Reading

Justice Vaillant, A. A., Goyal, A., & Varacallo, M. (2023). *Systemic Lupus Erythematosus*. StatPearls. Treasure Island (FL): StatPearls Publishing.

49.3

Myasthenia Gravis

Definition

Myasthenia gravis (MG) is a disorder of neuromuscular transmission.

Aetiology

Myasthenia gravis can occur as a congenital form with a reduced receptor density or as an autoimmune disease. Only the autoimmune disease will be discussed here. The aetiology corresponds to that of other autoimmune diseases. A genetic predisposition triggered by other factors is to be seen as causality. A connection with changes in the thymus is particularly striking. Thymomas, or lymphofollicular hyperplasia of the thymus, occur. The disease occurs almost exclusively in dogs. Cockers, terriers and retrievers seem to be overrepresented.

Pathogenesis

Myasthenia gravis is caused by autoantibodies that occupy nicotinic acetylcholine receptors (nAChRn) at the neuromuscular endplate of striated muscle, leading to a transmission disorder at the neuromuscular endplate.

Physiological transmission at the neuromuscular endplate begins at the presynaptic nerve terminal. This is a piston-shaped thickening at the end of the axon. Numerous vesicles are localised in the nerve terminal, each of which contains approximately 10 000 ($\pm$2000) acetylcholine molecules, which are synthesised from acetyl-CoA and choline by the enzymatic activity of choline transferase.

When an action potential reaches the motor end plate, there is a presynaptic influx of Ca^{2+} through the voltage-dependent Ca^{2+} channels. This influx of Ca^{2+} enables fusion of the vesicles with the presynaptic membrane. This process releases ACh into the synaptic cleft.

The synaptic cleft is about 70 nm wide and separates the presynaptic from the postsynaptic membrane of the muscle. The ACh in the synaptic cleft diffuses to an ACh receptor in the postsynaptic membrane. Reaction with the receptor opens a centrally located sodium channel and sodium can flow with the concentration gradient into the postsynaptic cell and trigger an action potential.

Acetylcholine is hydrolysed and inactivated by the activity of an acetylcholinesterase (AChE).

In MG, antibodies bind to the acetylcholine receptor. This leads to a structural change at the postsynaptic membrane, as well as a reduction of the acetyl receptors.

If the number of functional acetylcholine receptors falls below a critical level, the sodium influx at the postsynaptic membrane is not sufficient to generate an action potential. The result is clinically relevant muscle weakness (Figure 49.3.1).

Textbook of Small Animal Pathophysiology, First Edition. Stephan Neumann.
© 2025 John Wiley & Sons Ltd. Published 2025 by John Wiley & Sons Ltd.

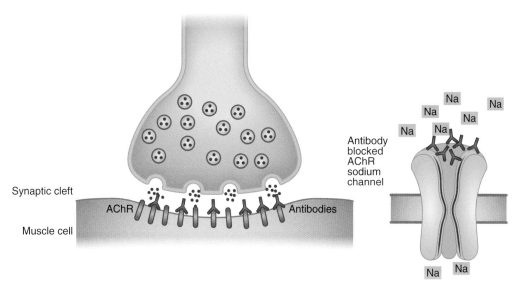

Figure 49.3.1 Pathomechanism of MG at the motor end plate.

Diagnostics

Clinical signs	Clinical pathology	Imaging	Histopathology	Microbiology
Progressive weakness	**AChR antibody**	X-ray	Not necessary	Not necessary
Regurgitation		Evidence of megaoesophagus		
Dyspnoea with aspiration pneumonia				
Improvement of weakness with Mestinon administration				

Pathophysiologic Consequences

The clinical changes of MG primarily refer to muscle weakness and thus affect the musculoskeletal system. In addition, muscle weakness of the striated oesophageal muscles is a common symptom.

Influenced organ system	Clinical symptoms
Respiratory system	Paresis
Gastrointestinal system	Regurgitation
Neuromuscular system	Dyspnoea

The clinical symptoms of **paresis** are not evenly distributed in MG, but occur more frequently in the hind limb.

Dyspnoea and **regurgitation** are associated with the development of megaoesophagus in MG. In dogs and cats, parts of the oesophageal wall are striated muscles and therefore sensitive to MG antibodies. In the case of megaoesophagus, regurgitation may occur. This can trigger aspiration pneumonia, causing **dyspnoea** and fever.

Therapy

Symptom	Therapy
Immunosuppression	Corticoids
Increased neuromuscular transmission	Mestinon

Further Reading

Mignan, T., Targett, M., and Lowrie, M. (2020). Classification of myasthenia gravis and congenital myasthenic syndromes in dogs and cats. *Journal of Veterinary Internal Medicine* 34 (5): 1707–1717. https://doi.org/10.1111/jvim.15855.

Uzawa, A., Kuwabara, S., Suzuki, S. et al. (2021). Roles of cytokines and T cells in the pathogenesis of myasthenia gravis. *Clinical and Experimental Immunology* 203 (3): 366–374. https://doi.org/10.1111/cei.13546.

Yi, J.S., Guptill, J.T., Stathopoulos, P. et al. (2018). B cells in the pathophysiology of myasthenia gravis. *Muscle & Nerve* 57 (2): 172–184. https://doi.org/10.1002/mus.25973.

50

Common Clinical Biochemical Parameters (Alphabetical)

50.1

Alanine Aminotransferase (ALT)

Physiology

Alanine aminotransferase (ALT) catalyses the transamination of alanine and is thus involved in the urea cycle and the gluconeogenesis. ALT is more or less liver specific; other organs in which ALT is detectable in low activity are heart, muscle and kidney tissue. Within the cell, ALT is present in the cytoplasm.

Liver cell damage and enzyme induction are considered to be the causes of increased serum activity of ALT. Increased enzyme induction as a trigger for increased serum activity is seen in connection with the administration of phenobarbital for the therapy of epilepsy.

Liver cell damage increases ALT serum activity mainly by bleb formation.

Blebs are membrane protrusions that can detach from the cell surface, leading to the release of intracellular contents into the bloodstream, including liver enzymes, such as ALT and aspartate aminotransferase (AST).

Bleb formation in hepatocytes can be a result of cytoskeletal disruption. Hepatotoxins can disrupt the cytoskeleton and destabilise the cell membrane, leading to the formation of blebs. Oxidative stress can also induce bleb formation in hepatocytes. Reactive oxygen species (ROS) can damage cellular components, including the cell membrane, leading to the formation of blebs.

Due to its localization in the cytoplasm, even slight increases in the permeability of the hepatocyte membrane lead to increased ALT activity in the serum. The serum half-life in dogs is a few days (3–4 days). Up to a threefold increase in serum activity is considered low grade and usually occurs with mild, chronic or secondary liver cell damage. Long-lasting high-serum activities, on the other hand, are observed in severe hepatocellular necrosis. No statement can be made about the genesis of the liver disease on the basis of increased ALT serum activity.

Variations

Increased Serum Activity

- Portosystemic shunt (mild increase)
- Metabolic disease: lipidosis, diabetes mellitus, feline hyperthyroidism, amyloidosis
- Neoplasia: lymphoma, metastasis of a neoplasia, hepatocellular carcinoma
- Nutritional: copper intoxication, haemochromatosis
- Inflammation:
  - Infectious: leptospirosis, feline infectious peritonitis (FIP), bacterial cholangiohepatitis
  - Non-infectious: chronic hepatitis, cirrhosis
- Toxic: steroid hepatopathy, anaesthetic drugs, tetracyclines, carprofen, phenobarbital
- Fever: mild elevation
- Trauma: car accident
- Genetic: copper storage disease, lysosomal storage disease

Textbook of Small Animal Pathophysiology, First Edition. Stephan Neumann.
© 2025 John Wiley & Sons Ltd. Published 2025 by John Wiley & Sons Ltd.

50.2

Albumin

Physiology

Albumin is a highly conserved protein found in the blood of dogs and cats and is composed of a single polypeptide chain. Albumin has a molecular weight of approximately 66 kDa and is the most abundant protein in blood plasma, accounting for 35–50% of total plasma proteins in dogs and cats. Albumin is synthesised in the liver and is released into the bloodstream, where it performs various functions.

Albumin is, in parts, responsible for colloid osmotic pressure in the blood plasma. Further, albumin has a high binding affinity for a variety of substances, including fatty acids, bilirubin and certain drugs, which can affect their distribution and metabolism in the body. The binding of albumin to substances, such as calcium, magnesium and copper can also affect their transport and availability in the body.

Variations

The concentration of albumin in the blood can be affected by a variety of factors. They can be differentiated into decreased synthesis and increased loss.

Decreased Synthesis

The steps of albumin synthesis in hepatocytes are:

1) Transcription: The gene that encodes albumin is transcribed into mRNA in the nucleus of the hepatocyte.
2) Translation: The mRNA is transported out of the nucleus and into the cytoplasm, where it serves as a template for the synthesis of albumin protein by ribosomes.
3) Post-translational modification: Once the albumin protein is synthesised, it undergoes several post-translational modifications, including glycosylation and disulphide bond formation, to ensure proper folding and stability.
4) Intracellular trafficking: The synthesised and modified albumin protein is then transported to the endoplasmic reticulum (ER) for further processing.
5) Folding and assembly: Within the ER, the albumin protein undergoes additional folding and assembly to form a stable structure.
6) Secretion: Once the albumin protein is properly folded and assembled, it is transported to the Golgi apparatus, where it is packaged into vesicles for secretion into the bloodstream.

Albumin synthesis in hepatocytes is regulated by hormones, cytokines and nutrient availability. Liver cell injury can inhibit the synthesis of albumin directly.

Hormones, such as growth hormone or insulin-like growth factor-1 (IGF-1), are important regulators of albumin synthesis in hepatocytes. An imbalance in these hormones can result in reduced albumin production. Inflammatory cytokines, such as interleukin-6 (IL-6), can inhibit albumin synthesis by hepatocytes. Finally, a lack of essential nutrients, such as amino acids, that are required for the synthesis of albumin can lead to a reduction in albumin production.

Textbook of Small Animal Pathophysiology, First Edition. Stephan Neumann.
© 2025 John Wiley & Sons Ltd. Published 2025 by John Wiley & Sons Ltd.

Increased Loss

Increased loss is mainly caused by renal and intestinal loss. The loss of albumin via **kidneys** is caused by glomerular alterations.

The following alteration of the glomeruli are associated with albumin loss.

1) Basement membrane damage: The glomerular basement membrane (GBM) is a thin, dense layer of extracellular matrix that acts as a barrier to prevent the passage of large molecules, such as albumin. Damage to the GBM can occur due to various reasons, including inflammation, immune-mediated disorders or genetic mutations, leading to increased permeability to albumin.
2) Podocyte dysfunction: Podocytes are specialised cells that wrap around the capillaries in the glomerulus and contribute to the formation of the filtration barrier. Podocyte damage or dysfunction can occur due to various causes, including autoimmune diseases, viral infections or medication toxicity. This dysfunction can result in increased permeability of the filtration barrier and leakage of albumin into the urine.
3) Endothelial cell dysfunction: Endothelial cells line the inner surface of the glomerular capillaries and play a critical role in maintaining the filtration barrier. Damage or dysfunction of endothelial cells can occur due to various reasons, such as infections, toxins or ischaemia, leading to increased permeability and leakage of albumin.
4) Increased hydrostatic pressure: Increased hydrostatic pressure within the glomerular capillaries can lead to stretching and damage to the filtration barrier, resulting in increased permeability to albumin.
5) Inflammatory cytokines: Inflammatory cytokines, such as TNF-α and IL-6, can trigger disruption of the glomerular filtration barrier and increase the permeability to albumin.
6) Oxidative stress: Increased levels of oxidative stress can cause damage to the glomerular filtration barrier, leading to increased permeability to albumin.

The **intestinal** loss of albumin can occur due to protein-losing enteropathy and malabsorption syndromes. The exact biochemistry of intestinal loss of albumin is thought to involve increased permeability of the intestinal barrier.

1) Increased intestinal permeability: The intestinal barrier is composed of a single layer of epithelial cells that prevent the passage of large molecules, such as albumin, from the gut lumen into the bloodstream. Increased intestinal permeability can occur due to various factors, including inflammation, bacterial overgrowth and medications, leading to the leakage of albumin into the gut lumen.
2) Inflammatory cytokines: Inflammatory cytokines, such as IL-1 and TNF-α, can trigger the disruption of the intestinal-barrier and cause intestinal loss of albumin.

Low albumin levels in dogs and cats can result in oedema, ascites and impaired wound healing, among other clinical signs.

High albumin levels as hyperalbuminaemia are caused by haemodilution, iatrogenic or in consequence of a shift of plasma in cases of oedema.

	Hypoalbuminaemia	Hyperalbuminaemia
Synthesis	Maldigestion	
	Malabsorption	
	Hepatic insufficiency (e.g. liver cirrhosis, portosystemic shunt)	
Loss	Nephropathy (glomerular loss, nephrotic syndrome)	
	Protein-losing enteropathy	
	burns/exudative skin diseases	
Inflammation	Negative acute phase	
Dilution	Hyperhydration	Dehydration

50.3

Alkaline Phosphatase (ALP)

Physiology

Alkaline phosphatase (ALP) is a membrane-bound enzyme that hydrolyses phosphoric esters to form organic phosphate. It is detectable in numerous tissues of the body. ALP is found in the form of various isoenzymes, some of which have short serum half-lives lasting only a few minutes (e.g. the intestinal wall isoenzyme). Due to their longer half-life, the liver isoenzyme (L-ALP), the bone isoenzyme (B-ALP) and the steroid-induced form of ALP (C-ALP) have clinical relevance. Due to its localization in the epithelia of the bile ducts, L-ALP is considered a so-called 'cholestasis marker'. Increased enzyme induction under the influence of cholestatic toxins is assumed to be the cause of the increase in L-ALP activity in the blood as a result of cholestasis. The steroid-induced form of ALP is formed under the influence of endogenous and exogenous corticoids. The steroid-induced form differs from the liver-specific isoenzyme primarily by its temperature stability at 65°C.

Variations

Only increased serum activity of ALP is of diagnostic relevance. It can be physiological in growing animals or based on cholestasis, bone lesions and cortisol induced in dogs.

Physiological:
Growth (in young animals, physiological values up to six times the reference ranges applicable in adult animals are measured because of the high osteoblast activity).

Cholestasis:
In cholestasis, hepatocytes can become directly damaged due to the accumulation of toxic bile acids and other substances. This damage can cause the release of ALP into the bloodstream. The cholestasis can also damage cholangiocytes, leading to the release of ALP into the bile ducts and subsequently into the bloodstream.

Bile acids can influence the production and activation of ALP in hepatocytes and cholangiocytes. Bile acids can bind to specific receptors, such as the farnesoid X receptor (FXR), and activate the transcription of ALP genes, leading to increased production and release of ALP into the bloodstream. Bile acids can also inhibit the uptake of ALP into hepatocytes, leading to the accumulation of ALP in the bloodstream.

Cortisol-induced ALP elevation:
The cortisol-induced elevation of ALP is only relevant in dogs. Mechanisms involved in the cortisol-induced elevation of ALP are:

Cortisol can stimulate bone resorption and reduce bone formation, leading to increased bone turnover. ALP is an enzyme that is produced by osteoblasts during bone formation, and its levels can be elevated in response to increased bone turnover.

Cortisol can directly stimulate the synthesis and secretion of ALP in hepatocytes. Cortisol can bind to glucocorticoid receptors in hepatocytes, leading to the transcription of ALP genes and the subsequent synthesis and secretion of ALP into the bloodstream.

Further cortisol can inhibit the uptake of ALP into hepatocytes, leading to the accumulation of ALP in the bloodstream. Finally prolonged elevation of cortisol levels can cause cholestasis.

Textbook of Small Animal Pathophysiology, First Edition. Stephan Neumann.
© 2025 John Wiley & Sons Ltd. Published 2025 by John Wiley & Sons Ltd.

Bone-induced ALP elevation:

The bone-induced ALP elevation is associated with osteoblast differentiation. During bone formation, osteoblasts differentiate and secrete ALP into the extracellular matrix.

ALP plays a critical role in bone mineralisation by hydrolysing inorganic pyrophosphate, a potent inhibitor of mineralisation. By breaking down pyrophosphate, ALP creates an environment favourable for mineralisation and the deposition of calcium and phosphate ions in the bone matrix. During bone turnover, osteoblasts resorb old bone tissue and replace it with new bone tissue. ALP is produced by osteoblasts during bone formation, and its levels can be elevated in response to increased bone turnover.

Various bone disorders, such as neoplasia can cause an increase in bone turnover and subsequently an elevation in ALP levels. In these conditions, the increased osteoblast activity results in the production and secretion of higher levels of ALP into the bloodstream.

Elevated serum activities are differentiated depending on the severity of elevation.

	Moderate elevation	Severe elevation
Hepatocytes	Hepatopathies with mild cholestasis	Hepatopathies with moderate to severe cholestasis lipidosis (cats)
Induction by hormones	Hyperthyroidism, diabetes mellitus, hypercortisolism,	Hyperadrenocorticism
Induction by drugs	Anticonvulsants, barbiturates, antibiotics	Glucocorticoids (dogs)
Bone diseases	Rickets, osteodystrophy, osteomalacia, hyperparathyroidism, bone tumours	

50.4

Ammonia

Physiology

Ammonia is a toxic product of amino acid breakdown. Non-toxic urea is synthesised from ammonia in the liver for detoxification. Liver diseases associated with loss of functional parenchyma, such as liver cirrhosis, can lead to elevations in blood ammonia. More commonly in dogs, vascular liver disease in the sense of portosystemic shunts is the cause of elevated blood ammonia concentrations. Ammonia is thought to play a major role in the development of hepato-encephalopathy. However, other possible triggers, such as γ-aminobutyric acid (GABA), short-chain fatty acids (e.g. octanoic acid), phenols and mercaptans are also discussed.

The detection of ammonium ions in the blood has acquired its special significance in the diagnosis of the portosystemic shunt. The sensitivity of ammonia measurement in serum can be improved by the so-called 'ammonium tolerance test'. In this test, not only the ammonia concentration is measured, but the ability of the liver to eliminate externally supplied ammonia from the portal venous blood is checked.

Variations

Increased Ammonia Serum Concentrations

- Portosystemic liver shunts
- Liver cirrhosis

Textbook of Small Animal Pathophysiology, First Edition. Stephan Neumann.
© 2025 John Wiley & Sons Ltd. Published 2025 by John Wiley & Sons Ltd.

50.5

Aspartate Aminotransferase (AST)

Physiology

The biochemical function of aspartate aminotransferase (AST), like that of ALT, is in the transamination. Under the catalysis of the AST, aspartate, an amino group donor for the urea cycle, is formed from glutamate. In contrast to ALT, AST is found in the cytoplasm and mitochondria of hepatocytes, although AST activity is also found in cells of the heart and skeletal muscles, as well as the kidneys and brain. AST is not liver-specific in dogs, it is useful for detecting liver disease when muscle disease has been ruled out. AST activity rises earlier after a liver insult than ALT, but falls off more quickly because of its half-life in serum of about five hours. Increased AST activity in serum occurs in various hepatopathies, such as degeneration, inflammation and neoplasia.

Variations

Increased Serum Activity

Hepatocellular damage, muscle damage, cardiac muscle damage

Hepatocellular damage

- Degenerative: hypoxia caused by anaemia or congestion;
- Portosystemic shunt (mild increase)
- Metabolic disease: lipidosis, diabetes mellitus, feline hyperthyroidism, amyloidosis
- Neoplasia: lymphoma, mctastasis of a neoplasia, hepatocellular carcinoma
- Nutritional: copper intoxication, haemochromatosis
- Inflammation:
  - Infectious: leptospirosis, feline infectious peritonitis (FIP), bacterial, cholangiohepatitis
  - Non-infectious: chronic hepatitis, cirrhosis
- Toxic: steroid hepatopathy, anaesthetic drugs, tetracyclines, carprofen, phenobarbital
- Fever: mild elevation
- Traumatic: car accident
- Genetic: copper storage disease, lysosomal storage disease

Muscle damage (mostly skeletal muscles, occasionally cardiac muscles, rarely smooth muscles)

- Degenerative: hypoxia due to exertion or seizures, exertional rhabdomyolysis
- Neoplastic: metastatic neoplasia
- Nutritional: Vitamin E/selenium deficiency
- Genetic: muscular dystrophy, myopathy due to hyper-, hypokalaemia
- Inflammatory: myositis caused by toxoplasma, neospora, bacteria
- Toxic: monensin
- Traumatic: intramuscular injections, car accident

Textbook of Small Animal Pathophysiology, First Edition. Stephan Neumann.
© 2025 John Wiley & Sons Ltd. Published 2025 by John Wiley & Sons Ltd.

50.6

Bile Acids

Physiology

Bile acids are steroids and are synthesised from cholesterol. In the hepatocytes, the so-called 'primary bile acids', cholic acid and chenodeoxycholic acid, are formed first. These are excreted into the intestine via the bile. There, under the influence of bacterial enzymes, hydroxyl groups are split off, which lead to the formation of the so-called 'secondary bile acids', deoxycholic acid and lithocholic acid.

In the intestine, bile acids perform an important function in the digestion of lipids and fat-soluble vitamins. The bile acids are involved in the formation of micelles, through which the absorption of lipids is made possible. The bile acid pool is constantly replenished by new synthesis of bile acids. Nevertheless, the organism behaves conservatively with regard to bile acids and tries to minimise enteral loss. This is done by returning 90–95% of the bile acids to the liver via the enterohepatic circulation. The bile acids contained in the portal blood are taken up in the liver predominantly by the hepatocytes on the sinusoidal membrane and secreted into the bile ducts at the basement membrane.

Processes in the liver that lead to vascular separation of the organ, such as portosystemic shunts, disrupt the bile acid circulation and lead to their increased serum concentration. The determination of bile acids has established itself as a parameter for the investigation of liver function and vascularisation. However, especially with regard to portosystemic shunts, the measurement of ammonia shows a higher sensitivity and specificity. In order to increase the significance of bile acids in relation to liver diseases, they can be measured in the fasting state and two hours postprandial, or after stimulation with ceruletide. However, a clear differentiation between different liver diseases is not possible on the basis of the bile acid concentration alone.

Variations

Increased Serum Concentration are of Medical Relevance

Decreased bile acid clearance from the portal blood

- Decreased functional liver tissue: diffuse hepatocellular disease
- Decreased portal blood flow to the liver: congenital or acquired portosystemic shunts

Decreased excretion of bile acids into the bile fluid

- Hepatic cholestasis: lipidosis, diabetes mellitus, steroid hepatopathy, lymphoma, cirrhosis, cholangiohepatitis
- Posthepatic cholestasis: cholangitis, bile duct carcinoma, pancreatitis, pancreatic carcinoma

50.7

Bilirubin

Physiology

Bilirubin is a breakdown product of haemoglobin metabolism. Its synthesis is a step in the breakdown of the porphyrin ring (haem) from haemoglobin. Initially, biliverdin is formed during this degradation, which occurs physiologically as part of cell moulting in the mononuclear phagocyte system (MPS). Under the catalysis of biliverdin reductase, biliverdin is reduced to bilirubin. Since it is hydrophobic, it is bound to albumin and transported from the site of its formation to the liver. There, the conjugation of water-insoluble to water-soluble bilirubin takes place within the framework of glucuronidation. The latter reaches the intestine via the bile duct system, where it is further reduced to stercobilin and excreted. A small amount returns to the liver via the enterohepatic circulation. Most of the bilirubin formed in the liver comes from haemoglobin breakdown; other sources include cytochromes.

An increase in the bilirubin concentration in the blood serum can be caused by hepatopathies or haemolyses. In principle, in the case of a haemolysis-related increase in bilirubin serum concentration (hyperbilirubinaemia), primarily hydrophobic bilirubin should be detected in the blood, and in the case of liver-related hyperbilirubinaemia, rather hydrophilic bilirubin. In practice, however, it has been shown that both are possible and can therefore be of little diagnostic use. Due to its colour, bilirubin produces the so-called 'icterus' at an increased blood concentration. From a serum concentration of about 2 mg/dl, this is clinically recognisable by the yellowing of the sclerae. Depending on the localisation of its development, prehepatic haemolytic jaundice is distinguished from intrahepatic jaundice, which is distinguished from posthepatic cholestatic jaundice.

Variations

Only increased serum concentrations of bilirubin are of medical importance. The reasons for this are the increased destruction of erythrocytes and cholestasis. The distinction between unconjugated and conjugated bilirubin based on the location of the lesion is not completely fixed, but only a bias.

	Unconjugated bilirubin	Conjugated bilirubin
Haemolysis	X	—
Decreased uptake of hepatocytes	X	—
Intrahepatic cholestasis	—	X
• Lipidosis, steroid hepatopathy, lymphoma, cirrhosis, cholangiohepatitis		
Posthepatic cholestasis	—	X
• Cholangitis, bile duct carcinoma, cholelithiasis, pancreatitis, pancreatic carcinoma		

Textbook of Small Animal Pathophysiology, First Edition. Stephan Neumann.
© 2025 John Wiley & Sons Ltd. Published 2025 by John Wiley & Sons Ltd.

50.8

Calcium

Physiology

Calcium is an essential mineral in dogs and cats. Calcium is required for the proper functioning of muscles, nerves and bones, as well as for blood clotting and enzyme activation.

The majority of calcium in dogs and cats is found in bone tissue, with a smaller proportion found in the bloodstream.

Calcium homeostasis in dogs and cats is tightly regulated by a complex system involving hormones, such as parathyroid hormone (PTH), calcitriol and calcitonin.

Parathyroid hormone is released by the parathyroid glands in response to low blood calcium levels and acts to increase calcium levels by promoting bone resorption and renal reabsorption of calcium. Calcitriol, the active form of vitamin D, is produced by the kidneys and acts to increase calcium absorption in the gut and promote bone mineralisation.

Calcitonin, which is produced by the thyroid gland, acts to lower blood calcium levels by inhibiting bone resorption and increasing urinary excretion of calcium.

Disorders of calcium homeostasis in dogs and cats can result in a range of clinical signs, including muscle weakness, seizures and bone fractures.

Variations

Hypercalcaemia	Hypocalcaemia
Increased Ca-mobilisation (bone and intestinal absorption)	**Hypoalbuminaemia (Hypoproteinaemia)**
• Caused by increased parathyroid hormone (PTH) or parathyroid hormone-like hormone (PTHrP)	**Decreased PTH-activity**
– Primary hyperparathyroidism	• Primary Hypoparathyroidism
– Neoplasia (lymphoma, carcinoma, anal sac carcinoma) (dog)	• Pseudohypoparathyroidism (reduced responsiveness of PTH receptors)
• Increased Vitamin D activity	**Insufficient Ca-mobilisation from bone or absorption from the intestine**
– Exogenous Vitamin D intake	• Hypovitaminosis
– Rodenticides (cholecalciferol)	• Exocrine pancreatic insufficiency
– Dietary oversupply	• Pregnancy, lactation
– Endogenous Vitamin D formation	• Eclampsia
– Granulomatous inflammation	
– Pulmonary angiostrongylosis	
• Bone neoplasia	
Myeloma, lymphoma, metastatic neoplasia	
Decreased renal excretion	**Excessive excretion of Ca via the urine**
• Renal failure	• Ethylene glycol intoxication
• Hypoadrenocorticism (dog, cat)	• Furosemide therapy
• Thiazides	

Textbook of Small Animal Pathophysiology, First Edition. Stephan Neumann.
© 2025 John Wiley & Sons Ltd. Published 2025 by John Wiley & Sons Ltd.

(Continued)

Hypercalcaemia	Hypocalcaemia
Other causes	**Other causes**
• Excessive intravenous Ca-infusion	• Acute pancreatitis (dog and cat)
• Haemoconcentration	
• Hypothyroidism	

50.9

Cholesterol

Physiology

Cholesterol is a lipid molecule that plays a critical role in various physiological processes in dogs and cats. Cholesterol is required for the proper functioning of cell membranes, as well as for the synthesis of hormones, bile acids and vitamin D.

The majority of cholesterol in dogs and cats is synthesised in the liver, with a smaller proportion obtained from the diet. Cholesterol homeostasis in dogs and cats is tightly regulated by a complex system involving hormones, such as insulin and leptin, as well as enzymes, such as HMG-CoA reductase.

Variations

Hypercholesterolaemia	Hypocholesterolaemia
Increased cholesterol production	**Decreased cholesterol production**
• By hepatocytes	• Decreased number of functional hepatocytes: portosystemic shunt (dog and cat)
• By enterocytes	• Liver cirrhosis
	• Protein-losing enteropathy (lymphangiectasia)
	• Hypoadrenocorticism
Decreased lipolysis or impaired lipoprotein metabolism	
• Hypothyroidism	
• Nephrotic syndrome	
• Protein-losing nephropathy	
Other causes	
• Acute pancreatitis	
• Cholestasis (obstructive)	
• Diabetes mellitus	
• Hyperadrenocorticism (excess glucocorticoids)	
• Hypercholesterolaemia (Briard, Doberman pinscher, Rottweiler)	
• Hyperlipaemia syndrome (Miniature Schnauzers, Beagles)	

Textbook of Small Animal Pathophysiology, First Edition. Stephan Neumann.

50.10

Creatinine

Physiology

Creatine is a molecule that plays a role in cellular energy metabolism in dogs and cats.

Creatine is synthesised in the liver and kidneys from amino acids, primarily arginine and glycine. Creatine is then transported to muscles, where it is stored as creatine phosphate. Creatine phosphate can be rapidly converted to ATP, providing energy for muscle contraction during exercise and other activities.

Creatine is metabolised to creatinine in dogs and cats as a natural process in muscle metabolism. Creatinine is a waste product of muscle metabolism that is produced in dogs and cats. Creatinine is produced in proportion to muscle mass and is primarily filtered from the blood by the kidneys and excreted in urine.

Variations

Increase

- Pre-renal
  - Dehydration, electrolyte imbalance
  - Circulatory insufficiency due to shock
  - Heart failure
  - M. Addison
  - Hypoalbuminaemia
- Renal
  - Acute renal failure
  - Chronic kidney disease
  - Glomerulonephritis
- Post-renal
  - Obstruction or rupture of the urinary tract (renal pelvis to urethra)

Textbook of Small Animal Pathophysiology, First Edition. Stephan Neumann.

50.11

Creatine Kinase

Physiology

Creatine kinase (CK) is an enzyme that plays a critical role in various physiological processes in dogs and cats. CK is found mainly in muscle tissues and brain tissue.

CK catalyses the transfer of a phosphate group from creatine phosphate to ADP, forming ATP, which provides energy for cellular processes. CK is released into the bloodstream following muscle damage or injury of the central nervous system.

Variations

Increase

Muscle damage (mostly skeletal muscle, occasionally cardiac muscle, rarely smooth muscle)

- Degenerative: hypoxia due to exertion or seizures, rhabdomyolysis after exertion
- Neoplastic: metastatic neoplasia
- Nutritional: Vitamin E/selenium deficiency
- Genetic: muscular dystrophy, myopathy due to hyper- and hypokalaemia
- Inflammatory: myositis caused by toxoplasma, neospora, bacteria
- Traumatic: intramuscular injections, car accident, seizures
- Urinary bladder obstruction (Cat).

Textbook of Small Animal Pathophysiology, First Edition. Stephan Neumann.
© 2025 John Wiley & Sons Ltd. Published 2025 by John Wiley & Sons Ltd.

50.12

Glucose

Physiology

Glucose is a major source of energy.

Glucose is primarily obtained from the diet, and excess glucose is stored in the liver and muscle tissues as glycogen. Glucose can also be produced by the liver through the process of gluconeogenesis. Insulin is a hormone that plays a key role in glucose metabolism by regulating the uptake and utilisation of glucose by cells in the body.

Glucagon is another hormone that plays a role in glucose metabolism by stimulating the breakdown of glycogen in the liver, releasing glucose into the blood.

Hyperglycaemia can lead to a range of complications, including neuropathy, nephropathy and retinopathy. Hypoglycaemia (low blood glucose levels) can also occur in dogs and cats, particularly if they have an insulin overdose or if they have not eaten for an extended period.

Variations

Increase

Physiological elevation: postprandial (up to 150 mg/dl), excitement, fear (up to 300 mg/dl), steroid-associated.

- Pathological hyperglycaemia
  - Type 1 diabetes mellitus (DM)
  - Type 2 DM
  - Drug-induced DM: glucocorticoids, thyroid hormones

Decrease

- Increased insulin secretion
  - Insulinoma (pancreatic neoplasia of the ß-cells)
- Decreased insulin antagonists
  - Hypoadrenocorticism (decreased cortisol)
- Exercise-induced hypoglycaemia (hunting dogs)

Textbook of Small Animal Pathophysiology, First Edition. Stephan Neumann.
© 2025 John Wiley & Sons Ltd. Published 2025 by John Wiley & Sons Ltd.

50.13

Glutamate Dehydrogenase (GLDH)

Physiology

Glutamate dehydrogenase (GLDH) catalyses the deamination of glutamate, thereby providing ammonia for the urea cycle. GLDH is considered liver-specific and shows highest activity in the area of centrilobular hepatocytes. Since the partial oxygen pressure is low in this area, hypoxia has a particularly negative effect on these hepatocytes, resulting in an increase in GLDH activity in the serum. The half-life of GLDH in humans is given as 18 hours. The mitochondrial localization of GLDH causes this enzyme to show a marked (over three times the upper reference range) increase in serum activity in severe liver cell damage.

Variations

Increase

- Hepatocyte damage

Textbook of Small Animal Pathophysiology, First Edition. Stephan Neumann.
© 2025 John Wiley & Sons Ltd. Published 2025 by John Wiley & Sons Ltd.

50.14

Lipase

Physiology

Pancreatic lipase assists in the hydrolysis of triglycerides in the small intestine. The half time in dogs is about two hours. Lipase has diagnostic significance for pancreatic diseases.

Variations

Increase

- Canine acute pancreatitis (values in the normal range or up to >10-fold increase of the reference value)
- Feline acute pancreatitis (values in the reference range or moderate increase < fivefold increase)
- Chronic pancreatitis (mild elevation)
- Neoplasia of the pancreas
- Decreased renal excretion or inactivation
  - Decrease in glomerular filtration rate (shock, dehydration)
  - Loss of functional renal parenchyma (acute or chronic renal failure) with elevation of lipase 2.5–4 times the reference value without damage to pancreatic acinar cells
  - Elevated lipase levels associated with renal disease may result from reduced inactivation of lipase

Textbook of Small Animal Pathophysiology, First Edition. Stephan Neumann.
© 2025 John Wiley & Sons Ltd. Published 2025 by John Wiley & Sons Ltd.

50.15

Phosphorus

Physiology

Phosphorus is an essential mineral. Phosphorus plays a critical role in bone metabolism, as well as cell signalling, energy metabolism and acid-base balance.

Phosphorus is obtained from the diet and is absorbed in the small intestine.

The kidneys play a key role in phosphorus metabolism by regulating the excretion of phosphorus from the body. In healthy dogs and cats, phosphorus homeostasis is maintained through a balance of dietary intake, absorption and renal excretion.

Variations

Increase

- Juvenile age (<1 year)
- Acute renal failure
- Chronic kidney disease
- Hypoparathyroidism
- Osteolytic bone tumour
- Hyperthyroidism
- Acromegaly

Decrease

- Hypovitaminosis D
- Hyperparathyroidism (primary, pseudo)
- Fanconi syndrome
- Glucocorticoid therapy
- M. Cushing
- Severe liver disease

Textbook of Small Animal Pathophysiology, First Edition. Stephan Neumann.
© 2025 John Wiley & Sons Ltd. Published 2025 by John Wiley & Sons Ltd.

50.16

Potassium

Physiology

The concentration of potassium in the extracellular fluid closely mirrors that in the serum. This balance depends on the total potassium content of the body and the continuous movement of potassium into and out of cells, particularly those rich in potassium. This dynamic interplay responds to fluctuations in the body's acid-base balance. To understand potassium concentration, its relationship to acid-base balance must be considered.

Several factors influence the interplay between potassium levels and acid-base balance. In cases of acidosis, caused by conditions, such as kidney dysfunction or diarrhoea, hyperkalaemia, an excess of potassium, can occur. This happens because potassium leaves the cells in response to the body's attempt to relieve acidosis by introducing hydrogen ions into the cells (inorganic or mineral acidosis).

However, acidosis caused by factors, such as L-lactate or ketoacidosis does not usually lead to hyperkalaemia. This different outcome results from the equilibrium between negative charges (from L-lactate or ketoacidosis) and positive charges (hydrogen ions) as they enter the cells, which prevents a significant increase in extracellular potassium levels. Understanding these nuanced interactions between types of acidosis and potassium movement highlights the complexity of maintaining potassium balance in relation to the acid-base status of the body.

Metabolic alkalosis causes mild hypokalaemia.

Respiratory acidosis or alkalosis is not associated with an increased serum potassium concentration.

The regulation of serum potassium concentration involves complex processes controlled by many factors:

Cellular distribution: Serum potassium concentration is influenced by its movement between intracellular and extracellular fluids. The actions of adrenaline (epinephrine) and insulin primarily drive the uptake of potassium into cells. In hyperkalaemia, where there is too much potassium in the blood, a regulatory mechanism initiates further uptake of potassium into cells. Conversely, hypokalaemia, characterised by low levels of potassium in the blood, causes potassium to leave the cells. Kidney function plays a crucial role in this by facilitating the reabsorption or excretion of potassium in the tubular apparatus of the kidney, thereby contributing significantly to potassium homeostasis.

The role of aldosterone in potassium excretion: Aldosterone, a hormone produced by the adrenal glands, plays a key role in regulating potassium levels. In particular, it promotes the excretion of potassium in the kidneys. When aldosterone levels rise, typically in response to factors, such as low blood pressure or high potassium levels, it increases the reabsorption of sodium and simultaneously increases the excretion of potassium. This mechanism helps to fine-tune serum potassium concentrations.

Variations

Increase

- Shift of potassium from intracellular to extracellular space
  - Metabolic acidosis, H^+ are transported into the intracellular space and in return a K^+ is transported to the extracellular space.

Textbook of Small Animal Pathophysiology, First Edition. Stephan Neumann.
© 2025 John Wiley & Sons Ltd. Published 2025 by John Wiley & Sons Ltd.

- Rhabdomyolysis/muscle damage
- Massive intravascular haemolysis
- Massive tissue necrosis
- Increased total potassium
  - Decreased renal excretion of potassium
    - Renal insufficiency or failure
    - Urinary tract obstruction or lesion with drainage into the abdominal cavity
    - Hypoaldosteronism
      - Hypoadrenocorticism
  - Increased uptake
  - Administration of potassium-rich fluids

Decrease

- Shift of potassium from extracellular to intracellular space
  - Metabolic alkalosis
  - Increased activity of insulin
- Reduced concentration of total potassium in the organism
  - Reduced oral uptake
  - Increased renal excretion
  - Hyperaldosteronism
  - Increased alimentary loss (vomiting, diarrhoea, excessive salivation)
- Hypokalaemia in renal failure in cats
- Myopathy with hypokalaemia e.g. in the Burmese cat

50.17

Sodium

Physiology

Sodium is found in both the intracellular and extracellular space. The concentration should always be assessed in the context of the hydration status.

Serum sodium concentration is regulated by two main mechanisms:

Blood volume

↓Blood volume (measured in the juxtaglomerular apparatus of the kidney).

    Activation of the renin-angiotensin-aldosterone system (RAAS).

    Reabsorption of Na^+, Cl^- and water in the proximal tubule system.

    Aldosterone stimulates active reabsorption of sodium in the collecting tubules.

↑Blood volume (measured at atrial baroreceptors)

    Reduction of Na reabsorption via atrial natriuretic peptide.

    Plasma osmolality

      Hyperosmolality

      Stimulation of thirst and release of antidiuretic hormone (ADH) to increase renal water reabsorption

      Hypoosmolality

      Reduction of water reabsorption and increased water excretion

Variations

Increase

- Water deficiency
  - Insufficient water intake
  - Disturbed thirst sensation
- Water loss without sufficient replenishment of losses
  - Through panting, hyperventilation or fever
  - Central or nephrogenic diabetes insipidus
- Water loss > Na loss (renal: osmotic diuresis; alimentary: osmotic diarrhoea)
- Increased sodium intake
  - Salt intoxication, administration of hypertonic saline solutions
- Decreased renal excretion of sodium
  - Hyperaldosteronism
  - Hyperadrenocorticism

Textbook of Small Animal Pathophysiology, First Edition. Stephan Neumann.
© 2025 John Wiley & Sons Ltd. Published 2025 by John Wiley & Sons Ltd.

Decrease

- Loss via the gastrointestinal tract
  - Vomiting, diarrhoea, excessive salivation
- Renal loss
  - Hypoadrenocorticism
  - Marked diuresis
  - Nephropathies
- Hypoaldosteronism
- Congestive heart failure (oedema)
- Liver cirrhosis
- Loop diuretics, aldosterone antagonists (e.g. Spironolactone)

50.18

Total Protein

Physiology

Total protein is a measurement of the concentration of all proteins in the blood, including albumin and globulins, and is an important diagnostic parameter in dogs and cats. Total protein levels are influenced by a variety of factors, including hydration status, liver function and immune status.

Albumin is the most abundant protein in the blood and plays an important role in maintaining oncotic pressure and transporting substances in the blood.

Globulins include a variety of proteins, such as immunoglobulins and transport proteins, and play an important role in immune function and protein transport.

Hydration status can have a significant effect on total protein levels, and interpretation of total protein levels should take into account the animal's hydration status.

Hypoalbuminaemia (low albumin levels) can occur in dogs and cats with certain medical conditions, such as liver disease, protein-losing enteropathy and chronic kidney disease.

Hypoalbuminaemia can lead to a range of clinical signs, including oedema, ascites and poor wound healing. For more details, see Chapter 50.2.

Hyperglobulinaemia (high globulin levels) can occur in dogs and cats with certain medical conditions, such as chronic inflammation, infection or immune-mediated disease.

Hyperglobulinaemia can help support a diagnosis of certain medical conditions but is not specific to any one disease process.

Variations

Increase

- Haemoconcentration, loss of water
- Increased protein synthesis
  - Inflammatory diseases
    - Infectious: bacterial, viral, fungal, protozoan
    - Non-infectious: necrosis, neoplasia, immune-mediated diseases
  - Neoplasia of B lymphocytes
    - Plasma cells: multiple myeloma, plasmacytoma
    - Lymphocytes: lymphoma, lymphocytic leukaemia

Decrease

- Increased protein loss via the vascular system
  - Blood loss
  - Protein-losing nephropathy
  - Renal glomerular damage (e.g. Amyloid or immune complexes)
  - Protein-losing enteropathy

  – Protein-losing dermatopathy
  – Protein loss due to peritonitis pleuritis
- Decreased protein synthesis or increased protein catabolism
  – Hepatopathy (reduction of functional liver cells <20%) e.g.: cirrhosis, hepatic necrosis or inflammation, hepatic atrophy in cases of portosystemic shunt, neoplasia
  – Malabsorption or maldigestion
  – Cachexia
  – Relative blood thinning due to hyperhydration

50.19

Urea

Physiology

Urea is a nitrogenous waste product that is produced in the liver. Urea is formed in the liver through a process called the 'urea cycle', which involves a series of enzyme-catalysed reactions. The cycle converts ammonia, a toxic byproduct of protein metabolism, into urea, which is much less toxic and can be safely excreted by the body.

After synthesis, urea is transported primarily unbound in the blood to the kidneys. In the kidneys, urea is freely filtered by the glomerulus, but some is reabsorbed in the proximal tubule. The amount of urea produced and excreted can be influenced by a number of factors, including diet, exercise and different diseases.

Urea levels are measured in the blood and are often used as a diagnostic tool to assess kidney function. High levels of urea in the blood can indicate kidney dysfunction, while low levels may be seen in cases of liver disease or malnutrition.

Variations

Increase

- Pre-renal
  - Dehydration, electrolyte imbalance
  - Circulatory insufficiency due to shock
  - Heart failure
  - M. Addison
  - Hyperthyroidism
  - Gastrointestinal bleeding
- Renal
  - Acute renal failure
  - Chronic kidney disease
  - Glomerulonephritis
- Post-renal
  - Obstruction or rupture of the urinary tract (renal pelvis to urethra)

Decrease

- Liver failure

Textbook of Small Animal Pathophysiology, First Edition. Stephan Neumann.
© 2025 John Wiley & Sons Ltd. Published 2025 by John Wiley & Sons Ltd.

Index

a

Abdominal enlargement 67, 398
ACE inhibitor 170, 179, 193, 302, 309, 325
Acetylcholine 44, 127, 157, 351, 514
Acetylsalicyl acid 174, 309, 448, 456, 486
Acidosis
    metabolic 22, 84, 92, 101, 102, 235, 304, 311, 319, 336, 346, 388, 493
    respiratory 26, 68, 95, 199, 205, 211, 215, 337
Acromegaly 68, 119, 140, 172, 352
ACTH stimulation test 398, 403
Acute renal failure 17, 101, 191, 316, 320, 497
Acute respiratory distress syndrome (ARDS) 16, 18, 94, 203–206, 288
Addison's disease 71, 227, 402, 404, 541
Adenylate cyclase 50, 61, 176, 379
Adiponectin 29, 30, 368
Adrenalin (Epinephrin) 64, 127, 182, 191, 255, 349, 350, 395, 399, 409, 535
Adrenocorticotropic hormone (ACTH) 16, 60, 63, 147, 349, 393, 403
Aelurostrongylus 79, 211, 213
Aerobic glycolysis 24, 93, 135, 169, 205
Alanine aminotransferase 517
Alkaline phosphatase 278, 279, 520
Alkalosis
    metabolic 75, 132, 136, 145, 230, 231, 235, 336, 338–339, 348, 535–536
    respiratory 84, 535
Alopecia 370, 398, 399
Alveolar cells 168, 203, 204, 217, 471
Aminoglycosides 72, 313, 429
Amlodipine 325, 407
Amylin 120
Anaerobic glycolysis 24, 33–34, 68, 101, 106, 158, 164, 199, 205, 215, 235, 261, 333, 338, 437
Anaplasmosis, 431, 433, 446, 480–483, 488, 490
ANA-titre 342, 510

Angiostrongylus 79, 211, 213
Angiotensin 30, 127, 134, 159, 176, 191, 204, 303, 314, 333, 344
Anticonvulsants 473, 521
Antithrombin 132, 246, 255, 257, 275, 307–308, 454–455
Anuria 84, 138–139, 316–317
Aortic stenosis 161–164, 172
Apoptosis 34–39, 54, 73, 139, 181, 192, 230, 260, 304, 314–315, 382, 399, 402–403, 438, 474–475, 500–501, 511
apTT 234–235, 447–448, 452–453
Aquaporine 62, 97, 139, 190, 222, 240, 246, 282, 302, 311, 314, 360, 366, 376–377, 398, 415, 492–493
Arachidonic acid 10, 44, 107, 132, 230, 394, 428
Aromatic amino acids 273
Arrhythmia 84, 92, 95, 130, 136–137, 145, 157, 160, 164, 173–176, 179, 181–183, 225, 234, 236, 251, 324, 333, 338, 347
Ascites 98, 159, 164–165, 169–170, 174–179, 206, 211, 245, 247, 258–259, 268, 309, 519, 536, 539
Aspartate aminotransferase 517, 523
Aspiration pneumonia 91–92, 125, 203, 213, 227–228, 515
Asthma 79, 94, 207–212, 441
Ataxia 70–73, 274, 391, 459, 472–473, 489
Atenolol 174, 179, 412
Atropine 183
Auerbach's plexus 81
Autoimmunity 52, 280, 487, 507–512
Autophagy 34–35, 39, 53, 149
AV-block 182
Axonopathy 429
Azathioprine 261, 433, 448, 512

b

Babesia 468, 495–498
Bacteroides 224, 280, 298
Basophilic granulocyte 8, 306
Bayliss effect 133
Benzodiazepines 273

Textbook of Small Animal Pathophysiology, First Edition. Stephan Neumann.
© 2025 John Wiley & Sons Ltd. Published 2025 by John Wiley & Sons Ltd.

Bile   67, 103, 113–115, 221–223, 244, 253–259, 264, 268, 273–274, 278–283, 289, 323, 364, 380, 393–394, 438, 493, 520, 524–525

Bile acids   27–28, 103, 114, 122–123, 255–158, 268, 273–274, 279, 371, 520, 524, 528

Bilirubin   113–115, 246, 255–256, 262–264, 268–269, 278, 289, 438, 493, 518, 525

Biliverdin   113, 255–256, 438, 525

Bisphenol A   55–56

Blebs   264, 282, 517

Blood pressure   30–31, 60–64, 131–134, 138–139, 157–159, 169, 186–195, 211, 215, 246, 251, 300–303, 311–314, 319, 324, 338, 340, 344, 349, 359–366, 384, 398–407, 411, 443, 477, 535

Borrelia   484–487

Bowman's capsule   300–301, 322, 333

Brachiocephalic   200–202

Bradycardia   111, 181–183, 316–319, 346, 370–371, 378

Bradykinin   9, 58–59, 77–79, 132, 243, 282, 289, 428

Brain oedema   117, 264

Brain tumours   420–421

Brown adipose tissue   61, 63–64, 106, 371, 373

Burmese cat   536

c

Cachexia   44–45, 99, 147–150, 169–170, 225, 227, 309, 322–323, 464, 504

Cadherin   117, 206–209, 492

Calcitonin   374, 526

Calcitriol   301–302, 324–325, 349, 353, 374–375, 378, 526

Calici virus   47

Campylobacter   83, 237, 280

Capsid   46–47, 49, 457–458, 461, 466, 472, 475

Capsule   50–51, 70, 117, 349, 374, 431, 463

Carbimazole   368

Cardiac neoplasm   185

Cardiomyopathy
   dilated   157, 176–177, 179–180, 405
   hypertrophic   157, 172–175

Carnitine deficiency   176

Caspases   36–37, 230, 499

Casts   316, 318

Catalase   367

Cataract   384–385

Catecholamine   60, 69, 130, 191–192, 199, 215, 269, 277, 337, 341, 344–345, 363–366, 379, 390, 393, 395, 399, 409–412

Cathepsin   6, 21, 23, 45, 210, 499

Caveoli   51

Cerebellar ataxia   71, 73

Cerebellum   70–71, 472

Ceruloplasmin   10–11, 246

Chaperones   53, 108

Chlorambucil   310, 312, 443, 512

Cholestasis   17–18, 114–115, 257–258, 264, 269, 278–279, 282–283, 294, 493, 520–521, 524–525, 528

Cholesterol   27–28, 140, 203, 222, 244, 253, 255–256, 264, 269, 275, 308, 365, 371–372, 384, 387, 393–395, 399, 499, 524, 528

Chondroitin   21, 426

Chromaffin cells   143–144, 231, 398, 409

Chronic renal failure   55, 139, 147, 191, 321–326, 341, 360, 376, 405, 430, 445, 533

Clopidogrel   174, 247, 309, 448, 456

Clostridia   237, 280

COLA amino acids   311

Cold receptors   61

Coma   43, 145, 252, 262, 264, 274, 341–342, 391, 497

COMT   409

Congenital cardiac diseases   161–166

Constipation   11–112, 74–77, 87–89, 92, 373, 377, 418

Copper   257–262, 266, 271, 517–118, 523

Coprophagia   297–298

Corneocyte   3

Corticotropin releasing hormone (CRH)   63–64, 394, 482

Cough   78–80, 125, 165, 168, 174, 177, 188, 195, 201, 204–208, 211–218, 472

C-reactive protein (CRP)   10–11, 17, 289, 414–415, 433

Creatinine   55, 101, 132, 177, 198, 301–302, 307, 313, 316–318, 322, 326, 332, 367, 403, 406, 492, 497, 529

Crystallisation hypothesis   330

Cubilin   310, 312

Cushing's disease   43, 67, 69, 191–193, 397–402, 420, 455–456, 534

cyclic AMP (cAMP)   10, 18, 50, 61–61, 83–85, 157, 176, 181, 238–140, 271, 279, 282, 284, 314, 350–351, 360–362, 374, 379–380, 399

Cyclooxigenase   463

Cyclosporine   433, 448, 512

Cytochrome C   36, 113

Cytoskeleton   3, 36–38, 50–56, 75, 85, 117, 204, 207, 230, 239, 264, 278, 282, 293, 314, 437, 457, 467–468, 517

d

Danger-associated molecular patterns (DAMPs)   9, 38–39, 266

Defensin   5–6, 12–13, 78, 196, 210, 221, 327

Delmadinone   418

Dendritic cell   5, 9, 11, 13, 51, 104, 203–204, 207, 223–224, 281, 318, 370, 471, 484, 507–508

Deoxycortone pivalate   404

Dermacentor   495–496

Detoxification   26, 253–254, 262–264, 522

Detrusor   138–141, 410

Dexamethasone suppression test   398

DGGR-lipase   287–290, 293
Diabetes
  insipidus   139, 340–342, 359–361, 493–494, 537
  ketoacidosis   110, 143, 336, 338, 387–389, 535
  mellitus   29–30, 119, 140, 190–193, 277, 293–294, 325, 327,
    336, 341, 354, 382–387, 517, 521, 523–524, 528, 531
Diarrhoea   82, 86, 477
Diazepam   425
Diazoxid   391
Diencephalon   61, 349
Diltiazem   174, 179, 183
Disc herniation   426, 428
Disseminated intravascular coagulation (DIC)   15, 18, 131,
    234–235, 450–452
Distemper   72, 107, 213, 471–474
Dopamin   105, 127, 231, 318, 350, 366, 393, 409, 482
Doxycycline   460, 482, 486, 490, 493, 498
Ductus arteriosus   162–166
Dwarfism   356–358
Dyschezia   87–88
Dysphagia   90–92, 125
Dyspnea   96
Dystroglycan   172–173
Dystrophin   172–175
Dysuria   138, 274–275, 328–329, 332–333, 418

e

E. coli   83, 213, 280, 413–414
Effusion   94, 97–102, 164, 174–175, 177–180, 184, 186–189,
    246 342, 462–463, 536
Ehrlichia   488–490
Eicosanoids   10, 227, 428, 477
Elastase   6, 19–20, 132, 198, 210, 285–287
Endocardiosis   167
Endolymph   70
Endothelin   21–22, 176–179, 191–192, 315, 317, 322, 454
Endotoxins   16, 50, 238, 254, 261–262
Enterobacter   280
Enteroglucagon   379
Eosinophilic granulocyte   7–8, 10–11, 15, 51–52
Epilepsy   129, 423–425, 517
Erythrocytosis   165, 441–434
Erythropoetin   100
Ethylene glycol intoxication   526
Exocrine pancreas insufficiency   82, 119, 296
Exotoxins   50
Extracellular matrix   3–4, 19, 22, 42, 45, 50, 53, 56, 167, 172,
    254, 267, 292, 314, 321–322, 462, 521

f

Factor II   225
Factor IX   225, 246, 257, 308, 451

Factor VII   225, 257, 275, 451
Factor X   225, 454
FAD   32
False neurotransmitter   258, 263, 275, 282
Fanconi syndrome   130–140, 310, 312, 534
Fas ligands   38
Fatigue   17, 60, 93, 95–96, 104–105, 145, 164, 169, 205,
    214–215, 259, 346, 372, 377, 497
Fatty Acid-Binding Protein   278
Fatty degeneration   25, 262
Feline immunodeficiency virus   466, 469–470
Feline infectious peritonitis   72, 99, 461–465, 517, 523
Feline leukemia virus   450
Ferroportin   439, 459
Fibroblast growth factor (FGF)   20, 357, 376, 426, 428
Fibrotic remodelling   12, 19, 22, 26, 139, 170, 173, 217, 281,
    293–294, 296, 306, 436
Flowing liver   253
Fludrocortisone   404
Folic acid   224, 254–255, 297–298
Formatio reticularis   93, 139
Fructosamine   383–385
Functio laesa   12
Furosemide   170, 174, 179, 247, 348, 526

g

Gastric dilatation volvulus   233–236
Gastrin   74, 220–221, 233, 256, 258–259, 263, 317, 323,
    326, 379–380
Gastritis   143, 229–232, 317, 325, 492
Ghrelin   62, 120, 258, 366, 368, 398, 400–401, 482
γ-hydroxybutyric acid (GABA)   58, 127, 258, 263, 282, 342,
    423, 429, 497, 522
Giardiasis   499–502
Glucagon   60, 62, 119, 134, 148, 243, 255, 277, 349, 379–381,
    386, 388, 390, 394, 531
Glucosaminoglycan   21, 102, 330, 371
Glucosuria   139, 311, 316, 318, 382, 384–385, 388
Glutamate   72–73, 127, 135, 137, 255, 298, 301, 304, 342, 346,
    399, 423–424, 482, 497, 523, 532
Glutamate dehydrogenase   532
Glutathione   33, 75, 215, 262
Glycine   58, 102, 127, 399, 529
Goblet cell   4, 78–79, 210, 225, 229
Gonadotropin releasing hormone (GnRH)   350, 395
G-protein   21, 61, 72, 157, 176, 190–191, 350, 360, 364,
    374, 379–380
Grand male   128, 423

h

Haematochezia   76, 88, 418, 453
Haematuria   328–329, 332–333, 417–418, 453

Haemophilia   451

Hansen type I and II   426–427

Haptoglobin   11, 246

HbA1c   383–385

Head tilt   71, 73, 421

Helicobacter   45, 229–232

Hepatic failure   260–265

Hepatic lipidosis   67, 113, 150, 277–279

Hepatitis, chronic   257–262, 266–272, 281, 517, 523

Hepatoencephalic syndrome   26, 268, 273–274

Hepatoses   262

Hepcidin   17, 439, 445, 449, 459–460

Hering-Breuer reflex   93

Herniation   188, 249, 426, 428

Herpes virus   71, 213, 261

High-density lipoprotein (HDL)   28

Histamine   5, 8, 58–59, 77, 79, 95, 114, 123, 127, 144, 207–208, 220, 256–260, 263, 332, 428, 463

Hydralazine   511

Hydropic swelling   25, 77

Hydroxyurea   165, 443

Hyperactivity   72, 134, 366–367

Hyperadrenocorticism   119, 122, 140, 190–191, 327, 347, 359, 397–401, 441, 521, 528, 537

Hyperaldosteronism   190, 192, 246, 257–258, 263, 338, 341, 405–408, 536–537

Hypercoagulability   247, 308, 454–456

Hyperpigmentation   357, 398

Hypersensitivity reaction   207, 459

Hyperthyroidism   55, 82, 94, 119–122, 139–143, 173, 175, 182–183, 190–191, 229, 327, 364–371, 405, 441, 517, 521, 523, 534, 541

Hypoadrenocorticism   82, 86, 110, 124–125, 138, 143, 182, 226–229, 342, 345, 402–404, 526, 528, 531, 536, 538

Hypocalcaemia   71–72, 98, 127, 133, 158, 182, 325, 375, 377–378, 388, 526–527

Hypoglycaemia   71–72, 127, 133–135, 263–264, 274, 358, 364, 379, 390–392, 403, 425, 531

Hypomotility   125, 226

Hypothalamic-pituitary axis   357

Hypothalamus   18, 49, 61–64, 93, 105–110, 119, 139, 308, 314, 349–351, 359–360, 364–365, 369–372, 380, 394–395, 398, 411– 463, 467, 477, 512

Hypothyroidism   72, 74–75, 117, 122, 124–125, 181–182, 226–227, 308, 364, 369–373, 430, 527, 528

Hypoxia-induced factor (HIF)   34, 206, 303, 437

i

Icterus   114–115, 268–269, 278, 281–282, 447–448, 463, 497, 525

Imidocarb   498

Inappetence   49, 84, 104, 110–112, 125, 230–231, 268, 287, 289, 323, 325, 376, 467, 481, 497

Incontinence   138–141, 361

Infertility   370, 459

Inflammatory bowel disease   82, 86, 105, 147, 237–242, 280, 283

Insulin-like growth factor (IGF)   29, 31, 41, 172, 268, 324, 352–358, 390, 434, 438, 518

Insulinoma   71, 119, 390–392, 531

Interferon   14, 17–18, 48, 223, 450, 462–466, 469, 472, 474, 510

Intussusception   43, 249–250

Ion channels   58, 61–62, 72, 126–127, 135–136, 154, 181, 230, 350, 399, 423

Ito cells   19, 253–254, 267

Ixodes ricinus   480, 484, 486

j

Jaundice   43, 103, 113–115, 262, 269, 281, 463, 494, 525

k

Keratinocyte   3–4, 16

Klebsiella   213, 280, 327, 414

Kupffer cells   254–255, 258, 266–269, 411

Kussmaul breathing   389

l

Lactate   24, 34, 101, 158, 235, 262, 304, 333, 336, 338, 387, 399, 535

Lactoferrin   196

Laminin   21, 37, 172–173, 267

Leishmaniasis   433, 503–506

Leptin   29–31, 62–63, 112, 120, 258, 313, 366, 368, 467, 477, 482, 528

Leptospira   491–494

Leucotriene   6

Levothyroxine   372

Lieberkühn's crypt   223

Lipase   27, 34, 61, 215, 221, 244, 277, 285–290, 293–294, 371, 379, 399, 488–489, 533

Lipoprotein   25–28, 81, 84, 255, 262, 308–309, 371, 484, 528

LPS   16, 50–51, 84, 107, 132, 167, 203, 323, 535

Lunge atelectasis   43, 197, 199

Lung emphysema   197

Lung fibrosis   217–218, 441

Lung oedema   79

Lymphangiectasia   243–248, 528

Lymphopenia   245–246, 411, 463–464, 468, 472–473, 476–478

Lymphotactin   14

Lysosomes   24, 39, 51, 53, 253, 362, 380, 488–489, 503

m

Major histocompatibility complex (MHC)   7–10, 13, 15, 223, 507–510

Malabsorption   82, 116, 119, 147–150, 159, 179, 239, 297, 501, 519, 540

Maldigestion   82, 120, 294, 297–298, 519, 540

Manganese   273

Marfan's syndrome   167

Maropitant   232, 265, 270, 279, 289, 325, 478, 493

Mast cell tumour   40, 122–123, 305

Matrix metalloproteinases   11, 19, 42, 434, 436

MDR   264, 278

Megalin   310, 312

Megaoesophagus   90–91, 124, 226–228, 371, 515

Meissner's plexus   81

Melanin concentrating hormone (MCH)   120

Melastatin   61

Melena   76, 231, 453

Mercaptan   273, 522

Mesangium cell   306

Mestinon   515–516

Metamizole   241

Metoclopramide   232, 279, 289, 325

Micturition   138–141, 329, 332

Midgut   480–481, 484–485, 495–496, 503

Mirtazepine   325

Mitotane   400

Mitral valve dysplasia   161–163

Modified transudate   67, 97–99, 170, 463

Molecular mimicry   382, 511

Monoaminooxidase (MAO)   409

Mucopolysaccharides   117

Multi-organ failure   77, 131, 288–289

Muscle atrophy   70–71, 93

Muscle spindle   70–71, 93

Myasthenia gravis   44, 124–125, 226–228, 514, 516

Mycoplasma   79, 211, 213, 459, 468

Myofibrils   61, 155

Myosin binding protein C   175

Myositis   91, 169, 226, 431, 493, 523, 530

n

NADH   32, 387

Natriuretic peptide   106, 173, 176–177, 190, 317, 393, 537

Nausea   17, 70, 95, 143–146, 230, 231–232, 252, 278, 325, 388, 412, 497

Necroptosis   38–39

Nectin   471, 473

Nephron   26, 30, 139, 191, 300–301, 307, 314, 317–318, 322–325, 331, 359–360, 393, 397

NETosis   6

Neuropathy   111, 370–371, 384, 429–431

NF-κB   150

Nociceptor   12, 58–62, 68, 231, 251, 282, 289, 294, 329

Noradrenaline (Norepinephrine)   64, 409

o

Obesity   27–31, 120–121, 192, 325, 370–372, 383–385, 400, 434, 531

Occludin   3–4, 223

Octopamine   258, 263, 282

Oedema

brain   117, 264

inflammatory   116–117, 280

myx   117

oncotic   116

Oestrogen   351, 357, 393, 396, 413, 417, 444, 511

Oliguria   15, 84, 132, 138, 316–317, 332, 341, 493

Omeprazole   265, 325, 493

Ondansetron   232, 265, 279, 289, 325, 478, 493

Opioid receptors   123, 257

Opsonising   50

Orexigenic neurons   111, 289

Organophosphates   429

Osmoreceptor   62, 314, 359

Osmoregulation   62, 64, 276

Osmotic pressure   97, 116–117, 185, 246, 255, 300, 384, 499, 518

Osteoarthritis   434–436

Osteodystrophy   376, 521

Osteomalacia   308, 521

Osteonectin   21

Oxidative phosphorylation   24, 34, 53, 148, 261

Oxytocin   349–350

p

Pancreatic duct   285–286, 289, 292, 294

Pancreatic enzymes

amylase   285–286, 290

carboxypeptidase A & B   285

chymotrypsin   16, 285–286

DNAsen   285

elastase   6, 19–20, 132, 198, 210, 285–287

lipase (*see* Lipase)

phospholipase   10, 38, 285, 287, 289, 428, 492

RNAsen   285

trypsin   222, 285–289

Pancreatitis

acute   287–294, 378, 527–528, 533

chronic   283, 290–297

Pancytopenia   444, 458–459, 489

Paneth cell   5, 223–224

Pannexin   79

Paralysis   145, 174–175, 251, 289, 318, 327, 346–348, 407, 418, 427–430, 455

Paraneoplastic syndrome   43–44, 397

Parathyroid hormone   302, 324, 374, 376, 526

Paresis   174–175, 427–428, 456, 459, 489, 515

Parvovirus   47, 83, 86, 107, 176, 237, 242, 475–479

Perforin   8–9, 507

Pericardium   153, 169, 184–188

Peroxisome   253, 278

Petit male   128, 423

Phenobarbital   261, 266, 422, 425, 473, 517, 523

Phenol   55–56, 102, 224, 273, 317, 522

Phenylethylamine   258, 263, 282

Pheochromocytoma   190, 192, 409–412

Phlebotomes   503

Phlebotomy   165, 443

Phosphates binders   325

Phosphorus   32, 177, 316, 318, 322, 326, 357, 375–376, 534

Pigmenturia   497

Pit cells, 253–254. 259

Plasmin   21, 23, 132, 491

Platelet-derived growth factor (PDGF)   20–21, 34, 267, 292, 306

PLI   293

Pneumonia   91–94, 109, 125, 203–204, 213–216, 219, 227–228, 337, 467, 469, 471, 473, 492–493, 515

Pollakisuria   138, 328–333

Polyarthritis   107, 431, 433, 486

Polycythaemia   95, 127, 132, 164–165, 211–212, 218, 441–443

Polyphagia   119–120, 297, 366, 384–385, 398, 400

Polyradiculoneuritis   429

Polyuria   138–142, 257, 263, 274–275, 311, 323–324, 360–361, 366, 377, 388, 401, 411, 415, 443

POMC   111, 394

Portosystemic shunt   257, 259–260, 264, 269, 272–276, 517, 519, 522–524, 528, 540

Potassium-bromide   473

Progesterone   350, 352, 383–384, 394, 413, 415–416

Prolactin   63, 349–350

Prolactin releasing peptide (PRP)   350

Prostacyclin   10, 454

Prostate   74, 87–88, 417–419

Proteasome   270

Proteoglycan   21–22, 51, 267, 357, 426

Prothrombin   10, 255, 331, 451, 463

Pseudohypoparathyroidism   526

PTHrP   44, 526

Ptyalism   92, 125

Purkinje fibre   71, 153, 155

Pyometra   139–140, 142, 413–416, 446

Pyridostigmine   228

Pyroptosis   39

r

Ranitidine   325

RANTES   14

Regurgitation   80, 125, 161, 165, 168–170, 213, 227–228, 515

Rheumatoid factors   432–433

Rhipicephalus sanguineus   480, 488, 496

Rickets   521

Rubber jaw   376–377

s

S-adenosylmethionine   283

Saliva   221, 457, 466

Samoyed   531

Sandfly   503

Sarcoglycan   172–173

Secretin   74, 221–222, 284, 380

Semaphorin   244

Sepsis   14–15, 17–18, 77, 107, 109, 198, 203, 204, 235, 282, 313, 320, 412, 452, 454, 456

Septal defect   162–163, 441

Serotonin   58, 105, 120, 127, 143–144, 174, 231, 238, 243, 256, 282, 289, 366, 393, 477, 482

Serum amyloid A (SAA)   10–11, 414–415

Shivering   62–63

Shock
    anaphylactic   130
    cardiogenic   130–132
    hypovolaemic   84, 100–101, 131, 234–235, 251
    neurogenic   130
    septic   18, 50, 77, 131–132, 235, 251

Sick sinus syndrome   182

Silimarien   270

SMAD-MAPK pathway   21

Smooth muscle actin   19, 267

Snoring   200–201

Somatostatin   147–148, 350, 379–381, 390

Somatotropin   349–350

Sotalol   174, 183

Spironolactone   170, 174, 407, 538

Status epilepticus   423

Stranguria   138

Stratum corneum   3–4

Substance P   58, 127, 143–146, 231

Surfactant   32, 196, 203–204, 214, 289

Swallowing   90–92, 110, 124, 220, 226–227

Sweating   62

Syncope 133–137, 164–165, 177, 179, 182, 187–188, 201–202, 346, 348, 377, 390

Systemic inflammatory response syndrome (SIRS) 131, 288–289, 294, 414

t

Tapasin 507

Taurine deficiency 176

Telomeres 53–54, 57

Tenesmus 87

Testosteron 52, 350, 357, 393–396, 417

Tetherin protein 466

Tetralogy of Fallot 161, 163

Theophylline 212

Thermoregulation 61–62, 107, 201–202

Thiamine deficiency 72

Thiazides 526

Thrombocytopenia 18, 234, 257, 263, 275–276, 447–451, 458–459, 472, 489–490, 492, 497, 504–505, 580–485

Thrombospondin 21

Thromboxane 10, 287, 333

Thyroid-stimulating hormone (TSH) 308, 349–350, 356, 362, 364, 367–371

Thyrotropin-releasing hormone (TRH) 364

Tight-junction 3–4, 77, 114, 150, 170, 222–223, 238–240, 244, 264, 278, 280–282, 284, 314, 411, 415, 445, 493, 499

TLI 290, 297

Toll-like receptor 9, 22, 131, 203, 223, 510

Torasemide 174

Toxoplasma 52, 72, 107, 280, 468, 472, 523, 530

Transcortin 393–394

Transferrin 254, 275, 282, 308, 439, 475, 478

Transforming growth factor (TGF) 7–8, 15–16, 19–23, 41, 171, 204, 206, 217–218, 267, 281, 292, 306, 321, 384, 386, 394, 434–435

Transudate 67, 97–100, 170, 185, 246, 463

Tricuspidal valve dysplasia 161–163, 165

Trigger-like 51

Trilostane 400

Trophozoite 499–501

Tubulointerstitial fibrosis 55

Tumor suppressor gene 36, 40–41

Turbid swelling 24

Turgour 84

Tyrosine kinase 16, 21, 29, 304, 350, 379, 426, 437

u

Ubiquitin 45, 147–148, 206, 268, 353–354, 368, 507

Ulcer 230–232, 466

Uraemia 26, 89, 102, 198, 231, 313, 332–333, 429, 445, 505

Uraemic toxins 313, 317, 324, 332, 429

Uria
    an- 84, 138–139, 316–317
    olig- 15, 132, 316–317, 332, 341
    poly- 138–142, 257, 263, 274–275, 311, 323–324, 360–361, 366 376–377, 388, 401, 411, 415, 443

Urine cortisol creatinine ratio 398

Urokinase 456

Urolithiasis 138, 327, 330, 334, 376

Uveitis 467–469, 489–492, 504–505

v

Vacuolar degeneration 24, 262

Vagus nerve 62, 79–80, 104, 143, 157, 206, 208, 220, 231, 362

Vascular endothelial growth factor (VEGF) 8, 17, 29, 31, 34, 244, 435, 445, 1084

Vasopressin (ADH) 361

Ventilation 93, 195, 197, 235, 317, 336–337, 339

Verapamil 183

Very-low-density lipoprotein (VLDL) 28, 277–278, 308

Vestibular ataxia 71

Viraemia 47, 457, 467, 471, 475

Virus replication 47, 461, 475–476

Virus spread 46

Vitamin B12 221, 223, 225, 254, 298

Vitamin K 188, 224–225, 255, 450–453

Von Willebrand factor 174, 451

w

Weight loss 60, 91–92, 111, 125, 147–150, 177, 227–231, 240–241, 268, 297–298, 307–308, 311–312, 354, 366–367, 384, 410–411, 463, 467, 489–490, 501, 504

z

Zipper-like 51

Zona
    fasciculata 393–394, 402
    glomerulosa 314, 344, 393–394, 402
    reticularis 393–395